A Practical Approach to
Measurement in
Physical Education

Health Education,
Physical Education, and
Recreation Series

RUTH ABERNATHY, Ph.D., Editorial Adviser
*Director, School of Physical
and Health Education
University of Washington
Seattle, Washington 98105*

A Practical Approach to Measurement in Physical Education

By Harold M. Barrow, P.E.D.
Professor of Physical Education, Wake Forest University,
Winston-Salem, North Carolina

and Rosemary McGee, Ph.D.
Professor of Physical Education, The University of North Carolina,
at Greensboro, Greensboro, North Carolina

Illustrated
SECOND EDITION

Lea & Febiger

Philadelphia . 1971

First Edition, 1964

Reprinted May, 1966, February, 1968 and March, 1970

Second Edition, 1971

ISBN 0–8121–0292–4

Library of Congress Catalog Card Number 72:152021

Published in Great Britain by Henry Kimpton Publishers, London

Printed in the United States of America

PREFACE

We are living in a burgeoning scientific age characterized by rapid changes and innovations to meet the needs growing out of those changes. The processes of education are challenged by these new demands as never before. As these processes have grown in complexity, the area of measurement has also undergone some marked changes. Measurement procedures have become more sophisticated during this last decade. More precise and exact instruments are being used to obtain more objective data on the one hand. At the same time, the educational emphasis has shifted toward some of the more qualitative aspects and teachers are no longer reluctant to use subjective techniques. One of the requirements of education today is accountability. Those school processes which expect to share in the budget, time, and space for their programs must demonstrate, through measurement, that these programs are bringing about desirable changes in students.

The second edition of this book has not changed materially in its philosophy. It is still designed for use as a practical approach to measurement. It has been brought up to date. The emphasis is still on the elementary and secondary school levels. New materials have been added in each of the four sections. The introductory chapters have been revised and expanded. History and trends have been added in Chapter 1 along with some new techniques in the statistical chapter. The second unit, concerning measurement of the product, has been thoroughly revised to parallel the emphasis now placed on the taxonomy of educational objectives—cognitive, affective, and psychomotor. Some new techniques have been presented in motor ability, fitness, and perceptual-motor awareness. More up-to-date sport skills tests have been included. The chapters on knowledge and understanding have been consolidated and new materials added on test construction. The affective domain has been stressed to a great extent and many new measures have been presented in this area. The third unit on process has been updated and emphasis has been placed on teacher evaluation. The last unit includes chapters on grading, classification, and rating scales. The new philosophy regarding grades has been reviewed as well as the concept of proficiency tests.

The authors are indebted to Mrs. Lamson Blaney and Mrs.

Emmy Mills, Jackson Library of the University of North Carolina at Greensboro, for valuable assistance with numerous requests on inter-library loan. Appreciation is expressed to Mrs. Wilson L. Stewart and to Mrs. Elizabeth Chafin for final manuscript preparations and to Mrs. Roger Taylor, artist for the second edition.

Winston-Salem, North Carolina
Greensboro, North Carolina

HAROLD M. BARROW
ROSEMARY McGEE

PREFACE TO THE FIRST EDITION

Several of the competencies which physical education teachers should possess are related to testing and measuring. It is our purpose to provide a text, in which these competencies may be learned, which is directed chiefly at the elementary and secondary school programs, and which is written for the undergraduate professional student and the teacher in service. Emphasis is placed on basic testing concepts and their application in terms of the product and process of education—the *student* and the *means* of educating him.

The text combines the traditional with the more practical, laboratory approach. It is conventional to the extent that concepts such as philosophy of testing, evaluation of tests, uses of tests, and administrative procedures are included. It has the laboratory approach to the extent that emphasis is placed on the application of the techniques presented.

The book is organized into four sections. The *first* section includes an introduction to testing. No attempt has been made to cater to the research worker, but simply to show that testing is a part of good teaching and good programming. The *second* unit employs the laboratory approach and is designed to measure the *student*. It includes tests to measure the physical, social, and mental learnings stressed in physical education. Emphasis is placed on the selecting of tests which are usable, which contribute substantially to the recognized uses of testing, and which can be included in complete enough detail to be administered and used. The *third* section contains the techniques to measure the various *means* of educating the student. The laboratory approach is used so the beginning teacher may have the necessary skill and knowledge to evaluate his program, leadership, facilities, methods, administrative procedures, and his own teachings. The *fourth* section handles certain problems connected with the construction of measurement devices. Since there are many missing links in testing at the present time, the teacher must frequently depend on his own initiative for evaluation.

A special indebtedness is acknowledged to Karl W. Bookwalter, M. Gladys Scott, Esther French, and Ethel Martus. Each is a stalwart leader of vision in the profession and each has given inspiration, direction, and encouragement to us in our pursuits in the areas of tests, measurements, and research.

Any endeavor of such scope is dependent upon helpful persons. Appreciation is expressed to Mrs. J. H. Walton, Mrs. Grace Barrow, and Miss June Galloway for studying the manuscript; to Mrs. T. M. McClelland, Miss Ruth Baity, and Mrs. Marie Teague for preparing it in final form; and to Miss Betty Gwynn Moore for illustrating the text.

Winston-Salem, North Carolina   HAROLD M. BARROW
Greensboro, North Carolina   ROSEMARY McGEE

CONTENTS

PART II. EVALUATION OF THE PRODUCT

PART III. EVALUATION OF THE PROCESS

Part I. Introduction and Background

Chapter 1
PHILOSOPHY OF MEASUREMENT

Evaluation is the art of judgment scientifically applied according to some predetermined standards. When it is applied to education, it is a distinct phase of a continuous, dynamic cycle. This cycle begins with the establishment of values and the formulation of goals growing out of philosophy, continues with the development of procedures to implement the goals, is related to the process of methodology and instruction, and culminates with the judgment and appraisal of results. Each of these phases is related to the other, although they follow each other in the sequential pattern shown in Figure 1–1 starting with the statement of goals and ending in judgments. These judgments are made with reference to two things: the individual to be educated and the means of educating him. In the light of results from judgments, goals are appraised and restated, the procedures are replanned, and the whole cycle is repeated. Thus, evaluation is a dynamic, never-ending process in education.

What is Education?

Since evaluation is a procedure of education, it would perhaps be well to review the nature of education. *Education can be defined as*

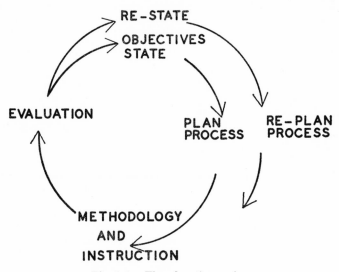

Fig. 1–1. The education cycle.

a change, a modification, or an adjustment on the part of an individual as a result of experience. It is associated with learning and is characteristically followed by some change in behavior. If the change has been good and in the right direction, it will help the individual to adjust more easily to his constantly changing environment and to understand more readily his experiences in that environment. This change is illuminated through growth, development, and achievement. It should be judged in terms of selected values and viewed as a continuous on-going process as it progresses from one level to another in a complex and interrelated pattern.

The Product. Society, through its philosophers and educators, examines and ultimately selects values considered to be essential. Among these values is the kind of a student who is judged to be best for that particular society. In the final analysis, this individual is the end of all educational endeavor. He will be referred to frequently in this textbook as a *product* and he will always be considered as an end. All measures of education which are used to accomplish a change in him are means to that end. This simple fact is a salient principle of education. Yet, in spite of its importance, it is frequently overlooked or ignored. All too often certain educational practices tend to become ends rather than means. For example, in some areas of extra-curricular activities, what originally was intended to serve as a means has now become an end. This is especially true in competitive athletics.

This idea of value selection through conceptualizing the type of individual needed by society is an important facet of the educational cycle. The achievement of this product is enhanced by the formulation of guides giving direction to the changes which are intended for his growth, development, and achievement. These points of reference are in the nature of goals. The remote goals are referred to as *aims*, and the more immediate ones as *objectives*. Objectives may be further broken down into specific goals called *outcomes*. Through aims, objectives, and outcomes, it is possible to give direction to the learning of the student and thereby to help bring about modifications which are desirable in terms of the selected values. Thus, educational direction is dictated by objectives and is inherent in their purpose.

The selection of values and the formulation of objectives becomes a problem of philosophy, since philosophy is pre-eminently the source of all goals, criteria, and standards. Furthermore, two salient purposes of philosophy have always been to interpret the broad aims of education and to furnish the frontier thinking which is necessary for new goals, re-direction, and different points of view. Out of principles and basic beliefs which have evolved from scientific fact and reasoned judgments, philosophy emerges and with this philosophy, values are established, and the course of education is charted.

The Process. When society has determined its values in terms of the kind of product it wants as a result of education, and when it has established objectives to serve as guides indicating the way toward the development of that product, the next logical step in educational planning concerns implementation. Implementation involves procedures, and the procedures of education will be referred to in this textbook as *process*. Basically, process concerns such matters as personnel, facilities, equipment, program of activities, methods and materials, supervision, and administrative devices. The teacher himself is one of the components. These procedures and aspects are means to ends—means by which, or through which, the desired product is achieved. It is necessary to plan this process in such manner that the already established objectives will be met. Goals in education are of vital importance. They relate process and product. Conditioned by philosophy, they become the criteria for the establishment of the process. They are the controls in a democracy, where the chief purpose of education is to teach the individual to live more fully and completely in his society. They furnish standards in the process of education. They foster methods and procedures which are in keeping with the demands of a democratic society and which guarantee laboratories in democratic living. Whereas objectives are primarily a responsibility of philosophy, process is chiefly a responsibility of science. Succinctly stated, through philosophy, society determines the type of product it desires, and establishes goals to indicate the direction that product is to grow and develop; and through science, it plans a program of implementation to achieve those goals.

What is Physical Education?

Physical education may be defined as an education by physical means where many of education's objectives are achieved through big muscle play activity. It is a vital phase of education and an integral part of the educational process. Values must be established in physical education just as they must in general education. This *product* in physical education is an ideal—a mythical individual with the qualities and characteristics of a physically educated person. The next step is the establishment of measurable objectives, including the social and mental aspects as well as the physical. Then, the physical education process must be determined to translate the established needs and values into experience and relate them to the objectives. These objectives, when achieved through the process, result in the previously established value—a physically educated person. Such a person has the qualities—sufficient skill and knowledge in sports and exercise, adequate physical fitness, sufficient emotional poise and control, and appropriate attitude toward participation in sports and exercise—to make him an intelligent and interested participant and to help him become a more effective member of society. Becoming a more effective member of society would mean that this person is prepared to live a useful and enjoyable life both for himself, for his community, and for his country.

Relationship of Physical Education and Education

There should be no conflict between education and physical education in the matter of either the product or the process. The product, objectives, and program of physical education must be in harmony with those of general education and must be recognized as a part of the educational cycle. Physical education programs are related to educational objectives. In fact, the aim of physical education itself is generally listed as one of the objectives of education. Modern programs of physical education have the same goals as education, although the physical educator must understand that his specialized area is just one of many disciplines which contribute to these goals. It can be shown that physical education serves most of education's objectives. For example, in the Seven Cardinal Principles of Education,[16] physical education can contribute directly to the objectives of *health, worthy use of leisure,* and *ethical character* and indirectly to the objectives of *citizenship, command of the fundamental processes, worthy home membership,* and *vocation.* In the four groups of objectives of the Educational Policies Commission[22]— self-realization, human relationships, economic efficiency, and civic responsibility—physical education can contribute its share toward the realization of these broad goals. For example, physical education may contribute to the objectives of *self-realization* in several ways. It contributes through the teaching of knowledges concerning health habits, through the teaching and development of skills and knowledges of sports and exercise, through the development of interest in and an appreciation for sports and exercise from both the participants' and spectators' standpoint, through an increased appreciation of one's own body and through a philosophy of life which includes play as an important aspect of the good life. Physical education may contribute to the objectives of *human relations* by providing a richer social experience for all students through games, sports, and dance, by teaching cooperation in the framework of competition, by providing training for leadership responsibilities, and by encouraging an increased emphasis on sportsmanship. Physical education may contribute to the objectives of *economic efficiency* by teaching that one's success in any vocation or profession is dependent on one's health and fitness, as well as one's industry, that one's work should have meaning and significance, and that one should buy and use many of the material things of life with a view to good health and fitness. Physical education may contribute to the objectives of *civic responsibility* through the teaching of democracy and citizenship. Sports and games offer fertile fields for the development of qualities of both leadership and "followership" which are necessary for living in a democratic society.

Thus the needs of the physical are inextricably related to the activities of the mental. At the same time movement does not take place without something happening to personality and social behavior. Also, perspiration is frequently related to inspiration. Thus, the product is an entity and the physical must take its place in the educational process along with the aspects of the mental, social, and spiritual. Each of these must make its contribution toward a unified, integrated, and effective individual. Succinctly stated, the ultimate end of physical education is the good of the whole individual and there can be no conflict between the aspects of the whole in either the direction or the process.

What is Evaluation and Measurement?

When the desired product has been established in physical education, when the objectives have been formulated, and when a program has been planned to produce that product, it is necessary to determine how well the objectives have been met, how efficient has been the process, and how good is the product. This phase of the educational process is concerned with tests, measurements, and evaluation. These techniques are important aspects of the on-going cycle of education. The formulated objectives are appraised by applying these techniques to student status, growth, adjustment, development, and achievement. The results of this application indicate the direction and the degree of change these aspects have taken. The three terms do not have the same connotation. The following definitions are suggested.

Evaluation is a process of education which makes use of measurement techniques which, when applied to either the product or process, result in both qualitative and quantitative data expressed in both subjective and objective manner and used for comparisons with preconceived criteria.

Measurement is a technique of evaluation which makes use of procedures which are generally precise and objective, which will generally result in quantitative data, and which characteristically can express its results in numerical form. It may be applied to qualitative procedures, however, when its techniques are objectified.

A *test* is a specific tool of measurement and implies a response from the person being measured.

From the definitions above, it is clearly evident that these terms are not synonymous, but that they are related. Evaluation is a part of the process of education, measurement is a technique of evaluation, and testing is a tool of measurement. Evaluation is broader in meaning than is measurement and its results are usually expressed in more qualitative terms. The definitions imply that measurement merely indicates status and its results have little significance in themselves. However, when status data are used for comparisons with predetermined criteria, evaluation occurs. The criteria referred to here are derived from the established aim, objectives, norms, standards, and perhaps previous measurements. Measurement answers specific questions related to quantity and quality, but evaluation appraises these answers in relation to the above criteria. Measurement is terminal in as much as there is no requirement that results be used. Evaluation, on the other hand, is a continuous process, for it determines the value or lack of value of a process, an action, a characteristic, or a device, and there is a follow-up. In the final analysis, evaluation becomes a technique for judging how effective the educational experience has been for the individual. It is related to philosophy, because it indicates the extent to which objectives are met. It is also related to science, since it employs scientific techniques and procedures. Measurement is merely fact finding in that it provides raw data. Evaluation implies the use of those data for assimilation of results, prescription for future use, and a follow-up. This statement is basic; it re-affirms the idea that evaluating is a continuous process.

Place of Evaluation and Measurement in Education

Evaluation and measurement are common everyday practices. They reflect man's ever-present curiosity about his environment and his concern about himself. His control over his environment improved as he found better ways of measuring. In fact, there is a high degree of relationship between measurement techniques in a field today and progress in that field in general. This is revealed best perhaps by the advancement in medicine.

Is a Universal Practice. Measurement is used in all fields of endeavor and is employed in its varied forms by all individuals. Much of the time the individual who is making evaluations is probably not consciously aware of his actions. In a sense, many evaluations are made daily in carrying out one's normal activities. For instance, in sports, evaluation occurs when a golfer chooses a five iron over a six in his approach to the green, when a basketball player passes off instead of shoots, when a batter takes a low pitch for a ball, or when the fielder of a bunt throws to first base rather than second. It may further occur in daily living when a professional student attends a movie rather than a professional meeting, or when the teenager elects to watch television rather than study his assignment, or when the over-weight person selects a dessert instead of a salad. All of these behaviors concern the establishment of some value and a subsequent follow-up involving judgment and a choice. Each individual faces a lifetime of such choices involving the values he has established for himself.

Provides for Self-Evaluation. An important facet of education is helping students to make the right choices by means of good evaluation. Invariably these evaluations are made in the light of criteria and standards which have been established out of scientific facts and past experience. The student takes a short-cut to this experience through his education. He becomes acquainted with desirable criteria and standards in those criteria which have been established over the years. On the basis of these criteria he is expected to make judgments and subsequently, if his standards are high enough, to make wise choices. In many ways these criteria and values substitute for trial and error experience and learning. If standards and values are lacking, unwise choices are made more than likely, resulting in unsatisfactory experiences. When this occurs, the individual learns the hard way. Without standards and subsequent evaluations, experience is a "dear school."

An important aspect of teaching and coaching is helping students make evaluations about themselves. Basically, they should be taught to establish their own values. In the motor skill area this could be a mental picture of the movements they want to make. The good teacher and coach projects this mental image in many ways. Then, the students, through self-evaluation and self-analysis, check on their progress. This self-analysis in physical education is not limited to the movement area. It can be applied equally well to attitudes and social behavior relating to sports. A most important aspect of teaching is helping students to make evaluations in this area which will result in choices that are socially acceptable and which will afford them an opportunity for achievement, success, and satisfaction both now and in the future. To this extent, evaluation is education and education is evaluation.

Relates the Product and the Process. Evaluation in education should aways be related to the ends desired or its loses its educational significance. Any values inherent in it depend on the benefits derived by the product. A good product results when a well-thought-out and skillfully planned program is developed in relation to formulated objectives, and when proper adaptation of methods and materials in instruction along with efficient administration occurs. These phases of the process should be followed by effective measurement and evaluation. Only when objectives have been defined, the program planned, and measurement made is it possible to fix the place of evaluation in the process. In the final analysis, its real justification is in the follow-up—the use of its results to improve the process and ultimately to provide for the needs of the product. This concept emphasizes once again the continuity of the educational cycle

Discovers Individual Differences. Another important facet of evaluation deals with the diversity of the student. Since each student is viewed as unique, the principle of individual differences must become a reality in education. If this principle is to become a functional principle, the needs of each individual must be established. One of the chief functions of education is to understand the student and an important purpose of measurement is to identify and recognize needs which will help in that understanding. Students differ in many ways. However, these differences can be translated into needs only when they have been revealed by measurement. It is as important to identify the gifted as it is the retarded and the average. When needs have been identified, a program can be planned to meet them. Thus, measurement is indispensable in planning a program to meet individual needs; it is also indispensable in recognizing when such needs have been met.

Serves the Needs of the Product Ultimately. This formal use of evaluation by the teacher is not a panacea for all of education's problems. It can be justified in the educational process only when it serves useful purposes. Its primary purpose, of course, is to serve the needs of the student just as any other procedure of the educational process. If this purpose is achieved, then evaluation occupies a significant place in education. When there is a proper follow-up after evaluation, it is generally reflected in the improvement of the process. Thus, the needs of the product and the needs of the process are inextricably interwoven. When the process is evaluated, it is possible that the outcomes desired in the product may be predicted to some degree. When the product is measured, it is equally possible that the process of education is also measured. The product should reflect the process. Worthwhile changes in the product are generally identified with the process. In the final analysis, society is ultimately interested in the product, and any change brought about in the process must be accompanied by desirable changes in the student or the value of the change is subject to question. The growth, development, and character of the product along lines considered to be valuable by society are the criteria of all educational practice.

Place of Measurement in Physical Education

In athletics and physical education, as in education and in life, the teacher and coach are constantly evaluating and measuring. He measures his students, his players, his associates, his opponents, his program and methods, himself, and many other things around him. The least valid form of evaluation he applies is a hunch or a guess. The most valid form is the use of well-established criteria as a basis for his comparisons. Usually this is done in the schools by means of tests and measures which have been validated against suitable criteria.

Measurement Applied to the Product. Since the teacher and coach must make evaluations in school situations, it follows that some planned program of evaluation will be put into operation. Effective utilization of evaluation occurs in physical education in two ways. *First,* it occurs when measurement procedures are applied directly to the *product* in order to measure accomplishment in a hierarchy of objectives which have been agreed upon by practically all authorities in the field[9] — (1) organic development including fitness, (2) psychomotor development with emphasis on sports skills, (3) cognitive area including knowledges and understandings concerning sports and exercise, and (4) affective area including social learnings involving sports with emphasis on sportsmanship.

Measurement Applied to the Process. *Second,* evaluation occurs when special techniques are used to measure the *process* of physical education itself. The teacher and administrator must know the degree to which the program and other aspects of the process meet acceptable educational standards. In evaluation of the process, techniques are used to measure the procedures of education and these procedures should be investigated according to the required program, the individual program, the intramural program, and the interscholastic program. Process measurement has several approaches, all of which provide the means for an improved service to the product. These approaches improve the over-all process by making instruction and administration more efficient and program more effective, and in the final analysis enhance the growth and development of the student.

How Measurements are Applied. Measurement and evaluation can be applied in several ways. In evaluating the product, the teacher and coach can do the evaluating or the student may evaluate himself. In some cases the students may evaluate each other. This student participation in evaluation is one of the great challenges in the field of teaching. In evaluating the process, evaluation techniques may be applied by the administrator, by teachers, or by an evaluation team. In some cases students participate.

Measurement in physical education can be applied for two basic purposes. It may be used first to measure *status*. However, when this same measurement is repeated one or more times, then achievement or *progress* may be noted. Generally both status and progress are compared with other values such as norms, standards, or criteria. Thus, a status measurement repeated at any given time will not only show how a student has progressed but also how he relates to his goals or to other students. In both the product and the process, measurement can show status, changes, and significances.

Some Basic Principles of Evaluation

A certain amount of planned evaluation has become essential to effective programming in physical education. If such practices are to be of most value, however, some competencies and guidelines should be established. The competencies have to do with knowledges which the physical educator must possess and practices which he must observe if his measurement program is to become effective. The guidelines concern principles from which he must form his basic beliefs concerning measurement. Effective evaluation is primarily based on observing these principles along with those which govern good teaching in general. The following principles should be understood by the teacher who is to engage in effective evaluation.

Determine Product. If evaluation is to be most productive, it must be related to the values which have been selected by society as being most desirable. The physical educator's first responsibility is to determine the *product* or to become aware of the product which has already been determined by society. In physical education, the desired product is the student who has the qualities and characteristics of a physically educated person. These are the values and this individual is the end of physical education and all other aspects are means to this end. This desired product is the ideal—the criterion of all physical education practices—and provides the criteria and the standards in those criteria for evaluation as well as a basis for the formulation of objectives. This is the underlying philosophy of all physical education practices.

Formulate Objectives. The place of evaluation cannot be fixed in the educational process until significant goals and purposes have been defined and direction established. Physical education objectives are formulated to serve as guides leading toward the attainment of the desired product. These objectives are important and will make a difference in teaching and learning. They enable the teacher to know what to teach and the student to know what to achieve. The procedures of measurement must relate the change in the product to the objectives. Evaluation is used to establish not only the direction of the change, but also the rate of change and its significance. If evaluation is to clarify direction, to identify rate of change, and to interpret significance, the objectives must be analyzed into specific outcomes. These objectives and outcomes become the points of reference for physical education process. Without them, evaluation is meaningless. Evaluation without objectives is like an "unguided" missile—out of control and no longer on target.

Establish Process. Just as the place of evaluation cannot be fixed in education until values are selected and objectives are formulated, neither can it be defined until the process itself is established. Physical education must establish its process and this process must be developed so that it will yield the values which have been determined. Process development occurs in the light of two things; the needs of the product which have been determined and the points of reference which have been established. Measurement technique is closely related to the procedures of the process. In fact, broadly speaking, it is one of the procedures. Measurement is indispensable in planning the process to help produce the desired product; it is also indispensable in determining the status and progress of that product. A good process is necessary if effective evaluation is to be expected. A physical education process under poor leadership and based on inadequacy of facilities and program will yield few positive results for evaluation to reveal.

Gather Data from Both Product and Process. Evaluation is a technique which is used to gather data for the appraisal of both the product and the process. This principle implies that both subjective and objective techniques will be used to collect both quantitative and qualitative data. It suggests that all traits, qualities, or characteristics possessed by the product and process exist in some amount or to some degree and can be measured.[30] This does not imply, however, that techniques are now available to measure all these characteristics. It does suggest that most subjective factors in the field can be evaluated to some degree. It is true that the less a quality or characteristic lends itself to identification, the more subjective the evaluation becomes. What cannot be measured can be judged, and there are tools and techniques to make these judgments even in the most qualitative aspects.

Necessary for Advancement in Scientific Education. Evaluation and measurement are necessary for advancement in scientific physical education.[30] Any part of education without evaluation is like a ship at sea without a chart and a compass. It is impossible to determine what the past and present positions are and even more impossible to predict or chart the course for the future. In its strictest sense, there can be no physical education and athletics without measurement of some type. For example, in the field of sports there would be little meaning to most activities without some form of measurement. The winner of the broad jump in a track meet is determined in terms of feet and inches. The winner of a basketball game is determined by a measure of the number of goals made. The winner of a diving event in aquatics is determined by a point scale. In its broadest sense evaluation becomes a major facet of education. Not only can the practice of measurement be educational to both the student and the teacher, but also its results are invaluable when they are applied to improving various phases of the process. Many times status can be improved only when it is revealed and it can be revealed only through measurement techniques.

Evaluation is Broader than Measurement. There is more to evaluation than measurement. Measurement merely identifies status, while evaluation assimilates status data and uses them to make comparisons with previously established criteria and to prescribe changes for future action. The importance of evaluation lies in the fact that after comparisons are made, there will be a followup. Objectives may be revised, programs replanned, personnel and facilities improved, and methodology changed. All of these changes would be brought about chiefly to create a better teaching and learning situation for the product. Successful evaluation is continuous and both the product and process need to be measured frequently with the ultimate purpose being to produce better physically educated students.

All Measurement is Not Objective. All measurement is not objective. Much of measurement is not as simple as are the tests which give results that can be recorded in inches, feet, times, and seconds. There are many characteristics which cannot be measured with objective techniques and their results cannot be expressed in quantitative terms. This sometimes makes measurement subjective and the subjective results are frequently less reliable than are objectively determined results. The problem in physical education is to objectify and systematize such measurements as much as possible, thereby increasing their reliability. Qualities and factors which can be identified and isolated lend themselves to quantitative measurement, whereas those components which are inexorably related to others and are not readily isolated or identified as distinct factors are difficult to measure and lend themselves only to qualitative techniques.

Does Not Take the Place of Teaching. Testing should not take the place of teaching, but should be used as a technique to help make teaching more effective. The basic function of the teacher is instruction and the instruction, like all phases of the process, should serve the needs of the student. The majority of the teacher's time should be devoted to this function. However, it is inevitable that some testing will be done and it follows that some phases of evaluation will probably be dynamic learning experiences. If measurement is organized as part of the instructional program, the teacher is frequently teaching while he is testing. After testing, of course, there must always be time left in the process for a follow-up or testing loses much of its educational force. Measurement and evaluation are valuable teaching techniques when they are related to instruction in this manner and when they provide motivation for the student to learn more readily. Furthermore, if the test has developmental value for the student, the administration of the test constitutes teaching in a direct sense. For example, if the skill tests provide training and practice in the fundamentals of an activity, they may be looked upon as drill techniques and many times are used as drills. The physical fitness test in most cases is an excellent means of developing fitness and may be used for that purpose, aside from testing. Also, in the area of self-evaluation, this principle is an important one. One tenet of evaluation is to lead the student to evaluate himself not only in the physical area, but also in the social and mental areas as well. Physical education is rich in opportunities for value judgments.

Used for a Specific Purpose. Testing for the sake of testing is wasteful of energy and time for both the teacher and the students. Measurement is definitely a means to an end and not an end in itself; therefore, it must be used for specific purposes. The application of this principle is assurance that measurement will be functional. In the light of measurement results gathered from the process, objective may be revised, new programs planned, and alterations made in methods. In the light of results gathered when measurement is applied to the product, there are such uses as classification, grading, guidance, and motivation. When measurement has been taken down from the ivory tower, where some professional people place it, and brought into the gymnasium, the playing field, and the classroom, it has been made *functional* for the average teacher. This is necessary, because if teaching is to become most effective, all teachers must make use of practical, scientific techniques of measurement which have been carefully selected for specific purposes.

Conducted by Qualified Personnel. If evaluation is to be effective, it must be conducted by qualified personnel who have training in its principles and procedures. It is axiomatic that many persons other than the specialist in physical education are concerned with evaluation. Among these are students, parents, administrators, auxiliary personnel, teacher aides, nurses and classroom teachers. All of these may share in some phase of the evaluation process in which they are qualified. In the final analysis, however, it is the specialist in physical education who must carry the load in conducting an effective evaluation program in physical education. He should have the following knowledges and competencies:

1. He must have knowledge of the availability of measurement instruments. This involves knowing what techniques are available and where the necessary information for their administration can be found.

2. He must know how to evaluate and select the tests for his specific purposes.

3. He must know the procedures of administration so that his test data are valid and reliable and so that time has not been wasted.

4. He must know how to interpret the results of his testing not only to himself but also to the student, the parent and the administrator.

5. He must have a purpose or purposes and use test results for these purposes for both his product and process.

6. He should be able to construct measurement techniques for his own use when none is available for his purpose. This would include not only physical performance tests, but also knowledge tests and social appraisal instruments.

7. He must have a knowledge of elementary statistics so that he can properly interpret his test results and so that he can construct his own tests and norms.

8. He must know how measurement relates to the total program and see the relationship between his curriculum, methodology, goals, and evaluation.

History of Measurement in Physical Education

History reveals that as man became more civilized, he also became more scientific and as he became more scientific, he sought more exact ways to measure. In America the history of measurement in physical education parallels the growth and development in research and the rise of physical education to a more respected position in the educational spectrum. Like medicine, physical education has gained a place of prominence and prestige only in proportion to the development and refinement of its measuring techniques. The history of tests and measurement in this country in physical education can be divided roughly into periods running from about 1860 to the present. These periods can be loosely divided into categories marked by the major emphasis which reflected the prevailing philosophy of the times. It is obvious, however, that these periods tend to overlap and run together and that there can be no clear cut lines of demarcation separating them. These periods are merely times when the specific measurement types came into prominence and were used most. To say they were used exclusively during these periods is not true. The first three periods reflected an emphasis on physical capacity and development, whereas the remaining ones were more indicative of the changing emphasis toward ability and efficiency to perform.

1. Anthropometric measurements	1860–1890
2. Strength tests	1880–1910
3. Cardiovascular tests	1900–1925
4. Athletic ability tests	1900–1930
5. Social measurements and intangibles	1920–
6. Sport skill tests	1920–
7. Process evaluation	1930–
8. Knowledge tests	1940–
9. Fitness tests	1940–

Anthropometric Measurements. While Quetelet, a French mathematician, was the first known person to use the term "anthropometric or anthropometry," the measurement of man dates back to ancient civilizations and is the oldest form of measurement. It was of interest in ancient India and later in Egypt where study was undertaken to find one part or component of the body which would predict or become a common measurement of all body parts. In Egypt, for example, the length of the middle finger was considered a common measure of all body proportions. For instance, five finger lengths to the knee, ten to the pubic arch, and eight the length of the arm reach.

The Greeks were experts in body proportions. Hippocrates was one of the first known test and measurement experts. He introduced a method of anthropometry by dividing the subject into two body types. His dichotomy, perhaps the forerunner of Sheldon's somatotypes, included the Phthesic dominated by the vertical dimension and Apoplectic dominated by horizontal dimension. This body typing was no doubt a prototype of others to follow. While Hippocrates studied physical types for medical purposes, Greek artists did so for aesthetic reasons.

The Greek sculptors particularly were concerned with the ideal of physical perfection. However, they changed their idea regarding body perfection over the centuries from the heavy broad body type with emphasis on strength to the more agile skilled type with emphasis on symmetry and grace. The Greek athlete alone rivaled the Gods as subjects for sculpturing. It was a custom in Greece for Olympic victors to have statues of marble carved in their honor. The Romans tended to follow the Greek canons in this regard. Over the centuries a similar type of anthropometry was carried on by other artists and sculptors—da Vinci, Michelangelo, and later

2

Joshua Reynolds were classic examples. In the early 19th century Rostan, a Frenchman, presented three physical types—Digestif, Musculataire, and Cerebral. These are definitely forerunners of Sheldon's somatotypes. However, purposes were different. Earlier measurements stressed body proportions for art sake, while more modern methods stressed social, emotional and intellectual facets of the unity mosaic.

The testing movement in America began with the work of Edward Hitchcock at Amherst in the science of anthropometrics. While body symmetry and proportion historically have been studied by artists and sculptors for aesthetic reasons, emphasis now shifted to educators for scientific reasons. In the beginning most of Hitchcock's measurements centered around such factors as height, weight, age, reach, girth, vital capacity, and some strength items. These measurements were repeated on the students at Amherst so that progress and gain could be shown. No doubt these first results were more of a concern for health as revealed through anatomical and physiological aspects since Hitchcock was a medical doctor and responsible for the health of his students. The fact that many pioneer physical educators were physicians had an impact on the advancement of the cause of measurement. It is thought by some that Hitchcock was probably influenced in these early years by the work of Archibald Maclaren of England who, in addition to developing programs in curriculum and methodology, also developed scientific techniques of measurements including anthropometric. The ultimate purpose of Hitchcock's measurement was to define the ideal physical proportions of man and, with the results of a quarter century of measurement, he was able to identify averages or the typical college man. In the famous 1885 meeting of pioneer physical educators, measurement was one of the chief topics for discussion.

To the work of Hitchcock was added the efforts of Dudley Allen Sargent. Sargent was no doubt influenced in his measurement work not only by Hitchcock, but also by Maclaren and William T. Brigham, an anthropologist, as he developed the body measurement idea even further. Starting in 1880 Sargent devised more than forty different measurements of the anthropometric types and used them with his students at Harvard. From these measurement results, he attempted to present a type of norm of the typical or the ideal man and woman. Also, through use of these measurements he attempted to prescribe a program of exercise for each student. His efforts to promote wider interest included the publication of a manual on measurement and testing and he also wrote articles for publication in journals. His system was adapted for use in both the public schools and colleges. These measurements emphasized symmetry and size and norms were established for each group with charts to

show how each individual compared with his norm.   The American
Association for the Advancement of Physical Education adopted his
measurement system for use in schools and colleges and the YMCA
adapted it to its uses.

Strength Measurements.   Around 1880 there was a shift in
emphasis of measurements away from size and symmetry to strength.
Even before the wane of interest in anthropometric measurement,
strength testing was being done.   Hitchcock had included such testing as a part of his early program at Amherst.   However, Sargent was
the real pioneer in strength testing and was the first to perceive beyond the tape measure and weighing scales and to recognize that
capacity for performance was a more important quality than size and
symmetry. Along with Brigham, Sargent experimented with the
dynamometer, a device invented in the 1880's, and devised a
strength test comprised of strength measures of the legs, back,
hand grip, and arms, along with a measure of vital capacity.   The
invention of the spirometer and the dynamometer undoubtedly
made this test possible.   The lung capacity item seems to have
remained vestigially a part of the strength testing field to this day
although vital capacity no longer is looked upon with the same confidence in regard to its relationship with actual strength.   However,
just as measurement evolved from size and form to strength, so it
evolved to another level where body efficiency with respect to movement became the center of attention rather than strength.   However, strength testing did return to a place of prominence in the
1920's as interest in it was revived and new tests developed.   The
best known of these was devised by Frederick Rand Rogers.[39]   His
scheme of testing was based on other strength test studies but he
differed from them in the manner of test construction.   His test was
devised in a scientific manner and was shown to have a high relationship with general athletic ability.   Rogers' ingenious use of the
Strength Index and the Physical Fitness Index makes this test one
of the true classics in the field.   It has been used, among other ways,
for purposes of classification.

Cardiovascular Measurement.   The shift in interest away from
anthropometry and strength took two directions.   Both were concerned with the efficiency with which movement took place.   Probably the most far-reaching of the two in terms of impact on testing
and programs of physical education was athletic ability testing.
However, the cardiac functional type test also became prominent.
Just as strength testing took on new meaning and accuracy with the
invention of the dynamometer, so did cardiovascular testing with
Mosso's invention of the ergograph in 1884.   The progress in this
area of testing was somewhat synonymous with the advancement
and rapid progress that has been made in the medical profession as

more and more was learned about the heart and circulation. As physiologists studied the effects of fatigue and the relation of muscles to the circulatory system, physical educators began to seek methods of testing the cardiovascular efficiency of the body. There appeared to be a relationship between the functioning of the body in movement and the condition of the heart and circulatory system. Tests in this area before 1930 merely laid the foundation for those which were to follow. All were developed through empirical methods and were somewhat less than adequate. Those developed after 1930 were devised according to the newer methods of test construction and were scientifically constructed.

The first test of cardiac function was published by Crampton in 1905.[20] This test set the pattern that was followed over the years by other similar tests including ones by McCurdy, Meylen, Foster, and Barach.[35,36,23,4] All of these tests proved less than adequate and it was not until later that a satisfactory instrument was devised. Such a test was devised by Schneider and was widely used during World War I to assess physical fitness of men for military duty.[40] However, the best test of this type was not developed until 1931 when Tuttle presented the Pulse-Ratio Test.[42] Tuttle's test has been shown to have value in measuring athletic condition and in detecting pathologic heart conditions. A few years later Brouha and fellow workers developed and presented the Harvard Step Test.[13] Succinctly stated, however, the use of cardiovascular testing in physical education has been limited.

Athletic Ability Testing. As strength testing fell into disrepute in physical education, emphasis began to be placed not only on cardiovascular tests, but also on testing the fundamental skills such as running, jumping and throwing. This category can be expanded to cover achievement tests, motor ability tests, motor capacity tests, and motor educability tests. Achievement testing had really already gotten under way before the turn of the century in the YMCA and the Turners when both developed pentathlon tests which were geared to track and field events. While Sargent had initially emphasized first anthropometry and then strength, he later shifted his interest to physical ability testing. In fact much of the initial research in motor ability, capacity and fitness by others was influenced by his pioneer work. Perhaps the booming growth in sports and games had something to do with the shift in attention and interest. Certainly behind the movement lay the new philosophy of Wood, Gulick, and Hetherington who emphasized these aspects as a part of the "new physical education." Another reason for the decline of strength testing was the cost of equipment needed for test administration. However, the most important reason for change was found in the new concept about strength. Leaders recognized that it was not strength but the way strength could be used that was important.

Sargent was a leader in the belief that strength tests did not measure endurance and speed, two of the qualities which seemed to make the most difference in performance. The movement away from strength tests spread and the public schools began to use achievement tests even before such devices were available in colleges. The Athletic Badge Tests were developed in 1913 by the American Playground Association with standards for both boys and girls. Test items were heavily weighted with track and field events along with a few items like the rope climb and vault. Colleges began to follow the lead of the YMCA and the public schools and the first such achievement tests for college were developed by Meylan of Columbia in 1907. These tests were used not only for grading purposes, but also classification where students might be permitted either to choose their activities or participate in some type of supervised program instead of class work.

The Sigma Delta Psi, a national athletic fraternity, was founded at Indiana University in 1912 and developed an ability test. Other physical ability tests were developed in a number of colleges and universities. All of these were for men, however, and it was not until the 1920's that such tests for women and girls were developed. Garfiel at Barnard developed the first listed motor ability test for women.[24] Somewhat later, Alden at Oregon and Collins and Howe at Wellesley also devised similar tests.[3,15]

The 1920's were particularly significant for the field of testing. Before this period much of the work done in measurement was unscientific and based on empiricism. Standards were arbitrarily established by the test maker in most instances and were not clearly identified. There was no provision for increments in scoring tables as performance reached the more difficult levels of attainment nor were there ways to equate scores on different tests. During this era, however, new statistical techniques became available and more scientifically constructed tests were developed. Validity and reliability of tests were improved and better means of developing scoring tables were used. The McCall T-scoring technique was employed for the first time. Pioneer work in the field of scientific test construction was done by C. H. McCloy of the University of Iowa. He developed achievement scales and the National Recreation Association also set up standards for boys in track, field, gymnastics, games, and swimming. Some new luminaries appeared on the scene with tests in the areas of motor ability and performance. David K. Brace of Texas developed his motor ability test which was later revised by McCloy and known as the Iowa Revision of the Brace Test.[12,33] McCloy recognized this revision at the time as a motor

educability test. Frederick Cozens devised a test of general athletic
ability for college men.[18] All of these tests have been used widely.
They were developed in accordance with the newest scientific
approaches in research and statistics and revealed insight into the
underlying variables to be measured and the interrelationships of
these traits. These early tests have served as models for modern
test construction. Strength testing was revived during this era.
Frederick Rand Rogers took Sargent's strength items and refined
them into a test giving a Strength Index and Physical Fitness
Index.[39] While all of the above listed tests were used as classification devices, better methods of classification were constantly being
sought. Both McCloy and Cozens developed classification indices
from weighted formula of age, height, and weight.[34,19] The initiating
of the Research Quarterly in1930 was not only a result of, but also a
stimulus to, the scientific era in research and measurement.

In the late 1920's and early 1930's the concept of measuring
general qualities was explored further and several well-constructed
tests were developed in general motor ability, motor capacity, and
motor educability. First, Brace using the latest scientific techniques,
developed a battery of motor ability tests. This battery was later revised by McCloy and adapted as one item for his Test of General
Motor Capacity.[32] This later test along with his test of General
Motor Ability, have become classics in the field. The General
Motor Capacity Test is presumably a test of innate performance
and gives a Motor Quotient which is the motor analogue of the
I.Q. In the same era, Humiston developed a motor ability test for
women which is still in use.[27]

Social Measurements. During the 1920's attention was first
directed toward some of the intangibles that had been attributed to
well-directed physical education programs. Since character, personality, and other social values had been considered outcomes of the
new sports and games program and were listed as objectives, it
seemed mandatory that status and progress in them be measured
in some way. McCloy and Van Buskirk pioneered in this area that
was later to provide many other efforts. Van Buskirk first used rating scales to appraise social and moral qualities. Later McCloy
developed a character inventory, and Blanchard devised a Behavior
Rating Scale.[31,6]

Sport Skill Testing. The initial use of sport skill tests was the
Athletic Badge Test in 1913. However, with the emphasis on sports
and games of the athletic type in the 1920's and early 1930's, it was
only natural that measurement should be slanted largely in this
direction. The early form of skill testing was more of the general or
fundamental skill type but as the new design in test construction
through statistical procedures became more prevalent, skill test

development became common. Brace presented one of the earliest skill tests on basketball.[11] Skill tests for achievement in specific sports were devised in great numbers during the 30's. The general procedure was to determine statistically a few simple test items to measure the total activity of that sport. Tests were developed for most sports, both team and individual, and in some cases norms were established for age and sex groups.

Knowledge Testing. No doubt knowledge testing has always been a part of physical education in the school programs. However, early attempts to measure knowledge were done through teacher-made tests. While these tests served an important function, they were not scientifically constructed and devised. Standardized tests are of recent vintage and most of these have been constructed since 1930 and the most used ones since 1940. Perhaps Snell and her co-workers at the University of Minnesota were among the first pioneers in scientific knowledge testing. The first knowledge tests reported in the literature, however, was by Bliss.[7]

Fitness Testing. In a sense a form of fitness testing has always been done. The individual has been assessed for his ability to meet the requirements of his environment. This was true in World War II which followed in the wake of two decades of scientific test making in physical education. Great stress was placed on fitness and this emphasis brought about a rush to develop fitness tests. These tests were geared to the needs of the war period. They could be mass administered, easily scored and interpreted. All branches of the armed forces—The Army, Air Force, Navy, Navy Aviation, Wacs, and Waves—devised fitness tests with appropriate norms. A number of other such tests were developed for school and college groups. Among the latter were Cureton's 14-item Motor Fitness Test at Illinois and Bookwalter's Indiana Motor Fitness Index.[21,8] Tests of this period, however, have now evolved into something more suitable for school and college use.

Process Evaluation. As programs of health and physical education grew in number and quality, there was a corresponding need to evaluate them. In the beginning the total process was broken down into parts and attention devoted to the evaluation of some areas more than others. It was not until the 1930's, however, that the subjective elements began to be quantified for purposes of evaluation. The first such quantitative device to receive wide recognition was devised by LaPorte and his committee.[28]

Trends in Measurement and Evaluation

History of any movement leads through the present and, when combined with the present, reveals trends for the future. Trends in measurement, like trends in any other aspects of education, are subject to change and are dependent on the new knowledge and research which lead the way for new emphasis and attention and to a change in philosophy. Today is an age of automation, sophistication, and technological wonders beyond man's wildest dreams of a few years ago. It is also an age of explosion of knowledge. Therefore, a trend today may become an accepted practice tomorrow, or what may appear a trend may be only a passing fancy and may fade in the light of new information and evidence. However, the following are some trends in measurement which seem to be shaping up and which are in various stages of fruition.

Refinement in Skill Testing. In the history of tests and measurements in this country, several stages have been experienced from anthropometric to fitness. Perhaps at the present time there is a renewed emphasis on evaluation of specific sport skills. This is a logical approach because if the student in physical education is to be educated, generally it must be done through the psychomotor domain. Therefore, there is a movement to develop better skill tests. An AAHPER Committee has developed a number of new tests and is in the process of developing others. If Franklin Henry and his colleagues are correct in their contention that skills are highly specific to the task, more and better skill tests are needed in this area.[25]

More Testing in the Cognitive Domain. There is a trend at the present for more standardized knowledge tests in physical education. These tests will, in the very near future, include not only rules, techniques, terminology, but also the growing body of knowledge that is developing and known as the cognitive domain. An AAHPER publication, "Knowledge and Understanding in Physical Education," presents this body of knowledge and the National Testing Service of Princeton, N.J. has developed standardized tests from this material.[2] This may not be the final answer by any means but it does mark a beginning and a trend.

More Use of Subjective Techniques. There seems to be a growing feeling that, if physical educators are to claim certain objectives, there must be an attempt to evaluate them or at least the progress students are making toward them. There are many qualitative elements in physical education and these facets of the program do not lend themselves to objective type measurement. If they are to be evaluated, then the commonly recognized subjective techniques such as the rating scale and inventories must be employed. More and more use is being made of rating scales even in measurement of more objective traits. This is a matter of expediency sometimes since skill testing is time consuming. It also may be partly a reaction against some of the traditional skill tests which are cumbersome and unwieldy. There is definitely a move from the quantitative to the qualitative but first the qualitative must be quantified.

More Sophisticated Techniques. The age of automation is an age of exactness when a space ship can be sent to the moon, land, and return and only be off time schedule and course a couple seconds and a few hundred yards. In physical education this trend will call for a re-evaluation of some time-honored tests which have been looked upon as classics. Many of them were designed years ago with limited knowledge and techniques. Many of them do not provide validities and reliabilities and some which do have used questionable criteria for validation purposes. Many of them need refinement, adaptation and updating. Testing might become the wellspring out of which evolves a rare individualized program for all.

Testing Will Become More Practical in Public Schools. Testing needs to be taken from the laboratory where research people have placed it to the classroom, the gym, and the playfield. There are signs this is being done. Testing means statistics to some teachers and this frequently leads to mental blocks. As professional training courses become more proficient, all teachers will know more about the philosophy and techniques of testing and will use tests more often.

Use of More Diagnostic Tests to Determine Individual Needs. Diagnosis and prognosis will become necessities and programs will have to serve many purposes. If teachers are to take advantage of the many possibilities for diagnosis of students, then purposes must be identified and the degree of refinement and sophistication of techniques will depend on these many purposes. Maybe physical educators are just beginning to see that testing has broader purposes than grading.

Continued Emphasis on Cardiovascular Testing for Fitness. This is the day and age of the jogger and the running of five miles per day. Whether this is a fad or not, only time will tell, but hopefully it is not. The very fact that medical people support the idea that man must literally run for his life may be enough to make this small start a movement. There are many training programs in colleges and universities and now doctors are starting their own clinics. Perhaps the persons most responsible for the movement are Cureton of Illinois and Karpovitch of Springfield. Cooper of the Air Force has done a lot to glamorize the field with his Aerobics.[17] The 5-minute treadmill run and the 12-minute run are now standard procedures.

Emphasis on Perceptual-Motor Evaluation. Much more must be learned about the field of perception and movement. There is a need for better measurement of perceptual-motor abilities, whenever it is learned what these are. Also, a better means of assessing the programs designed to improve dysfunction in this area is needed.

In the past most programs have been directed at those with learning difficulties and the 4-5-6 year age groups, but this area may well have something to offer all students.

Emphasis on Teacher Evaluation.   This is an area that is returning with or without merit.   In spite of the history of difficulties and controversy in evaluating the teacher, an effort must be made to implement such evaluation in a more effective manner.   College administrations are beginning to get tougher where tenure is concerned and, in the future, will apply the merit system at least in this one respect.   However, basically the overriding purpose of teacher evaluation will be improvement in instruction.

Greater Use of Proficiency Tests.   There is a decided movement toward the development and use of proficiency tests.   Studies show that many institutions either have some type of proficiency tests or are developing them.   Such programs are of two kinds: proficiency tests for the basic instructional program and proficiency tests for the professional training program.   There is no doubt the idea of permitting some of the more competent students to pass out of the program, or at least some of it, is due to two things.   First, it is in keeping with the practices in other disciplines which do it either for credit or advanced placement.   Second, it is a way to combat the explosion of the college population by permitting the most competent to be phased out of the program so that more of the time, staff, and facilities can be devoted to the less competent who need it most.   In generalizing about such schemes, it is the usual procedure to employ both knowledge and skills testing.

Emphasis Away From General Motor Ability.   A number of researchers including Franklin Henry of California and Slater-Hammel of Indiana think that motor tasks can no longer be considered as general but rather as highly specific entities.   Henry believes that each skill pattern is a stored program in man's brain—he calls it the "memory drum theory."[25]   Thus, the skill is specific to the activity.   There is no general quality of speed; a given individual might possess speed in football and a different kind in basketball.   Frankly, this trend has not gotten well under way yet and many traditionalists still consider that there could be a general motor ability.

Measurement of Motivation.   One last trend has to do with motivation.   It is a day when many people know what to do or what is best for them to do.   They still don't do it so there is need to study and measure motivation.   More should be known about what motivates people so when it can be identified through measurement, some use can be made of it.   If men in a training program are going to continue to exercise throughout life, they will need to have some type of motivation.

References

1. AAHPER, CPEA, and NAPECW: Physical Education for College Men and Women (report of joint conference, 1954 and revised 1959). Washington, D.C.: AAHPER, 1959.
2. AAHPER: *Knowledge and Understanding in Physical Education.* Washington, D.C.: AAHPER, 1969.
3. Alden, F. D., *et al.*: A Motor Ability Test for University Women for Classification of Entering Students into Homogeneous Groups, Research Quarterly, *13*, 85–120, March, 1932.
4. Barach, J. H.: The Energy Index (SDR) of the Circulatory System, Arch. Int. Med., *20*, 829, 1917.
5. Barrow, H. M.: The "What" and "How" of Testing. The Physical Educator, *12*, 8–9, March, 1955.
6. Blanchard, B. E.: A Behavior Frequency Rating Scale for Measurement of Character and Personality in Physical Education, Research Quarterly, *7*, 56, May, 1936.
7. Bliss, J. C.: *Basketball*, Philadelphia, Lea & Febiger, 1929.
8. Bookwalter, K. W.: Test Manual for Indiana University Motor Fitness Indices for High School and College Age Men Research Quarterly, *14*, 356–365, December, 1943.
9. Bookwalter, Karl W., and Carolyn W. Bookwalter: Purposes, Standards, and Results in Physical Education, Bulletin of School of Education, Indiana University, *38*, 1–6, September, 1962.
10. Bovard, J. F., F. W. Cozens, and E. P. Hagman: *Tests and Measurements in Physical Education,* 3rd Ed., Philadelphia, W. B. Saunders Co., 1949.
11. Brace, D. K.: Testing Basketball Techniques, American Physical Education Review, *29*, 159–165, April, 1924.
12. ———: *Measuring Motor Ability,* New York, A. S. Barnes and Co., 1927.
13. Brouha, L.: The Step Test: A Simple Method of Measuring Physical Fitness for Muscular Work in Young Men, Research Quarterly, *14*, 31–36, March, 1943.
14. Bucher, C. A.: *Foundations of Physical Education.* St. Louis, The C. V. Mosby Co., 1960.
15. Collins, V. D., and E. C. Howe: The Measurement of Organic and Neuromuscular Fitness, American Physical Education Review, *29*, 64–70, February, 1924.
16. Commission on the Reorganization of Education: Cardinal Principles of Secondary Education. Department of Interior, Bureau of Education, Bulletin No. 35, 1918. Washington, D.C., United States Printing Office, 1928.
17. Cooper, K. H.: *Aerobics,* New York, Bantam Book, Inc., 1968.
18. Cozens, F. W.: *The Measurement of General Athletic Ability for College Men.* Eugene, Oregon, University of Oregon Press, 1929.
19. Cozens, F. W., and N. P. Neilson: Age, Height, and Weight, as Factors in the Classification of Elementary School Children, Journal of Health and Physical Education, *3*, 21, December, 1932.
20. Crampton, C. W.: A Test of Condition, Medical News, LXXXVIII, 529, September, 1905.
21. Cureton, T. K.: *Physical Fitness Appraisal and Guidance.* St. Louis, The C. V. Mosby Co., 1947, p. 397.
22. Educational Policies Commission: The Purpose of Education in American Democracy. Washington, D.C. National Education Association, 1938.
23. Foster, W. L.: A Test of Physical Efficiency, American Physical Education Review, 632, 1914.
24. Garfiel, E.: The Measurement of Motor Ability, Arch. Psychology, *62*, April, 1925.
25. Henry, Franklin M.: Increased Response for Complicated Movements and a Memory Drum Theory of Motor Reaction, Research Quarterly, *31*, 448–458, 1960.
26. Hetherington, C. W.: *The School Program in Physical Education.* Yonkers, World Book Co., 1922.
27. Humiston, D.: A Measurement of Motor Ability in College Women, Research Quarterly, *8*, 181–185, May, 1937.
28. LaPorte, William R.: *The Physical Education Curriculum.* Los Angeles, College Book Store, 1955.

29. Larson, L. A., and R. D. Yocom: *Measurement and Evaluation in Physical Health, and Recreation Education.* St. Louis, The C. V. Mosby Co., 1951.
30. McCall, W. A.: *Measurement,* New York, The Macmillan Co., 1939.
31. McCloy, C. H.: Character Building Through Physical Education, Research Quarterly, *1,* 41–61, October, 1931.
32. ———: The Measurement of General Motor Capacity and General Motor Ability, Research Quarterly, *8,* 46–61, March, 1934.
33. ———: An Analytical Study of the Stunt Type Test as a Measure of Motor Educability, Research Quarterly, *8,* 46–55, October, 1937.
34. McCloy, C. H., and N. D. Young: *Tests and Measurements in Health and Physical Education.* 3rd Ed., New York, Appleton-Century-Crofts, Inc., 1954, p. 59.
35. McCurdy, J. H.: Adolescent Changes in Heart Rate and Blood Pressure, American Physical Education Review, 421, June, 1910.
36. Meylan, G. L.: Twenty Years Progress in Tests of Efficiency, American Physical Education Review, 441, 1913.
37. Nash, J. B.: *Physical Education: Interpretation and Objectives.* New York, A. S. Barnes & Co., 1948.
38. Oberteuffer, Delbert, and Celeste Ulrich: *Physical Education,* 3rd Ed., New York, Harper & Row, 1962.
39. Rogers, F. J.: Physical Capacity Tests in the Administration of Physical Education. New York, Teachers College, Columbia University. Contribution to Education No. 173, 1925.
40. Schneider, E. C.: A Cardiovascular Rating as a Measure of Physical Fatigue and Efficiency, J.A.M.A. *74,* 1507, May, 1920.
41. Staley, S. C.: *Curriculum in Sports.* Philadelphia, W. B. Saunders Co., 1935.
42. ———: *Sports Education.* New York, A. S. Barnes & Co., 1939.
43. Tuttle, W. W.: The Use of the Pulse-Ratio Test for Rating Physical Efficiency, Research Quarterly, *2,* 5–8, May, 1931.
44. Williams, J. F.: *The Principles of Physical Education.* 7th Ed., Philadelphia, W. B. Saunders Co., 1959.

Chapter 2

THE INTERPRETATION AND USE OF TESTS

Basic to the realization of the full potential of a testing program is an underlying relationship between the teacher and the students. Testing time is often a time of anticipation and anxiety. The development of ideal teacher-student relationships and a healthy learning environment come when the student realizes that, in testing, the teacher is doing something *for* him rather than *to* him.[3]

Testing can be justified when it is conducted for the good of the students and for the improvement of instruction. The latter is so directly related to the former that the student becomes uppermost in importance. The teacher, however, is the focal person to implement the program and to help the students establish positive attitudes about measurement procedures. He is the one who explains the purposes of the tests, how they will be used, and the meanings they have. The student should receive the ultimate benefit from tests but, too often, the student is not aware of this. The burden of responsibility falls to the teacher to set the proper mental stage for his students. Then he reaps optimum cooperation and enhances the value of the entire testing program throughout the school year.

Interpretation of Results

The interpretation of test results is of importance to everyone related to the educational process: the teacher, the student, the parent, and the administrator. This discussion will consider why the interpretation is important and, briefly, some of the ways it can be accomplished.

The Teacher. The teacher uses test results to guide his program through the year and to determine if his objectives are being reached. Without some realistic indication of attainment he is proceeding at random to present a curriculum. Are the students more fit? Do they know more about watching a football game? Is their skill level appropriate to their age? Is their attitude about physical activity developing in a mature and positive way? Are there special areas of weakness which need attention? These may be some of the specific questions to be answered. They can be answered, to a much fuller and more reliable point by what the teacher *knows*. This can be done by administering and interpreting appropriate and objective measures throughout the year.

The teacher plays the role of the interpreter so his job is one of communication. Students and parents are informed about the reasons for giving certain tests and the meanings they reveal. The administrator is told about the units of instruction presented and the ways in which the tests serve as meshing and integrating parts of that program.

Occasionally a teacher may feel the need of test results as a defense for a program or, more specifically, for giving a certain grade. Generally, however, the teacher should look upon tests as instruments to help him measure the overall progress of his students. They are more wisely used to sustain a good program carried out by a teacher with a positive professional attitude than to justify a program carried out by a teacher who is not sure of his own belief in the worth of the program. The point is a basic, philosophical one concerning the teacher. He determines the effectiveness or the ineffectiveness of tests as they become instruments for implementing his basic philosophy concerning physical education.

The teacher's role of interpretation never ceases. He must talk, explain, present results graphically, use the bulletin boards, send letters of explanation home, have conferences with students and with parents, and use every means at his disposal to impart a basic *understanding* of test results. Whenever he succeeds, an even more important concept concerning an understanding of the total physical education program is realized.

The Student. The student is interested in the meaning of test results because he is learning about himself. He wants to know if his achievement is comparable with others of his age and physical development. He wants to know if he has improved in skills, in fitness, and in understandings. Furthermore, his knowledge of these facts makes him more interested in his physical education classes. Students are becoming more self-directed and need to know as much about themselves as possible. This information will help them with the decisions they make about the conduct of their lives.

The implementation falls to the teacher. He should use tests periodically and follow-up promptly with their interpretation. He should be careful to post test scales for the class as a whole and not for any individuals. He thus avoids embarrassments and minimizes an excessive emphasis on a competitive feeling among the members of the class. He should be objective and impartial and should convey to the students that the tests are also objective and impartial. He should let the students know the standards he expects and the requirements for promotion. He should solicit the cooperation of the students by a full explanation of the tests given and the uses to which they will be applied. Only when a full understanding is evident can the teacher expect optimum cooperation and performance from the students.

The Parent.   Parents are inherently interested in the performance of their children.   Understanding test results helps them to understand their children.   They want to know if their children are developing physically as might be expected, if they are learning to play with classmates, if they are improving their skills, and if they are assuming leadership roles.   This type of information is indirectly apparent through grades, but much more specifically evident through test scores of various kinds.   Such scores provide concrete evidence of student performance.   The parents then understand the children better and indirectly they fathom what a physical education program can contribute to the over-all growth and development of their children.   This informational contact can be good public relations.   As parents understand the program and its benefits they are more supportive of the school in general and of the physical education program in particular.

The teacher is aided greatly by the students interpreting to the parents.   Together they help parents understand the program of physical education as well as the test scores.   Various materials sent home such as profiles, letters, and program and test plans for the year help in this endeavor.   Parents can be invited to demonstrations, to regular classes, to conferences with the teacher, and to PTA programs focusing on the physical education program.   All of these forms of communication supplement the report card and put it into proper perspective as just one of many kinds of information which the school shares with the parent about the student.

The Administrator.   The school administrator is in touch with the educational procedures throughout the school.   The program balance, the methodology, and the implementation all reflect the role of the testing program.   The responsibility of the administrator to be aware of all that occurs in the school is two-fold; he must use his initiative to seek information and teachers must use their initiative to supply it to him.   Lack of administrative support often reflects a lack of understanding.   Therefore, the teacher should discuss the program with the administrators and elicit their help in making it a worthwhile educational experience.

The teacher should discuss with the administrator the program for the year, the testing that is incorporated in it, and how it will be used.   He should discuss his philosophy about grading and how he structures the factors to be considered.   He should invite the administrator to watch some of the testing sessions during the school year and he should share with him copies of all materials which are given to students and to parents.

In summary, it may be said that the industry, initiative, creativity, and communicative skill of the physical education teacher will be employed as an understanding of tests and their uses and interpretations are made apparent to all those whose interest is vested in the students.

The Uses of Test Results for Measuring the Product of Physical Education—the Student

The primary use of test scores is to assess status and thereby to identify progress or achievement. The secondary uses are varied. The discussion will encompass five general areas, each having adjunct ones: grading, classification, guidance, motivation, and research.

Grading. Test scores are used more often for grading purposes than for any other reason. In one way this appears sound because it assures at least some objectivity in the assessment of grades. In another way it may be questionable if this is the sole application of test scores. Grades probably should not be based exclusively on test scores, and furthermore, test scores should not be relegated to this one narrow purpose.

Grades reflect attainment, improvement, and a standard of excellence. They are educational indices to help the student understand his position of competency. Grades are relative to a degree because they must be interpreted in relation to the tests used, the group tested, and the standards which the teacher considers appropriate to a particular group (see Chapter 16, p. 536). Philosophy concerning grades is in a state of flux. Learning and achieving seem justifiable goals which should not have to be coerced because of the pressure of grades. Students and educators alike are re-thinking the role of grades in education. It may be that grades will not continue to be used in the traditional ways for promotion and graduation. Students and teachers will always want to know about achievement, however. So status of achievement will need to be ascertained even if the use of the information changes.

Classification. Classification implies a grouping of students for certain educational purposes. At times, students of similar skill level are grouped to enhance instruction and to meet the needs of the highly skilled student, of the poorly skilled student, as well as the student of average skill. This practice is also considered justifiable for competitive purposes. Sometimes students are grouped in mixed ability levels. Then the poorly skilled students can experience competition challenging enough to aid their own skill development (see Chapter 15, p. 517). Groupings are used occasionally to enhance interpersonal relationships. The activity program is one vehicle for causing changes in the social structure of the group and of each individual in it.

Classification can be accomplished by using motor ability tests, fitness tests, skills tests, social scales, attitude scales, or by a combination of these tests. The tests used depend on the purpose of the grouping. Ideally, motor ability and fitness groupings encompass large groups. For example, all the boys with similar motor ability scores would be scheduled for physical education at the same time in their school program. More realistically, the practicality of scheduling enables the students on just one grade level to meet together. Then the classification process occurs within the class and permits subgroupings for more individualized instruction. Conceivably, such groupings might be re-shuffled several times within the semester.

Classification is one application of test scores which is not used to its fullest because of the inconvenience of testing. The benefits in better instructional groupings, however, are usually worth the time and effort.

Guidance. The guidance aspects are so interwoven throughout the whole realm of test scores and their uses that it is difficult to delineate them. In its broadest sense, all of testing is used in some type of guidance capacity for all students. The permanent records of the school should provide a place for recording, periodically, various kinds of physical education test scores such as fitness scores, motor ability scores, and grades. These cumulative records accompany the student throughout his academic life and should provide a complete picture of his status, including the physical and social as well as the academic aspects of his achievement. The teaching and administrative personnel of the school should make use of the information in the cumulative folder to plan, cooperatively, courses of action which would be helpful to any student under consideration.

Counseling is employed frequently for students requiring special help. A handicapped child or a student with a social adjustment problem would be examples. The more complete the information on all aspects of the student's education, the more effective the counseling can be. The physical education teacher should contribute to this information with test scores and anecdotal observations.

Related more specifically to the physical education program, there are diagnostic tests, prognostic tests, and proficiency tests which have a part in the guidance of students. Diagnostic tests are designed to identify weak areas. Such batteries should be comprehensive to sample as many aspects of a sport as possible. A teacher might want to determine the weaknesses in the softball playing ability of her girls. She should test their batting, base running, fielding, stealing, throwing, and catching abilities and from these results determine where her emphases should be placed. This process can work for individual students as well as for a whole class.

Such tests of knowledges as well as skills are used little. They are given primarily for the guidance of the teacher so he may focus on the weak areas to be taught or coached.

Prognostic tests are designed for determining levels of potential skill development. Such tests deal with concepts of capacity and ultimate skill attainment. As predictors of skillful players, they are of importance to coaches. They are limited in number, questionable in meaning, and little used. This area of testing is one in which much work needs to be done.

Proficiency tests are beginning to receive more attention. Proficiency in skills and in knowledges might excuse a student from some sports so that he can enroll for activities in which he is less proficient. This concept once evoked scheduling problems for secondary schools. Flexible and modular scheduling have remedied this situation and have, indeed, made proficiency testing even more essential. Proficiency testing is pertinent, as well, to the proper functioning of the non-graded school. Placement at appropriate activity levels and exemptions from activities are uses in which proficiency tests in both skills and knowledges are making meaningful contributions. Proficiency tests may find more use in the future as a standard for promotion at the elementary, junior high school, and secondary school levels. It is feasible that certain levels of achievement in physical skills should be attained for promotion just as specified levels of achievement are considered in other subjects within the curriculum.

Motivation. The use of test results for motivational purposes is somewhat nebulous but nevertheless quite significant. This use is closely related to the teacher-student rapport covering the whole area of testing. Students can be motivated to perform at their maximum because of their inherent competitive spirit, because they are anxious to make the best possible showing, and because the subject itself is important to them.

They should be motivated to perform well as they compete with themselves and not always with other members of the class. Self-improvement and self-realization are the sounder approaches to the motivational concept.

Research. The research uses of test results are many and varied. The teacher who has a research interest will usually be experimenting with various approaches, new methods, and possibly new activities. The effectiveness of these pursuits can be measured by applying research techniques to testing procedures. The appropriateness, the value, and the comparable results of the research endeavors can become evident. A research project can stimulate a teacher and add to his professional growth. It can serve to keep alert an inquiring mind. A word of caution should be stated about overuse of the research idea. It can be very time-consuming and interest-capturing at the expense of the total program. The other extreme is probably the more prevalent one, however, so it would be appropriate to encourage research endeavors by teachers. Through research they can improve their programs, develop more objective tests in some areas, devise tests in areas heretofore undeveloped, and learn to make better use of the test scores available to them.

All of the uses of test results are designed to enhance the fullest development of the student by assuring him the best possible program of physical education in keeping with his individual needs.

The Use of Test Results for Measuring the Process of Physical Education—The Program. (See Chapters 13 and 14)

The Program. Program evaluation is a long-range project usually culminating at the close of a semester or of a school year. This is the time for a close look at the program to spot weaknesses and to re-evaluate objectives. Measures of status and progress, comparisons with established standards, and identification of strengths and weaknesses are some of the possible uses of program evaluation. Have the objectives been met? Were they appropriate? Did the activities provide for a progression of skill and were the skills difficult enough to challenge? The junior high school program should not be a repetition of the elementary school program, just as the college program should not be a repetition of the secondary school program. Were suitable achievement levels reached and if not, why not? What were the students' reactions to and suggestions for the program? Such broad and fundamental questions as these can be answered about a program just completed. Often, scores from a variety of measures will show whether achievement levels have been reached and surpassed, whether fitness levels have been sustained, whether new activities have been learned, and whether changes in program are indicated. This is a continuous process. (See Chapter 13, page 475.)

The Methods. The approaches used by the teacher can be studied also. If changes have been made, he can assess their effectiveness. If progress has been minimal, he can examine his methods as a possible source of explanation. If great strides have been made, the impact of various methods can be studied. Methodology is continually changing so this end-of-the-year review provides an ideal time for the teacher to look at the complete program and to evaluate the methods used.

The Teacher. In addition to evaluating the program and the methods used to implement it, the teacher should include evaluation of himself. This can be done by the administrator, by the teacher, and by the students. Check lists, conferences, and self-appraisals are some of the techniques used. The teacher must maintain an objective viewpoint. The students and the program should be foremost in his mind and, if they are, his personal evaluation should serve as a professional experience for growth. (See Chapter 14, page 512.)

This discussion ends with an emphasis on the teacher and his competence to provide a good program for the benefit of the students. All the effort is focused on the students. Worthwhile experiences for them come from a good program. Before this can be realized, the responsibility of the teacher as planner, user, and interpreter of tests and test results must be fulfilled.

References

1. Bovard, John F., Frederick W. Cozens, and E. Patricia Hagman: *Tests and Measurements in Physical Education*. 3rd Ed. Philadelphia, W. B. Saunders Co., 1950.
2. Larson, Leonard, A., and Rachael Dunaven Yocom: *Measurement and Evaluation in Physical Health, and Recreation Education*. St. Louis, C. V. Mosby Co., 1951.
3. Lennon, Roger T.: Testing: Bond or Barrier Between Pupil and Teacher? *Education, 75*, 38–42, September, 1954.
4. Scott, M. Gladys, and Esther French: *Measurement and Evaluation in Physical Education*. Dubuque, Iowa, Wm. C. Brown Co., 1959.

Chapter 3
EVALUATION OF PERFORMANCE TESTS

The Need for Selecting Appropriate Tests

Selection of appropriate tests is necessary if wise application of results is to be realized. The little time allotted for measurement activities should be spent wisely. The choices of tests should be made in light of the objectives sought. If the tester is a researcher, he may be interested in a detailed, technical measurement. The teacher will be just as concerned about the accuracy and honesty of the results, but he will need to find a test which will be easy to use and appropriate to the group situation present in schools. The theme of this text is centered on the teacher and on helping him get the best answers with the best tools. This chapter will present some criteria for selecting measurement devices.

The pressure of time probably should not be the deciding factor but it must be considered. A test should serve the student directly and indirectly, but it must do so with efficiency. Some selection has been made in choosing the tests to be included in this book. Further selections will need to be made by the teacher in light of each teaching situation. Judgments will continue to be needed as new tests become available.

Such questions as, "Why give a test?," "What information is needed?," and "To what use will the results be put?" are the kinds of considerations which will help in making appropriate test selections. If these questions cannot be answered, the job of selection will be difficult and the measurement program likely will be ineffective. Further, an aimless program without direction and focus will be evident. With a good concept of what physical education is and what the teacher is hoping to accomplish, and with some definite objectives and plans in mind, the measurement program can be a real force for good.

Criteria for Test Selection

Technical Standards. Standards for judging tests which are of a technical nature will have been established during the development of the tests, and certainly prior to the publication and general use of them by the teaching public. These standards involve the application of some technical and statistical steps which should accompany each test when published.

1. Objectivity

Objectivity is the *first* of the technical standards to be considered. Objectivity is the degree of uniformity with which various persons score the same test.[17] It refers to the lack of any personal influence of the scorer on the test results. If the test is well standardized and is administered properly, the role of the scorer should not have a noticeable influence on the results. Objectivity is a measure of the worth of the scores and is inherent in the test. If a test is scored by two instructors, concurrently and independently, the results should be similar. The correlation coefficient produced from the two sets of scores should be high. This measure, which is similar to reliability, changes only one condition in the testing procedure and that is the scorer.

The statistical technique employed for ascertaining objectivity is a correlation. This tool is described in Chapter 5 on statistics. For the present it is sufficient to know that a correlation results in a coefficient which ranges from 0 to either + or −1.00. Further delineations of the coefficients and their relative values are presented in Table 3–1. Objectivity coefficients are higher for scores which are precise and numerical and they are lower for scores which are subjectively determined. For example, the agreement of two timers on a 100-yard dash should be very good. The agreement of two judges rating a gymnastics routine will be less stable. This is one reason rating scales have been devised to objectify, as much as possible, subjective observations. The motivation, clarity of directions, organization, scoring accuracy, and the like provided by one instructor should not be so different from that given by another as to influence the scores appreciably. If such is the case, however, the test is said to be lacking in objectivity. Objectivity is enhanced by

Table 3–1.   Arbitrary Standards for Interpreting Correlation Coefficients

Coefficients	Validity	Reliability and Objectivity
.95 to .99		excellent
.90 to .94		very good
.85 to .89	excellent	acceptable
.80 to .84	very good	acceptable
.75 to .79	acceptable	poor
.70 to .74	acceptable	poor
.65 to .69	questionable (except for very complex tests)	questionable (except for groups)
.60 to .64	questionable	questionable (except for groups)

clear test directions, precise scoring methods, and adherence to them. Table 3–1 presents some coefficients and some arbitrary standards which have been reported by various writers. Because of the multitude of factors which influence coefficients but cannot be controlled, it probably is safe to say that the arbitrary standards are too high and that tests with slightly lower coefficients would be acceptable for use and could be relied upon to produce meaningful measurement information.

2. Reliability

a. *Definition.* Reliability is the *second* technical standard which the teacher can use when selecting tests. A test is said to be reliable if it is dependable, if similar results will occur when the test is repeated by the same group under like conditions. Reliability is related to the test performance itself. The tester is the same, the students are the same, and the test is the same. It is administered and then re-administered. If the students fall in the same positions on the scale, the test is perfectly reliable. The student who performed best the first time is still best, the poorest performer is still poorest, and all in between are approximately in the same order. A test is given to position students on a ladder, so to speak. If their positions are true indications of their skill, then the test is said to be *valid;* if their positions are dependable and consistent, then the test is considered to be *reliable.*

Countless factors influence reliability. The equipment used in the test may not be of sufficient quality to produce consistent results —a poorly inflated ball or a mutilated badminton shuttlecock. The instrument recording the measurement may be too gross, such as a 100-pound spring scale used to measure dorsal flexion of the wrist. The number and length of the trials needed to get a stable measure are important. Usually the best of three broad jumps is considered adequate, whereas most accuracy tests require about twenty trials. The longer the test, the more reliable it will be. Averaging scores usually produces more reliable results than taking only the best score. Averaging has a leveling influence on the scores.

The directions may be so complicated that the student cannot remember the procedure. The test may be so long as to introduce a fatigue factor. The student may be in a different motivational frame from one day to the next. The teacher may present the test in a different way. But if all things are standardized as much as practically possible, the test should prove to be reliable and therefore worthy of confidence.

b. *Methods of Establishing Reliability.* Reliability is also interpreted by using the statistical technique called a correlation coefficient. The reliability coefficient is obtained by correlating one measure of the test with another measure of the same test and thus is judged by an internal and dependent measure. Consequently, reliability coefficients are generally higher than validity coefficients. Reliability coefficients may be derived either by the interclass method suggested by the product-moment correlation or by the intraclass approach employed in analysis of variance.

(1) TEST-RETEST. One method of establishing reliability is to administer the test completely one time and then to give it another time. Usually the second administration is on the next day or two and under very similar conditions and certainly before forgetting, practicing, and learning factors become too influential in the results. This method is time consuming and sacrifices some of the interest factor of the students during the second administration. The coefficients would be derived from the Pearson Product-Moment method of arriving at correlation coefficients.

(2) SPLIT HALVES (odd and even). A time saving and creditable method is to administer the test only once and then correlate the total of the even-numbered trials with the total of the odd-numbered trials. In a 10-trial test, the 1, 3, 5, 7, and 9th trials totaled would provide one score and the 2, 4, 6, 8 and 10th trials totaled would provide the second score for the correlation problem. This method requires the subsequent use of the Spearman-Brown Prophecy Formula to predict what the reliability would be had the test-retest method been used instead. The Prophecy Formula predicts the reliability of the whole test on the basis of only half of it. This formula is also useful to predict what effect additional trials or longer trials or even reduced trials would do to the reliability of a test. The resultant coefficient is usually referred to as a "stepped-up" one.

Spearman-Brown Prophecy Formula[9]:

$$r_x = \frac{nr}{1 + (n-1)r}$$

r_x = stepped-up coefficient
n = proportion of increase in the test
r = split-halves coefficient

Split-halves coefficient = .55

$$r_x = \frac{2(.55)}{1 + (2-1).55} = \frac{1.10}{1 + .55} = \frac{1.10}{1.55} = .7096 \text{ or } .71$$

A particular test yielded an odd-even coefficient of .55 which, when stepped-up by the Spearman-Brown Prophecy Formula, produced a reliability coefficient of .71 for the entire test. The researcher might want to recommend additional trials to achieve a higher reliability coefficient. To double the length of the total test on the basis of the split-half or odd-even coefficient, the formula would read as follows:

$$r = \frac{4\,(.55)}{1 + (4-1).55} = \frac{2.20}{2.65} = .83$$

Even this does not produce a really high reliability coefficient, so some other methods of refining the test might be required. The common practice is to estimate the coefficient for twice the number of trials because of the split-halves situation so Table 5–7, page 104, is included for convenience in making conversions. The split-halves method is appropriate for use with knowledge tests because of the large number of items. This application is discussed in Chapter 11 on Knowledge Testing.

(3) ANALYSIS OF VARIANCE. The analysis of variance technique for establishing reliability has been recommended in the research literature and has some merit over the other two methods. This intraclass method permits the identification of sources of variability in performance that are used in estimating reliability. These sources of variability are usually day-by-day differences in performance and trial-by-trial differences in performance. The Spearman-Brown Prophecy formula will permit the manipulation of the number of trials to arrive at an acceptable coefficient of reliability. The analysis of variance technique will permit the additional manipulation of the number of days to determine adequacy of the coefficient. For example, the researcher would report several reliability coefficients representing various combinations of days and trials of test performance. The subsequent user of the test would then select the version of the test with an acceptable coefficient yet efficient to administer. A coefficient of .99 might be possible if a test were given 4 days with 5 trials on each day. This same test might give a reliability coefficient of .90 given 2 days with 1 trial on each day. The research report would show the matrix of possible reliability coefficients and the teacher would select the plan most appropriate to his situation. Baumgartner[3] states that the intraclass correlation method (estimated from the analysis of variance) is the most preferable method of establishing reliability, the test-retest is the second best, and the split-halves method is least desirable. For the student of Measurement, it is sufficient to recognize the method used just as the method of establishing validity is important. The coefficient alone is not nearly as meaningful as the coefficient accompanied by the method of attaining it.

(4) PARALLEL FORMS. This type of reliability is used generally with written tests. The object is to construct two tests of similar difficulty and content. The students take both tests. If they per-

form similarly on them and *if* the two forms of the test really are parallel, then the test may be considered reliable.

Some authors make a distinction between reliability coefficients required for tests used in group measurement and for tests administered on an individual basis. Group measurement reliabilities can be lowered because so many uncontrollable factors are present in mass administrations which adversely influence reliability indices. The standards presented in Table 3–1 are not definite. The type of test and the type of group taking it should be considered when trying to assess the value of the validity and reliability coefficients reported for a particular test.

3. Validity

a. Definition. Validity is the most important of the technical standards because it tests the *honesty* of a test. The teacher will want to have confidence that a test he has selected to use as a measure of the tennis serve, for example, is indeed just that and not a test of shoulder girdle strength or of general motor ability. It must be a measure of a rather specific skill—namely, the tennis serve. It would be unfair to use a fitness test as one basis for assigning grades if the test were so complicated that an intelligence factor weighed heavily in the performance score of each student. If a test is presented as a measure of the volleyball volley, then, to be valid, it must measure volleying ability and, ideally, it must measure it to such a degree that other influencing factors such as height and weight are incidental to the final results. A test may be considered valid if it is measuring, as accurately as possible, what it is described as measuring. Validity is inherent in the purpose of the test.

b. Methods of Establishing Validity. There are several ways of ascertaining validity. Each way involves the comparison of the new test with some standard, called a criterion, which has already been established. This results in two sets of scores: one for the new test being developed, and one for the criterion measure. These sets of scores, one for each student, are correlated. If the relationship is close, the test is considered valid. If the standard chosen for making the comparison is poor, then the validity reported is often misleading. The standard or criterion used as the comparison factor must be the best possible. Several have been used to establish the validity of various motor tests and each will be discussed. They may be used in combination as well as separately. For example, a new test may be compared with tournament standings as well as with subjective ratings. This multiple use of criterion measures is an attempt by researchers to make doubly sure that the new test is valid.

(1) SUBJECTIVE RATINGS. Subjective ratings sometimes are

given by the teacher to use in grading. When used for establishing validity, they are given by at least three judges and often five or seven. Ratings generally involve judgments on the form of a performance. The tennis serve will provide an example. The technique of the serve, its execution, force, form, accuracy, and the like will be noted for each student by three judges. They evaluate on the basis of a rating scale which defines carefully the distinguishing points between a performance worth five points and one worth only two points, for instance. As a second step, these same students are given a service placement test. Then the composite or average of the three judges' ratings is compared with the objective service placement test score for each student. Two assessments are available for each student; they are correlated, and the resultant coefficient is used as the basis for interpreting the validity of the service placement test. If the scores on the test *rank* the students in approximately the same order that the judges evaluated them, the coefficient will be relatively high and the service test will be said to be valid on the basis of the criterion of judges' ratings.

The opinion of experts—knowledgeable observers—is often a more accurate measure than is a poor test. No apologies need be made for the use of subjective ratings. Care should be taken that the skill is well defined, that the rating scale is refined, and the raters are competent (see Chapter 17, p. 555). Ratings can be poor criteria, but if carefully done, they may be relied upon to yield dependable results.

Many of the motor tests in the professional literature have been validated on the basis of subjective ratings. Many others have been validated on the basis of other objective measures. The teacher needs to realize that the objective test used as a criterion was probably itself validated by subjective ratings. It is possible that some of the early subjective ratings were poorly executed and this emphasizes the need for constant re-evaluation of the objective tests that are available in the measurement literature.

(2) PREVIOUSLY VALIDATED TESTS. Some skill tests are created as refinements of other tests already available. The test may be simplified, shortened, or revised in some way. The old form of the test is administered to a group and then the new form is given to the same group. If the standings of the people in the group remain similar, then the new test may be said to be measuring appreciably what the old test was measuring. And, if the old test was reputed to be a measure of the badminton clear, for example, then the new test may assume validity for the same measure. Researchers seem to favor the use of previously validated tests as criteria for establishing validity because the tests yield objective scores as opposed to subjective ones. Care should be taken that the previously validated

test was itself carefully and accurately validated before it is accepted as a standard for measuring the validity of a new test.

(3) COMPOSITE SCORES. Composite scores are used generally as a criterion when a broad general type of ability (such as fitness or motor ability) is being measured. They are used also when a test battery is anticipated. The researcher may realize that he is not likely to find one skill test which will give an ample measure of football playing ability, for example, but that several tests sampling the essential skills of football will be needed.

A composite score is achieved by administering a gamut of tests, each supposedly related to the measurement area in question. The scores are put into some type of comparable form, such as T-Scores, and are added to get one total or composite score. Other tests or perhaps even some which were in the composite listing are then correlated with the composite score, each in turn, and in various combinations. The composite score is then used to help select the battery of tests which comes closest to measuring whatever all the individual tests were attempting to cover in their measurements.

The composite score uses the "buck shot" theory implying that if enough related tests are given, surely some of them will be measures of the skill in question. This particular standard for establishing validity is somewhat in question for this reason. It may encompass too broad a base of skills to identify anything but very general types of ability. If, on the other hand, the test items are carefully selected, the composite score theory has some merit.

(4) TOURNAMENT STANDINGS. Tournament standings serve as adequate standards for establishing validity when a high level of skill is anticipated. Some tests are designed for beginning players, others for advanced players, some for young players, and others for more developed players. This is taken into account when planning a test. Tournament standings for advanced players are rather reliable and serve as good indications of playing ability. They are less dependable when the tournament players are beginners or when the sport involved is a team sport instead of an individual one.

A round robin tournament is a good style to use, as is some type of ladder tournament. These are longer tournaments requiring more contests, and may be counted on to put the players in their proper order of playing excellence. Once this standing is set and assigned some numerical value, it can be compared with various tests which measure the fundamental skills in a game. For example, tennis tests for the service, and forehand and backhand drives could be validated against tournament standings *if* these strokes are considered important to overall tennis playing ability.

This particular criterion is not used often because of the length of time required to complete the tournament, but it should be considered a good criterion especially for developing skills tests for players above the beginning levels of skill.

(5) FACE VALIDITY (Empirical Judgment). Face validity is another standard for validating tests and it is a useful one at times. The 50-yard dash is considered to be a measure of running ability if speed of running also means excellence of running. The tester considers the dash and arbitrarily says it is a measure of running. He concludes this on the basis of logic, common sense, judgment, and so-called face validity; that is to say that one can look at a test and see inherently what it is measuring. The basketball wall pass may be a measure of shoulder girdle strength, reaction time, ball handling ability, basketball playing ability, height, and on and on. It is perhaps related to each of these factors to some degree. The dash, on the other hand, while influenced by reaction time, weight, and the like, is basically a measure of running ability and there is very little quarrel with that belief. It is generally accepted to be such a measure and thus the dash is an example of a test which is said to have face validity.

The teacher should evaluate the available tests by looking first at their validity. Not only the coefficients but also the criteria which were used as the bases for computing the coefficients should be examined.

4. Norms

a. Definition. Norms are the *fourth* of the technical standards to be discussed. If a test is accompanied by norms, its usefulness is enhanced. A norm is a scale which permits conversion from a raw score to a score capable of comparisons and interpretations. Its characteristics of average and range are known. A raw score of 16 is quite meaningless, but if that 16 falls at the 78th percentile or is equivalent to a T-Score of 58, it becomes capable of comparisons and interpretations.

b. Characteristics and Comparisons of Various Normative Scales. A word of caution should be stated about norms. They should not be accepted at face value. Norms are representative of some larger population. They should be based on a particular type of group which is well identified. For example, Percentile Norms on the Basketball Wall Pass for High School Girls, or T-Scores on the AAHPER Fitness Test for 11-year-old Boys label the norms. Age and sex are usually the two essential classifications. Other factors might be geographic location, race, and skill level. Norms should be based on large numbers of cases. Adequate cases alone do not make good norms but, coupled with proper sampling, they provide a symmetrical distribution.

If the performance of a group is not similar in range and average to the normative group then the norms are not appropriate and should not be used for interpretative purposes. It would be far better for the teacher to construct norms based on the scores of his own students.

Chapter 5 on statistics discusses the computational procedures and characteristics of various kinds of normative scales. Familiarity with the various kinds of norms will help the teacher interpret the scores that accompany many tests. Their usefulness is without question but their appropriateness for use with any particular group should be checked carefully. Tables 3–2 and 3–3 are included to help the teacher compare the range, center score, and relative standings of various normative scales. These comparisons are appropriate only when the scores used to establish the norms are normally distributed.

Table 3–2. Conversion Table for Seven Normative Scales*

Percentiles	T-Scale	Six Sigma Scale	Stanines	Hull Scale	Standard "z" Scale	C-Scale
99.9	80	100			3	
99.75	78	97		90		
99.5	76	94				
99.25	75	92	9	85		10
99.0	74	91				
98.5	72	87				
98	70	84		80	2	9
97	69	82				
96	68	80	8	75		
95	67	79				
94	66	77				
93	65	75				8
92	64	74		70		
91	63	72				
90	62.5		7			
89	62	70				
88	61.5					
87	61	69		65		
86	60.5					
85	60					
84	60	67			1	7
83	59.5					
82	59					
81	59	65				
80	58.5					

* Smithells, Philip A., and Peter E. Cameron: *Principles of Evaluation in Physical Education.* New York, Harper & Brothers, 1962. The Percentile and T-Scale columns are taken from p. 227 and used by permission of Harper & Row.

Table 3–2. Conversion Table for Seven Normative Scales (Continued)

Percentiles	T-Scale	Six Sigma Scale	Stanines	Hull Scale	Standard "z" Scale	C-Scale
79	58					
78	58	63				
77	57.5					
76	57	62		60		
75	56.5					
74	56	60	6			
73	56					
72	55.5					
71	55					
70	55	59				6
69	54.5					
68	54.5					
67	54	57		55		
66	54					
65	53.5					
64	53.5					
63	53	55				
62	53					
61	52.5					
60	52.5					
59	52	53				
58	52					
57	52					
56	51.5					
55	51.5					
54	51	52				
53	51					
52	50.5					
51	50					
50	50	50	5	50	0	5
49	50					
48	49.5					
47	49					
46	49	48				
45	48.5					
44	48					
43	48	47				
42	47.5					
41	47.5					
40	47					
39	47	45				
38	46 5					
37	46 5					
36	46	43		45		
35	46					

Table 3–2.   Conversion Table for Seven Normative Scales (Continued)

Percentiles	T-Scale	Six Sigma Scale	Stanines	Hull Scale	Standard "z" Scale	C-Scale
34	45.5					
33	45.5					
32	45	42				4
31	45					
30	44.5					
29	44.5					
28	44	40				
27	44					
26	43.5		4			
25	43	38		40		
24	43					
23	42.5					
22	42	36				
21	42					
20	41.5					
19	41	35				
18	41					
17	40.5					
16	40					
15	40	33			−1	3
14	39	32		35		
13	38.5					
12	38	30				
11	37.5		3			
10	37	28				
9	36	27		30		
8	35	25				2
7	34	24				
6	33	22				
5	32	20		25		
4	31	19	2			
3	30	17			−2	1
2	29	15		20		
1.5	28	14				
1.0	26	10				
.75	25	9	1	15		0
.5	24	7				
.25	22	3		10		
.1	20	0			−3	

Table 3–3. Characteristics of Various Normative Scales

Type of Scale	Range	Center Score
1. Percentile	0 to 100	50
2. Six Sigma Scale	0 to 100	50
3. Hull	approx. 10 to 90	50
4. T-Scale	approx. 20 to 80	50
5. C-Scale	0 to 10	5
6. Stanine	1 to 9	5
7. Standard "z" Scale	approx. −3 to +3	0

Practical Standards. The practical standards to be considered when selecting tests are more immediate than the technical ones. They are important when preparations are being made to give a test, when it is actually administered, and when the results are used.

1. Administrative Considerations

a. Equipment. The equipment and supplies should be readily available and inexpensive. A test which requires an elaborate and expensive piece of equipment will not be used often in a school situation. Most tests require the use of some equipment, but it should be the kind that is either on hand or can be easily and economically constructed. Sports equipment such as balls, rackets, and the like should be of good quality to help the performance of the students.

b. Time. The equipment, floor and wall markings, and all preliminary arrangements should be refined to such a degree that they can be efficiently readied with a minimum of extra preparations. A test which requires many intricate markings calling for an excessive amount of the teacher's after-school time will seldom be the test he will select to administer.

The time required to administer the test will be a factor to consider. Group testing, partner testing, and station testing illustrate the efficient use of personnel to streamline the time requirements for administering tests. Not many tests will be used which require an individual performance of several minutes while the remaining students wait their turns. Most test batteries can be administered to an entire class in one or two class periods if well planned and organized.

c. Money. The cost of measurement equipment need not be prohibitive. Equipment can be collected from year to year in most school systems. The teacher should collect high quality and accurate measurement tools over a period of time and refrain from making large investments for highly specialized and expensive equipment. A budget allotment should be designated for measurement equip-

3

ment just as for sports equipment, supplies, uniforms, records, first aid supplies, and the like.

d. Utility. The test results should be readily usable. If norms are available and appropriate, the raw scores should be converted quickly. No complicated formula should be necessary for each step of the conversion. The quicker the results are available to the students in some meaningful form, the more educational application they will have. Profiles, graphs, and charts can be used by the instructor to help the students understand their performance.

Often a teacher will find a test which suits his needs after he makes some revisions and adaptations. Caution should be used in making revisions because they will influence the validity and reliability of the test and may make the norms inappropriate. Adjustments can be made to make the test into a drill or a practice test, but little leeway should be assumed by the teacher in making appreciable adjustments. Deviations from the prescribed directions may make the test a measure of something quite different from what was intended.

e. After Effects. The instructor should be reluctant to use a test which will have negative after effects on his students. Some fitness items are administered to the point of exhaustion and may cause nausea. All out performance on some items will cause muscle soreness and discomfort lasting two or three days. Items inappropriate for a certain group might cause a student to develop a mental block against all testing. Such traumatic experiences are unnecessary, uncalled for, and the teacher should be on the alert to prevent them.

2. Developmental Values

These values are nebulous and intangible but nevertheless quite vital to the over-all decision of selection. Tests can influence the program, the instructor, and the student. But the effects on the students are most important, and these indirectly influence the program. The student reacts to tests in various ways which should be considered when selecting tests.

a. Physical. Scott and French[15] relate various criteria for effective tests especially in the area of skill measurements. They state that tests should be game-like, they should encourage good form, they should test important skills, they should be of suitable difficulty, and they should meet various statistical standards.

Most test descriptions state that the tests are constructed for a specific sport and for a certain grade level. It would be unfair to the test and certainly to the students to administer a college fitness test to junior high school boys and to expect of them a comparable performance. A skill test should challenge the student to perform to the best of his ability. Tests which require no effort are not meaningful to students and contribute little to their physical development. Appropriateness should be the key word for selection. If the tests are geared to the skill area involved and designed for that age group, then the student should have a meaningful and satisfying physical experience. A boy is challenging himself while taking a fitness test. He is not wasting time. A student continues to practice and train in the fundamentals of basketball during a skills test. Tests can be just as much a part of the instructional plan as drills and games.

b. *Mental.* The attitude of the student is closely related to his physical performance. If a test is of appropriate difficulty and presented to the student in an educationally sound manner, he should be motivated to perform well. The test should interest him, be sensible, and meaningful. A test which is too complicated, too difficult, or which is unrelated to the skill area for which it is used, will fail to provide a sound educational experience. The student will lose respect for the measurement program in physical education. A poor performance could very well be the result of poor test selection. The student is penalized because the teacher has not made a competent test selection. Testing can be a worthwhile mental practice because, through it, students learn concepts about interpretations, comparisons, reasons for various kinds of performance, individual differences, growth, and personal reactions.

c. *Social.* Testing in a school situation is a group experience. Not often is it appropriate or feasible to administer tests in a solo fashion. Groupings, waiting turns, helping score and administer tests, tolerance, patience, cooperation, and competitiveness are some of the factors which are present. The student has time for introspection as he relates to his place in the group, to his role in the testing procedures, to his performance in relation to his classmates, and to his interpretation of the entire process. If poorly used, testing opportunities and follow-up sessions can be negative social experiences; or they can be vehicles for better interpersonal relationships. This must be structured, however, by the teacher and students.

There are so many factors for the teacher to consider when selecting tests that, at first, it may seem a formidable job. Test selection is one way for the teacher to approach his objectives. When a test is over, the student should be a better student. With program objectives well understood and with the development of the students uppermost in his mind, the teacher should be able to include appropriate measurement tools in his program. Good decisions on test selections will help create desirable psychological, sociological, and physiological results for each student.

References

1. AAHPER: *Research Methods in Health, Physical Education, Recreation.* 2nd Ed. Washington, D.C., AAHPER, 1959.
2. Baumgartner, Ted A.: Estimating Reliability When All Test Trials Are Administered on the Same Day, Research Quarterly, *40*, 222–225, March, 1969.
3. ———: Stability of Physical Performance Test Scores, Research Quarterly, *40*, 257–261, May, 1969.
4. ———: The Application of the Spearman-Brown Prophecy Formula When Applied to Physical Performance Tests, Research Quarterly, *39*, 847–856, December, 1968.
5. Carlson, R. Robert, and Walter Kroll: The Use of Analysis of Variance in Estimating Reliability of Isometric Elbow Flexion Strength, Research Quarterly, 41, 129–134, May, 1970.
6. Feldt, Leonard S., and Mary E. McKee: Estimating the Reliability of Skill Tests, Research Quarterly, *29*, 279–293, October, 1958.
7. Guilford, J. P.: *Fundamental Statistics in Psychology and Education.* 4th Ed., New York, McGraw-Hill Book Co., Inc., 1965.
8. Kroll, Walter: A Note on the Coefficient of Intraclass Correlation as an Estimate of Reliability, Research Quarterly, *33*, 313–316, May, 1962.
9. Larson, Leonard A., and Rachael Dunaven Yocom: *Measurement and Evaluation in Physical Health, and Recreation Education.* St. Louis, The C. V. Mosby Co., 1951.
10. Lindquist, Everett F. (ed.): *Educational Measurement,* Chapter 15, Reliability, Washington, D.C.: American Council on Education, 1951.
11. Malina, Robert M.: Reliability of Different Methods of Scoring Throwing Accuracy, Research Quarterly, *39*, 149–160, March, 1968.
12. Mathews, Donald K.: *Measurement in Physical Education.* 3rd Ed., Philadelphia, W. B. Saunders Co., 1968.
13. Phillips, Marjorie, and Karl W. Bookwalter: Three Little Words, The Physical Educator, *5*, 21, March, 1948.
14. Safrit, Margaret Jo Anne: Construction of Skill Test for Beginning Fencers, MSPE, University of Wisconsin, Madison, 1962.
15. Scott, M. Gladys, and Esther French: *Measurement and Evaluation in Physical Education.* Dubuque, Iowa, Wm. C. Brown Co., 1959.
16. Smithells, Philip A., and Peter E. Cameron: *Principles of Evaluation in Physical Education.* New York, Harper & Brothers, 1962.
17. Willgoose, Carl E.: *Evaluation in Health Education and Physical Education.* New York, McGraw-Hill Book Co., Inc., 1961.
18. Winer, B. J.: *Statistical Principles in Experimental Design.* New York, McGraw-Hill Book Co., Inc., 1962.
19. Zabik, Roger M., and Andrew S. Jackson: Reliability of Archery Achievement, Research Quarterly, *40*, 254–255, March, 1969.

Chapter 4
ADMINISTRATION OF TESTS*

In the past, one of the glaring weaknesses in measurement has been an inadequate preparation on the part of the teacher in the knowledges and techniques concerned with the organization, administration, and interpretation of a testing program. Proper selection of tests is of no avail unless the testing program is conducted in an efficient manner. Efficient test administration should guarantee maximum accuracy for valid and reliable results, and insure that time has been used to the best advantage. Also, the results must have meaning and the teacher must be able to interpret the test data which are obtained.

Efficiency in testing does not just happen. It is the result of step-by-step planning and preparation. There must be an understanding of the techniques to be used, a competence in the actual administrative procedures, proper utilization of space, effective use of leadership, and an adequate follow-up. It is essential that the teacher have an understanding and an appreciation of the need to conserve time. Physical tests generally are more involved than mental tests, and the time alloted to the physical education class generally is shorter than for most other subjects. Unless special attention is devoted to conserving time, testing might consume more than its proportional share of the total allotment, and might result in excessive loss of instruction. However, time should not be saved at the expense of accurate scores.

The program of measurement should be organized as a part of the instructional program, and with certain definite purposes in mind. When it is so organized, the time devoted to testing is not wasted; testing becomes a part of teaching and is thereby an educational activity in itself like any other procedure. While there is no arbitrary rule in the matter of time allotment, it is a generally accepted principle that testing should take no more than 10% of instruction time.[4] If tests are used as teaching devices, however, and if they are made to serve a number of purposes, this time may be greater than 10%. In reality, most good teaching involves testing in one form or another and, in the same way, most testing is teaching.

The very nature of testing calls for supervision by highly qualified personnel. Test results are only as valid as the basic data which

* Adapted from the following source: Barrow, H. M.: The ABC's of Testing, Journal of Health, Physical Education and Recreation, *33*, 35–37, May-June, 1962.

have been collected through testing techniques. Tests carelessly administered, or tests administered to a group of students who are not properly motivated, provide results which have little meaning or value. A student has not been tested until he has given maximum effort, nor is his score accurate if the test has been improperly administered, judged, or scored. Since tests will vary according to objectives, purpose, and type, no set rules may be established to cover all administrative procedures. More specific suggestions are made for particular tests in the chapters where those tests are presented. However, for purposes of simplicity, some general suggestions can be made. These suggestions are listed under three headings: (1) Advance Preparation, (2) Duties During Testing, and (3) Duties After Testing.

Advance Preparation

Selection of Tests. The proper selection of measurement techniques is the first consideration in administering tests. Selection of the exact test will depend upon the type of information which is sought by the teacher. Tests should be selected with certain considerations in mind. *First,* it is necessary to know whether the product of education, or the process is to be measured. *Second,* if the process is to be evaluated, it is necessary to know what education procedure is being considered and for what purpose the results will be used. It is possible to evaluate the teacher and staff, the methodology, the curriculum, or the total program. If the product is to be measured, it is necessary to have in mind the purpose for which the results will be used, such as classification, grading, or diagnosis. *Third,* tests must be selected in the light of certain administrative procedures. Such procedures are especially significant. Tests should be chosen with a view to the time available, the size and age of the group, the number of qualified leaders, the difficulty in administering the test, and the amount of equipment and facilities which are on hand. One or more of these factors might eliminate an otherwise highly desirable and valid test. *Fourth,* the tests must have high standards in the other selective criteria of validity, reliability, objectivity, utility, and norms. These criteria should be accompanied by good physiological and psychological reactions on the part of the student.

Knowledge of the Test. The director of testing should have a sound knowledge of the test which is to be used and a thorough understanding of its administrative procedures. Procedures and techniques should be studied carefully. The inexperienced teacher would profit by writing out all the necessary details. Frequently this can be done on 3 by 5- or 5 by 8-inch cards. The cards can then be shuffled at the convenience of the instructor. It is a good plan for a diagram to be drawn of the complete lay-out. This lay-out could be posted at a convenient place for the benefit of the students.

Equipment and Facilities. A study should be made of the space need, special equipment, courses, special markings, and supplies. The proper use of space, equipment, and materials can reduce the amount of time needed for conducting tests. Proper space planning reduces confusion and avoids crowding and congestion. The following suggestions should be helpful:

1. Courses and Markings. Most tests give specific directions for the lay-out of test stations. All directions in regard to courses, courts, special designs, and markings should be observed carefully. They should never be modified by the inexperienced tester, and by the veteran tester only when he is assured that the proposed changes will in no way affect the scores or the use of scores. The field or floor should be laid out properly and marked for rapid scoring in such events as throws, jumps, and kicks for distance. A football field which has been marked off into 5-yard zones provides an excellent lay-out for throwing and kicking events for distance. A mat marked at 1-, 2-, 3-inch intervals with parallel lines can be used for the standing broad jump. Perhaps the simplest way to set up the standing broad jump station is to use an already established line on the floor for the take-off line and fasten a tape measure to the floor at right angles to this line. Lines on walls or floors can be put on with rapid-drying washable paint or with masking or adhesive tape. Targets can be made in the same manner or they may be painted on canvas, oil cloth, plastic, mats, or plywood. The latter methods provide more flexibility in their use.

2. Equipment. All equipment such as horizontal bars, parallel bars, chinning bars, targets, ropes, poles, jumping standards, and special devices should be available and put in place before testing is begun. Safety is an important consideration in the placement and use of equipment. Common sense should prevail in the placement of testing stations. Some logical order should be selected. Overlapping of areas and overcrowding is dangerous and is not conducive to best results. However, testing is expedited when as many testing stations are set up as leadership, space, and equipment permit.

3. Materials. Some of the tests require a great many supplies and materials. Most test directions will indicate the type and amount. If they are not indicated, the director of testing should determine the kind and amount needed and secure them prior to the testing period. These materials might include such items as stop watches, balls, tape measures, signs, string, cord, chalk, pencils, score cards, and tongue depressors for markers. If students are to do their own recording or if partners are to score, pencils in quantity should be provided. The novice should make out a list of the needed supplies and check them off as he provides them. The important thing is to have them on hand and ready for use.

Preparation of Score Cards. Scoring forms should be designed and prepared in advance. Sometimes students may even prepare their own from a pattern made available to them. There are several types of score cards and various methods for recording scores. The particular situation will dictate the type of card to be used. Each of the types described below has its strong points.

1. Class Roll Sheet. This score sheet has names of all class members in alphabetical order with spaces for their scores and other pertinent data which may be needed. This type of score card can be used more readily when there is one examiner who administers and scores all test items, or when the station-to-station method is used and each station has class roll sheets. Sometimes such score cards are used as cumulative records for the group when scores from individual score cards are transferred to them. In any event this method expedites the conversion of raw scores to scale scores and presents an over-view of class performance (see Fig. 8–12, p. 239).

2. Squad Cards. The squad card is used sometimes when the squads rotate from station to station and the squad leaders carry the squad cards with them. It is a smaller version of the class roll sheet and has the same characteristics. It is more flexible, however, and permits the squads to score themselves under the direction of squad leaders or a trained tester.

3. Individual Score Cards. Perhaps the best method for recording scores and certainly the most flexible, since the student can move about independently of his group, is the individual score card. Each student carries his card with him from station to station and must assume responsibility for its care. This card usually is designed for the specific test and generally provides space for such information as the student's name, class, date, age, weight, height, raw score, and converted score. If the scores can be summed, there should be a place for a composite score. Generally a 3 by 5 card will serve the purposes for most score cards but in some cases the 5 by 8 is better. This individual card, or "carry type" as it is sometimes called, is generally used when the students score for each other, or when they rotate from station to station independently of their groups and are scored by a trained examiner. Since the student must assume responsibility for his card, he shares to a greater extent in the measurement program. Also, he can see his score and he has a better idea about his status. If the score cards are cumulative, he may easily see his progress and achievement. One disadvantage of the "carry type" card is that the student frequently loses it, or if the card is used more than once, it tends to become mutilated. (See Chapters 7 and 8 for examples.)

When individual score cards are used, scale score conversion tables with scale scores for all possible raw scores should be posted at some convenient spot for the benefit of the student. With a minimum of training, the student is then able to convert his own raw score in terms of the posted norms. These norms answer many questions for the student such as "How good was my throw?" or "Which was my weakest event?" Scale scores may even be printed on the obverse side of the individual card, a practice which implements considerably the conversion of scores by the students themselves. Conversion tables should be constructed so they are easy to read at a glance since the instructor may have to convert all raw scores for all students on all test items.

Scale scores for each item of the battery sometimes are placed directly on the individual score card along with the corresponding raw scores. This permits the student to convert his raw scores immediately to scale scores by merely encircling his raw score or indicating it in some manner. He may then connect the circles with lines and construct a profile directly on the card (see Fig. 4–1). This enables the student to see in a graphic way his status in the various test items and when a second administration of the same test is plotted along with the first, progress may also be noted.

Preparation of Standardized Directions. In the administration of most tests there will be two types of directions necessary. One set should be prepared for the trained test administrators so that

	BOYS										GIRLS									
GRADE 6	BALL BOUNCE	JUMP ROPE	JUMP FOR HEIGHT	WALL BALL	ACCURACY THROW	SIDE STEPPING	DISTANCE THROW	KICK AND RUN	CLIMB	CHINNING	BALL BOUNCE	JUMP ROPE	JUMP FOR HEIGHT	WALL BALL	ACCURACY THROW	SIDE STEPPING	DISTANCE THROW	KICK AND RUN	CLIMB	CHINNING
NUMBER OF CASES	100	100	100	100	100	100	100	100	100	100	100	100	100	100	100	100	100	100	100	100
90	6.6	49	19.5	35	6	25	60	9.1	3	13	7.7	61	17.5	33	4	23	37	10.0	3	11
80	6.9	41	18.0	34	5	24	50	93	3	12	8.4	56	16.0	31	3	22	32	10.2	3	10
70	7.2	38	17.0	32	5	23	48	9.5	3	11	8.8	53	15.0	30	2	21	29	10.4	2	9
60	7.5	35	15.5	31	5	22	46	9.8	3	10	9.1	49	14.0	28	2	20	26	10.6	2	8
50	8.0	31	15.0	30	4	21	44	9.9	3	9	9.4	47	13.0	27	1	20	24	10.8	2	7
40	8.4	27	14.0	29	4	21	40	10.1	2	9	9.8	44	12.5	26	1	19	23	11.0	2	7
30	9.0	21	14.0	28	4	20	37	10.3	2	8	10.3	42	12.0	24	1	18	21	11.2	1	6
20	9.7	17	13.0	27	3	19	35	10.6	2	7	11.2	38	10.0	24	0	17	20	11.6	1	4
10	10.7	9	11.0	24	2	17	31	11.1	1	6	12.4	33	9	20	0	16	17	11.9	1	3

(PERCENTILE)

Fig. 4–1. Score Card showing profile for individual student achievement. (Courtesy Greensboro Public Schools, Greensboro, N.C.)

they will know exactly how to explain, demonstrate, administer, and score their particular test items. The second set of directions concerns the instructions given to the students for taking the test. These two sets of directions may differ somewhat. The directions should be standardized and prepared in written form. They should create interest and stimulate maximum performance. If possible, they should be memorized by the examiner. If they are not memorized, they should be placed in written form on appropriate size cards which can easily be shuffled as the tester gives directions. They should be read exactly as they are written. The following suggestions are made with reference to test directions for students: they should be as brief and concise as possible; they should accompany or precede the demonstration; they should be adapted to the age level of the subjects; and they should emphasize the correct procedure rather than the incorrect. Sometimes it is possible to combine into one set the directions both to the students and to the test administrator. The directions for the student might be placed in italics or bold type on the instructor's cards. In this way the directions will stand out and can be more easily read by the examiner.

Preparation of the Testing Area. Careful planning in setting up the testing area is important. If the test instructions call for a specific arrangement, that pattern should be followed. If not, the instructor should make his own arrangement with certain principles in mind. *First,* the stations should be arranged to accommodate the flow of traffic. A diagram of the area should be drawn showing the floor plan and space requirements. *Second,* the stations should be placed from the least strenuous to the most strenuous, or spaced so that alternate sets of muscle groups are tested unless otherwise specified. *Third,* the station should be clearly identified by a name or a number. *Fourth,* a factor of safety should be a consideration in the placement of events which might be dangerous if they are permitted to overlap. Sometimes by careful placement an entire test battery can be administered from a central location (see North Carolina Fitness Test, Chapter 8, p. 249). In this example, each station has a trained scorer, but one person in a central position can administer all five items at the same time. A requisite here is for all items to consume about the same amount of time. If one item tends to move more slowly than the others, two or more stations may be employed for that particular item. This system has more recently been called circuit testing.[1]

Selection of Organization and Administration Procedures. Nothing should be left to chance. The tester should carefully plan all procedures for organizing the subjects in advance. The question of when and how the demonstration will be done is important. When the order of test items in a battery is not suggested by the test maker, an order must be established. Ways and means for economical administration of tests should be studied. The way a class is organized for testing will depend to a great extent on the type of test and the characteristics of the group to be tested. No one plan can be adapted to all situations. There are three main ways to organize the class.

1. *Mass Testing.* The most effective use of time allotment is made when a large number of students are tested at one time. Many tests can be administered on a mass basis. In this method one examiner can explain and demonstrate all test items and administer them to all the students. There are two variations of this method. First, the students may be paired into partners, and while one half of the group is being tested, the other half acts as scorers and recorders. This method is time saving and should be used whenever the test items are adapted to its use. In the second variation, all members of the class can be given the test at the same time which makes it a greater time saver than the first-mentioned method. This system is used when it is feasible for each student to score himself.

2. *Squad Method.* Another method involves all of the students at the same time, but the class is divided into squads and each squad works independently. This method works best when each station operates on a comparable time basis so that all the squads may rotate together. If squads are already organized for instruction it is a simple matter to have each squad tested on a particular test item by the squad leader or by a trained assistant. Either squad cards or individual cards may be used to record scores. After each squad member has been tested, the squad can rotate to another test station and begin testing there. As was pointed out above, this method works best when all stations require about the same amount of time for administration or when multiple stations are used for the slower-moving items. If squads are not already organized, some simple method of dividing the group may be used. For instance, if there are thirty pupils and five test items and individual score cards are used, the cards may be divided into five groups and each group can be marked with a different color. As the class assembles, all students holding red cards are designated as one squad and can report to one station, the green to another, the blue to another and so on. See the North Carolina Fitness Test for circuit testing (page 249).

3. *Station-to-Station Method.* Sometimes in large groups where the order of events is not important or where some stations require more time than others, the best method of organization is on a station-to-station basis. Here the student rotates from one station to another as an individual and does not remain with any particular

group or squad. He is scored by a trained assistant and must have an individual score card to carry with him. In this system sometimes it may be that one or more test items are slower to administer than the others. In this case, two testing stations may be set up for the slower-moving items. This prevents a piling up of subjects at any one station. The age of the student will have some influence on the use of this station-to-station approach. The method is sometimes not feasible when younger children are tested.

4. Combinations. Sometimes it may be best to combine two of the above methods. In many cases, for example, the squads can rotate from one test to another on a station-to-station basis. On occasions the mass technique may be used for one or two items, and then a shift made to the squad or station-to-station method for the other test items. No one plan of organization will fit all situations. In any event each test item should be explained and demonstrated to all of the members of the class before testing is actually started. Frequently it is possible to set up one or more testing stations adjacent to the playing floor or field. The instructor may then test one group, squad, or team while the others participate in the regularly scheduled activity. For example, if a class is divided into five squads or teams, one group may be tested while the other four compete or engage in drills.

Scoring. One of the most important considerations in testing is the observation of performance and the recording of results. Results must be observed carefully and recorded quickly and accurately. Many tests require the scorer to have specialized training. For example, if the assistant is to operate a stop watch, he should have some instruction in its use. Sometimes test administration is implemented in events like the throws and jumps when two people, a spotter and a recorder, assist with the scoring. Time is saved if only the best out of three trials is actually measured. This method usually works best when the contestant takes his three trials in succession. When markers are used, such as tongue depressors with the thrower's name on them, a number of students, perhaps an entire squad, can take their throws and each one be marked. When all members of the group have completed their throws, they can be measured at the same time. In judging scores and recording results there are three main methods. Naturally, there is some relationship between the way a class is organized for testing and the method of scoring.

1. By Instructors. This method is perhaps the most time consuming and should be used only when the situation dictates. The instructor may do the scoring when one squad is being tested while the other squads are participating in regular class activity, or when the nature of the test is such that only a highly specialized person can administer it. Posture and nutrition type tests would be in this category.

2. By Partners. This method is generally used when the tests are administered on a mass basis. The class is divided into partners and, while an examiner administers the tests and supervises them, scores are judged and recorded by the partner who is not taking the test at the time. Partners may also do the scoring within the squad. When this partner method of scoring is employed, the director of testing, in his explanation, must emphasize the scoring techniques to be followed.

3. By Squad Leaders. When tests are administered on a squad basis, generally they are administered and scored by a squad leader. The training of this squad leader may be done at a training session prior to the period of testing. This system works especially well where a student leadership program is in operation and where leaders are already trained in the techniques of leadership.

4. By Trained Testers. When tests are administered on a station-to-station basis, scoring is generally done by trained examiners who have been instructed in methods of judging and scoring at a training session prior to the day or period of testing. These trained individuals may be students, faculty members, professional students from a teacher-training institution, or interested non-school personnel.

Orientation of Students. The students should be instructed in the purpose of the tests and the manner in which the test results will be used by the teacher. In general, students should be told what they are striving for and the outcomes to be achieved. If practice is desirable or necessary, the test items may be explained and demonstrated days in advance of the actual testing period. Special directions should be given the student regarding equipment, dress to be worn, shoes, pencils, score cards, *etc.* Students are frequently motivated when they are told that test scores will be posted. In some cases, however, this might be bad psychology. Poor student attitude is not conducive to best performance. A student's past experience with tests may influence his attitude toward taking them. For example, he may have suffered nausea, or he may have become extremely stiff and sore following testing. Also, he may have learned that his scores were not being used and there was no purpose behind the testing. If the students receive proper orientation, however, they will know that the tests will have a useful purpose and that the test results will be used. Furthermore, they will know something about the testing procedure—how the scoring will be done, the general lay-out of the testing area, and what is expected of them. All of these factors should contribute to a more positive attitude on their part.

Training of Student Leaders and Scorers. If highly qualified people are available, they should be used to assist in the testing program. Experienced assistants are especially important when the test procedures and techniques are more complicated and difficult. Experience is mandatory in the use of such equipment as stop watches or such techniques as counting of pulse rate in a cardio-vascular-type test. However, many times it will be necessary for students to assist in administering tests and keeping records. The use of student leaders is not only a necessity from the administrative standpoint, but also an educationally sound procedure. It is one of the ways students can share in the measurement program. A great deal more training is required to administer tests than to judge results and record scores. When students are used to assist in the test administration process, some training is necessary. One or more training sessions are necessary if the students are to have a complete understanding of the test and the testing procedure. Student assistants must be trained in the procedures for administration, the techniques for the individual test items, the techniques of demonstration, and the method of scoring. They should be impressed with the necessity for being accurate, uniform, explicit, and alert. The standardized directions mentioned previously should be followed implicitly. Instructions should be so simple and definite that any examiner might carry on the testing procedure at any station. If it is possible, the student assistants should go through the entire test as subjects. This makes it easier for them to learn the correct techniques. At the same time it gives them an opportunity to share in the taking of the test. Special emphasis should be placed on scoring procedures. This is especially true when specialized equipment is to be employed, such as stop watches and dynamometers. Some practice in the use of these instruments is essential.

Duties During Testing

Last Minute Check. Time is one of the most valuable factors in a physical education class. A good instructor is always trying ways to gain valuable minutes for teaching and instruction. When the testing period is at hand, the instructor should begin by making a last minute check of equipment, supplies, and facilities which are to be used. When the class has assembled, everything should be ready and in place so the testing procedure may start immediately without loss of time. If the group to be tested is unorganized, such as a group from study hall or a group during orientation or pre-registration, some effort should be made to see that they report to the testing area in an orderly and punctual manner. If the group is quite large, the students should be staggered according to alphabetical order or some comparable way.

Explanation. The standardized directions which have previously been discussed in this chapter should be prepared, made available to the examiners, and followed exactly as written. The directions for the instructor will serve as a guide in the demonstration, and the directions for the student should be read or given to the student in an interesting and enthusiastic way. Generally it is best if the instructor has memorized the explanation so the directions to different groups may be consistent. Combining the explanation with the demonstration is an effective and time-saving method of presenting a test battery.

Demonstration. A demonstration of each test item is usually desirable. Techniques to be demonstrated should be planned and learned in advance; otherwise, it may be like the blind leading the blind. The demonstration may accompany the explanation or follow it. The examiner who is doing the demonstrating should first present the test battery as a whole in the order of item occurrence if there is an order, and then he should stress the more important details. He should gain the attention of the entire class by arranging all members so they can see the demonstration and hear the explanation. It is usually well to demonstrate all the items before testing is done. Students should be given an opportunity to ask questions.

Warm-up. As soon as the explanation and demonstration are completed and testing is to begin a short warm-up exercise period should be administered to everyone. This is not only a safety precaution, but it also seems to insure better performance on the tests. Many tests require a special warm-up—the softball throw for distance, the running broad jump, or the sprints. It is the responsibility of the trained assistant to see that each student is properly warmed up for his specialized event before that student is tested. In certain tests it is possible to provide space for warm-up or practice.

Administration. This is the period where all the planning and preparation is brought to fruition. The testing period should always be conducted in a positive and efficient manner. The matter of student discipline is an important consideration. Administration should be planned so that all the students may be kept active most of the time. Crowding around a particular station is an invitation to behavior problems. In situations where leadership is limited or facilities lacking so that only a few students can be tested at a time, the rest of the group could be organized into some activity which would occupy them while they are waiting their turns to be tested. Multiple stations may be set up if leadership is available and practice areas set up for those waiting. If the planning has been thorough and the preparation of the tests and students adequate, then test administration should proceed in a smooth and efficient manner. However, certain matters will inevitably arise which will need immediate attention, such as a broken piece of equipment repaired, a chalked line replenished, new masking tape put in position, a missing score card replaced, or over-crowding at one or more stations relieved.

Motivation. Mention has been made of the fact that the student has not been tested until he has done his best. In the first place, the tests should be presented in such a manner that the student will be stimulated and will want to excel. On some age levels, however, it is sometimes necessary to encourage the student to exert greater effort. Older girls particularly tend not to care about excelling. After the onset of puberty, especially, they are more concerned about their personal appearance than physical prowess. In general, a student will do better when he is told the purpose of the test and the method of scoring. He will also want to know the various levels of achievement, and he will try harder when he sees the importance of a test as part of the over-all program. All students should be instructed in the reasons for the test and the way test results will be used. Proper attitude and genuine enthusiasm on the part of the teacher are usually reflected in a good attitude by the students. Assistants should be given some definite suggestions on how to motivate the students to greater effort during administration. Some suggestions are: showing an interest in a student's performance, encouraging greater effort, praising good performance, and reminding students of the correct technique and rules. For example, the student may be reminded in the medicine ball put to put the ball rather than to throw it or to keep behind the restraining line. The poorly skilled should not be embarrassed by having attention called to his poor performance or by being ridiculed for his form or effort.

Safety. Testing is accompanied by excitement and enthusiasm on the part of students. They like self-testing activities and the challenge of most physical tests. They are stimulated and are eager to excel and test themselves. Safeguards must be observed to prevent accidents. There are a number of ways this can be done. Safety precautions may be emphasized during the orientation period. Class discipline must be maintained. A warm-up period is essential to prevent pulled muscles. If students have weak joints at the knee or ankle, certain tests like the squat jumps or the dodge run may be contraindicated. Leaders should be warned to look for certain hazards and trained to prevent accidents. The entire class must be instructed in any special precaution which may be necessary due to the nature of a particular test or facility. Precautions are necessary not only for particular stations, but also on the route of traffic between stations. As a rule, medical examinations should precede the administration of all strenuous physical tests. In the event such medical examinations have not been given, any student who is permitted to schedule a class in the instructional program may take the test. When there is a doubt, however, a student should be excused. Proper conditioning should precede the administration of those tests which require great efforts of strength and endurance.

Duties After Testing

Collecting Score Cards. If the class or squad card is used, the collection of score cards presents little problem. When individual score cards are used, they may be collected by the squad leader from his respective squad members, by the trained assistants at the last station where the student was tested, or at the door by one assistant as the students go to the dressing room.

Converting Raw Scores. When tests are administered and the results scored, a raw score is obtained. These raw scores are generally meaningless so it becomes necessary in most cases to convert them to something more meaningful, or to compare them with some predetermined standard. The most common methods of conversion are to percentiles, some type of standard score, or a weighted score. The actual conversion itself is usually accomplished through use of norms in the forms of scoring tables. These tables should be made available in advance and in such manner that scores can be identified and converted quickly. Score cards should have spaces for the recording of these converted scores. Some raw scores are compared with a single predetermined standard. This standard is usually established on a pass-or-fail basis and is set at some level which can be met by a certain percentage of a group.

Comparing Results with Norms and Constructing Profiles and Graphs. Sometimes converted scores are more useful when they in turn are compared with additional standards. Many tests are accompanied by these. For example, in the Morrison Test of Basic Sports Skills in Chapter 7, the raw scores for both batteries are first related to norms as they are converted to T-Scores. These T-Scores from each battery are summed into composite scores. These composite scores in turn are referred to a composite norm table for placement of each student into levels or categories. This provides a norm for the composite scores.

If it is feasible, the score cards should contain the norms so the student's rating can be checked directly on the card. Also, when there are several items in the test battery and especially when the items seem to have diagnostic value, scale scores may be placed directly on the card and a profile constructed of the student's achievement (see Fig. 8–15, p. 255). Process evaluation scores frequently may be placed in profiles, also.

Constructing Norms. In some cases the test administrator must analyze his test results and prepare his own norms (see Chapter 5, p. 95). He must have a knowledge of statistics so he may effectively analyze test results. This analysis generally includes finding the average and spread of scores and is usually followed by the establishment of some appropriate type of norm, generally a percentile or a standard score of some type.

Interpreting Results. The next step in the testing program is the interpretation of results in terms of the norms according to either the *product* or the *process*. The student should always be informed of his score and his score should be interpreted to him. Interpretation should be made to enable him to know his status, progress, weakness, or need. If time is available, it is well if he can be told how his needs can be met. Scale scores are perhaps the easiest type of norms to interpret. It is desirable for the student to receive this information in private, but this is time-consuming and rarely feasible. Ordinary physical test scores can be interpreted in several ways—by the student himself, by his squad leader, by a trained class leader, or by the teacher. With the probable exception of the I.Q., no score need be withheld from the student. In addition to the student himself, results of product measurement may need to be interpreted to parents, administrators and others.

The evaluation of the process is always done for a purpose and this purpose generally needs to be known and understood by someone— the staff, the administration, the board of education or trustees, other faculty members, the PTA, and the general public. Therefore, the results of process evaluation should be interpreted fully to the appropriate groups in order to achieve one's purposes. Many times present status is needed in order to show the gap between what is needed and what is available.

Using Results and the Follow-up. In effective evaluation, there is always measurement, followed by analysis, followed by use. Test data have many uses, but in the final analysis, if they are to be of most value, they must be applied to improve either the product or the process. The most significant phase of evaluation is what happens after results are used. Regardless of whether measurement is applied directly to product or process, a follow-up is indicated. The follow-up is usually revealed through a re-direction of aims and objectives, a re-planning of the process by a prescription of change in some process factors, and a general raising of standards in all areas of process. All of this requires further evaluation. Thus, the follow-up implies that evaluation is a continuous, on-going process.

References

1. Annarino, Anthony: Utilizing Circuit Testing Programs, Journal of the American Association for Health, Physical Education and Recreation, *40*, 73, May, 1969.
2. Barrow, H. M.: The ABC's of Testing, Journal of Health, Physical Education and Recreation, *33*, 35–37, May–June, 1962.
3. Bovard, J. F., F. W. Cozens, and E. P. Hagman: *Tests and Measurements in Physical Education*. 3rd. Ed., Philadelphia, W. B. Saunders Co., 1949, pp. 366–381.
4. Clarke, H. H.: *Application of Measurement to Health and Physical Education*. Englewood Cliffs, N.J., Prentice-Hall, Inc., 1959, p. 384.
5. ————: *Application of Measurement to Health and Physical Education*. Englewood Cliffs, N.J., Prentice-Hall, Inc., 1959, pp. 377–399.
6. Mathews, Donald K.: *Measurement in Physical Education*. 2nd. Ed., Philadelphia, W. B. Saunders Co., 1963, pp. 329–343.
7. Meyers, Carlton R., and T. E. Blesh: *Measurement in Physical Education* New York, The Ronald Press, 1962, pp. 136–137.
8. Scott, M. Gladys, and Esther French: *Measurement and Evaluation in Physical Education*. Dubuque, Wm. C. Brown Co., 1959, pp. 465–488.
9. Wilgoose, C. E.: *Evaluation in Health and Physical Education*. New York, McGraw-Hill Book Co., Inc., 1961, pp. 366–387.

Chapter 5
STATISTICAL TECHNIQUES

Many teachers are reluctant to give tests because they feel inadequate to administer and interpret them. Other teachers give tests and then either misinterpret or fail to use the results. It is bad enough to have a poor plan for evaluating the physical education program, but a more serious error is the failure to make use of the information that is available. This chapter will attempt to prepare the teacher for efficient and effective use of data of various kinds. Careful statistical work and basic statistical procedures should help provide the scientific evidence for program improvement and enrichment.

Getting Ready to Handle Data

Innate neatness and orderliness are qualities which will be of great value to the teacher when he begins to handle data. Many of these preliminary admonitions, if put to use, will make for more accurate and faster computational work. The teacher should make them a part of his habitual procedures whenever analyzing any kind of evaluative material.

Mechanical Details. 1. It is a good practice to label and date every sheet of paper with data on it. The upper right hand corner is a good location for labeling.

For example:

8th grade girls
AAHPER fitness test scores
October, 1971

or

9th grade boys
Sportsmanship Inventory
October, 1971 and April, 1971

or

Tennis knowledge test
12th grade boys
May, 1971

Comparisons may be made between new data and that of past years. Well-labeled data will be easy to find and can be used with confidence. Even within the year, records for each class should be labeled

and dated so there is no possible chance of error in the use or interpretation of them.

2. It is good practice to double check the tallies on the frequency
distributions or on a scattergram before starting the computation
(see page 98). Catching errors at this stage will prevent re-doing
of the entire problem. A re-tally on another frequency distribution
is a check plan which works. Another good way is to dot each tally
or to "light every little candle,"

i.e.; Tally = ||||
Re-checked tallies = ïïïï

Each mark should be dotted when re-tallying is complete and if not,
another check is necessary. Such safety procedures may seem time
consuming but they are habitual for the careful and thorough tester.

3. It is a good practice to use a ruler to help read the data from
the right line and column. This is especially important if working
with a data sheet full of columns of figures for a long list of names.
One finger on the ruler should guide the reader to the correct column
and the ruler will keep him reading across on the correct line.

4. The use of colored pencils will help distinguish different
columns of data. This, too, will make for accuracy in tallying; *i.e.*
first column in red; second column in green; third column of data
in blue, *etc.* Colored pencils may be useful also to draw lines and
double lines to denote sectioning and totaling situations.

These mechanical details, and others that the teacher will devise
himself, may seem minor, but they may make the difference between
inaccurate and accurate statistical analysis.

Arithmetic Refreshers. This section will serve as a review of
some of the basic rules for using numbers.

1. Signs. Some examples will serve to illustrate the rules concerning signs in adding and subtracting and in multiplying and
dividing. Exercise 5–1 will provide a good check after reviewing
these procedures. Reference to a basic mathematics text will further
supplement this review.

Rules for the use of signs:[13]

1. To add numbers with like signs, add the values and use the common sign.
2. To add numbers with unlike signs, find the difference in their
   values and use the sign of the larger value.
3. To subtract one number from another, change the sign of the
   number to be subtracted and then add algebraically.
4. To multiply or divide two numbers with like signs, the answer is
   positive.

5. To multiply or divide two numbers with unlike signs, the answer is negative.

Examples: Addition:
$$(\ 6) + (\ 7) = \ \ \ 13$$
$$(-6) + (-7) = -13$$
$$(\ 6) + (-7) = - \ 1$$
$$(-6) + (\ 7) = \ \ \ 1$$

Subtraction:
$$(\ 6) - (\ 7) = - \ 1$$
$$(-6) - (-7) = \ \ \ 1$$
$$(\ 6) - (-7) = \ \ \ 13$$
$$(-6) - (\ 7) = -13$$

Multiplication:
$$(\ 6) \ . \ (\ 7) = \ \ \ 42$$
$$(-6) \ . \ (-7) = \ \ \ 42$$
$$(\ 6) \ . \ (-7) = -42$$
$$(-6) \ . \ (\ 7) = -42$$

Division:
$$(\ 6) \div (\ 7) = \ \ \ .86$$
$$(-6) \div (-7) = \ \ \ .86$$
$$(\ 6) \div (-7) = -.86$$
$$(-6) \div (\ 7) = -.86$$

EXERCISE 5–1

SIGNS

Answers may be found on page 111.

Add these numbers:

1. $(+ \ 6) + (-14) =$ 6. $(-10) + (+ \ 4) =$
2. $(+ \ 9) + (+ \ 3) =$ 7. $(-10) + (-10) =$
3. $(+ \ 3) + (- \ 4) =$ 8. $(+ \ 7) + (- \ 4) =$
4. $(+ \ 4) + (+ \ 4) =$ 9. $(- \ 6) + (-11) =$
5. $(- \ 4) + (+ \ 9) =$ 10. $(- \ 3) + (- \ 2) =$

Subtract these numbers:

1. $(+ \ 4) - (+ \ 3) =$ 6. $(+ \ 7) - (+ \ 4) =$
2. $(- \ 4) - (- \ 7) =$ 7. $(- \ 9) - (- \ 3) =$
3. $(+ \ 6) - (- \ 4) =$ 8. $(+ \ 9) - (- \ 7) =$
4. $(+ \ 6) - (- \ 9) =$ 9. $(- \ 4) - (- \ 9) =$
5. $(+13) - (+ \ 6) =$ 10. $(- \ 4) - (+10) =$

Multiply these numbers:

1. $(+ \ 6) \ . \ (+ \ 9) =$ 6. $(- \ 4) \ . \ (+ \ 3) =$
2. $(+ \ 3) \ . \ (- \ 2) =$ 7. $(+ \ 5) \ . \ (- \ 6) =$
3. $(- \ 4) \ . \ (- \ 6) =$ 8. $(+ \ 9) \ . \ (+ \ 4) =$
4. $(- \ 9) \ . \ (+ \ 4) =$ 9. $(- \ 9) \ . \ (+ \ 8) =$
5. $(- \ 4) \ . \ (-10) =$ 10. $(+ \ 3) \ . \ (+ \ 7) =$

Divide these numbers:

1. $(+12) \div (+ \ 4) =$ 6. $(- \ 4) \div (\ \ 0) =$
2. $(+10) \div (- \ 2) =$ 7. $(+ \ 9) \div (- \ 3) =$
3. $(- \ 8) \div (- \ 4) =$ 8. $(- \ 3) \div (- \ 3) =$
4. $(-10) \div (+ \ 5) =$ 9. $(- \ 4) \div (+ \ 8) =$
5. $(+ \ 4) \div (- \ 4) =$ 10. $(+ \ 0) \div (- \ 4) =$

2. Squares and Square Roots. The most efficient procedure to use when dealing with squares and square roots is to consult a prepared table. These are usually found in the back of statistics books and are available also in paperback editions of statistical tables Such an investment for a professional library would be quite worthwhile.

The computation of squares involves simple multiplication and requires care only in proper placement of decimals. The answer can be checked by dividing by the number squared. Such double checking is excellent procedure.

$$\text{Example: } 24^2 = (24)\ (24)\ =\ 576$$
$$\text{Check: } 576 \div 24\ =\ 24$$

The computation of square roots is more involved. The numbers should be marked off by 2's on each side of the decimal point before beginning the computation.

$$\text{Examples: } \sqrt{4\ \overline{63.94}\ \overline{32}\ \overline{10}}$$
$$\sqrt{\overline{39.43}\ \overline{11}}$$
$$\sqrt{\overline{3.64}\ \overline{3}}$$

Every coupling line inside the radical $(\sqrt{\ \ })$ will result in one number above the radical. The habit of estimating the answer or checking the feasibility of the answer before accepting it is a good one to form. In the first example, there will be two numbers in the answer to the left of the decimal mark and the first one will be a 2. This estimate of the answer will prevent the error of connecting $\overline{46}\ \overline{3}.$ and placing a 6 above the radical as the first number. In the answer to the second example there will be one number to the left of the decimal and it will be a 6. In the third example, the answer should begin with a 1. and so on.

The coupling of numbers has another use because the problem is solved by progressively adding two numbers at a time to the remainder after each step. After starting with the first number, it is always necessary to double the partial answer to get a new divisor. Then the next coupled pair of numbers is dropped into the dividend. An example to outline the steps should help:

Step 1 $\sqrt{24.60\ \overline{16}\ \overline{00}}$ (1) Mark off by 2's from each side of the decimal mark.

Step 2 $\sqrt{\dfrac{4}{24.60}\ \overline{16}\ \overline{00}}$
            $\underline{16}$

(2) Select the largest number that will go into 24 squared (4) and place it first in the answer.

Step 3
$$\begin{array}{r} 4. \\ \sqrt{24.60\ \overline{16}\ \overline{00}} \\ 16 \\ \hline 8?\diagup\ 8\ 60 \end{array}$$

(3) Drop the next two numbers into place by the 8 and double the partial answer to start a new divisor.

Step 4
$$\begin{array}{r} 4.\ 9 \\ \sqrt{24.60\ \overline{16}\ \overline{00}} \\ 16 \\ \hline 89\diagup\ 8\ 60 \\ 8\ 01 \\ \hline 59 \end{array}$$

(4) Estimate how many times 8? will go into 860 and use this number, (9) in the answer and in the divisor to replace the .?. Whatever number goes in the new divisor must also go in the answer.

Step 5
$$\begin{array}{r} 4.\ 9 \\ \sqrt{24.60\ \overline{16}\ \overline{00}} \\ 16 \\ \hline 89\diagup\ 8\ 60 \\ 8\ 01 \\ \hline 98?\diagup\ 59\ 16 \end{array}$$

(5) Double the 49 for the new divisor. Drop the next two numbers into the dividend.

Step 6
$$\begin{array}{r} 4.\ 9\ \ 6 \\ \sqrt{24.60\ \overline{16}\ \overline{00}} \\ 16 \\ \hline 89\diagup\ 8\ 60 \\ 8\ 01 \\ \hline 986\diagup\ 59\ 16 \\ 59\ 16 \end{array}$$

(6) Estimate how many times 98? will go into 5916 and fill in this number (6) into the answer and into the divisor.

Continue no further because the answer comes out even.

The square root of 24.6016 is 4.96. Here, too, a checking procedure is recommended. As a check, it is possible to divide 24.6016 by 4.96 to see if 4.96 is also the answer. Or a square root table may be consulted. A square root table should be used initially if one is available. However, at first it would be advantageous to work a few square root problems. It is well to know the correct procedures in case the specific square root needed is not in the table.

EXERCISE 5–2

SQUARES AND SQUARE ROOT

Answers may be found on page 111.

Find the Square:

1. 16.34 =
2.   .04 =
3. 103.00 =
4.   3.94 =
5.   .736 =

Find the Square Root:

1. $\sqrt{19.43}$ =

2. $\sqrt{.0346}$ =

3. $\sqrt{426.9362}$ =

4. $\sqrt{.74}$ =

5. $\sqrt{6.3974}$ =

3. Units of Measure.

(a) Minutes and Seconds. Many skill tests are timed and thus result in a slightly different notation for analysis. For example, 1:15.03 means that a certain act was performed in 1 minute, 15 seconds, and 3 hundredths of a second. Seconds will usually be the significant number because many physical tests terminate in less than a minute. The smaller number will indicate the faster performance. In preparing a frequency distribution to tally timed scores, the best score should be at the top; thus, if the data are in seconds or some interval of time, the fewer number of seconds should be at the top.

Example: 16–17 (seconds)
18–19
20–21
etc.

(b) Feet and Inches. Distance measures are usually recorded in either feet or inches. The Standing Broad Jump is frequently recorded to the nearest inch, i.e. 68 inches. This is better than recording 5 feet 8 inches because the chance of error in preparing the frequency distribution is lessened. On the other hand, if the tape or the mat is marked off in feet and inches a recording of 5 feet 8 inches would be more accurate. It is desirable to avoid transposing from one scale to another. A throw for distance might be recorded in feet and inches but accuracy to the nearest foot is about as precise a measurement as can be expected, i.e. 78 feet, 54 feet, etc.

(c) Days, Months, Years. Some norms are recorded by age groupings. Years alone may be used. A 12-year-old is a 12-year-old until the date of his next birthday. Or a 12-year-old is one whose age is anywhere from 11 years and 6 months to 12 years and 6 months. This latter pattern is sometimes used, but it is more difficult to compute. The former plan is recommended, but consistency in following the same plan, whichever is adopted, is even more vital.

Occasionally norms will be listed by months. For example, the interval 144–149 would designate students from 12 years to 12 years and 6 months. This plan usually requires conversion of ages from years to months. A better plan is to report norms as the common practice dictates. The custom is to speak of a 12-year-old, not of a 144-month-old.

Machines. The use of various computational aids is recommended highly. They provide a more accurate and a more efficient method of computation than can be accomplished by hand. Adding machines are readily available from other departments in the school. Small, hand adding machines are inexpensive and make a worthwhile investment for anyone engaged in this type of work. Calculators are more scarce, but should be sought if a sizable statistical analysis is anticipated. In addition to adding, subtracting, multiplying, and dividing, calculators can be used to expedite such computational problems as square roots and T-scales, and correlations.

Treating Data

Statistical analysis is a method of adding meaning to various types of data. Characteristics of the data can be determined— averages, ranges, spreads, relationships, comparisons, proportions, and the like—and thus the data become capable of interpretation in practical terms. A class of 12-year-old boys recorded scores, in inches, for the Standing Broad Jump. Jerry, a member of this class, jumped 65 inches. How well did the boys, as a class, perform? What is their range? What is their average performance? What does Jerry's 65-inch jump mean in relation to his class, to other standards, to his previous performance? Is it good, poor, or average? Just such questions as these can be answered by some organization and analysis of the scores.

Ungrouped Data. The treatment of ungrouped data is usually relegated to small groups of scores unless a calculator can be used. Otherwise unwieldiness results and the analytical process is lengthened. As an example, assume that only 10 12-year-old boys performed the Broad Jump and that the following scores, in inches, were recorded for them:

71, 52, 44, 58, 68, 57, 76, 61, 65, 49

As listed, the scores are meaningless. The teacher is unable to tell his students the average performance, the ranks, or the range. By quick examination the teacher can see that the 76-inch jump is the longest one and that the 44-inch jump is the shortest. This also represents the range of jumps. By adding all the raw scores and dividing by 10 (the number of students) the teacher can determine the arithmetic average; *i.e.* 601 ÷ 10 = 60.1 inches. Now each score can be interpreted in relation to the average, either above or below 60 inches. Jerry will know that his 65-inch jump is above the average and approximately 5 inches better than the average for these 10 boys.

Ranking of the ungrouped data will add a little more light to the interpretation.

Score	Rank
76	1
71	2
68	3
65	4
61	5
58	6
57	7
52	8
49	9
44	10

Now Jerry also knows that his 65-inch jump was the fourth highest in the class.

These simple techniques of organizing the data changed Jerry's 65-inch score from an isolated, unrelated number to one of relative standing possible of interpretation. These statistical techniques also made interpretations possible which 12-year-old Jerry is capable of understanding.

Grouped Data. More often than not the teacher will want to organize a considerable amount of data. In such cases the data are placed into intervals or grouped to make the computation more efficient. The identity of the individual score is lost, but the slight loss in precision will be minimal and will not unduly influence the results. Throughout this chapter, data on the Standing Broad Jump for 12-year-old boys will serve as the example. Hopefully some advantage can be gained in understanding the various procedures if the same set of data is used throughout.

A frequency distribution must be prepared first because all other steps stem from it. From 10 to 20 intervals are desirable in a frequency distribution to avoid groupings that are too gross. Around 15 intervals are considered ideal.

Step 1. Consider the range of scores. If the jumps range from 42 to 80 inches, a 36-point spread is provided.

Step 2. Decide on the size of the interval. Dividing by three would give about 12 intervals, dividing by 2 would give around 18 intervals, and dividing by 5 would provide about 7 intervals. On the other hand, if about 15 intervals are desirable, dividing the range by 15 would give the appropriate size interval. Fifteen would go into 36 about $2\frac{1}{2}$ times so an arbitrary decision would need to be made selecting either 2 or 3 as the size of the interval in the frequency distribution. Usually the decision should be made which will provide too many intervals instead of too few. Intervals the size of 1, 2, 3, 5, 7, or 10 points are used most commonly. An interval of size three seems appropriate here and is used in the example given (see Table 5–1).

Step 3. Prepare the frequency distribution. The lower limit of the interval is divisible by the size of the interval. The longest jump was 80 inches. Three will not go into 80 even but it will go into 78. So 78–80 becomes the top interval. It has two characteristics: the lower limit is divisible by three and the complete interval encompasses the top score. The size of the interval can be checked by going up the frequency distribution in 3's on both sides; *i.e.* 42, 45, 48, etc. and 44, 47, 50. This is a wise check procedure to prevent either omitting an interval or getting off the proper sequence.

Step 4. Once the frequency distribution has been prepared (see Column (1) in Table 5–1), the tally of the raw scores is made in Column (2) and then the tallies in each interval are summarized in an "f" (frequency) column designated as (3) in Table 5–1.

Organizing the data to just this point allows certain analyses: the jumps range from approximately 42 to 80 inches, the scores are fairly well distributed along the scale, and the mode (the most prevalent or popular score) is represented by a jump of 64 inches. This is the midpoint of the 63 to 65 interval where 11 cases fall, the most for any interval. The mode is a type of average which sometimes gives a rough estimate of average performance.

Table 5–1. Frequency Distribution for Calculating the
Mean and Standard Deviation

Inches (1)	*Tally* (2)	*f* (3)	*d* (4)	*fd* (5)	*fd²* (6)
78–80	‖	2	6	12	72
75–77	‖	2	5	10	50
72–74	‖‖	4	4	16	64
69–71	╫╫ ‖‖	8	3	24	72
66–68	╫╫ ╫╫	10	2	20	40
63–65	╫╫ ╫╫ ‖	11	1	11	11
60–62	╫╫ ‖‖‖	9	0	—	—
57–59	‖	2	—1	— 2	2
54–56	‖	1	—2	— 2	4
51–53	╫╫ ‖	7	—3	—21	63
48–50	‖‖	3	—4	—12	48
45–47	‖	1	—5	— 5	25
42–44	‖	1	—6	— 6	36
		61		+93	487
				—48	
				+45	

Types of Distributions. There are basically two different types of distribution which are commonly analyzed. *First*, there is the normal curve which includes in its statistical family the mean, standard deviation, T-Scale, and other related scales such as standard scores, sigma scores, *etc.* The normal or bell-shaped curve, in which the standard deviations are equally distributed, is characterized as follows:

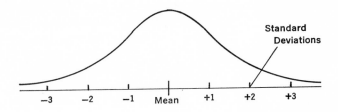

Second, there is the percentile distribution which places all the cases proportionally along the scale and uses in its analysis the median, quartile deviation, percentiles, and other related scales to percentiles such as quartiles and deciles. The percentile distribution is characterized by deciles that are not evenly distributed and by the frequency of cases proportionally distributed along the scale:[1]

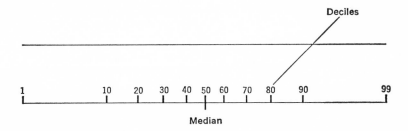

Collectively both types of distributions have measures of central tendency or average, *i.e.* mean, median; and both have measures of dispersion or spread, *i.e* standard deviations, quartile deviation; and both have norms which are representative, *i.e.* T-Scales, and percentiles. Instead of discussing and describing the various techniques in the traditional way just mentioned, they will be covered according to the type of distribution. This latter plan permits the development of the techniques as they build progressively from one step to the next. The same sample of data already introduced will continue to illustrate the various techniques as they are developed. A larger sample representing the same group will be introduced for developing the norms.

Statistical Techniques Related to the Normal Curve.

1. Mean (see Table 5–1 on page 76).

The mean is the value in the distribution which represents the average performance.

Step 1. Columns (1), (2), and (3) have already been prepared to show the preliminary steps.

Step 2. In Column (4) a zero is placed arbitrarily toward the center of the distribution. This is the *A*ssumed *M*ean or an estimate of where the mean will fall. From the zero in the deviations, Column (4), (d), the *d*istance or *d*eviation of each interval from the zero mark is written in. Below the zero, the deviations will be negative.

Step 3. To fill in Column (5), the "fd" column, Columns (3) and (4) are multiplied. Often these 2 numbers are added instead of multiplied so caution should be exercised at this step. Then this column is totaled, using the appropriate sign.

Step 4. The appropriate values are substituted into the following formula to compute the mean of this distribution:

$$M = AM + \left(\frac{\Sigma fd}{N}\right) i$$

$$= 61 + \left(\frac{45}{61}\right) 3$$

$$= 61 + (.74) 3$$

$$= 61 + 2.22$$

$$M = 63.22 \text{ inches or}$$

63″ rounded to the nearest inch.

AM = Assumed Mean—midpoint of the interval

Σfd = sum of the "fd" Column (5)
N = Number of cases
i = size of the interval

This group of boys jumped an average of 63 inches. Jerry is a member of this group and his 65-inch jump is just a little above average.

2. Standard Deviation. Step 1. Columns (1), (2), (3), (4), and (5) have already been finished.

Step 2. Column (6) in Table 5–1 is completed by multiplying Columns (4) and (5). A common error is to square Column (5), so again caution is recommended.

$$(d) (fd) = fd^2 = \text{right}$$

$$(fd) (fd) = f^2d^2 = \text{wrong}$$

Step 3. All the numbers in Column (6) are positive and are totaled.

Step. 4. The following formula is used by substituting the appropriate values to compute the standard deviation of this distribution:

$$\text{SD or } \sigma = i \sqrt{\frac{\Sigma fd^2}{N} - \left(\frac{\Sigma fd}{N}\right)^2} \qquad i = \text{size of the interval}$$

$$= 3 \sqrt{\frac{487}{61} - \left(\frac{45}{61}\right)^2} \qquad \sqrt{} = \text{radical—find square root}$$

$$= 3 \sqrt{7.983 - (.74)^2} \qquad \Sigma fd^2 = \text{sum of fd}^2 \text{ Column (6)}$$

$$= 3 \sqrt{7.983 - .485} \qquad \Sigma fd = \text{sum of fd Column (5)}$$

$$= 3 \sqrt{7.435} \qquad N = \text{Number of cases}$$

$$= (3) \ (2.73)$$

$$\sigma = 8.19$$

The standard deviation indicates the spread of the scores that might be expected to encompass all the scores on the Broad Jump performed by this group. Plus and minus three standard deviations will cover 99.7 per cent of all the cases. Figure 5–1 will illustrate the point using rounded whole numbers of a Mean of 63 and a Standard Deviation of 8.

It would be unusual for anyone in this group to have jumped fewer than 40 inches or more than 87 inches. This spread coincides roughly with the range of scores for this particular distribution; *i.e.* 42 to 80.

Back to Jerry and his 65-inch jump. Now it is known that 68 per cent of the boys will jump between 55 and 71 inches and that

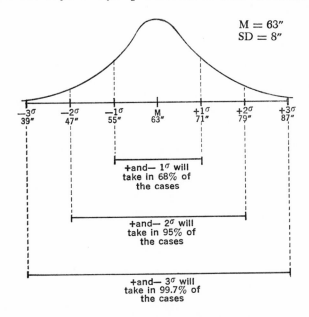

Fig. 5–1. Area under the normal curve.

Jerry's 65-inch jump is close to the mean and therefore an average performance.

A picture of the spread of scores is helpful in evaluating the particular test as well as the performance. If the scores for a group were distributed in the following manner,

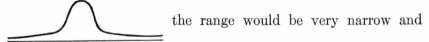 the range would be very narrow and

everyone would be performing at approximately the same level. The test is not making any distinction between various levels of performance. If the curve were skewed it would indicate that the test was either too difficult or too easy for a particular group.

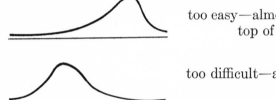

too easy—almost everyone toward the top of the scale

too difficult—almost everyone toward the bottom of the scale

Ideally, the curve should be symmetrical and fairly well spread if the test is to distinguish average performance from good and poor performance.

3. T-Scales. A T-Scale is a normative scale, which means that raw scores may be converted for comparison and ease of interpretation. Several tests using different measurements such as inches, seconds, *etc.* could each be converted to T-Scales. Then comparisons between the tests are possible and relative levels of performance are evident. Generally, a T-Scale can be characterized by a mean of 50, a Standard Deviation of 10, and a range of from approximately 20 to 80 points. Such identifying points make intelligible a T-Score of 73, for instance. A score of 73 in terms of 100 might not seem so good but, when identified as a T-Score and interpreted in light of T-Scale characteristics, it is quite respectable.

There are two methods of computing T-Scales which will be presented here. Either is quick, easy, effective and acceptable. The larger the sample and the more normal the curve, the closer the two methods will approximate each other.

More than the usually accepted number of intervals in the frequency distribution is desirable in order to obtain as much precision and discrimination as possible. The example distribution will still be based on 12-year-old boys and their performance on the Broad Jump. Many more cases are used as is customary for establishing norms. Data representing at least 100 cases are minimal and many more cases are desirable for establishing norms of any kind. It will be interesting to see how Jerry's 65-inch jump looks in relation to the performance of many boys of his age and similar geographic location.

The following formula can be used to compute the T-score for any individual score.

$$\text{T-Score} = 50 + \frac{10(X - M)}{\sigma}$$

		X =	Any raw score
Raw Scores	= 65 "	M =	Mean of raw scores
M	= 60.62 inches	σ =	Standard Deviation of
SD	= 8.50		raw scores
		50 =	Mean of T-Scale
		10 =	Standard Deviation of T-Scale

$$\text{T-score for 65} = 50 + \frac{10(65-60.62)}{8.50}$$

$$= 50 + \frac{43.80}{8.5}$$

$$= 50 + 5.15$$

$$\text{T-score}_{65} = 55.15 \text{ or rounded to } 55$$

Jerry's jump of 65 inches is equal to a T-score of 55 which is a little above average for this group of 12-year old boys. Usually, however, the whole scale is needed and not a conversion for an isolated score.

(a) T-Scale by a Graph Method.

Step 1. At least 3 scores are plotted on a sheet of graph paper. (See Figure 5–2.) Prepare the 2 axes to represent the raw scores (jumps in inches) and the T-scores.

Step 2. We know that the mean of the Broad Jump data for 600 cases is 60.62 inches. Plot the mean T-score of 50 to coincide with the mean Broad Jump of 60.62 inches.

Step 3. The standard deviation of a T-scale is 10 and the standard deviation of this Broad Jump data is 8.5. Next plot the 40th and 60th T-scores (which represent 1 standard deviation above and below the mean T-score of 50) by subtracting and adding 8.5 from the mean of 60.62 (which represents 1 standard deviation above and below the mean raw score of 60.62).

T-scores	Raw Scores
60	69.12
50	60.62
40	52.12

See Figure 5–2.

Step 4. A line is drawn through the three dots on the graph paper resulting in a straight line. This line will permit the conversion of jump distances into T-scores for every step on the raw score scale.

4

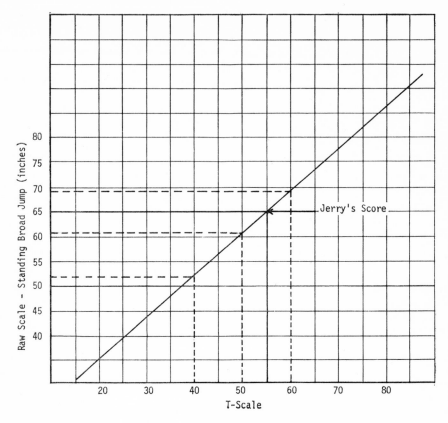

Fig. 5–2. Graph for Plotting T-Scale (600 12-year-old boys)

If the line covering from about 20—80 on the T-scale does not encompass the raw score range then some skewness in the raw scores is indicated. This might result in T-scores either below 20 or above 80.

Jerry's 65–inch jump results in a T-Score of 55.

(b) T-Scale by the Successive Method.[5] The standard deviation of the raw-score distribution is divided by the standard deviation of the T–Scale distribution. This constant value is used to either add or subtract successively from the mean of the raw score distribution to get each step along the T-Scale. For the 600 cases in Table 5–2 such a procedure would yield these results:

$$SD = 8.50, \quad \text{Mean} = 60.62, \quad N = 600$$

$$\text{Constant value} = \frac{SD}{10} = \frac{8.50}{10} = .85$$

Raw Score	T-Score
.	.
.	.
.	.
64.87	55
64.02	54
63.17	53
62.32	52
61.47	51
60.62	50 Mean
59.77	49
58.92	48
58.07	47
57.22	46
56.37	45
.	.
.	.
.	.

Several decimal places should be carried in the constant value so as not to compound slight rounding errors at the extremes of the distribution.

A conversion table should be prepared which shows the inches rounded into whole numbers to correspond with appropriate T-Scores. Such a table is easier for the students to read and eliminates the necessity to round to whole numbers each time reference is made to the normative table.

T-Score Norms—Broad Jump
12-year Old Boys
N = 600

Raw Scores (inches)	T-Scores
.	.
.	.
.	.
65	55
64	54
63	53
62	52
61	51
60	49
59	48
58	47
57	46
56	45
.	.
.	.
.	.

4. *Other Normative Scales.* There are other normative scales derived from the distribution of the normal curve. Several will be presented because of their possible application and because of their addition to general background knowledge concerning norms.

(*a*) Standard "z" Scores. Standard scores, sometimes referred to as "z" scores, are computed by converting a raw score into its respective position on the base of the normal curve in terms of standard deviations. Consequently, standard scores range generally from +3 to —3 but can extend as far as from +4 to —4. Reference to a Table of Proportions of the Area Under the Normal Distribution Curve will indicate the percentage of cases above and below a certain standard score (see Table 5–2).

The following formula is used to compute the standard score for each raw score:

$$\text{Standard "z" Score} = \frac{X - M}{SD}$$

X = any raw score

M = Mean of the raw score distribution

SD = Standard Deviation of the raw score distribution

Jerry's score of 65 inches converted to a standard "z" score would be as follows:

Raw Score   = 65

Mean   = 60.62

Standard Deviation =   8.50

$$\text{Standard "z" Score} = \frac{65 - 60.62}{8.50} = \frac{4.38}{8.50} = .515 \text{ or } .52 \text{ rounded}$$

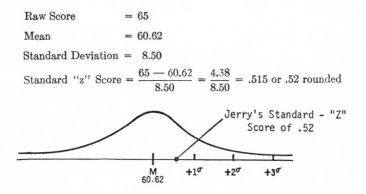

Jerry's Standard - "Z"
Score of .52

M   +1σ +2σ +3σ
60.62

Referring to Table 5–2, it is evident that a standard "z" score of .52 represents an area from the mean covering 19.85 per cent of the cases. This, plus the 50 per cent below the mean, indicates that Jerry's 65-inch jump places him at a point on the scale where 69.85 per cent of 12-year-old boys could be expected to make shorter jumps and 30.15 per cent of this same age group could be expected to do better. Standard "z" scores relate directly to the standard deviations and to the normal curve. They are used little because of

Table 5–2.* Percentage Parts of the Total Area under the Normal Probability Curve Corresponding to Distances on the Base Line between the Mean and Successive Points from the Mean in Units of Standard Deviation†

Units	.00	.01	.02	.03	.04	.05	.06	.07	.08	.09
0.0	00.00	00.40	00.80	01.20	01.60	01.99	02.39	02.79	03.19	03.59
0.1	03.98	04.38	04.78	05.17	05.57	05.96	06.36	06.75	07.14	07.53
0.2	07.93	08.32	08.71	09.10	09.48	09.87	10.26	10.64	11.03	11.41
0.3	11.79	12.17	12.55	12.93	13.31	13.68	14.06	14.43	14.80	15.17
0.4	15.54	15.91	16.28	16.64	17.00	17.36	17.72	18.08	18.44	18.79
0.5	19.15	19.50	19.85	20.19	20.54	20.88	21.23	21.57	21.90	22.24
0.6	22.57	22.91	23.24	23.57	23.89	24.22	24.54	24.86	25.17	25.49
0.7	25.80	26.11	26.42	26.73	27.04	27.34	27.64	27.94	28.23	28.52
0.8	28.81	29.10	29.39	29.67	29.95	30.23	30.51	30.78	31.06	31.33
0.9	31.59	31.86	32.12	32.38	32.64	32.90	33.15	33.40	33.65	33.89
1.0	34.13	34.38	34.61	34.85	35.08	35.31	35.54	35.77	35.99	36.21
1.1	36.43	36.65	36.86	37.08	37.29	37.49	37.70	37.90	38.10	38.30
1.2	38.49	38.69	38.88	39.07	39.25	39.44	39.62	39.80	39.97	40.15
1.3	40.32	40.49	40.66	40.82	40.99	41.15	41.31	41.47	41.62	41.77
1.4	41.92	42.07	42.22	42.36	42.51	42.65	42.79	42.92	43.06	43.19
1.5	43.32	43.45	43.57	43.70	43.83	43.94	44.06	44.18	44.29	44.41
1.6	44.52	44.63	44.74	44.84	44.95	45.05	45.15	45.25	45.35	45.45
1.7	45.54	45.64	45.73	45.82	45.91	45.99	46.08	46.16	46.25	46.33
1.8	46.41	46.49	46.56	46.64	46.71	46.78	46.86	46.93	46.99	47.06
1.9	47.13	47.19	47.26	47.32	47.38	47.44	47.50	47.56	47.61	47.67
2.0	47.72	47.78	47.83	47.88	47.93	47.98	48.03	48.08	48.12	48.17
2.1	48.21	48.26	48.30	48.34	48.38	48.42	48.46	48.50	48.54	48.57
2.2	48.61	48.64	48.68	48.71	48.75	48.78	48.81	48.84	48.87	48.90
2.3	48.93	48.96	48.98	49.01	49.04	49.06	49.09	49.11	49.13	49.16
2.4	49.18	49.20	49.22	49.25	49.27	49.29	49.31	49.32	49.34	49.36
2.5	49.38	49.40	49.41	49.43	49.45	49.46	49.48	49.49	49.51	49.52
2.6	49.53	49.55	49.56	49.57	49.59	49.60	49.61	49.62	49.63	49.64
2.7	49.65	49.66	49.67	49.68	49.69	49.70	49.71	49.72	49.73	49.74
2.8	49.74	49.75	49.76	49.77	49.77	49.78	49.79	49.79	49.80	49.81
2.9	49.81	49.82	49.82	49.83	49.84	49.84	49.85	49.85	49.86	49.86
3.0	49.865									
3.1	49.903									
3.2	49.93129									
3.3	49.95166									
3.4	49.96631									
3.5	49.97674									
3.6	49.98409									
3.7	49.98922									
3.8	49.99277									
3.9	49.99519									

* Adapted from: *Biometrika Tables for Statisticians.* Vol. 1, 1954. Edited by E. S. Pearson and H. O. Hartley.

† Located in Mathews, Donald K., *Measurement in Physical Education.* 2nd Ed., Philadelphia: W. B. Saunders Co., 1963, p. 36, and reprinted by permission of the publisher and the author.

the negative and positive values that result and because of their small size. However, it is well for the teacher to understand their computation and interpretation in case he encounters norms reported in standard "z" scores.

(b) Six Sigma Scores.[2] The Six Sigma Scale is likewise based on the mean and standard deviation of the raw data. It provides a scale from 0 to 100 with 50 indicative of the mean. Various norms using this scale are reported as "standard scores," "scale scores," "six sigma scores," and "sigma scores." This practice results in some confusion with standard "z" scores. However, if the scale ranges from 0 to 100 instead of from + and − 3 or 4, the reader knows the norms are based on the six sigma scale.

Step 1. The Mean and Standard Deviation are determined.

Step 2. The Standard Deviation is multiplied by 3 and divided by 50.

Step 3. This index (constant) number is used to add to or subtract from the mean of the raw scores to arrive successively at a Sigma Score for every value from 0 to 100.

$$\text{Example: Six Sigma Score Constant} = \frac{3(\text{S.D.})}{50}$$

$$\text{Mean} = 60.62$$

$$\text{S.D.} = 8.50$$

$$\frac{3\,(8.50)}{50} = \frac{25.50}{50} = .51$$

$$\text{Constant} = .51$$

Raw Score	Six Sigma Score	Inches (Rounded)
.	.	
.	.	.
.	.	
65.21	59	65
64.70	58	
64.19	57	64
63.68	56	
63.17	55	63
62.66	54	
62.15	53	62
61.64	52	
61.13	51	61
60.62 Mean	50 Mean	
60.11	49	60
59.60	48	
59.09	47	59
58.58	46	
58.07	45	58
.	.	.
.	.	.

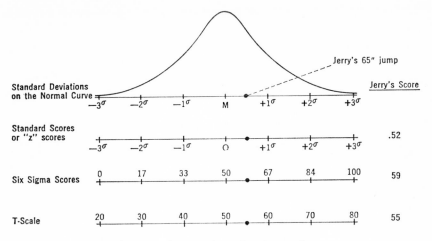

Fig. 5–3. A comparison of various scales.

The final preparation of the norms would show the raw scores rounded to inches to correspond to the Six Sigma Scores. Where a distance is equal to more than 1 score along the normative scale, the student is credited with the higher value.

Statistical Techniques Related to Proportions. The percentile concept requires interpretation in terms of the *proportion* of cases above or below a certain point. It does not reveal the distance of a certain score from the average. It merely tells what proportion performed better and what proportion performed poorer with indirect regard for evaluating the excellence of the performance.

1. Median. The median is a measure of central tendency which indicates the score above and below which 50 per cent of the cases fall. It is the middle score of the distribution when all of the scores are ranked in order. Unlike the mean, this measure of central tendency is unaffected by extremes in scores. The size of the score is immaterial. The rank of the score is the determining factor. Once again the Broad Jump data for the 61 12-year-old boys will serve as the example. The frequency distribution is repeated here to illustrate the steps in computing the Median, Quartiles, *etc.* The formula for computing the median follows:[3]

$$\text{Mdn} = ll + \left(\frac{(N)(50\%) - fc}{f\,i} \right) i$$

ll = exact *l*ower *l*imit of the interval containing the median

fc = sum of all frequencies *below* this interval

fi = frequency in the interval containing the median

N = number of cases

i = size of interval

Step 1. The cumulative frequency column is filled in and re-checked to see that the top number equals the N. See Table 5-3.

Step 2. The Median is the 50th percentile. So it is necessary to multiply 61 times 50 per cent or divide it by 2 to get the exact half of the cases—30.5.

Step 3. Then the formula is used by making the appropriate substitutions.

$$\text{Mdn} = 62.50 + \left(\frac{(61)(.50) - 24}{11} \right) 3$$

62.50 is the exact lower limit of the interval containing 30.5.

$$= 62.50 + \left(\frac{30.5 - 24}{11} \right) 3$$

24 is the cumulative frequency up to (but not including) the interval containing the median. This number should always be the smaller number in the numerator.

$$= 62.50 + \left(\frac{6.5}{11} \right) 3$$

11 is the frequency of the interval containing the median

$$= 62.50 + (.59)\,3$$
$$= 62.50 + 1.77$$
$$\text{Mdn} = 64.27 \text{ inches}$$

A score of 64.27 is the exact middle of the distribution. Fifty per cent of the group have made higher scores and 50 per cent have made lower scores.

2. Quartile. Quartiles denote the points on the scale represented by 25, 50 and 75 per cent of the cases. A slight adjustment in the formula for the median will prepare it for solving the values for Quartiles 1 and 3. Quartile 2 is the same as the Median or the 50 per cent point.

Table 5-3.   Frequency Distribution for Proportional Calculations

$i = 3$	f	$Cum.\,f$
78–80	2	61
75–77	2	59
72–74	4	57
69–71	8	53
66–68	10	45
63–65	11	35
60–62	9	24
57–59	2	15
54–56	1	13
51–53	7	12
48–50	3	5
45–47	1	2
42–44	1	1

N = 61

$$Q_1 = ll + \left(\frac{(N)\ (25\%) - fc}{fi} \right) i$$

25% of 61 is 15.25 so the ll must be the *lower* *limit* of the interval containing 15.25. Refer to Table 5-3.

$$Q_1 = 59.5 + \left(\frac{15.25 - 15}{9} \right) 3 = 59.5 + \left(\frac{.25}{9} \right) 3 = 59.5 + (.028) 3 = 59.5 +$$

.084 = 59.58.

75% of 61 is 45.75 so the *lower* *limit* must be for the interval containing this value. Again refer to Table 5-3.

$$Q_3 = 68.5 + \left(\frac{45.75 - 45}{8} \right) 3 = 68.5 + \left(\frac{.75}{8} \right) 3 = 68.5 + (.094) 3$$

$$= 68.5 + .282 = 68.78$$

75% of the boys jumped farther than 59.58 or 60 inches.

50% of the boys jumped farther than 64.27 or 64 inches.

25% of the boys jumped farther than 68.78 or 69 inches.

3. Quartile Deviation. This statistical procedure will indicate the spread of scores for this type of distribution.

$$QD = \frac{Q_3 - Q_1}{2} = \frac{68.78 - 59.58}{2} = \frac{9.2}{2} = 4.6$$

This value of 4.6 extended above and below the median will include 50 per cent of the cases.

59.67   Mdn   68.87
64.27

4. Percentiles. Percentiles are probably the most frequently used scales in the educational field for reporting norms. They show relative rank but not relative excellence even though the two are related and are often considered synonymous. Since proportions are used to compute percentiles instead of standard deviations, it is usual for the distances between various deciles to be uneven. Ten per cent of the cases must fit into every decile. In some instances all 10 per cent of the cases may have made identical scores, while in other cases scores ranging over several points may have been included to get 10 per cent of the cases.

> Quartiles divide the distribution into 4 parts.
> Deciles divide the distribution into 10 parts.
> Percentiles divide the distribution into 100 parts.

Two methods for computing percentiles will be explained. One will be designated as the interpolation method and the other as the smoothed ogive or graphic method. Both methods are acceptable.

The graphic method involves less computation and is more easily read to determine every percentile step along the scale. It is also preferable for reading percentiles at the extremes of the scale. The same normative scores used to compute T-Scales will be used to illustrate these percentile methods so various comparisons can be made.

(a) Smoothed Ogive Method of Computing Percentiles. The same broad jump scores are presented in a frequency distribution in Table 5–4. The interval has been changed because here, as in the T-Scale development, as many intervals as possible are desirable. Fewer intervals cut down on the amount of computation but also sacrifice some of the precision of the resulting scale.

Step 1. The cumulative frequency (cum. f.) is computed in relation to the exact *upper* limit of the interval. In this way, everything up to that point "on the ladder" of the frequency column is included in the cumulative frequency column. Consequently, the top number in the cumulative frequency should equal the number of cases. Establish a pattern of adding the last recorded cumulative frequency to the next frequency and writing the total straight across on that line. As a check it is wise to add all the frequencies up to a certain point and see if the cumulative frequency recorded on the same line corresponds to the same number. *e.g.* $1+1+4+4+7 = 17$ and 17 does appear directly across from the interval 42–44 on Table 5–4.

Table 5–4. Frequency Distribution for Percentile Norms

	f	$Cum\ f$	$Cum\ \%\ f$
90–above	1	600	100.00
87–89	–		
84–86	2	599	99.83
81–83	2	597	99.50
78–80	11	595	99.17
75–77	17	584	97.33
72–74	30	567	94.50
69–71	42	537	89.50
66–68	56	495	82.50
63–65	85	439	73.17
60–62	91	354	59.00
57–59	75	263	43.83
54–56	71	188	31.33
51–53	51	117	19.50
48–50	34	66	11.00
45–47	15	32	5.33
42–44	7	17	2.83
39–41	4	10	1.67
36–38	4	6	1.00
33–35	1	2	.33
30–32	1	1	.17
	600		

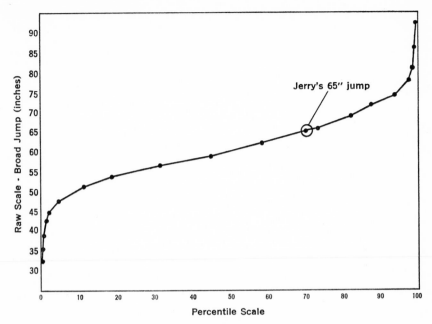

Fig. 5–4. Percentiles by the Smoothed Ogive Method.
(600 12-year-old boys.)

Step 2. The percentage of cumulative frequency column (% cum/f) is obtained by dividing each cumulative frequency value by N.

$1 \div 600 = .17$

$2 \div 600 = .33$

$6 \div 600 = 1.00$

$10 \div 600 = 1.67$ and on up the column. The decimal point is moved two places to the right to convert the answer to a per cent. An alternate method to find these values is accomplished by finding the constant of $100/N = 100/600 = .167$. Then each cumulative frequency is multiplied by this value. For example, in the fifth interval up, $(17) (.167) = 2.839$ so approximately the same value results as reported in Table 5–4.

Step 3. Next the cumulative percentage frequency and the corresponding *upper limits* of each interval are plotted on a sheet of graph paper. Then the smoothed ogive (pronounced ojive) is made by sketching in lines to join the dots. See Figure 5–4. Now each centile and decile can be read from the graph. It would be time-saving in the long run to prepare a raw-score—percentile scale so the same numbers would not have to be read from the graph repeatedly. This is especially true if large numbers are involved. For example, there are 85 cases that scored jumps of from 63 to 65 inches. The conversion scale prepared from the smoothed ogive will be more efficient to use than recurrent references to the graphic picture of the percentile scale.

Raw Scores	Percentiles
.	.
.	.
70	87
69	84
68	81
67	78
66	75
65	71
64	66
63	61
62	57
61	52
60	46
.	.
.	.

Percentiles are usually reported in round whole numbers which require some rounding of percentile numbers as the scale is prepared in this final form. The distance between each raw score is not always the same number of percentile points; from 46 to 52 is 6 points, from 71 to 75 is 4 points; from 81 to 84 is 3 points. This would not be possible on a T-Scale where each step of the scale is approximately identical in size. This fact is one of the main distinguishing points between the two types of norms—T-Scales and percentiles.

(b) Interpolation Method of Computing Percentiles. The interpolation method of computing percentiles utilizes the same procedures that were employed to detect median and quartile values. Instead of the 50 per cent, and the 25 and 75 per cent values, the various decile values will be used. A review of the procedures for obtaining the median and quartiles will be helpful in clarifying these procedures. The frequency distribution and cumulative frequency columns shown in Table 5–4 will be used to find the various decile points along the percentile scale. Following is the formula for computing deciles or percentiles:

$$\text{Percentile}_? = ll + \left(\frac{(N)(P_?) - f_c}{f_i} \right) i$$

Percentile$_?$ or P$_?$ = the specific percentile sought, $i.e.$ P$_{80}$, P$_{34}$, P$_{19}$, etc.

(N)(P$_?$) = Number of cases multiplied by the exact percentile sought

ll = lower limit of the interval where the (N)(P$_?$) number is located

f_c = cumulative frequency up to the interval containing the percentile

f_i = number of cases in the interval containing the percentile

i = size of the interval in the frequency distribution

The following illustrations will show the various steps taken for each decile figured. The 95th and 5th percentiles were computed to fill in the extremes of the distribution. Any specific percentile, *i.e.* 43rd, 92nd, 15th, *etc.* may be found by following the same procedures.

$P_{95} = (N)(.95) = 570$

$= 74.5 + \left(\dfrac{570-567}{17}\right) 3 = 74.5 + \left(\dfrac{3}{17}\right) 3 = 74.5 + (.18) 3 = 74.5 + .54 = 75.04$

$P_{90} = (N)(.90) = 540$

$= 71.50 + \left(\dfrac{540-537}{30}\right) 3 = 71.50 + \left(\dfrac{3}{30}\right) 3 = 71.50 + (.1) 3 = 71.50 + .3 = 71.80$

$P_{80} = (N)(.80) = 480$

$= 65.50 + \left(\dfrac{480-439}{56}\right) 3 = 65.50 + \left(\dfrac{41}{56}\right) 3 = 65.50 + (.73) 3 = 65.50 + 2.19$
$= 67.69$

$P_{70} = (N)(.70) = 420$

$= 62.50 + \left(\dfrac{420-354}{85}\right) 3 = 62.50 + \left(\dfrac{66}{85}\right) 3 = 62.50 + (.78) 3 = 62.50 + 2.34$
$= 64.84$

$P_{60} = (N)(.60) = 360$

$= 62.50 + \left(\dfrac{360-354}{85}\right) 3 = 62.50 + \left(\dfrac{6}{85}\right) 3 = 62.50 + (.07) 3 = 62.50 + .21$
$= 62.71$

$P_{50} = (N)(.50) = 300$

$= 59.50 + \left(\dfrac{300-263}{91}\right) 3 = 59.50 + \left(\dfrac{37}{91}\right) 3 = 59.50 + (.41) 3 = 59.50 + 1.23$
$= 60.73$

$P_{40} = (N)(.40) = 240$

$= 56.50 + \left(\dfrac{240-188}{75}\right) 3 = 56.50 + \left(\dfrac{52}{75}\right) 3 = 56.50 + (.69) 3 = 56.50 + 2.07$
$= 58.57$

$P_{30} = (N)(.30) = 180$

$= 53.50 + \left(\dfrac{180-117}{71}\right) 3 = 53.50 + \left(\dfrac{63}{71}\right) 3 = 53.50 + (.89) 3 = 53.50 + 2.67$
$= 56.17$

$P_{20} = (N)(.20) = 120$

$= 53.50 + \left(\dfrac{120-117}{71}\right) 3 = 53.50 + \left(\dfrac{3}{71}\right) 3 = 53.50 + (.04) 3 = 53.50 + .12$
$= 53.62$

$P_{10} = (N)(.10) = 60$

$= 47.50 + \left(\dfrac{60-32}{34}\right) 3 = 47.50 + \left(\dfrac{28}{34}\right) 3 = 47.50 + (.82) 3 = 47.50 + 2.46$
$= 49.96$

$P_{05} = (N)(.05) = 30$

$= 44.50 + \left(\dfrac{30-17}{15}\right) 3 = 44.50 + \left(\dfrac{13}{15}\right) 3 = 44.50 + (.87) 3 = 44.50 + 2.61$
$= 47.11$

If the deciles (every 10 steps) provide enough refinement these values can be rounded off and used to interpret the raw score standings.

Deciles	Raw Scores
95	75
90	72
80	68
70	65
60	63
50	61
40	59
30	56
20	54
10	50
5	47

If more refinement is needed, these 10 or 12 points can be plotted on a graph and then the intermediate points can be read more accurately. Or the intermediate points can be estimated. Figure 5–5 shows the plotted scale using the decile values reported above. A few check points will be illustrated with the P_{80} problem.

$$P_{80} = ll + \left(\frac{(N)(.80) - fc}{fi} \right) i$$

the (N) (P_{80}) is always larger than the f_c. the subtraction always results in a positive number

$$= 65.50 + \left(\frac{480-439}{56} \right) 3$$

$$= 65.50 + \left(\frac{41}{56} \right) 3$$

$\frac{41}{56}$ of the scores in this interval are needed to reach the 480 mark.

$$= 65.50 + (.73) 3$$

the quotient is always less than 1.00. Here it is .73

$$= 65.50 + 2.19$$
$$P_{80} = 67.69 \text{ or rounded to } 68''$$

the amount added to the lower limit is always less than the size of the interval— in this case, less than 3. Here it is 2.19.

The two methods presented for computing percentiles will approximate each other if there is absence of skewness in the distribution— if it is normal, that is—and if there is sufficient number of cases. The two factors are interrelated.

(c) Interpretation of Percentile. A percentile is a point on the scale above or below which a certain proportion of the cases fall. Jerry's jump of 65 inches is interpreted to fall at the 70th or 71st percentile. Seventy per cent of the boys of the same age and general background as Jerry will jump shorter than 65 inches and 30 per cent of them will jump farther.

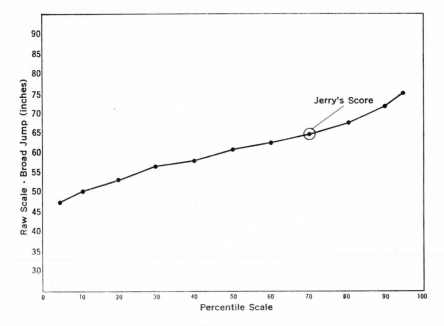

Fig. 5–5. Percentiles Plotted by Interpolation Method.

Norms. A norm is a standard point of reference that can provide a basis for judgment.[15] Norms are used to interpret relative standing, to compare scores or groups, and either to combine or average scores. The T-Scale and the Percentile scales remain the most widely used. The preparation of these scales as well as standard "z" scales and six sigma scales has been illustrated in the preceding pages. Norms imply a large number of cases. One hundred cases is minimal. Several hundred is more desirable. Such numbers can be collected by conducting testing programs in several schools in several different communities. They can be collected by combining the scores for certain tests given in a particular school over several years. Teachers who can find no appropriate norms already established will want to prepare their own. Such a practice is highly recommended. Appropriate norms are interpreted as those representing a group similar to the one for which they are used. If the mean and standard deviations for the group are similar to the mean and standard deviation of the normative group, the norms are appropriate usually. The characteristics of the normative sample should parallel the traits of the group using them for interpretation. For example, the performance of 12-year-old boys should not be interpreted on a scale prepared on the basis of performance of 15-year-old boys. Geographic location, racial origin, educational background, age, and sex are some of the factors which are considered when selecting a normative scale as a means of interpreting and comparing a specific group. Similarity of the groups is essential.

Measures of Relationship. Several statistical techniques are available for indicating the relationship of one variable to another. For example, is there a relationship between weight and ability to throw a ball? Can it be said generally that a heavy person can throw a ball a greater distance than a lighter person? Do the two characteristics seem to go together? When one is present is the other likely to be present also? Such relationships are measured by correlation coefficients which indicate relationship—but not cause and effect. If there is some likelihood that the heavy boy will throw farther, this is not to say that the heaviness is what *causes* the boy to throw farther. The farther throw might be the result of previous training, diet, height, attitude or even of the weight factor mentioned, but the exact *reason* is *not* identified by the correlation. The correlation coefficient simply indicates that there might be a tendency to expect a certain performance when a certain other factor is present. These are positive relationships, but lack of relationship and inverse relationship are possible of identification also.

Correlation coefficients range from +1.00 to −1.00. Coefficients of .86, .94, *etc.* for example, indicate a sizeable relationship; such coefficients as .16, .03, −.01, −.23, *etc.* would be so small, probably, as to indicate no appreciable relationship or no tendency for the two factors to be present simultaneously; coefficients such as −.73, −.86, *etc.* would show an inverse relationship. A negative or inverse relationship would mean that just the opposite to what was expected occurred, *i.e.* the heavy boys are likely to throw the ball the shorter distances.

Table 5–5.   Calculation of Rank-Difference Correlation

Case No.	Broad Jump	Height	R_1	R_2	D	D^2
1	76	66	1	1	0.0	0.00
2	71	62	2	2.5	.5	.25
3	68	58	3	7	4.0	16.00
4	65	59	4	6	2.0	4.00
5	61	57	5	8	3.0	9.00
6	58	56	6	9	3.0	9.00
7	57	60	7	4.5	2.5	6.25
8	52	52	8	10	2.0	4.00
9	49	60	9	4.5	4.5	20.25
10	44	62	10	2.5	7.5	56.25

$$\Sigma D^2 = 125.00$$

1. Rank Difference Correlation.[3] This method of computing an
estimate of a correlation coefficient is appropriate for small numbers
of cases—say less than 25 or 30. It is called the Spearman Rank-
Difference Correlation method and is designated as Rho (ρ). An
example will illustrate the computational steps. Two measures are
needed for each person.

Step 1. One scale is arranged in descending order. The Broad
Jump in this case (see Table 5–5).

Step 2. The corresponding height of each boy is listed opposite
his own Broad Jump score.

Step 3. Rank values are assigned to the Broad Jump scores (R_1).

Step 4. Rank values are assigned to the Height scores (R_2). If
two values are tied, like the same number for both fourth and fifth
places in the rank order, the two places in the rank that they would
occupy are added and divided by two. That rank value is then
assigned to both the tied values. For example, two students have
a height of 60 inches and they should occupy rank positions 4 and
5. Each is assigned rank 4.5.

Step 5. The differences between the two ranks are recorded (D).
Signs do not matter.

Step 6. The differences are squared (D^2).

Step 7. The D^2 Column is totaled.

Step 8. The following formula is used to solve for rho:

$$\rho = 1 - \frac{6\Sigma D^2}{N(N^2-1)} = 1 - \frac{6(125)}{10(10^2-1)} = 1 - \frac{750}{990} = 1 - .758$$

$$\rho = .242 \text{ or } .24$$

A ρ of .24 is not sizeable so it is possible to say that, for these ten
boys, there is not much relationship between the length of their
jump and their height.

Rho is an approximation of r. The difference between the two

**Table 5–6.* Table for Converting a Spearman Rho Coefficient Into
Its Equivalent Pearson r**

ρ	r	ρ	r	ρ	r	ρ	r
.05	.052	.30	.313	.55	.568	.80	.813
.10	.105	.35	.364	.60	.618	.85	.861
.15	.157	.40	.416	.65	.668	.90	.908
.20	.209	.45	.467	.70	.717	.95	.954
.25	.261	.50	.518	.75	.765	1.00	1.000

* Located in Guilford, J. P., *Fundamental Statistics in Psychology and Education.*
1st ed., New York: McGraw-Hill Book Co., Inc., 1942, Table 68, p. 229, and reprinted
by permission of the publisher.

CORRELATION CHART FOR COMPUTATION OF

X SCALE REPRESENTS *Sit-Ups*

Y SCALE REPRESENTS *Broad Jump*

						4-5	6-7	8-9	10-11	12-13	14-15	16-17	18-19	20-21	22-23	24-25
	-100	-90	-80	-70	-60	-50	-40	-30	-20	-10		10	20	30	40	50
	-90	-81	-72	-63	-54	-45	-36	-27	-18	-9		9	18	27	36	45
	-80	-72	-64	-56	-48	-40	-32	-24	-16	-8		8	16	24	32	40
	-70	-63	-56	-49	-42	-35	-28	-21	-14	-7		7	14	21	28	35
78-80	-60	-54	-48	-42	-36	-30	-24	-18	-12	-6		6	12 II (24)	18	24	30
75-77	-50	-45	-40	-35	-30	-25	-20	-15	-10	-5		5 I (5)	10	15	20 I (20)	25
72-74	-40	-36	-32	-28	-24	-20	-16	-12	-8	-4		4 II (8)	8	12 I (12)	16 I (16)	20
69-71	-30	-27	-24	-21	-18	-15	-12	-9	-6	-3		3 I (3)	6 I (6)	9 III (27)	12 III (36)	15
66-68	-20	-18	-16	-14	-12	-10	-8 I (-8)	-6	-4	-2 I (-2)	I	b 2 III (6)	4	6 III (18)	8 I (8)	10
63-65	-10	-9	-8	-7	-6	-5	-4	-3	-2 I (-2)	-1 I (-1)	I	1 I (1)	2 II (4)	3 III (9)	4	5
60-62							I			I	I		I	I	III	
57-59	10	9	8	7	6	5	4	3	2	1		-1	-2	-3 I (-3)	-4 I (-4)	-5
54-56	20	18	16	14	12	10	8	6	4	2	I	-2	-4	-6	-8	-10
51-53	30	27	24	21	18	a 15 I (15)	12	9 I (9)	6 I (6)	3	II	-3 I (-3)	-6	-9	-12 I (-12)	-15
48-50	40	36	32	28	24	20	16	12	8	4	I	-4	-8 I (-8)	-12 I (-12)	-16	-20
45-47	50	45	40	35	30	25	20	15	10	5		-5	-10 I (-10)	-15	-20	-25
42-44	60	54	48	42	36	30	24	18	12	6		-6	-12	-18	-24 I (-24)	-30
	70	63	56	49	42	35	28	21	14	7		-7	-14	-21	-28	-35
	80	72	64	56	48	40	32	24	16	8		-8	-16	-24	-32	-40
	90	81	72	63	54	45	36	27	18	9		-9	-18	-27	-36	-45
	100	90	80	70	60	50	40	30	20	10		-10	-20	-30	-40	-50
f						1	2	1	2	3	7	9	8	13	12	-
d	-10	-9	-8	-7	-6	-5	-4	-3	-2	-1		1	2	3	4	5
x′						-5	-8	-3	-4	-3	-	9	16	39	48	-
x′²						25	32	9	8	3	-	9	32	117	192	-

Fig. 5-6. Scattergram.

PEARSON PRODUCT-MOMENT COEFFICIENT OF CORRELATION

12-yr. old. Boys
N = 61

$$\frac{\Sigma x'}{N} = \frac{109}{61} = 1.787$$

$$\left(\frac{\Sigma x'}{N}\right)^2 = (\ 1.787\ )^2 = 3.204$$

$$\frac{\Sigma x'^2}{N} = \frac{561}{61} = 9.197$$

$$\frac{\Sigma y'}{N} = \frac{45}{61} = .738$$

$$\left(\frac{\Sigma y'}{N}\right)^2 = (\ .738\ )^2 = .545$$

$$\frac{\Sigma y'^2}{N} = \frac{487}{61} = 7.984$$

$$\frac{\Sigma x'y'}{N} = \frac{157}{61} = 2.574$$

$$\sigma_x = \sqrt{\frac{\Sigma x'^2}{N} - \left(\frac{\Sigma x'}{N}\right)^2} = \sqrt{9.197 - 3.204}$$
$$= \sqrt{5.993} = 2.44$$

$$\sigma_y = \sqrt{\frac{\Sigma y'^2}{N} - \left(\frac{\Sigma y'}{N}\right)^2} = \sqrt{7.984 - .545}$$
$$= \sqrt{7.439} = 2.72$$

$$r = \frac{\frac{\Sigma x'y'}{N} - \left(\frac{\Sigma x'}{N}\right)\left(\frac{\Sigma y'}{N}\right)}{\sigma_x \cdot \sigma_y}$$

$$= \frac{2.574 - (1.787)(.738)}{(2.44)(2.72)} = \frac{2.574 - 1.319}{6.637}$$

$$\frac{1.255}{6.637} = \boxed{.189 \text{ or } .19}$$

Correlation Chart by E. F. Lindquist, copyright, 1938, published by Houghton Mifflin Co., Boston. Reprinted by permission of the author and the publisher.

never exceeds .018 and most generally r is larger than ρ as shown in Table 5–6.[3] Jerry's broad jump was 65 inches and his height at the time was 59 inches but there doesn't seem to be much relationship between the two facts.

2. *Pearson Product-Moment Correlation.*[3]

a. *Scattergram Method:* The data for the 61 12-year-old boys will serve to illustrate this statistical technique. On the basis of a very limited sample of 10 cases there seemed to be little relationship between performance on the Broad Jump and the height of these 10 boys. Perhaps there is more relationship between the Broad Jump and the number of Sit-Ups done by the boys. This question will be explored for this relatively small group of 61 boys to illustrate the Pearson Product-Moment method of computing a correlation coefficient. Step by step, the procedure is outlined below. See Figure 5–6 to follow the development of the problem.

Step 1. The scores are tallied on the scattergram. The two axes represent the frequency distribution for the two variables being correlated. For example, a boy who jumped 53 inches and scored 4 Sit-Ups would be represented by a tally in the square designated as "a". A re-plotting of the tallies should be made by dotting each tally. Each tally should be dotted, showing agreement of the 2 plottings, before the computational work continues.

Step 2. The "f" column and row are filled in. These should be identical to previous tallies if mean and standard deviation problems have been worked.

Step 3. The y' and y'[2] and the x' and x'[2] are identical to the fd and fd[2] symbols used in the Mean and Standard Deviation problems illustrated on pages 78 and 79. The x and y are used here to distinguish between the two distributions. These columns and rows are filled in and totaled in the spaces provided.

Step 4. The moment values are filled in. The values printed in the upper right-hand corners of each little box are the product-moments. They show the extent of deviation from the approximate mean of each distribution. The number of tallies in the box is used to multiply the moment value. For example, "b" in Figure 5–6 shows that 3 cases fell within this box and the moment value of 2 is multiplied by 3 to get the 6. Circling these values with red pencil makes them easier to pick out as they are added together. The lower left side and the upper right side of the scattergram are positive. The upper left and lower right quarters are negative. These values are obtained by multiplying the deviations (d) from the axes which converge on a certain box. See "c" as an example in Figure 5–6, $(-8)\,(9) = -72$ and this is the value printed in the box. This procedure for determining the product-moment will be necessary whenever a printed scattergram form is not available.

Step 5. All of the encircled product-moments are added cross-wise to the x'y' + and — columns. This procedure can be done vertically as a check against the horizontal record. The columns are totaled and the correct algebraic sign is noted.

Step 6. Once the scattergram is plotted and all the columns and rows are added, the problem is solved by simple substitution in the formulas given.

The information available at several steps in the process can be used to compute Means and Standard Deviations for each distribution. The following formulas will indicate the substitutions needed.

$$M_x = AM + \left(\frac{\Sigma x'}{N}\right) i \quad \text{same as} \quad M = AM + \left(\frac{\Sigma fd}{N}\right) i$$

$$SD_x = i \sqrt{\frac{\Sigma x'^2}{N} - \left(\frac{\Sigma x'}{N}\right)^2} \quad \text{same as} \quad SD = i \sqrt{\frac{\Sigma fd^2}{N} - \left(\frac{\Sigma fd}{N}\right)^2}$$

This procedure should be used for computing Means and Standard Deviations if a correlation is planned anyway, thus avoiding duplication of much of the mechanical work.

The correlation coefficient in this particular problem of .19 is not sizable at all. It would be safe to conclude that there isn't much indication that the boys who performed well on the Broad Jump also performed well on the Sit-Ups.

A few pictures of scattergrams will illustrate the approximate answer to expect. After working several correlation problems, the teacher will be able to estimate the approximate coefficient from the plotting.

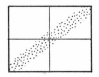 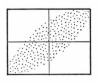 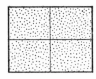 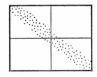

| a high correlation, positive, about .90 | an average positive correlation, about .45 or .50 | no pattern no correlation r is about .00 | a high negative correlation about −.90 |

The same problem in Figure 5–6 shows well-scattered plotting with some tendency toward the positive diagonal. Thus, the coefficient of .19 seems feasible.

Jerry jumped 65 inches and also did 28 Sit-Ups. The 65-inch jump is a little above average. The 28 Sit-Ups fall at about the 97th percentile. The correlation coefficient of .19 between these two variables indicated that similar levels of performance would not be expected. Jerry is an isolated case in point.

b. Formula Method for Ungrouped Data. This method is used when a calculator is available. It eliminates the plotting of the scattergram and solves the coefficient directly from the raw scores for each person. The same data for 61 12-year old boys on Broad Jump and Sit-up performances will be used to illustrate.

Step 1. Set-up the data sheet and compute multiplications and totals.

Let No. = student number or name
X = Sit-up scores
X^2 = Sit-up scores squared
Y = Broad Jump scores
Y^2 = Broad Jump scores squared
XY = Product of Sit-Up and Broad Jump scores.

The data would look something like this and each column would be totaled:

No.	X	X^2	Y	Y^2	XY
1	22	484	44	1936	968
2	20	400	57	3249	1140
3	23	529	71	5041	1633
4	17	289	76	5776	1292
5	15	225	61	3721	915
.	.	.	.	.	.
.	.	.	.	.	.
.	.	.	.	.	.
61	28	784	65	4225	1820
	1103	21399	3858	247708	70191

Step 2. Substitute the totaled values into the following formula[3]:

$$r = \frac{N\Sigma XY - (\Sigma X)(\Sigma Y)}{\sqrt{N\Sigma X^2 - (\Sigma X)^2}\ \sqrt{N\Sigma Y^2 - (\Sigma Y)^2}}$$

$$= \frac{61(70191) - (1103)(3858)}{\sqrt{(61)(21399) - (1103)^2}\ \sqrt{(61)(247708) - (3858)^2}}$$

$$= \frac{26277}{(297.8751)(475.4198)}$$

$$= \frac{26277}{141616.0610}$$

$$r = .1856$$

This method results in an answer very close to the one yielded by the scattergram method, *i.e.* r = .189. The size of the numbers makes it apparent why a calculator is recommended for this procedure. It would be more efficient and more accurate than hand calculations.

4. Spearman-Brown Prophecy Formula.[3] One additional correlation will be discussed because it is used often in test construction. This particular application relates to reliability coefficients. Often it is difficult, practically speaking, to administer as many trials of a test as desirable to establish the reliability coefficient. This formula will enable the teacher to estimate what the reliability would be on either a longer test or a shorter test. Usually it is the question of lengthening that is under consideration.

The regular Pearson Product-Moment correlation is computed on the basis of $\frac{1}{2}$ of the trials *vs.* the other $\frac{1}{2}$ of the trials. The odd-numbered trials are added for one score and the even-numbered trials are added for the other score. These two scores for each individual are correlated by the Pearson Product-Moment method.

Then the following formula is applied:

$$r_x = \frac{nr}{1 + (n-1)\,r}$$

Example — To double the length:

$$r_x = \frac{(2)(.68)}{1 + (2\text{-}1)\,.68}$$

$$= \frac{1.36}{1.68}$$

$$= .81$$

n = increase in the length of the test. Twice its length would be a 2. Three times would be a 3, $\frac{1}{2}$ as long would be a .5, etc.

r = correlation coefficient obtained on the 2 halves of the test.

The reliability coefficient of .68 computed on halves would increase to .81 for the full length of the test. Such a coefficient would be acceptable. This procedure made it unnecessary to administer the full test once and then a second time to obtain the data for establishing the reliability coefficient for the full length of the test.

Use of Table 5–7 will convert the split-halves coefficient to its full strength if the test were doubled in length. This table can be used in place of the formula method. The formula method, however, is useful if the reliability estimate for other than twice the length of the test were desired.

Comparing Groups. *1. Using Norms.* Another word of caution should be expressed regarding the proper use of norms to interpret raw scores. If the sample is not representative, if it is too limited, if it is not fairly normal, if it is not similar in its characteristics to the group being interpreted by it, then it would be misleading and perhaps even erroneous to translate raw scores to scaled scores from a normative scale.

If appropriate norms are not available for interpreting certain raw scores, the teacher would do well to prepare his own scale. Comparing the mean and standard deviation of the raw scores with

Table 5–7.   Coefficients Stepped Up by the Spearman-Brown Prophecy
Formula as an Estimate for Twice the Number of Trials*

Odd-Even	Spearman-Brown	Odd-Even	Spearman-Brown	Odd-Even	Spearman-Brown
.60	.75	.70	.82	.80	.89
.61	.76	.71	.83	.81	.90
.62	.77	.72	.84	.82	.90
.63	.78	.73	.84	.83	.91
.64	.78	.74	.85	.84	.91
.65	.79	.75	.86	.85	.92
.66	.80	.76	.86	.86	.93
.67	.80	.77	.87	.87	.93
.68	.81	.78	.88	.88	.94
.69	.82	.79	.88	.89	.94

* Located in Scott, M. Gladys, & Esther French, *Measurement and Evaluation in Physical Education.* Dubuque, Iowa: Wm. C. Brown Publishers, 1959, p. 87, and reprinted by permission of the authors.

the mean and standard deviation of the raw scores used to prepare the norms would be one way of testing the appropriateness of a certain normative scale. If the means and standard deviations are similar, the norms may be used with some degree of assurance.

2. Testing Significance of Difference. There are some statistical tests for judging the differences between groups. These will be discussed in concept only.

(*a*) Unrelated Groups. Perhaps a teacher wants to know if his 6th period class performed significantly differently from his 7th period class on a certain test. One mean may be 56.93 and the other may be 53.13. Are these significantly different or are they merely a difference produced by chance? If the latter is true then it is possible to say that probably there is no difference between the groups even though the means differ a little. Perhaps the teacher wants to know if the mean for his group is the same as the mean for a normative group. This would help him to know if it would be appropriate to use the norms. Just such a case would be another example of testing the significance of difference between groups. Perhaps the teacher wants to know if the students performed better on one item in the test battery than on another. Once transposed into comparable scores, this question can also be answered. Statistics books discussing the Significance of Difference between Unrelated Means would be helpful in solving such problems.

(*b*) Related Groups or Matched Pairs. Perhaps the teacher administers a fitness test early in the school year and then gives it again late in the spring. He will want to know if there has been any improvement in the fitness level of his students. Such a comparison as this involves two scores for each person and is based on the *difference* between these two scores for each person in the group. This is an analysis of matched pairs of scores and is discussed in statistics books as the Significance of Difference between matched pairs or correlated samples, or related groups.

This discussion of concept is included to alert the teacher to the possibility of making erroneous conclusions about the significance of various means. Some means which seem very close may, in truth, be significantly different and some, which seem distinctly different, may not be. Most often such questions are asked about the *means*, but tests of significance are also available for proportions (percentages), correlations, variances, *etc.* The teacher should be aware that there are statistical tests to determine the significance of differences between tests and between groups.

Presenting Data

Once the statistical calculations are complete they are more meaningful if put into some sort of tabular or graphic form. This permits a pictorial presentation which is easier to interpret.

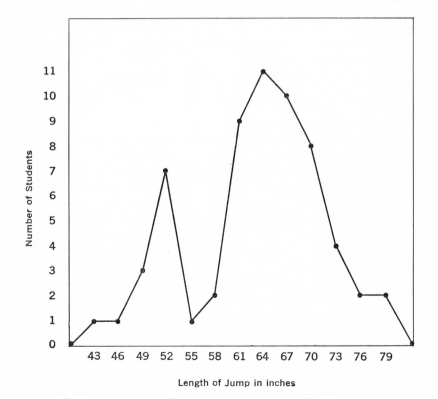

Fig. 5–7. Frequency Polygon. Broad jump for 61 12-year-old boys.

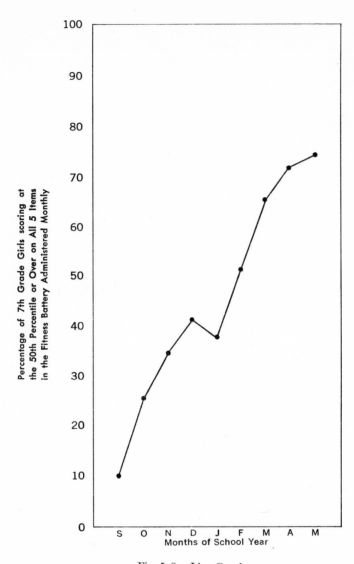

Fig. 5–8.   Line Graph.

Graphs.   Graphs are designed to show two types of information:
(1) continuous data such as depicted in a frequency polygon,
smoothed ogive and line graph; and, (2) discrete data such as can
be effectively shown in a bar graph, pie graph, or histogram.   These
will be illustrated.

Some hints for effective use of graphs follow:

Graphs should be well labeled.

Each axis should be well defined and marked off in equal
intervals.

Graph paper with sufficient number of squares should be used.
Do not try to conserve paper in graphic presentations.
Dark markings on the graph paper in units of 5 are desirable.
The axes should begin with zero whenever possible to avoid
misleading the reader.

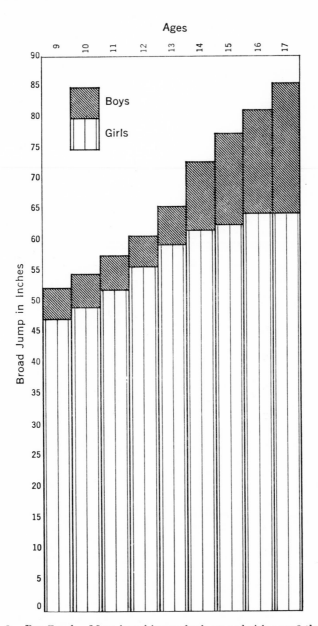

Fig. 5–9. Bar Graph. Mean broad jumps for boys and girls ages 9 through 17.

1. The *frequency polygon* is plotted at the midpoint of each interval (see Fig. 5–7). One interval above and one below the frequency distribution are included to provide beginning and ending lines when the dots are connected. This is a picture of Table 5–1.

2. The *line graph* seen in Figure 5–8 is good to show the influence of a time element on a particular variable.

3. The *smoothed ogive* has already been presented in Figure 5–4. It represents the cumulative frequency in percentages.

4. The *bar graph* can be used for comparisons. Sectioning within the bar is also possible. Figure 5–9 is an example of this type of graph.

5. The *histogram* is plotted at the midpoint of the interval and then extended to the exact limits of the interval to determine the width of the column. This is shown in Figure 5–10 and is another illustration of Table 5–1.

6. The *pie graph* shows the proportions that make up the whole. Figure 5–11 would be one application.

7. The *profile* is another type of graphic presentation which can be plotted to show achievement in several areas and to make comparisons within certain groups. The sample profile plotted in Figure 5–12 for Jerry shows he is especially good at Sit-Ups. He is very weak in Pull-Ups. He does above average in Side Stepping, Broad Jump, and Squat Thrusts. If the teacher wished to study each

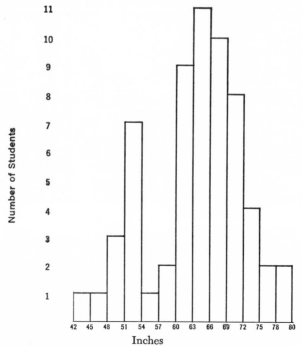

Fig. 5–10.   Histogram. Broad jump record for 61 12-year-old boys.

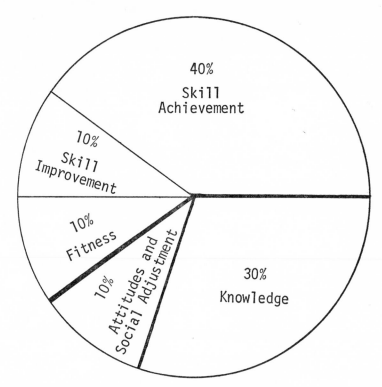

Fig. 5–11. Pie Graph. Possible percentage weightings for arrving at a grade.

student this way he would know how to design the program to fit the individual needs of his students. Just such a profile as this could be plotted for the class averages to show the areas in which the class as a whole needed to concentrate to improve its over-all fitness. Another testing period later in the school year could be devoted to the fitness tests and those scores could be plotted on the same profile to show changes in development. The profile has an additional application as a device which is of interest to parents.

Tables. Tables, like graphs, make clear points which would be very involved if described in words. It is helpful to present the summary of data in tabular form and then to discuss the points of emphasis which the table reveals.

Tables should be well labeled and independently self-explanatory. They should be carefully spaced to provide clear reading. They should be sectioned by vertical and horizontal lines and double lines to denote appropriate sectioning. They, like graphs, provide a condensation of a vast amount of information into a small space and an intelligible form. The use of tables is recommended to help interpret and apply the information gained from a good program of measurement.

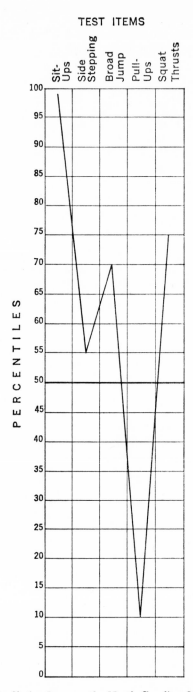

Fig. 5–12.   Profile for Jerry on the North Carolina fitness battery.

References

1. Campbell, W. R., and N. M. Tucker: *An Introduction to Tests and Measurement in Physical Education.* London, G. Bell and Sons Ltd., 1967.
2. Clarke, H. Harrison: *Application of Measurement to Health and Physical Education.* 4th Ed., Englewood Cliffs, N.J., Prentice-Hall, Inc., 1967.
3. Guilford, J. P.: *Fundamental Statistics in Psychology and Education.* 4th Ed., New York, McGraw-Hill Book Co., 1965.
4. Johnson, Joan D., and David L. Kelley: *A Workbook for Tests and Measurements in Physical Education.* Palo Alto, California, Peek Publications, 1967.
5. Mathews, Donald K.: *Measurement in Physical Education.* 3rd Ed., Philadelphia, W. B. Saunders Co., 1968.
6. McNemar, Quinn: *Psychological Statistics.* 4th Ed., New York, John Wiley and Sons, Inc., 1969.
7. Meyers, Carlton R., and T. Erwin Blesh: *Measurement in Physical Education.* New York, The Ronald Press, 1962.
8. Neilson, N. P.: *Statistics, Tests and Measurements in Physical Education.* Palo Alto, California, National Texts, 1960.
9. Scott, M. Gladys, and Esther French: *Measurement and Evaluation in Physical Education.* Dubuque, Iowa, Wm. C. Brown Co. Publishers, 1959.
10. Stroup, Francis: *Measurement in Physical Education.* New York, The Ronald Press, 1957.
11. Townsend, Edward Arthur, and Paul J. Burke: *Statistics for the Classroom Teacher* (*A Self-Teaching Unit*). New York, The Macmillan Co., 1963.
12. Votaw, David F., and Clarence T. Gray: *Statistics Applied to Education and Psychology.* New York, The Ronald Press, 1939.
13. Walker, Helen M.: *Mathematics Essential for Elementary Statistics.* New York, Henry Holt & Company, 1951.
14. Weber, Jerome C., and David R. Lamb: *Statistics and Research in Physical Education.* St. Louis, C. V. Mosby Company, 1970.
15. Willgoose, Carl E.: *Evaluation in Health Education and Physical Education.* New York, McGraw-Hill Book Co., 1961.

ANSWERS TO EXERCISES

Exercise 5–1, page 70.

Add:		Multiply:	
1. − 8	6. − 6	1. +54	6. −12
2. +12	7. −20	2. − 6	7. −30
3. − 1	8. + 3	3. +24	8. +36
4. + 8	9. −17	4. −36	9. −72
5. + 5	10. − 5	5. +40	10. +21

Subtract:		Divide:	
1. + 1	6. + 3	1. + 3	6. − 0
2. + 3	7. − 6	2. − 5	7. − 3
3. +10	8. +16	3. + 2	8. + 1
4. +15	9. + 5	4. − 2	9. − .5
5. + 7	10. −14	5. − 1	10. 0

Exercise 5–2, page 72.

Find the Square:		Find the Square Root:	
1.	266.9956	1.	4.41
2.	.0016	2.	.186
3.	10609	3.	20.65
4.	15.5236	4.	.86
5.	.541696	5.	2.528

Part II. Evaluation of the Product

Chapter 6
INTRODUCTION TO MEASUREMENTS OF ALL TYPES

Introduction

All modern philosophy and most educational practices now view the student as a unity. This unified and integrated individual is made up of many elements and is the result of many forces which play upon him. As a product he is acted upon not only by his own nature, but also by the forces found in his environment. His nature has evolved into such components as mental, physical, social, and spiritual. His environment includes not only his physical surroundings but also his fellow students, teachers, and associates and the traditions, folkways, and mores of his society. However, there is more than just the action of these diverse elements upon him. There is an interrelatedness between the components of his nature and the varied forces of his environment to produce what he is at any given time. This action, reaction, and interaction is experience, and by its very nature it can never be all physical, all mental, or all social. It has been traditional in education to classify experience into the intellectual and physical. While formal discipline made this classification because of the belief in the dichotomy of the individual, modern education does it chiefly for convenience. Modern education views the student as an entity and recognizes the interrelationships of his parts.

The experience inherent in the action, reaction, and interaction of man and his surroundings takes many forms and produces many changes. Such changes differ from one person to another. These changes have been identified as education. Since physical education has been defined as education through physical means, it implies something more than the physical. Like education in general, its hierarchy of objectives takes into account the organismic nature of the student. These objectives include much more than the training of the physical. Traditionally, they cover the three domains of learning commonly referred to in physical education as psychomotor, cognitive, and affective. When these objectives have been achieved through these areas of learning, they result in a physically educated person. This person has been described as one who has attained reasonable skill in a wide variety of activities, a high level of fitness, adequate knowledge of sports and exercise, and sufficient emotional poise and attitude to become a good participant in sports and exercise. A physically educated person is one aspect of the totally integrated and effective citizen. When this aim of physical education has been achieved along with the many other objectives of education, a liberally educated person results.

It has been said that whatever exists, exists in amounts; and if it exists in amounts, it can be measured.[11] When this principle is applied to the *product* of physical education, it suggests the evaluation of various traits or components of the student. Broadly speaking, these components include such qualities as organic fitness, fundamental skills, sport skills, knowledges and understandings associated with sports and exercise, and the various types of social learnings taught in physical education. This concept suggests that in the process of evaluation of the product, the student must be divided into parts and each part evaluated separately. This practice has become traditional in education. Since educators now view the student as a whole but understand that he must grow, develop, and learn specifically, this part method of evaluation is an educationally sound procedure. However, it is recognized as an educationally sound procedure only if the teacher fully comprehends the unity concept and understands that, contrary to a well-known mathematical thesis, the sum of the parts does not always add up to the whole when dealing with the human entities. It is relatively easy to analyze the students in parts or elements, but when the process of synthesis is used to combine these same elements into a whole, there are not enough elements to do the job. The whole is something more than the sum of its parts.

For instance, this total concept of the individual is exemplified by the term "fitness." Much stress is placed on "total fitness." Total fitness is then broken down into several aspects, including physical, mental, social, and emotional. Physical fitness is reduced to the still narrower concept of motor fitness. Then, of course, it is necessary to proliferate still further by analyzing motor fitness into its various components, such as endurance, strength, power, flexibility, etc. Thus, virtually all of these items involve measurements of specifics. However, when all these specific elements are measured and the results are placed in a profile, the parts do not add up to the whole. Something of this "wholeness" is not measured. In the process of synthesis, some of the parts of the fitness mosaic are inevitably missing.

When dealing with his *product*, the physical educator does measure specific aspects in most instances. It might be well before he starts his process of analysis and divides the student into parts, to view him as a whole. It is equally important to look at the parts in relation to the whole after measurements. The wholeness and the unity of the individual is divided into segments partly for better understanding and partly for convenience. However, as has been pointed out, these separate components do not operate independently as entities in themselves. They are not separate and diverse items but are inextricably related. They are like threads in the loom as they are woven into fabric by man's experience. They have meaning only when viewed in this context, which is one of synthesis rather than analysis. Eventually they must be reviewed in relation to the whole student. These qualities and the factors which are associated with them can generally be measured by one means or another. In this chapter the major qualities or factors will be enumerated and defined. Also, the different types of tests and measures used to evaluate them will be presented. This over-view into the factors to be measured and the various procedures and techniques to be used is basic to understanding the subsequent chapters.

The Domains of Learning

It is possible to classify learning in physical education in a number of ways. Such learning may be listed under the recognized learning areas, or under the objectives inherent in these areas. In the former, learning has traditionally been classified into *technical, associated,* and *concomitant* indicating respectively motor performance, mental learnings, and psychosocial patterns of behavior. This tripartition is really not all-inclusive since associated learning refers to incidental learning and concomitant to learning without intent. A more modern approach to learning categories is through classification according to the taxonomy of educational objectives.[4, 8] Taxonomy means a set of classifications and has been used successfully in the sciences for clarity of understanding and for communication. More recently it has been applied to educational objectives.

When taxonomy is applied to the goals of education, three broad areas or domains are revealed. They are: *cognitive, affective,* and *psychomotor* domains. All educational objectives presumably can be fitted into this tripartite framework, although admittedly such classification is chiefly for convenience, since there can be no clear-cut lines of demarcation between them. In the learning process, once these objectives have been achieved by the learner, a liberally educated person is more likely to result. By the same token, if the physical education objectives are accomplished for any given learner, the result will probably be a better physically educated person. Perhaps the most important one of these domains to the physical educator is the *psychomotor* (technical) because it is the medium through which the *cognitive* (associated) and *affective* (concomitant) domains are achieved. However, it must be pointed out once again before man is empirically divided into these parts or domains, recognition must be given to the unity, holistic, or whole-man concept. These three domains do not exist as separate entities but are inexorably related and interrelated with each other. No learning is all physical, or mental or social. Sometimes it is difficult to tell where one begins and another leaves off.

Each of these tripartite areas is unique in that in some respects one is inexorably related with the other two. They are different to the extent that one cannot be predicted from another but they are related to the extent that learning in one area is affected by learning in another, and they are inextricably intertwined. Being physically educated involves the whole person and learning is never singular. Learning in physical education comes through movement in the form of sports, games, dance and gymnastics, but it encompasses far more than skills and fitness. The learner learns specificities but his whole being is affected. When he learns a skill specifically, he acquires other learnings as well, although the teacher-coach may be totally unaware of their presence, or at least he may not have planned for them in his process. Motor skill development is dependent on some knowledge and understanding. One of the great challenges in teaching and coaching is how to project learning in order to assist the student to transcend mere skill in movement.

These three domains do not lend themselves to the process of taxonomy with the same facility. Because of its quantitative nature and the great amount of previous work in the area, the *cognitive* domain lends itself best to a structural classification. The *affective* domain, because of its intangible nature and the dearth of previous measurement lends itself to structuring somewhat less readily. The third domain, the *psychomotor*, is still in the formative stages of taxonomy. Few attempts have been made by educators to classify learning in this area and physical education scholars have only recently begun work in this field. For purposes of this book, all of those learnings which make up movement and which have an influence on it and which are not classified under either of the other two domains will be classified under psychomotor. No attempt is made to suggest that this system of classification is final. It is presented here chiefly for convenience with the recognition that it is perhaps a traditional scheme of classification.

Psychomotor Domain. A great deal has been said in recent years about human movement, and *psychomotor* is concerned with movement and other closely related factors which influence it. Movement is inevitable as man's changing life processes interact with and react to his dynamic and constantly changing environment. Through sports, exercise, and the dance, the individual overcomes both his own forces and the forces of the universe. Movement is associated with muscular contraction and all motor performance involves muscle action in its myriad forms. It is also associated with neural mechanisms; hence *psychomotor* or sometimes *neuromotor* or *neuromuscular*. There are levels of utilization of the body's forces. There are many restrictions or limitations on movements, some of which are variable and change as man's experiences change. The factors of fitness, for instance, are dynamic and changeable and are directly related to the experience the individual has had or is having. There also are factors which aid and help make more effective such man-made forms of movement as sport and exercise. The purpose of this unit is to deal with the aspects and factors which make up movement and which influence it. For purposes of measurement in physical education, the forms of movement may be classified into a number of categories.

Movement is a complex quality and is influenced by many forces. *First*, there are those *physical performance factors* which underlie the action for all movement. These factors include speed, agility, strength, power, etc. and are revealed through the fundamental skills of running, jumping, throwing, climbing, hanging, etc. *Second*, there are certain *structural factors* which either help or hinder movement.[9] These factors include age, height, weight, body type, and structure. *Third*, there are certain *sociopsychological* factors which influence behavior and ultimately affect movement to a marked degree. These factors will be discussed under the affective domain.

The physical educator generally measures the first of these when he is interested in evaluating movements, although indirectly he may concern himself with the second if he establishes norms for those movements based on age, weight, or height, or combinations. The coach and teacher must also be cognizant of the third group consisting of certain mental, emotional, and social factors. These do have great influence on movement, but they are not usually measured directly in tests of physical performance.

The physical performance factors are the ones most influential in this area. They are of three kinds. *First*, there are those factors which are basic to all performance, such as agility, power, speed, arm and shoulder coordination, balance, flexibility, etc. *Second*, there are fundamental movements, such as running, jumping, throwing, climbing, and hanging. These are called racial activities and are common to the performance of all people since they make up the basic patterns of motor movement.[21] *Third*, there are highly specialized movements which are the result of training and experience and which are not common to all individuals. These are acquired through practice and specialization. They include athletic or sports activities and skills, gymnastics, and dance. These highly specialized movements represent the result or the influence of the factors which are basic to all performance and also the fundamental movements.

The fundamental skills are both cause and effect since they are the result of the basic factors and are themselves basic to the specific sport skills.[9] The factors which are basic to all motor performance are causal and represent the first level of performance. In subsequent paragraphs these basic factors are elaborated upon in order to increase understanding of such qualities as motor ability, motor fitness, and sport skill.

In addition to these, there are the processes of perception which now appear to be inexorably related to movement. Therefore, *perceptual-motor* learning is another facet of the psychomotor domain. Also, since one of the characteristics of the taxonomy scheme of classification is that all objectives and areas of learning will fall within the parameters of these three domains, the structural factors of *posture, nutritional status,* and *body types,* too, will be discussed as a part of the psychomotor domain. These come within the province of this domain because they are factors which may significantly influence movement.

PHYSICAL PERFORMANCE FACTORS. *a. Strength.* All of the factors of motor performance described in this unit depend in varying degrees on muscular movement and thus, strength. Strength is a prerequisite to all activity since it takes a certain amount of it to be agile, to have power, and to run fast. Strength is related to a type of endurance since the more efficient the muscle is in its work load, the longer it can function. However, while strength as a factor is inextricably related to other motor performance factors, it remains an entity in itself and is a salient element of the whole. Strength of and in itself is not an indicant of capacity, nor fitness, nor educability, but merely the ability to apply force. *Strength may be defined as the capacity of the individual to exert muscular force.* This force is revealed by the individual's ability to pull, push, lift, or squeeze an object, or to hold the body in a hanging position. Maximum strength is applied in these ways with a singular muscular contraction, and the strength of the muscle is in proportion to its effective cross section.

Strength of muscle is necessary if the student is to perform his normal daily activities in an efficient manner. Strength in excess of this amount will enable him to perform them more easily and effectively. This excess over daily demands is needed for two reasons. First, it is needed for emergency situations where survival is a factor. Second, after one's daily normal activities are completed, he should have sufficient strength to live his life more fully and completely in leisure time pursuits. Strength can be measured by such test items as the chins, dips, push-ups, and hanging, and by pulling, pushing, and lifting various devices, such as scales, dynamometers and weights. More and more, strength has come to play a part in athletics. If everything else is equal, the stronger player or team usually prevails. This has been true for many years in such sports as football, boxing, and wrestling. Recently, however, the idea has become popular in other activities. In sports like baseball, basketball, golf, and swimming, coaches seek first to recruit the strong boys and then develop more strength in them through strength-building activities. Strength is one of the most dynamic factors of motor performance and is subject to improvement. The amount can be negligible or dramatic, depending on the amount of the resistance used and the duration of the training program.

b. *Speed.* An essential for successful performance in many motor activities is speed. Generally, when speed is discussed, one thinks of leg speed in running activities. But speed, like reaction time, concerns many body parts and may vary from one part to another. In general, *speed may be defined as the capacity of the individual to perform successive movements of the same pattern at a fast rate.* Speed of muscle contraction would appear to be an innate quality, but certainly speed of movement used in running the sprints or running in any game such as football, can be improved through training in the proper techniques and through continued practice in the coordination of movements.

Strength is highly related to speed. This fact might indicate that improving the strength of the moving part might result in a corresponding increase in speed. In any event, speed is an important element in most athletic performances. It is a valuable ingredient in such sports as football, baseball, basketball, and track. Many times in football the lighter team wins because it is the faster team. Generally, speed can be measured by a short dash of from 40 to 60 yards. The distance depends on the age and condition of the person being tested. Sometimes a shuttle run is used where space is limited for sprints. As in all motor performance, there are limiting factors to speed. The rapidity of movement is affected by body weight, body density, muscle viscosity, and such mechanical and structural features as length of limbs and flexibility of joints.

c. *Power.* Power is recognized as one of the most basic components of movement. It is the *capacity of the individual to bring into play maximum muscle contraction at the fastest rate of speed.* Power is an explosive action and it is equal to the product of force times velocity, where force has to do with muscle strength and velocity with the speed with which strength is used in motor performance. Power is a mechanical principle which is concerned with propelling the body or projecting its parts in a forceful, explosive manner in the shortest period of time. It is the ability to release maximum muscular force at maximum speed. This power factor is a characteristic of the superior athlete. Speed and force are combined in athletic performance for high standards of excellence. The most successful athlete, of course, would be the individual who has superior strength, exceptional speed, and the ability to effectively coordinate them or integrate them into explosive action for excellent performance. This athlete can be described as the power athlete who hits the home runs in baseball, clears the backboards in basketball, drives through the line in football, tosses the shot great distances in track and field meets, and hits the long drives off the golf tee. Power is frequently measured by some type of jump, charge, or throw. The vertical jump and the standing broad jump are most commonly used to measure leg power. A shot put or medicine ball put may be used to indicate power in the arms and shoulder. A charge at a blocking sled may measure body power. Power is required for efficiency in such activities as jumping for height or distance, kicking a soccer ball or football, throwing or putting a ball or weight, striking with a bat or club, charging an opponent, and sprinting with short bursts of speed. In addition to the factors of speed and strength, power is limited by such factors as weight, muscle viscosity, and body structure.

d. *Endurance.* Endurance *is the result of a physiological capacity of the individual to sustain movement over a period of time.* Endurance is of two kinds. One is associated with the factor of strength, whereas the other is associated with the circulatory-respiratory systems. The two types are related, however.

In the first type, associated with strength, the individual with endurance has the ability to continue successive movements in situations where the muscles or muscle groups being used are loaded heavily. Naturally, the stronger person is able to work over a longer period of time than the weaker person. However, strength in itself does not provide the entire answer to muscular endurance. A strong muscle can be improved in endurance by developing more efficiency so that its recovery rate will be faster. This phenomenon of recovery is related to the number of functioning capillaries which are present within the muscle, as well as the strength of the muscle itself. Such endurance is characterized by the ability to continue repetitious actions with a heavy load at a maximum speed for a short period of time. Such endurance can be improved by increasing rength through the application of some form of the overload inciple. As muscles are taxed beyond the point of comfort, or are overloaded, endurance is developed. This endurance can be measured in several ways. An example is the chin-ups.

The type of endurance associated with circulatory-respiratory systems is characterized by a physiological fitness and is related to the phenomenon of "wind." In this instance, exercise is carried on with sufficient duration and intensity to place stress on the heart, circulatory, and respiratory systems. In this type of endurance there is an adjustment in the circulatory-respiratory systems to prolong action. Such endurance enables the individual to sustain moderate contraction of the skeletal muscles over a comparatively long period of time. The adjustment in the heart, lungs, and circulatory systems which has just been mentioned can be made more efficient through training. The best type of test to measure this facet of motor performance is distance running.

e. Agility. One of the most important factors influencing movement is agility. This factor is revealed by *the ability of the body or parts of the body to change directions rapidly and accurately.* Measures of this quality test the ability of the student to move quickly from one position in space to another. Agility involves coordinating quickly and accurately the big muscles of the body in a particular activity. These rapid changes in movement patterns by the whole body or by some of its parts have been measured by such test items as dodge run, obstacle run, zigzag run, side step, and squat thrust. One's level of agility is probably a result of both innate capacity and training and experience. Certainly agility plays an important role in physical education activities, especially in such events as gymnastics, diving, basketball, pole vaulting, hurdling, high jumping, and in the maneuvering of the ends and backs in football. It is revealed to a great extent in sports involving efficient footwork and quick changes in body position. Agility is more effective when it is combined with high levels of strength, endurance, and speed. While it is somewhat dependent on one's heritage, it can be improved.

f. Balance. Balance is an important aspect of efficient motor response and is one of the basic motor factors. *It is the ability of the individual to maintain his neuro-muscular system in a static condition for an efficient response or to control it in a specific efficient posture while it is moving.* The first type of balance is referred to as static balance and the second as dynamic. Both are basic to movement under varying conditions. Each is perhaps made up of the same constituents but in varying amounts. Both indicate a certain amount of steadiness and stability and are characterized by a certain amount of ease and poise in maintaining position.

The factor of balance is founded in several elements. First, it is related to the functioning of the organs of the inner ear where the semicircular canals are located. These are commonly recognized as the organs of balance. Second, it is definitely related to kinesthetic sense located in the muscles and joints. One must have the "feel" of an activity for stability. Third, it is partly dependent on visual perception. One is able to maintain a pose or control stability of movement much better with the eyes open. This is probably shown most clearly in the item known as the "stork stand." This is a stunt which requires the placement of one foot against the opposite knee and the hands on the hips. When the eyes are open, balance may be maintained rather easily, but it becomes much more difficult to maintain when the eyes are closed.

Good balance plays its part in daily normal activities, and is especially significant in many sport activities. In daily life it prevents falls and helps maintain equilibrium in carrying out many tasks. In the area of sports and exercise, it is an important aspect of motor performance and more specifically motor ability. It is related to other factors of movement but significantly to agility and coordination.

Dynamic balance is revealed by one's ability to move from one point or space to another and maintain equilibrium. For such efficient movement a certain amount of steadiness and stability is required. This is the same quality displayed by the lumberjack as he jumps from one log to another. Such activities as tumbling, stunts, apparatus, dancing, skiing, skating, and swimming depend to a high degree on good balance. Static balance is actually the same measure but to a different degree. In this instance the range of movement is much less or perhaps there is very little range. This type of balance is revealed through such activities as standing on a rail or beam, doing a hand stand, or maintaining equilibrium after a fast ride. In both static and dynamic balance, stance is of vital importance in maintaining stability after the body has been placed in an unfavorable position by movement.

g. Flexibility. Another factor which is recognized as basic to proficiency in motor movement is flexibility. It is significant in the performance of many skills and as a motor fitness factor. *Flexibility may be defined as the range of movement in a joint.* It concerns degree of movement and limits the degree to which the body or body parts can bend or twist by means of flexion and extension of muscles. This degree of movement depends on the flexibility and extensibility of the muscles and the ligaments surrounding the particular joint. The degree of flexibility needed by any student has not been determined. One generally thinks in terms of a full range of movement but this full range of movement is desirable only when it can contribute to better performance.

Flexibility is a specific quality more than it is a general one. For example, flexibility must be considered in terms of specific joints and for specific uses. There may even be variability from one joint to another. Within the same joint, flexibility may vary from time to time depending on such factors as warm-up, temperature, effort, relaxation, and pain-tolerance. A good range of movement in general has several advantages for the student. A high level of flexibility fosters a saving in energy during vigorous movement because of the better mechanical adjustment. Also, because of this better physiological and mechanical adjustment of the joint and muscles, the individual may be less vulnerable to injury. Flexibility, like balance, plays its part in maintaining good posture and it is related to such components as endurance, speed, and agility. Flexibility negates tension and thus is a positive force in motor ability.

Flexibility may be measured by testing the range of movement at specific joints. A great many devices have been used to do this, such as flexometers and tests which require touching the finger tips to the floor. These tests measure the ability of the body or parts of the body to extend or flex.

h. Coordination. Coordination is another of the factors which is basic to performance and especially to highly complex movements. *It may be defined as the ability of the performer to integrate types of movements into specific patterns.* The requirements for different activities may be quite different. Coordination, like several other components, is interrelated with other factors. Performing integrated patterns of movement with good coordination involves agility, balance, speed, and kinesthetic sense. Interestingly enough, strength and endurance are not especially significant in coordination except to the extent that coordination is impaired after fatigue sets in. This integration into skill patterns not only plays an important part in sports, but also in one's daily, normal activities.

The essential quality of this factor concerns the capacity of the student to perform specific movements in a series quickly and accurately. In this case a performer understands and can perform each part of the total movement and can change rapidly from one pattern to another for efficient execution. Such movements are revealed in activities like a golf swing, pole vault, the complicated pivot in the discus throw, and certain gymnastic stunts. The more complicated the movement, the greater is the requirement in terms of coordination. Good coordination is associated with insight into the nature of the movement, with kinesthetic sense, and with a learner's perception of relationships and it can be improved through training and practice. The bar snap for distance has been used to measure this factor.

i. Kinesthetic Sense. A factor which is very much involved in movement and especially in learning specific skills is kinesthetic sense. *Kinesthesis may be defined as the sense which gives the individual an awareness of position of the body or parts of the body as it moves through space.* As a result of this information received from the senses, the individual is able to control his movements more accurately. This position sense is found in receptors located in the muscles, fascia of muscles, tendons, and joints. These receptors act as feedback mechanisms for making the individual aware of the intensity of stretch or contraction of the muscle, or the stress placed on the tendon, muscle fascia, or joint. With this information, the performer can tell with varying degrees of accuracy the position of the body and/or body part as it moves in space.

This awareness of movement position is an important factor in learning a movement. It operates to a degree each time the body or part of it is called upon to challenge the forces of gravity in sports, exercise, and daily tasks. It is significantly related to balance, and plays a dynamic part in establishing and maintaining patterns of good posture. In the highly complex skills which are encountered in diving, gymnastics, trampolining, and some forms of the dance, this sense enables the performer to distinguish his position in space with a degree of accuracy and consistency. As a result of this awareness, the performer can acquire the ability to execute the designated movement more accurately and effectively. The factor is fundamental and must be exercised if it is to be developed. Certainly the knowledge of where one is in a complicated skill can be facilitated by having a mental picture of the whole movement. Also, in the learning process, learning occurs more rapidly when the sensations can be retained in memory and used again in practice to achieve greater perfection. There are a number of devices which have been used to measure kinesthetic perception.

j. Hand-Eye-Foot-Eye-Coordination. One of the most important factors in the performance of many sport skills is concerned with the coordination of the eyes with either the feet, hands, or head. Skillfulness in this area of movement is characterized by control, accuracy, and steadiness. Many of these movements involve a ball or a similar object. All such movements involve a primary objective, and the performer must keep his eyes trained on this primary objective while he carries out the initial part of the movement. This is frequently referred to as "keeping your eye on the ball." This is good advice to the performer and is necessary for him to judge such variable factors as speed, distance, direction, and size.

This factor is closely related to several other qualities, such as depth perception, kinesthetic sense, rhythm, insight into learning, agility, and relaxation. The quality is evidently a combination of the innate and the acquired. Skills involving this factor can be developed through practice. There are myriads of skills involving coordination of the eyes with hands. All activities involving hitting, batting, catching, fielding, and throwing belong in this category. While there are not so many activities for the eyes and foot, they are still coordinated in many activities involving kicking skills. Even the head and eyes are coordinated in the soccer skill of heading. In all cases, the quality involves the ability of a performer to judge accurately the speed and direction of some object and, in most sports, it further involves the ability to adjust the body or parts of the body in relation to the object. These adjustments take several forms: (*a*) Hitting or kicking an object from a stationary position, such as hitting a golf ball from a tee, or kicking a football from a tee. (*b*) Fielding, catching, hitting, or kicking a moving object, such as catching a pass in football, or making a pass from a moving ball in soccer. (*c*) Throwing, shooting, or kicking at a goal or distant target. In this case, the primary objective is the goal or target and not the ball.

FUNDAMENTAL SKILLS. Man's basic patterns of movement are embodied in the fundamental skills. These are frequently referred to as the immemorial racial activities of man since they are racial in nature and are common to all mankind. These fundamental patterns of movement are expressed as walking, running, jumping, throwing, striking, hanging, and carrying. Such activities with minor variations have no boundaries either geographically or racially. They are gross motor activities and are made up of most postural and locomotor movements as well as some manipulative. Their quality and efficiency are dependent on the underlying physical performance factors such as power, speed and the like which were discussed in the preceding section.

These fundamental skills have formed the basis of man's work and play since time immemorial. They were prime instigators of the evolutionary processes and were the catalyst that lifted man to higher and higher levels. They were the basis for his survival activities and they later developed into his more purposive work. His play, games, gymnastics and dance are adaptations, modifications, and elaborations of these basic patterns. In the process of evolution an inextricable relationship was set up between these big muscle movements and man's organic and nervous systems. The development and maintenance of these systems are dependent on man's movements through these patterns. These patterns may be engaged in directly by running, for example, or indirectly through participation in work, play, dance and other activities which are organized and integrated out of the basic patterns and adapted to specialized purposes. It is these fundamental skills which are frequently measured in physical tests such as a dash, a throw for distance, a jump, and the like. These fundamental skills are universal in nature and common to all races, whereas their adaptation into games and dance makes a new product which is unique and specific and as different as the mores and customs of people.

GENERAL ABILITIES. It has been traditional for man's motor behavior to be divided into categories. In the light of more recent research some doubt now exists concerning the generality of movement. Some scientists believe that all movement is highly specific to the task and there can be no such thing as a general motor ability or capacity. The issue has not been settled clearly, however, so for purposes of this text the traditional general qualities of *motor capacity, motor educability, motor ability,* and *motor fitness* will be presented.

a. Motor Capacity. Motor capacity is defined as the general overall quality which is indicative of an individual's potential or innate ability. As an isolated quality, the factors which undergird it have been difficult to identify. Such factors must not be subject to modification through education since they are indicants of maximum potential. McCloy did pioneer work in this area and presented a test of General Motor Capacity with a Motor Quotient which presumably was the motor analogue of the I.Q.[12] McCloy isolated four elements which he considered indicative of capacity: size and maturity, power, motor educability, and agility and coordination. While tests of capacity would be desirable, the ones which have been developed have been used very little.

b. Motor Educability. It is obvious that some individuals learn skills more readily than others and that there are varying degrees of ability to learn. There appears to be an inherent aptitude for motor learning in the same way that there is for mental learning. This quality has to do with educability. *Motor educability may be defined as the ease and thoroughness with which one learns new motor skills.* Since it is undoubtedly related to insight, it is perhaps as much psychological as physiological. This might suggest that it is not a factor of motor learning in the same sense as the factors described in the preceding paragraphs, but rather a combination of many factors. However, the presence or lack of it has a great deal to do with how quickly and effectively motor skills can be learned.

In the past this quality has been evaluated by presenting motor problems which are new to the student. Traditionally, this has been done through stunt-type activities where stunts involving performance of unfamiliar motor patterns are presented. One who possesses a high level of this quality is generally called a "natural," as he responds to teaching and coaching quickly and usually has levels of achievement in the championship class. Motor educability, like both motor ability and motor fitness, is affected by body size, body build, and most of the factors described previously. Maturation undoubtedly plays its role in the improvement shown by different individuals. Strangely, however, this quality is influenced very little by strength and endurance. Most of the items which have been used to test motor educability are capable of being improved through practice. Therefore, if the test is to be valid, the individual must not have previously practiced the event. Naturally, it would improve these tests if items could be found which were not subject to improvement through practice. This is hardly possible since all motor performance seems to improve with specific practice.

c. *Motor Ability.* Motor ability is made up of factors which are basic to all movement. To some degree all the factors which have been discussed in the preceding paragraphs concern motor ability. These factors are indicative of abilities which underlie, or which form the basis for movement and are causal to both fundamental body movements such as running, jumping, and throwing, and specific skills as applied to sports. Motor ability may be defined as *the present acquired and innate ability to perform motor skills of a general or fundamental nature, exclusive of highly specialized sports or gymnastic techniques.* This definition has several pertinent implications. First, it implies that motor ability is a result of two things, innate capacity and diverse training and experience. Second, it also implies that a valid measure of it must avoid highly specialized skills as revealed in sports. For example, executing a kip-up on the parallel bar or making the overhead serve in tennis are highly specialized skills and thus would not be appropriate measures of motor ability. Third, it would further imply that motor ability is made up of factors which are relatively static and enduring in contrast to factors which are dynamic and changeable. Change in motor ability status would come about relatively slowly, and only to the extent that one's potential and his ability to practice enter the picture. Thus, motor ability is relatively static since its more dominant factors seem to become a part of muscle memory and persist for a fairly long span of time.

Improvement in the more dominant motor ability factors—at least those which lend themselves more easily to measurement—would come about more slowly than in the dominant factors of fitness, and only as the individual approached closer to his potential through training and practice. This progress would continue at a diminishing rate. Also, the principle of "overlearning" holds true with motor ability factors and achievement in them is not lost quickly through disuse once they are "overlearned." Naturally, factors like strength and endurance are reflected in motor ability, since it is a well-known principle that strength serves as a basis for the operation of many other factors in motor performance. It is fairly obvious that an individual must have a certain amount of strength and endurance to be agile, to run fast, and to jump far. Strength and endurance, however, are not the dominant factors in motor ability that they are in motor fitness. Progress in motor fitness is more easily observed since it is more dynamic and changeable; whereas progress in motor ability is observed to occur more slowly since it is by nature more static and enduring.

Motor ability is a mosaic comprised of many components. Test items are generally used in a battery to measure as many of these components as possible. Test administrative feasibility prevents measurement of each factor independently. In most cases, however, test items cut across factors and measure more than one. A valid test item of motor ability would presumably be a primary measure of at least one specific factor and perhaps a secondary measure of several others. The ability to measure more than one factor generally gives a test item a broader relationship with motor ability. This characteristic is desirable, but at the same time, somewhat lessens the use of the battery for diagnostic purposes. To compensate for this loss, however, some batteries are made up of items which measure different areas or muscle groups. These test results might clearly indicate weakness in various areas and this knowledge could be used for diagnostic purposes.

Motor ability tests have many uses, but in general they have been employed for classification of students into homogeneous groups, diagnosis of weaknesses, motivation, and guidance. The most common of these uses, however, is classification into ability groups (see Chapter 15, p. 517).

d. *Fitness.* The term "fitness" is perhaps one of the most controversial in the field of measurement in physical education. It is a most elusive quality and frequently has been defined in rather abstract terms. An acceptable definition of it has long eluded the experts. In the dictionary, fitness is defined as "having the necessary qualities; or a readiness or preparedness." These seem to imply that fitness is a preparation for something or that fitness has the necessary qualities for something. The question which first comes to mind is "preparation for what?" or "necessary qualities for what?" It is obvious that these "necessary qualities" and "preparations" will vary with the individual. No single set of standards for fitness is possible. The continually changing life processes cause a different need and emphasis for different individuals as they grow older. There is an optimum level of fitness for age groups. The 50-year-old needs a different type of fitness from the 18-year-old. Also, the needs and requirements of an ever-changing environment interacting with the on-going life processes of the individual dictate amounts and degree of fitness necessary. This implies that vocation and avocation will play their parts in determining adequate fitness, along with age. The longshoreman needs a different quality of fitness from the office worker, and the mountain climber needs a different degree of fitness from the bowler. Sex and body type are factors which alter the body needs. Women's needs are not necessarily the same as men's for the corresponding age, and the extreme endomorph has needs and requirements that differ from the mesamorph. Thus, part of the elusory character of the term "fitness" lies in the purpose for which it is needed, and these purposes vary. This is a moot question and makes it difficult to resolve fitness into a single concise definition. The American Association for Health, Physical Education and Recreation arrived at the following definition.

Fitness is that state which characterizes the degree to which the person is able to function. Fitness is an individual matter. It implies the ability of each person to live most effectively with his potential. Ability to function depends upon the physical, mental, emotional, social, and spiritual components of fitness, all of which are related to each other and are mutually interdependent.[1]

In this definition, the reference is to "total fitness" and refers to the individual's capacity to survive and live effectively in his environment. Much has been said concerning total fitness where the total person or whole person is involved—the spiritual, mental, emotional, social, and cultural, as well as the physical. When viewed in this light, physical fitness is a limited phase of total fitness. However, it is one which is basic to other forms of fitness. Physical fitness, as one aspect of total fitness, is a means to an end; the end is the good of the whole individual. Physical education has long accepted its obligation with regard to this principle of the human entity. This does not imply that physical fitness is not a significant aspect of total fitness and a highly desirable means. As a means directed toward the whole individual, it should become an important objective of the over-all physical education program. Physical fitness, while it is not so broad in its meaning as total fitness, would include adequate degrees of health, posture, physique, proper functioning of vital organs, nutrition, and good health habits, along with an adequate amount of endurance, strength, stamina, and flexibility.

A more limited phase of physical fitness is *"motor fitness"* and since it is limited in its scope, it becomes a less elusive quality and can be defined more easily than total fitness or physical fitness. *Motor fitness may be defined as a readiness or preparedness for performance with special regard for big muscle activity without undue fatigue. It concerns the capacity to move the body efficiently with force over a reasonable length of time.* Motor fitness, as a limited phase of physical fitness, would seem to be the aspect that most fitness tests actually measure. Motor fitness, while it does not assess the factors of physical fitness directly, does reflect them to a degree. Furthermore, it is highly related to total fitness in the same manner. This interpretation is in keeping with the principle that the individual is an integer and cannot be divided into divisible units for education and training.

Motor fitness is gauged by performance and this performance is based on a composite of many factors. The most commonly mentioned fitness factors are strength, endurance, power, speed, agility, balance, flexibility, and stamina. Some of these factors evidently are more dominant than others and thus have a higher relationship with motor fitness. It is interesting to note how closely these factors resemble the list experts have used to analyze motor ability. Furthermore, although experts have assigned to motor ability and motor fitness definitions which seem to distinguish one from the other, the same factors have been used to describe them and, in many cases, the same test items have been used to measure the same factors in each. In contrast to motor ability whose dominant factors are relatively static and enduring, motor fitness is made up of factors which seem more dynamic and changeable, such as strength and endurance. Improvement in some of the more dominant ones might be quite rapid as exhibited by the results achieved in an accelerated physical training program during World War II. Minimum standards of motor fitness may be achieved over a short period of time. By the same token, fitness is lost unless it becomes a product of day-to-day living.

It is possible, according to the interpretation of motor fitness and motor ability in this chapter, for an individual to have an adequate amount of fitness but be lacking in motor ability. It is equally possible for him to have the coordinated skills in muscle memory and the agility and power to perform them. However, he might lack the necessary endurance and strength to perform them over a period of time. This is evident in the basketball player who is out of condition after a few months of idleness but who still maintains general and specific skills. There are numerous tests designed to measure fitness. Most of these are similar in design and measure similar factors. The AAHPER Fitness Test has been the most widely used test.[2]

SPECIALIZED ABILITIES. One of the most fundamental aspects of physical education is the teaching and acquisition of specialized skill. Most of the "education through the physical" takes place by means of those skills which include sports or athletic activities as well as the dance and gymnastics. Development of these skills in sports and dance has long been recognized as one of the major objectives of physical education. These specialized skills may be defined as *those physical activities constituting each sport which are distinctive to that sport.* They are unique in this respect. Skills will vary according to the sport and measurement must be made on a specific basis. The particular skill techniques involved are not common to all people as are the fundamental skills but will vary according to the customs, mores, nationality, and geography of a people. They result from training and experience and are acquired through specialized practice.

A sport skill is a unit and, when compounded with other units into a group, along with certain rules, a sport or athletic game results. These units are based on the fundamental skills such as running, jumping, throwing, etc. Proficiency in these skills depends upon the basic factors which underlie them, such as agility, speed, power, coordination, etc. Thus, specific skills are the effect of both the fundamental skills and the basic factors which have been previously described. Combinations of these fundamental skills in various sequences along with the functioning of the basic factors result in skills that are specific for each sport or activity.

Naturally, a measurement program for sport skills is specifically related to the activity of which it is a part. Sport skills may be evaluated in two ways. First, subjective methods may be used. Where the skills involved are complex and present problems in accurate measurement, these techniques may be employed. In this event, rating scales are used and judgment of the rater is indicative of the level of the student's ability. Second, objective skill tests may be used. Most skill tests have been devised by analyzing a sport into component parts, identifying each fundamental separately, and devising a test to measure each. Sometimes the skill itself becomes the best measure and it is standardized as a test item in the over-all battery. Naturally, all test items used to measure skill should meet certain requirements with respect to validity either on a logical basis or a statistical basis, or both.

Sport skills are the heart of the physical education program and the key to future participation. Most of the objectives of physica education, remote and immediate, are dependent on the development of skill. Without skill there can be little, if any, satisfying participation in physical activities, and without participation, the lasting values—organic, neuromuscular, mental, and social—sought through a comprehensive physical education program are impossible to achieve. In the final analysis, skill provides the medium through which all the objectives of physical education can more nearly be

attained. There are skill tests for practically all sports. One of
the most classic examples is the Dyer Tennis Test[7] (see Chapter 9,
p. 331).

PERCEPTUAL-MOTOR LEARNING AND PERFORMANCE. Perceptual-
motor refers to the ability of the individual to receive, interpret
and react properly to a multitude of stimuli which are impinging
on him not only from outside himself but also from within. This
linking of perceptual abilities to movement and motor learning
has become a new dimension in learning theory and only recently
has physical education become involved with its processes. Psy-
chologists, optometrists, and special education people and others
have pioneered in this work.

Perception has been defined as "the total pattern arising from
many sensations and resulting in a meaning which is more than the
sum of its parts."[6] *Motor learning* is the integration of movement
into a pattern for a purpose as a result of training procedures or
environmental conditions.[10] Proponents in this area maintain that
perception and movement are but two sides of the same coin and
that they cannot be separated in the learning and performance
processes. The impinging stimuli are called *input* and made up of
sensations from the senses of sight, hearing, touch, taste, and smell
from outside and from the kinesthetic or proprioceptor senses from
within. The uniqueness of perceptual-motor performance is that
emphasis is now placed on sensations which influence performance
and the interpretation of these sensations along with the motor
activities which succeed and precede them called output. Thus, in
perceptual-motor learning there is input (stimuli from all the sense
organs), and output (overt response or movement) along with a
control system to integrate the input and a storage system for
memory. Modern theory holds to the view that input-output cannot be separated and are inexorably related as they occur in a
closed loop system controlled by feedback.

The current ideas surrounding perceptual-motor behavior are
primarily based on the new *information theory* which views the mind
and human behavior as a computer. This computer analogy for the
mind is sometimes called the cybernetic theory or the feedback
theory. A great deal of research in this area has been done with the
dysfunctioning youngster. The slow learner in the classroom and
particularly the poor reader have been the subjects for much of the
research. Also, more recently the mentally retarded have been
studied in relation to perceptual-motor learning programs. It has
been shown through research that these programs result in positive
effects for many of the dysfunctioning children. An important

question still unanswered concerns the value of such programs for the normally functioning child.

One of the major obstacles in studying perceptual-motor behavior has been the lack of instruments to evaluate status and progress. Not only are standards lacking in what is considered normal but the area is so complex that the many aspects of perceptual-motor behavior have not yet been identified. Most evaluation schemes are highly subjective, lacking in validation, and few have established reliabilities. There are some surveys and check lists that are presently in use.

STRUCTURAL FACTORS. *a. Posture.* The body, with its approximately 200 bones and 700 muscles, is subjected repeatedly to the forces of the universe. Man's environment is filled with stresses and strains as gravity is incessantly pulling the body downward. In addition to the forces of gravity itself, the human body also has to overcome strains growing out of its own movement, tensions, and inertia. Even the body at rest in a sitting or reclining position is vulnerable to these intrinsic and extrinsic forces. There also appears to be a relationship between the position of the body and certain psychological factors. The study of posture and its evaluation comes within the province of physical education since it concerns a knowledge of body mechanics and a maintenance of muscle tone. Also, while it has not been proven objectively, most authorities concede there is probably a relationship between posture and health.

Posture is concerned with the position of the whole body and its segments. It may run the gamut from good to bad with all shades in between. Good posture is the proper alignment of the important segments of the body so they are balanced over their base of support to produce an effective, functioning body. Two facts concerning posture should be clearly understood at this point. First, there is no one, single, ideal posture, but many postures. The human body is not a static organism. It is dynamic as action produces change. This action results in such postures as standing, sitting, reclining, walking, and exercising. Second, posture is an individual matter. No two students will be entirely alike in the relationship of their body parts. With respect to the first fact, most posture tests use standing posture as a basis for their evaluation. Yet in one's daily normal activities, standing posture is used relatively little by the average person. In regard to the second fact, there are individual differences in anatomical parts and body build and these relate to posture. Yet posture standards have not been devised in accordance with these differences.

In fact, there are no universal posture standards of a functional nature. Present posture tests are chiefly of standing posture. Most measures have been largely of the subjective type, although many objective techniques do exist. It might be pointed out, however, that even when objective devices are employed, they are based to a great extent on subjective judgment. This is true because objective devices must be based on certain standards which in turn are based on criteria. In the final analysis these criteria revert to subjective judgment as do all criteria, since they are based on expert opinion.

It is obvious that precise techniques for posture measurement are lacking for the average teacher. This lack of precision in measurement does not prevent posture evaluation, however. If evaluation is to occur, it must start with a norm or standard. Present posture standards are not universally agreed upon by experts, but most of the recognized posture standards reflect the consensus of experts relative to the make-up of good standing posture. This ideal has come to be recognized as an erect straight-line body position with all main segments of the body—head, neck, chest, abdomen, and knees—balanced over their bases of support. Certainly the ability to stand in the designated position does reflect how well the above ideal can be met.

While many objective methods are available to evaluate this position, perhaps the best approach for the average teacher is through the use of a simple inspection-type measurement. Much progress has been made the last few years in the use of such subjective devices. These observational techniques can be objectified with the use of suitable rating scales or check lists, and observers can be trained in their use. Valid results can be obtained when the rater observes carefully and knows what he is looking for, and, at the same time, has learned how to use the particular device properly. The rater also must be aware of the pitfalls of rating (see Chapter 17, p. 555). While objective devices might be more valuable in motivating the student, the subjective devices probably yield results which have far more value to the teacher. The objective devices can record posture only one time, whereas the subjective devices may be projected and the subject rated more than one time and in terms of several postures: for example, standing, sitting, walking, and exercising. In any event, the results of such observation should be interpreted in terms of the student's age, skeletal structure, sex, nutritional status, etc. (see Chapter 10, p. 347).

b. Nutrition. Another area which seems to come within the province of the physical educator is the evaluation of the nutritional status of his students. He has responsibilities here because of the important role that nutrition plays in physical fitness and health. Nutrition is related to the body's intake and consumption of food and it affects growth and development. It also is related, through its various processes, to posture, fatigue, body size and physique, mental health, organic development in general, and resistance to disease. There is an indirect relationship with one's ability in motor learning and performance, and there is even some evidence to show a relationship with personality development.

Nutrition may be defined as the sum of the processes by which the body takes in, assimilates, and utilizes food substances. It is directly related to growth, development, maintenance, and repair of the body and its parts. Nutrition, like health, may be good or bad. Good nutritional status implies that all the processes mentioned above are operating efficiently and that each part of the cycle is performing its function. Poor nutrition or malnutrition implies a breakdown or failure somewhere in the process. A nutritional deficiency interrupts normal growth and development cycles, especially in children and youth. This breakdown may be due to a shortage in the total food intake itself, or of some basic elements. Malnutrition may be present because the body is not able to assimilate and use the essential nutrients due to breakdown in the physiological processes.

The physical educator is in an excellent position to observe nutritional status of his students and has a special opportunity and a demanding obligation to detect cases of malnutrition. He works in close intimacy with his students and can watch for the revealing symptoms. He should have a knowledge of the characteristics of both good and poor nutrition and know how measurement techniques can be employed to screen those students in need of help. The primary purpose of such screening is to identify the malnourished. The next step after identification is referral of the cases of possible malnutrition to the health specialist. Measurement of nutritional status has been done for many years. The original methods of appraisal were anthropometric and consisted chiefly of age, height, and weight measurement. These techniques were not valid chiefly because they failed to recognize the principle of individual differences. They attempted to make all individuals of the same sex, age, and height conform to the same mold regardless of the size and proportion of the skeleton, muscles, and fat. More recent techniques recognize there are differences in body type and provide norms for them. At the present time there are two approaches to the appraisal of nutritional status. One approach involves subjective opinion and is made in terms of the signs and symptoms of good or poor nutrition. The inspection technique is used with a check list. This device can be used at any time during the gym period and inspection can take place in the locker room, shower-room, gymnasium or playground. The second approach is through objective measurement where special devices and forms are used (see Chapter 10, p. 347).

c. *Body Type.* The belief that body type is related to health and personality as well as physical performance dates back to ancient times. The physical educator in America since 1860 has always been interested in this subject. While body type is no doubt a result of hereditary factors, what is commonly recognized as physique is partly a product of environmental influences and comes as a by-product of exercise, diet, and good health habits. It is also true that occupation and climate have played a role in long term body type modification for races. Since body type is a result of combinations of genes and subject to chance for any given individual, there are infinite possibilities for individual differences. For the population in general this law of chance is operative and body types tend to fall along a curve of normal distribution. Thus, it would seem that body type, like other human traits, follows along a continuum rather than into readily quantified and well-defined categories. However, in the past body types have been categorized into dichotomies and trichotomies for the sake of convenience.

The physical educator should be concerned with body types for several reasons. First, since there is now objective evidence indicating a relationship between body type and success in physical education activities, the curriculum must be adapted to meet the different needs which are presented because of the great variation in body types. Also, it has been further shown that there is a low positive correlation between physical structure and both mental and social traits.[18] Probably the most important reason for the physical educator to understand this area is so he may help his student to understand and appreciate the nature of his own body type, to accept it as a part of his heritage, and to learn to live happily with it.

Since there are basic differences between the sexes in the way modern culture views the ideal male and female figures, it behooves the physical educator to know what these characteristics are. However, it is equally important for him to know that even within one sex there are wide differences from the norm. Such variation within one sex may be greater than the differences between the sexes. Each sex exhibits degrees of the secondary characteristics of the other. Such bisexuality in body type is referred to as Gynandromorphy. As a part of careful guidance by the physical educator the point can be made that body type or physique is not a test of either masculinity or femininity.

Appraisal for body type has been highly subjective and but little used in physical education. There are several techniques or methods of classification but the concept of Somatotype by Sheldon is the best known.[18] Somatotyping divides individuals into three types as follows: endomorph rated as 7-1-1, mesomorph rated as 1-7-1, and ectomorph rated as 1-1-7. Somatotype rating involves categorizing subjects according to the three numbers listed above.

Cognitive Domain. A physically educated person is more than one educated in movement. There are the intellectual abilities and skills. In traditional education the acquiring of these has become the most important and common objective in American education. Learnings in the cognitive area in physical education about sports, dance, other movement activities and the self may either be directly a part of the school curriculum or they may be projected as outcomes of the activities themselves as associated learnings. However, the cognitive domain generally speaking has become an important facet of the physical education curriculum and is evaluated along with the psychomotor domain. Just as the learner acquires specific skills in the psychomotor domain, he also learns particulars in the cognitive domain. In the taxonomy of educational objectives Bloom *et al.* have classified this cognitive domain into the following six levels: *knowledge, comprehension, application, analysis, synthesis,* and *evaluation.*[4] Knowledge and comprehension are the bases for cognition and higher cognitive processes. Beyond these parameters come the higher intellectual abilities and skills. There is a hierarchical arrangement from the simple to the more complex in these cognitive processes as shown in Figure 6–1.[4]

1. *Knowledge* is defined as an awareness of specific facts, universals and information and involves remembering and the ability to recall. The most common knowledges in the cognitive domain of sports, exercise, dance and related activities are: (1) terminology; (2) rules governing the activity; (3) techniques involved in performing the activity; (4) historical background; (5) strategy; (6) equipment and facilities; (7) game courtesies and etiquette; and (8) values inherent in the activity for the participant. Satisfying and effective participation in an activity cannot be experienced until the student has learned much of this information. However, learning in physical education does not stop here. There are certain other areas which seem essential if physical education is to achieve its objectives of continuing and intelligent participation. In addition to learning motor skills, the learner to be physically educated also must have knowledge and understanding regarding such facts as: (1) the importance of fitness; (2) how fitness may be achieved; (3) the need for systematic activity; (4) the values derived from systematic activity; (5) how to achieve neuromuscular relaxation; and (6) the techniques of using the fundamental skills.

2. *Comprehension* is the lower level of understanding and implies the abilities to interpret knowledge and to determine its implica-

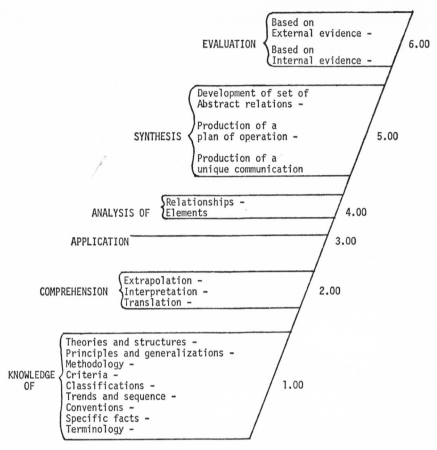

Fig. 6–1. The Taxonomy Continuum for the Cognitive Domain. Adapted by permission from the following source: Bloom, B. S., *et al.*: *Taxonomy of Educational Objectives: The Classification of Educational Goals. Handbook I: Cognitive Domain.* New York, David McKay Company, Inc., 1956.

tions, consequences, and effects. An example would be knowing the facts and principles concerning the effect of exercise on the heart and circulatory systems and understanding the necessity of exercise for survival.

3. *Application* is a higher level cognitive structure which enables the learner to use his knowledge and understanding in a particular concrete situation. It is possible for one to know and understand the facts but still not apply them. In this case there is no doubt of the close relationship between the affective and cognitive domains. This is why it has been said that every cognitive behavior has its affective counterpart. Cognitive skills are essential for affective adjustment. Knowing and understanding in physical education have much more significance if they enable the student to participate

more effectively in his motor skills and movement activities, and this involves one's value system.

4. *Analysis* involves a higher level cognitive process than application. It is based on knowledge and understanding but implies the ability to identify the elements or parts of the whole, to see their relationships, and to structure them into some systematic arrangement or organization.

5. *Synthesis* involves a similar level to that of analysis but is a reverse process. As a process it moves from the specific elements, or parts to form the whole. Once again knowing and understanding become the basis out of which facts and information are combined into wholes or some patterns that are different and larger than any part.

6. *Evaluation* is the highest level of the cognitive domain because it is used to form judgments with respect to the value of information made available through the other cognitive processes. Again it is obvious that the cognitive cannot be separated from the affective domain at this point since values and adaptive behavior are involved.

Some cognitive learning may be looked upon in physical education as psychomotor learning extended. For example, once the facts and ideas are known and understood by the learner, they may influence skill learnings and enhance further efficiency in performance of these skills. For example, in learning to play a sport the athlete is given directions by his coach on training procedures. This knowledge has value for the conditioning and fitness of the athlete, but it also reverts to the skills of the sport which are themselves improved as a result of the knowledges.

Since these knowledges and understandings of the cognitive domain comprise one of the major objectives of physical education, they must be planned for in the educational process. The physical education curriculum should include the cognitive domain involving these knowledges and understandings of man and his movements as they are concerned with sports, dance, gymnastics and exercise. It should also include the ideas which are necessary for a better understanding of relationships and significances in the conduct of the activities so the student will not only become a better participant but also will have a greater intellectual appreciation of the world of movement. The first textbook concerning this cognitive domain has now been made available by the AAHPER and should serve as a springboard for more work in this area.[3]

If the cognitive domain is to be included in the curriculum as an important objective, it must be evaluated in the same manner as all other objectives and for the same reasons. The most valid method for appraising achievement in these areas is through observation to determine whether knowledges and understandings have become functional. A student's application of knowledge and understanding through performance in an activity is the best test of his achievement. Another method is through oral response as the student answers questions asked by the teacher. As a "steady diet" for evaluation both of these methods are impractical, chiefly because of the time element involved and the lack of an adequate sampling of the material for all the students.

The generally accepted way of evaluating cognitive learnings is by the more formal approach of written tests. These tests take many forms but in the final analysis they may be classified in two ways. First, from the standpoint of test format, the test may be either the essay type or the objective type. The essay test enables the student to discuss the questions involved and is probably best to appraise understanding and higher levels of learning. The objective test makes use of short answers which can be graded objectively and makes use of simple recall and recognition type questions. It is weak in measuring higher level learning but can measure knowledges quite adequately. Second, from the standpoint of construction, tests may be classified as teacher-made or standardized. The standardized test is constructed by a test expert who presents the reliability and validity coefficients as supporting evidence and may present norms. The teacher-made tests, while they may follow similar lines in their construction as the standardized tests, do not provide validity and reliability coefficients. However, they are constructed by teachers according to some systematic procedure so the test will measure the knowledges and understandings taught in the activity.

The National Testing Service has developed standardized tests from the material in "Knowledge and Understanding in Physical Education."[3] By means of these tests it is now possible to test for achievement in the cognitive domain at the elementary, junior high school, and senior high school levels.

Affective Domain. A student is not physically educated by simply developing psychomotor and cognitive skills. There is still another aspect of learning inherent in the teaching of physical education activities. This is the *affective* domain which includes *attitudes, interest, values, appreciations,* and *adjustments*.

This domain may become the most important one of all in the years ahead. Education in the past has placed emphasis on cognitive and psychomotor areas and in most instances has left the affective area to chance. Emphasis on the affective domain is no longer evident in the objectives of most disciplines. Most courses now being taught are directed entirely in the cognitive and the psychomotor areas. Yet, the sociopsychological patterns are inevitably present and are being shaped for better or worse regardless of whether or not emphasis is given to them in the objectives. They can be learnings that come about in a casual manner without the intention to learn because they are inexorably a part of psychomotor and cognitive learnings.

That there has been an erosion of the affective objectives in the schools is apparent. In society there seems to be a similar erosion in man's system of values, particularly in the young. Could there be a relationship? Perhaps the reason for the erosion of the affective objective is not singular. With the fall of the doctrine of formal discipline, many disciplines dropped the affective domain from their goals because many presumed objectives were no longer applicable anyway. Also, there has been no clear-cut curricula content and methodology whereby these areas could be taught as a part of a course. Perhaps the most important reason is that the affective domain area is highly subjective and intangible; it could not be explicitly evaluated for purposes of determining status and achievement and of course grading. Our more scientific age seems to place greater emphasis on objectivity and quantification in measurement and hence these intangible objectives were dropped.

In this area of the affective domain the student learns particulars just as he does in the cognitive and psychomotor domains. These learnings, while they may be less precise and definite than skills and knowledges, do have specificity. The specific factors concerned here are *interest, appreciation, attitudes, values,* and *adjustments.* These are the basic elements in the psychosocial picture. They are the ways in which the individual makes his adjustments to himself and to the society in which he lives. In the Taxonomy for educational objectives it is suggested that these elements have too broad a meaning to lend themselves to a continuum of hierarchical arrangement from simple to complex.[8] Unlike the cognitive domain where the categories seem to have this hierarchical arrangement, *interest, appreciation, attitude, value,* and *adjustments* do not lend themselves to ordering from low to high on a continuum. Therefore, another dimension has been proposed and employed in connection with these basic elements. See Figure 6–2.[8]

The affective domain continuum is a structure which provides an order of difficulty. Behavioral components are structured in a simple upward hierarchy to more complex patterns. As shown on the continuum the parts are *receiving, responding, valuing, organization,* and *characterization by a value complex.* These can be ordered from the simple to the more complex and can be structured as shown on Figure 6–2 into a single continuum.[8] There is provision made on the continuum for the appearance of the basic elements of *interest, appreciation, attitude, value* and *adjustment* and these elements are distributed along the scale. Thus, the affective domain continuum

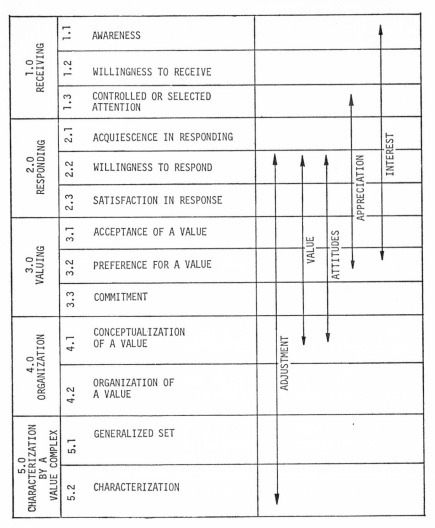

1.0 RECEIVING	1.1	AWARENESS					
	1.2	WILLINGNESS TO RECEIVE					
	1.3	CONTROLLED OR SELECTED ATTENTION					
2.0 RESPONDING	2.1	ACQUIESCENCE IN RESPONDING					INTEREST
	2.2	WILLINGNESS TO RESPOND				APPRECIATION	
	2.3	SATISFACTION IN RESPONSE					
3.0 VALUING	3.1	ACCEPTANCE OF A VALUE		VALUE	ATTITUDES		
	3.2	PREFERENCE FOR A VALUE					
	3.3	COMMITMENT					
4.0 ORGANIZATION	4.1	CONCEPTUALIZATION OF A VALUE	ADJUSTMENT				
	4.2	ORGANIZATION OF A VALUE					
5.0 CHARACTERIZATION BY A VALUE COMPLEX	5.1	GENERALIZED SET					
	5.2	CHARACTERIZATION					

Fig. 6–2. The Taxonomy Continuum for the Affective Domain. Adapted by permission from the following source: Krathwohl, D. R. *et al.*: *Taxonomy of Educational Objectives: The Classification of Educational Goals. Handbook II: Affective Domain.* New York, David McKay Company, Inc., 1964.

provides for a means of ordering and relating the different elements or factors of psychosocial behavior. The simple kind of behavior would be achieved before the categories above it could be learned. It is obvious from the continuum that some of the elements run concurrently while some of them—interest and adjustment—occupy some space on the scale alone. As the individual ascends the social and emotional continuum through the levels of *receiving, responding, valuing, organizing, and characterization by value complex,* he uses the elements of *interest, attitude, appreciations, values* and *adaptations* to achieve psychosocial maturity. This process may be similar to what the sociologist calls *socialization* or the cultural anthropologist calls *enculturation.* Krathwohl *et al.* identify the process as *internalization.*[8]

Internalization starts with receiving and responding but unless the individual becomes fixated at these levels, he establishes values and moves to a hierarchy or cluster of values through conceptualization into a value system. He ultimately behaves consistently with this value system which becomes his philosophy of life, or perhaps on an even higher level, he behaves as an autonomous, self-actualizing person. Thus, it can be seen that the individual can move on the scale from a state of compliance directed by external sanctions through a stage of identification with acceptable behavior until he achieves the highest level of *internalization* where his actions are guided by his own internal sanctions. This stage represents a position on the continuum in the upper quartile and perhaps few people ever achieve it completely. It corresponds pretty much to the higher level of character development identified by Peck and Havinghurst as the *rational-altruistic* stage, or Piaget's stage where the individual moves from restraint through rules to the upper level where the individual becomes an autonomous self-actualizing citizen.[14,15]

In this psychosocial or affective continuum several things become evident. First, it seems that each aspect of affective behavior has a cognitive counterpart. This is where the unity concept enters the picture again, and the two domains are inextricably related just as they are both related to the psychomotor. It is interesting how each of these domains may serve as a means of reaching the others. A learner does not act without thinking and feeling, or think without acting and feeling, or feel without acting or thinking.

A person at any given period of his life is a product of all the psychosocial forces on the affective continuum combined with all the other forces of his culture and heredity. In keeping with the unity concept, none of these forces operates in closed circuit channels. They are highly interrelated and interdependent. In the area of the affective domain the student is continually making adjustments and there is always action, reaction, and interaction between these social and emotional forces as well as all other facets of the whole person. Through psychomotor skills the students learn certain affective learnings such as interest, attitudes, appreciation or values. If these affective learnings are of the right type, they will have reverberations and will affect skills, and help improve them. The improved skills will then again serve to enhance the affective domain. Thus, out of the processes of interaction between the psychomotor and the affective along with the cognitive, will come

6

those learnings at the most positive end of the *internalization* continuum.

Hence, from the original learning of a psychomotor skill, there will come as by-products both cognitive and affective learnings, increased psychomotor learnings and perhaps even some other influences in the areas of fitness, posture, and nutrition. For example, the obese girl takes part in a modern dance class for a requirement and learns some basic dance skills. Her interest is aroused and her attitude is improved as a result of her participation. With improvement in her attitude comes appreciation along with further improvement in her dance skills. Along with the more improved dance skills come increased emphasis on the values she established concerning not only her movement image but also the image she has of her own body. With the better body image might come an increased interest in posture and nutrition along with a determination to do something about it. The improvement in the body image enhances the self-image and both have been shown to be forces in personality development. Thus, the extent of learning in any domain frequently depends on the influence of the other domain processes and one might say in physical education that the learner may enter the palace of cognitive and affective domains over the draw-bridge of the psychomotor.

Perhaps this is the point at which to discuss the influence of such terms as *body-image, movement-image,* and *self-image.* Since these modalities are related to each other and have all been shown to have a relationship with the development of the personality, they come within the province of the educator in the affective domain. If there is a hierarchical arrangement of these concepts, it would be in the order they are discussed below.

Body-image is the way the body and its parts are perceived in space—a sort of self-picture of oneself.[17]

Movement-image is the way the moving body is perceived in sport skills, dance and fundamental skills.[17]

Self-image is the way the total abilities of social, mental and emotional are perceived.[17]

The process of *internalization* culminates in the formation of a self-image for each person as he appraises himself in relation to how he thinks he is perceived by others. There is another facet which parallels this process or accompanies it. Along with the *self-image* there is formed what is known as the *ideal-self* which is a composite of the expectations of society, the aspirations of the self, and the perfectability of models in the form of other people. If there is too much distance between these two, there is generally psychological repercussions which have overtones for all the domains.

The process of developing the *self-image* then is related to *self-*

identification and the identification of the self through the process of *internalization* structures human personality. A part of the total process and basic to it is the development of an acceptable *body-image* with its accompanying *movement-image*. The process of personality development is a complex of many interacting forces. The process of socialization creates the *self-image*. It has been shown that this self concept starts with the *body-image* at an early age. Since the world of the young is a movement world, body movement cannot be divorced entirely from the *body-image*. Thus, *movement-image* is related to *body-image* and they both lead to the development of the *self-image* and this identification of the self through the processes of *internalization* creates the human personality. Body types and perceptual-motor skills discussed under the psychomotor domain have a direct relationship with this area of learning in the affective domain because they are both value-infused processes and as such relate to the *internalization* continuum.

This affective domain is an important facet of the physical education matrix as shown by its objectives. It is clear the teacher-coach has an obligation to teach these concepts and principles both by precept and example. If such psychosocial traits are to be taught as a part of the school curriculum and if they are listed in the hierarchy of objectives, they must be evaluated. It would be inexact and misleading to imply that these facets can be measured with the same scientific techniques which are somewhat freely used in the domains of the cognitive and psychomotor. Measurement becomes exceedingly difficult in this area because of the complexity of the factors and the lack of reliable measurement techniques. There has been no systematic attempt to measure status and achievement in this domain as there has been in the cognitive domain. Since the domain does occupy a place of significance in a child's learning, qualitative techniques are now being devised and beginning to be used more widely. The professional student should be aware of some of the pitfalls in connection with the use and interpretation of these evaluation techniques. If the student answers the responses himself, it does not take an especially bright person to detect the answers which will bring him the rewards of acceptance and positive sanctions of his reference groups. However, he may really behave in a different way in practice. On the other hand, if the teacher makes the response about the student, he must bear in mind that modern culture brings certain rewards to those who keep their feelings to themselves and to observe and evaluate the deep underlying emotion is difficult to do through behavior. This becomes more of a problem as the one who is being observed achieves higher levels on the *internalization* scale. Krathwohl *et al.* seem to think that it is possible in a school situation to evaluate the changes which take place at the lower end of the continuum but much more difficult to assess those at the top.[8] If these can be changed at all in the schools, such changes would come about over a long period of time and no one teacher would have access to students long enough to measure such change.

This social objective is one of the four major objectives in physical education. It is clear that the teacher and coach has an obligation to teach these concepts by both precept and example. If traits are to be taught as a part of the school curriculum, measurement becomes necessary. It would be inexact and misleading to imply that these traits can be measured by the same scientific techniques which are used freely in the area of technical and associated learnings. Measurement becomes exceedingly difficult in this area because of the complexity of its factors and because objective measurement techniques are not available to any great degree. Since the area does occupy a place of great importance in learning, qualitative evaluation techniques have been developed and widely used for evaluation purposes. Perhaps the best technique is the rating scale, but check lists, questionnaires, autobiographies, self appraisal, and anecdotal records have been employed.

Overview of Measurement Techniques

In the preceding sections of this chapter the major factors or traits of the product of physical education have been enumerated and defined. This seemed necessary in order for the student to have a better understanding of these many variables to be measured and to have an insight into how they are related to the whole individual. The relationship and interrelationships of these variables have been explained and it has been clearly pointed out that each of these factors does not exist as an entity to itself. The remainder of this chapter will be devoted to a brief overview of the various type tools, procedures, and techniques which are commonly used in measuring the listed qualities and factors. Specific tests will not be identified, but the general areas will be discussed. Over the years a great many techniques and procedures have been developed for measuring the various aspects of the *product*. Many of these were developed for purposes of research and are not practical for use in the physical education class. Since emphasis in this textbook concerns tools and techniques which are usable in practical situations, only those types will be presented which are readily adaptable to class use. No claim is made that these are all the types of techniques in use for the collection of data. If the student is to understand the succeeding chapters in this text, however, he should know the nature of the most commonly used techniques and instruments which are available to measure the various types of learnings. Some of these techniques are used more in one area than others.

Anecdotal Record. The anecdotal record is a means of evaluating the actual behavior of students and perhaps its techniques apply best in the area of concomitant learnings, although its use is certainly not limited strictly to this area. *It may be defined as a written objective record of an incident in the life of a student as observed by a teacher or leader.* The information becomes much more meaningful when a number of observations are made, since it is always dangerous to draw conclusion from too few samples. When a number of successive observations are made, patterns of conduct begin to stand out and behavior trends become quite evident. The teacher then has greater insight into the problems and social adjustments of the student who is under observation. This anecdote should never be a time-consuming task for the teacher since the usual form of the report is a short, concise description of significant incidents in the student's behavior. When observations are made carefully and when records are kept accurately, the teacher is then in a position to summarize the findings and interpret results. After interpretation, there should come a follow-up. In addition to giving valuable insight into patterns of behavior exhibited by certain students, this device can also be used as a means of validating certain inventory results. Students do not always behave in actual situations as they say they would have behaved or do behave in their answers on the inventory. This technique in physical education would probably not be applied to an entire class, but would be used only in special cases to better understand certain students with special problems.

Autobiography. Various means are used by the teacher to understand his students. If the physical educator is to make fullest use of his opportunities for guidance, he should understand more about each individual, his needs, his problems, and his ambitions. A device which is designed to obtain some of this information is the autobiography. It is similar to the anecdote except it is written by the student instead of the teacher. *An autobiography is a self-written story about some phase of the writer's own life and experience.* It may be directed toward any particular phase of the student's experience from which the teacher may wish to draw information. Its emphasis is generally limited to a certain topic over a specific period. If the student's story is well done, it will give the teacher a good picture of his attitudes, feelings, and actions concerning the indicated phase or area. For instance, the teacher may want to learn something about Jerry's past experience in fitness activities and his attitude toward fitness. Jerry's autobiography will reveal much insight into what he has done to become fit and the importance he attaches to fitness.

Check List. A tool frequently used to gather information about the product of physical education which cannot be obtained from any of the usual objective sources is the check list. It is sometimes combined with one or more other techniques such as the interview, observation, and inventory. In its simplest form, it is a list of things to look for as observations are being made. The general procedure in the construction of a check list is to select a list of items for which appraisal is to be made in terms of certain traits or criteria. Generally, there are columns in which the observer or the student places his check mark. Yes or no, absence or presence, and for or against, etc., are the usual categories for checking. Sometimes the check list takes the form of an incidence chart where the number of times an incident occurs is checked or where the reverse is true and the absence of a particular behavior or action is noted. Check lists are useful in assessing behavior in the area of affective learnings and they may be applied in the area of psychomotor learnings. The latter is especially true where an activity as a whole is being measured. For instance, in evaluating tennis ability a list of tennis skills and activities can be established which combine to represent the skilled tennis player. These items can be placed in check list form and the observer can check their presence or absence.

Interview. The interview is a tool quite similar in nature to the questionnaire and might be rightfully termed an oral questionnaire. The purposes for the two are the same, and much of the same information found by one can be duplicated by the other. However, the nature of the interview is such that it is better adapted to obtaining the more personal data of a confidential nature although its use is definitely not restricted to this purpose. Frequently, the two techniques are used to complement each other, and they have both been used to supplement the information supplied by observation techniques. The success of this procedure depends on several factors. First, the interview has to be directed toward a specific purpose and this purpose should be made known to the student prior to the time of the interview. Second, the physical climate for the interview should be adequate, with some thought being given to sufficient time allotment and a private setting in a friendly atmosphere. Such a climate can help create the rapport which has to be established between the teacher and student if the student is to talk freely about his feelings, aspirations, and problems. Third, the interview should be structured to some extent in order for the discussion to be kept in line with the purpose of the interview and to help objectify the results as much as possible. The structuring could be done in the form of a check list. The information obtained through the interview technique is only as valuable as the skill which is displayed by the interviewer.

Inventory. Another tool which can be used by the physical educator in assessing the product is the inventory. It is used essentially for the same purposes as the anecdote and the autobiography but can be focused a bit more definitely and can be controlled to a greater extent with regard to the information which it can reveal. The inventory, as its name implies, usually consists of a list of qualities, traits, or characteristics. It is frequently used in measuring health attitudes and also evaluating concomitant learnings. In design it may be general in nature or specific. For instance, its design may be such that the student has to analyze his behavior, attitudes, or feelings in terms of general qualities; or he may be called upon to respond in a specific way to actual situations which arise in class. In any event, the information found is about what the student does, or feels, or likes, or is interested in. Inventories might be classed as practice, attitude, or interest inventories and all reveal the student's social adjustment to a degree. Most inventories do not have the validity for such purposes of testing as grading and diagnosis, but their results may frequently be used to reveal certain strengths and weaknesses and conceivably could be used as screening devices for the maladjusted.

Observations. One of the most extensive means of evaluating the product is through observation. Not only is it extensive from the standpoint of the kinds of information which it can reveal, but also from the point of view of the ways observations can be taken. *Observation in physical education may be defined as the act of watching the behavior, actions, or status of students for a specific purpose by a trained observer.* This implies that the teacher must have training and practice not only in the act of observing, but also in recording the findings and interpreting them with accuracy. One of the big problems in the use of this technique is to objectify the procedures as much as possible, because without an acceptable degree of objectivity, the results do not have great value. It is probably due to this apparent subjectivity of observations that many persons question its validity. However, suitable objectivity may be obtained if the observer knows his subject, concentrates on the specific problems outlined in his purpose, and applies the suggestions of how to make ratings more valid (see Chapter 17, p. 555). The teacher, just as the learner of technical skills, must have a mental picture of the traits, qualities, or acts he is specifically observing. It is valuable to have a list of things to look for as observations are made. The use of check lists, rating scales, and charts helps to objectify observation results. The scout in basketball games frequently makes use of charts to guide him in his observations and to record them.

Mechanical means are often used to observe and record certain activities. In fact, this is now a common procedure in scouting athletic games. Formerly, football scouts observed opponents and recorded their observations. They still do this, but the most effective technique in present day scouting is the study of the actual game films which record action far more accurately than the scout and do it more inclusively. Also, the films serve as a permanent record for reviewing questionable situations.

Observations are generally made in a normal setting where the observer makes no attempt to control the situation or the students being observed. However, under certain circumstances, he may wish to control one or both of these variables.

Physical Performance Tests. Skills and fitness are the very heart and core of the physical education program. This is true because it is through physical activities that all the other learnings and accomplishments attributed to physical education become possible. This is the unique approach that physical education has to character development, social growth, and mental learnings. This area of the physical is best measured through what is empirically called physical performance tests. *The physical performance test may be defined as those objective tests used to measure technical learnings which include motor ability, motor fitness, sport skill, posture, and nutrition.* Naturally, these qualities are made up of many variables. Measurement of each presents a somewhat different problem. In general, all of them are developed along similar lines. In fact, they follow very closely the methods of construction for written tests. All test makers have made use of scientific and statistical techniques to improve the validity of their tests. There are several important considerations in planning these tests. They are listed in their logical order below. However, the order may vary just a bit in some cases. The logical steps are: (1) choosing the criterion, (2) selecting the test items, (3) establishing the reliability and objectivity of individual test items, (4) establishing the validity of the test, (5) developing the norms, and (6) writing the test report. There is no cut-and-dried way of arriving at any of these steps. Rather, there are a number of ways which are considered acceptable procedures for each. The type of test planned and the nature of the variables will dictate the choice of procedures to a great extent.

Questionnaire. One of the most frequently used methods of obtaining information directly from the individual about his present status and practices is the questionnaire. However, this tool should be employed only as a last resort when the information desired can be obtained in no other way. This technique is especially adapted to large groups when factual information is sought. It is a quickly applied technique and when the items are well constructed, it can reveal valuable data. This method of obtaining data has probably been overworked, especially in the area of research, and its use has frequently been employed when other techniques would have served the intended purpose better. This has brought some justifiable criticism and has cast some reflection on its use. However, in measurement areas other than for research it has proven a valuable tool for obtaining information about the student. When it is intelligently constructed and properly employed, and its results accurately interpreted, it can lead to valuable conclusions. The conclusions revealed should lead to follow-up procedures in relation to the original purposes of the test.

The questionnaire is especially useful in gaining information about the attitude and interest of students, an area where objective measurement is not feasible anyway. The success of the questionnaire depends on how well each question is constructed. There are approved criteria which can be applied to questions both regarding their form and their function.

Rating Scale. One of the most valuable techniques in measuring the product is the rating scale. Like the check list, the rating scale brings order to the processes of observation and self-appraisal but goes a step farther by providing for degrees of the quality, trait, or factor being examined. It frequently serves as a recording device for observation, but on many occasions it is used for discrimination and interpretation. This is especially true in research when criteria are being developed for performance tests through the jury technique. A survey of the physical education objectives will show that many desirable outcomes are of an intangible nature and do not lend themselves to objective techniques of measurement. Also, a survey of the tools and techniques used to measure certain factors will show that many of them are too time-consuming and impractical to use in a measurement program. The rating scale is the best means of measuring these subjective areas and factors where no adequate objective techniques are available or where existing techniques are administratively not feasible. It is possible also to use the rating scale to supplement objective measurement. In some cases, such scales may be used as the primary means of measurement while the objective measurement may be used to supplement it.

In function, the rating scale is a subjective estimate but if it is properly constructed and used, it will help to narrow the gap between the subjective and the objective in physical education. Rating scales are excellent means of objectifying the many hard-to-measure variables in physical education. They make observation far more accurate and serve as a means of focusing the attention of the teacher and the student on the important outcomes of the program. There are numerous types of rating scales (see Chapter 17, p. 555).

The type to be employed will be dictated by the nature of the information desired and the characteristics of the individuals being rated. On occasion, it may be desirable to combine two or more types of scales to obtain the needed data. There are certain basic principles for the construction of rating scales and guides on how they are to be used (see Chapter 17, p. 555). When these principles and guides are followed and when the teacher knows the area that is being rated, the rating scale will enable the rater to ascertain more accurately and precisely the degree to which the trait, factor, or quality under examination is present. Such ratings are in common use in the measurement of attitudes and appreciations, sportsmanship, form in sports and dance, and when the activity is being measured as a whole. The pattern is generally the same. A criterion is established, type of rating scale is selected, factors to be rated are identified, categories are defined, and observation and rating take place.

Sociometry. A technique which has come to occupy an important place in the area of concomitant learnings is sociometrics. All physical education activity has been described as a social experience and through its activities of sports and dance, socialization and personality development may occur in students. In any group of students, there are social forces at work which tend to produce certain relationships and interrelationships between students within the group. The role the child plays in his group and his relationships with other members of that group are significant factors in how nearly he realizes his potential. It is human nature to work for significance and to desire prestige in one's group. Sociometrics is a technique or method of measuring the amount of organization of a social group in order to show the patterns of relationships and interrelationships. It is a practical means of objectifying to some degree these relationships and interrelationships within the group.

The sociometric test starts with asking the group members to indicate their feelings about each other. It simply and graphically shows who would like to be with whom for a particular activity. It is carried one step further and permits the students not only to choose those with whom they want to be but also to reject others they do not want. In the final analysis, it indicates which individuals are accepted and which are not. On the basis of these findings a follow-up should be made. The analysis indicates several things. Leaders are located; the rejected, isolated, and unwanted are identified; and a basis for classification into cooperative and productive units is found. It further can identify gangs and cliques which tend to promote social disintegration in the group rather than integration. When all of these facts are revealed, the teacher can select techniques and experiences to help each student adjust more readily in his social relationships. One of the most important of these is to arrange the students into harmonious groups, since they tend to reach their potential much more readily when they work with those they like. Also, the rejected and isolated students can be given special help in making acceptable social adjustments.

The sociogram is a tool used to show graphically these relationships and interrelationships within the group mentioned above. It diagrams the group organization and shows graphic patterns of who accepts whom, who is rejected by whom, and the other forces which tend to prevent social integration in the group.

Written Tests. If the individual is to be evaluated as a whole, measurement techniques should be applied to all three domains of learning—psychomotor, cognitive, and affective. In the area of cognitive learnings, oral tests and observation of the student in actual performance have been used, but in general both methods are too time-consuming for practical use. Written tests are the best means of measuring knowledges and understandings in evaluating the mental objective in physical education. It might be well for the student to keep in mind that these cognitive learnings are interrelated with psychomotor and affective. Even the test results in these areas tend to have some relationship.

Written tests may be classified two ways. From the standpoint of format they may be grouped into essay and objective. From the standpoint of construction they may be grouped into standardized or teacher-made.

References

1. AAHPER: Fitness for Youth, Statement Prepared and Approved by the 100 Delegates to the AAHPER Fitness Conference, Washington, D.C., September, 1956.
2. ———: Youth Fitness Test Manual. Washington, D.C. AAHPER, 1961 (Revised).
3. ———: Knowledge and Understanding in Physical Education, Washington, D.C., AAHPER, 1969.
4. Bloom, B. S. et al.: Taxonomy of Educational Objectives: The Classification of Educational Goals. Handbook I: Cognitive Domain. New York, David McKay Company, Inc., 1956.
5. Clarke, H. H.: Application of Measurement to Health and Physical Education. Englewood Cliffs, N.J., Prentice-Hall, Inc., 1959.
6. Cratty, B. J.: Movement Behavior and Motor Learning, Philadelphia, Lea & Febiger, 1964, p. 24.
7. Dyer, J. T.: The Backboard Test of Tennis Ability, Research Quarterly (Supplement), 6, 63–65, March, 1935.
8. Krathwohl, D. R., B. S. Bloom, and B. B. Masia: Taxonomy of Educational Objectives: The Classification of Educational Goals. Handbook II: Affective Domain. New York, David McKay Company, Inc., 1964.
9. Larson, L. A., and R. D. Yocom: Measurement and Evaluation in Physical, Health and Recreation Education. St. Louis, The C. V. Mosby Co., 1951.
10. Lawther, J. D.: Directing Motor Skill Learning. Quest, VI, 68–76, May, 1966.
11. McCall, W. A.: Measurement. New York, The Macmillan Co., 1939.
12. McCloy, C. H., and N. D. Young: Tests and Measurements in Health and Physical Education. 3rd. Ed., New York, Appleton-Century-Crofts, Inc., 1954, p. 114.

13. Oberteuffer, Delbert: *Physical Education*. New York, Harper & Brothers, 1956.
14. Peck, R. F., and R. J. Havinghurst *et al.*: *The Psychology of Character Development*. New York, John Wiley and Sons, 1960.
15. Piaget, J.: *The Moral Judgment of the Child*. Glencoe, Ill., The Free Press, 1948.
16. Rich, J. M.: *Education and Human Values*. Reading, Mass., Addison-Wesley Publishing Co., 1968.
17. Sakers, A. E.: The Relationship Between a Selected Measure of Motor Ability and the Actual-Ideal Self-Concept, Body-Image, and Movement-Concept of the Adolescent Girl. Unpublished Master's Thesis, University of Maryland, 1969.
18. Sheldon, W. H.: *Atlas of Men*. New York, Harper and Bros., 1954, p. 19.
19. Staley, S. C.: *Curriculum in Sports*. Phildelphia, W. B. Saunders Co., 1935.
20. ———: *Sports Education*. New York, A. S. Barnes & Co., 1939.
21. Williams, J. F.: *The Principles of Physical Education*. 7th Ed., Philadelphia, W. B. Saunders Co., 1959.

Chapter 7
TESTS OF MOTOR ABILITY AND ACHIEVEMENT

Barrow Motor Ability Test*

Purpose: To measure general or fundamental skills for the purpose of classification and guidance.

Evaluation: Multiple R of .92 with a standard error of 3.968.

Level and Sex: College men and junior and senior high school boys.

Time Allotment and Number of Subjects: A class of 30 to 35 subjects can be tested in a 45-minute period.

Floor Plan and Space Requirement: If only one station of each test is employed, a single gymnasium provides ample space. Figure 7–1 shows the floor plan.

Class Organization: This battery is best administered by the station-to-station method. Since the three items are not strenuous the order of events is unimportant. The students should be given individual score cards and asked to rotate from one station to another alone or with a squad. To facilitate administration, more than one station may be set up if enough

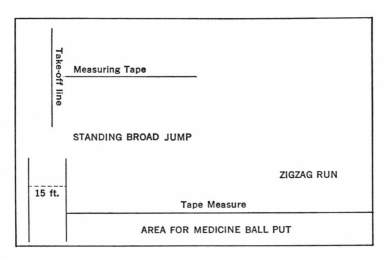

Fig. 7–1. Floor plan for Barrow motor ability test.

* Adapted from the following source: Barrow, H. M., *Motor Ability Testing for College Men.* Minneapolis, Burgess Publishing Co., 1957.

leadership is trained to administer them. The zigzag run moves somewhat slower than the other events. Scoring can be done either by a trained squad leader or a trained assistant who administers a particular station.

General Procedure: 1. All three items should be explained and demonstrated before testing begins.

2. The purpose of the test should be made known to the students.

3. The scores on the zigzag run are more reliable if tennis shoes are worn.

4. Student leaders can be trained in advance to administer these items.

Uses: The results of this motor ability test may be used as a basis for classifying students into ability groups. If the student's rating is "Excellent," he should be placed in an advanced group and a program designed to challenge the gifted. If the student's rating is "Inferior," he should be assigned to a remedial or fundamental class and a program designed to care for his individual needs. If the student scores in the remaining three categories, he should be assigned to the regular required program.

Where it is necessary for intra-class grouping, class members may be grouped on the basis of these motor ability scores into both homogeneous groups for teaching and heterogeneous groups for playing (see Chapter 15, p. 517).

Test Description

ITEM NUMBER I—STANDING BROAD JUMP Figure (7–2A)

Purpose: To measure power primarily, and agility, speed, and strength secondarily.

Facilities and Equipment: One 5 by 12-foot tumbling mat marked with a take-off line and parallel lines two inches apart indicating distance from the take-off line. If the mat is not available, the floor can be used with a take-off mark and a tape measure.

Directions: The subject assumes the starting position behind the take-off mark with his feet parallel. He takes a preliminary movement by bending his knees and swinging his arms and jumps outward as far as possible. Three trials are permitted in succession.

Instructions: You should crouch before you jump and swing your arms downward. As you jump outward, the arms should be swung forward and upward. Take off from the mark with both feet simultaneously and try not to fall backwards after landing.

Scoring: The final score is the distance of the best jump measured to the nearest inch.

Testing Personnel: One trained assistant to supervise the testing station and measure and record the score.

ITEM NUMBER II—ZIGZAG RUN (Figure 7–2B)

Purpose: To measure agility primarily and speed secondarily.

Facilities and Equipment: Stop watch, five standards which are commonly used for high jumping, volleyball, or badminton. (If these are not available, chairs may be used.) Space for the zigzag course (Fig. 7–2B) placed on the gymnasium floor with the standards placed at the indicated spots.

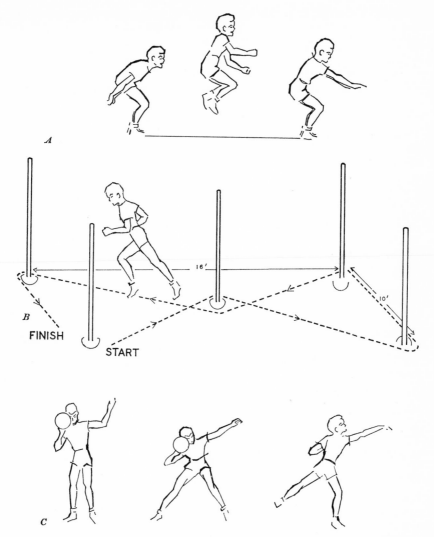

Fig. 7–2. Test items for the Barrow motor ability test. *A*, Standing broad jump *B*, Zigzag run. *C*, Medicine ball put.

Directions: The event should be explained and demonstrated. The subject begins at the start and follows the prescribed course for three complete laps. The watch is stopped when the subject finishes his run at the end of the third lap.

Instructions: For the start of your run you may use a standing start. On the command to go, you run the prescribed course in a figure-of-eight fashion. Do not grasp the standards as you round them and do not misplace them in any way. You complete three circuits of the course and continue to run past the finish mark. If you foul or fail to run the prescribed course, you will be asked to run again.

Score: The final score is the elapsed time to the nearest tenth of a second which is required to run the prescribed course three times.

Testing Personnel: One trained assistant to supervise the testing station and to time and record the scores.

ITEM NUMBER III—SIX POUND MEDICINE BALL PUT (Figure 7–2*C*).

Purpose: To measure arm and shoulder girdle strength primarily, and power, agility, arm and shoulder girdle coordination, speed, and balance secondarily.

Facilities and Equipment: A space in a gymnasium approximately 90 by 25 feet. A restraining line is clearly marked with a second line fifteen feet to the rear. The throw must be made from between these lines. The event may be measured with a tape measure but it will facilitate administration if concentric circles are placed.

Directions: The event must be explained and demonstrated since the try must be a put and not a throw. The subject stands between the two restraining lines and puts the ball straight down the course. He takes three trials in succession. Fouls count as a trial but in the event that all three trials are fouls, the subject must put until he makes a fair put.

Instructions: You must take up a position in the throwing area with the side opposite the throwing arm toward the line of throw. You must put the ball and not throw it. You must not step on or over the restraining line during the throw.

Scoring: The final score is the distance of the best put measured to the nearest foot.

Testing Personnel: One trained assistant to supervise the testing station and to measure the throws and record the scores. Student assistants are needed to mark the spot of the throws and to return the balls to the throwing area.

Johnson Fundamental Skills Test*

Purpose. To measure achievement in the fundamental skills.

Evaluation. All test items for all age levels and both sexes were found to have a statistically significant validity coefficient when actual test scores were correlated with expert ratings.

Level and Sex. Boys and girls grades 1 through 6.

Time Allotment and Number of Subjects. A class of 20 to 25 pupils can be tested in a 45-minute class period.

Floor Plan and Space Requirement. A single gymnasium or a large play room provides enough space. Figure 7–3 shows the floor plan.

* Adapted by permission of the author from the following source: Johnson, R. D., *Measurement of Achievement in Fundamental Skills of Elementary School Children.* Unpublished Thesis, State University of Iowa, Iowa City, Iowa, 1960.

Score Card

BARROW MOTOR ABILITY TEST
SCORE CARD

Name _____
          Last   First   Middle

Grade	Classification Excellent____
Age	Good ____ Average ____
Height	Poor ____ Inferior ____
Weight	

Test Events	Raw Score	T-Score
1. Zigzag Run		
2. Medicine Ball Put		
3. Standing Broad Jump		

Total T-Score_____

Norms

Table 7–1.   T-Scores for College Men

T-Score	Standing Broad Jump (Inches)	Zigzag Run (Seconds)	Medicine Ball Put (Feet)	T-Score
80	113 Up	20.8 Up	58 Up	80
75	109–112	21.6–20.9	55–57	75
70	105–108	22.4–21.7	52–54	70
65	101–104	23.2–22.5	48–51	65
60	97–100	23.9–23.3	45–47	60
55	93–96	24.7–24.0	42–44	55
50	89–92	25.5–24.8	39–41	50
45	85–88	26.3–25.6	35–38	45
40	81–84	27.1–26.4	32–34	40
35	77–80	27.8–27.2	29–31	35
30	73–76	28.6–27.9	26–28	30
25	69–72	29.4–28.7	23–25	25
20	68 Down	29.5 Down	22 Down	20

Table 7–2. Standing Broad Jump T-Scores For High School and Junior High School Boys

Grade	7	8	9	10	11	
T-Score						T-Score
80	90 Up	97 Up	103 Up	105 Up	112 Up	80
75	86–89	92–96	98–102	101–104	107–111	75
70	82–85	88–91	93–97	97–100	103–106	70
65	77–81	83–87	88–92	92–96	97–102	65
60	73–76	78–82	83–87	88–91	93–96	60
55	69–72	73–77	79–82	83–87	88–92	55
50	65–68	69–72	74–78	79–82	83–87	50
45	61–64	64–68	69–73	75–78	78–82	45
40	56–60	59–63	64–68	71–74	74–77	40
35	52–55	54–58	59–63	66–70	69–73	35
30	48–51	50–53	54–58	62–65	64–68	30
25	44–47	45–49	49–53	58–61	59–63	25
20	43 Down	44 Down	48 Down	57 Down	58 Down	20

Table 7–3. Zigzag Run T-Scores for High School and Junior High School Boys

Grade	7	8	9	10	11	
T-Score						T-Score
80	20.1 Down	17.8 Down	20.2 Down	21.6 Down	21.5 Down	80
75	21.4–20.2	19.5–17.9	21.3–20.3	22.7–21.7	22.6–21.6	75
70	22.7–21.5	21.2–19.6	22.4–21.4	23.8–22.8	23.7–22.7	70
65	24.0–22.8	22.8–21.3	23.5–22.5	24.8–23.9	24.7–23.8	65
60	25.2–24.1	24.5–22.9	24.6–23.6	25.8–24.9	25.8–24.8	60
55	26.5–25.3	26.2–24.6	25.7–24.7	26.9–25.9	26.8–25.9	55
50	27.8–26.6	27.8–26.3	26.8–25.8	27.9–27.0	27.8–26.9	50
45	29.0–27.9	29.5–27.9	27.9–26.9	28.9–28.0	28.9–27.9	45
40	30.3–29.1	31.2–29.6	29.0–28.0	29.9–29.0	29.9–29.0	40
35	31.6–30.4	32.8–31.3	30.1–29.1	31.0–30.0	31.0–30.0	35
30	32.8–31.7	34.5–32.9	31.2–30.2	32.1–31.1	32.0–31.1	30
25	34.1–32.9	36.2–34 6	32.3–31.3	33.1–32.2	33.0–32.1	25
20	34.2 Up	36.3 Up	32.4 Up	33.2 Up	33.1 Up	20

Table 7–4. Medicine Ball Put T-Scores for High School and Junior High School Boys

Grade	7	8	9	10	11	
T-Score						T-Score
80	43 Up	45 Up	49 Up	50 Up	54 Up	80
75	38–42	43–44	46–48	47–49	51–53	75
70	35–37	40–42	44–45	44–46	48–50	70
65	33–34	37–39	41–43	42–43	46–47	65
60	30–32	34–36	38–40	39–41	43–45	60
55	27–29	31–33	35–37	37–38	40–42	55
50	25–26	28–30	32–34	34–36	37–39	50
45	22–24	25–27	29–31	32–33	34–36	45
40	19–21	23–24	27–28	29–31	31–33	40
35	17–18	20–22	24–26	27–28	28–30	35
30	14–16	17–19	21–23	24–26	25–27	30
25	12–13	14–16	18–20	22–23	22–24	25
20	11 Down	13 Down	17 Down	21 Down	21 Down	20

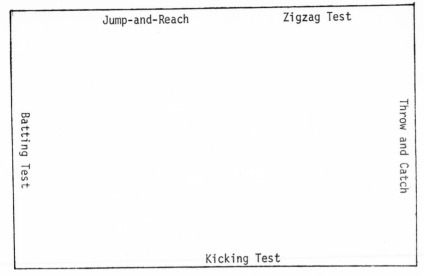

Fig. 7–3.   Floor plan for Johnson fundamental skills test.

Class Organization. The station-to-station plan can be used if assistants are trained for administering and scoring the various items. The students can be issued individual score cards and asked to rotate from one station to another either alone or in squads. Scoring can be done by a trained assistant.

General Procedure. 1. All four items should be explained and demonstrated before testing begins.
2. The purpose of the test should be made known to the students.
3. Student leaders must be trained in advance to administer and score.

Uses. The results of the tests could be used to measure status in the fundamental skills and to show progress if given at the end of the year. The results could be used for purposes of classification into either heterogeneous or homogeneous groups.

Test Description

ITEM NUMBER I—ZIGZAG TESTS

Purpose: To measure the fundamental skill of running.

Facilities and Equipment: Four folding chairs and one stop watch. The course is marked as follows:
    Four folding chairs are placed 6 feet apart on a gymnasium floor, between a starting line and an X placed on the wall of the gymnasium. The first chair is placed 6 feet from the starting line, and the last chair is placed 6 feet from the wall. The X, 6 inches in size, is four feet from the floor and placed on the wall. The length of the starting line is one foot. There should be an area 20 feet long behind the starting line that is free from obstruction.

Directions: The student is instructed to stand behind the middle of the starting line and, on the command, "Go," to run either to the right or to the left of the first chair, to zigzag around the three remaining chairs, to touch the X, to return in the same manner, and to touch the starting line with his foot.

Scoring: Time to the nearest tenth of a second required for running the course. Three trials are given, with the shortest time being the score. For any of the following fouls the subject is required to run the course again: having any part of the forward foot over the starting line when the command is given; not zigzagging around the chairs in the prescribed manner; and not touching the X on the wall before returning toward the starting line.

Testing Personnel: One trained assistant to supervise the testing station and to time and record the scores.

ITEM NUMBER II—JUMP-AND-REACH

Purpose: To measure the fundamental skill of jumping.

Facilities and Equipment: Chalk dust and one piece of construction paper, 6 inches wide and three feet high, ruled off in half inches. Horizontal lines are made on the construction paper at one-half inch intervals. The paper is fastened to the wall at such a height that the O line on the chart is just below the point that represents the standing reach of the shortest performer.

Directions: The subject stands with one side of his body parallel with the wall chart. He dips his forefinger in chalk, reaches as high as possible, and makes a chalk mark on the chart. He then jumps upward as far as possible and makes a mark on the wall at the peak of his jump (on the construction paper).

Scoring: The score is the inches (to the nearest half inch) between the two chalk marks. The subject is given five jumps, with the highest jump recorded on his score card. The subject is not allowed to make any preliminary steps forward before the jump.

Testing Personnel: One trained assistant to supervise the testing station and to measure and record the scores.

ITEM NUMBER III—KICKING TEST

Purpose: To measure the fundamental skill of kicking.

Facilities and Equipment: One soccer ball and an area in the gym marked as follows:

On a flat wall space, a target area 5 feet high and 10 feet wide is marked with one-half inch tape. This area is divided into five equal rectangles placed perpendicular to the floor. The number 5 is taped in the center rectangle of the target, number 3 is taped in the rectangles adjacent to the center rectangle, number 1 is taped on the two remaining rectangles. On the floor three lines 3 feet long are marked: one is 10 feet from the wall; one, 20 feet; and one, 30 feet from the wall.

Directions: The subject places the soccer ball behind the 10-foot line marked on the floor. From that position he attempts to kick the ball in such a manner that it may hit the wall target. The subjects kick three times from each of the lines marked on the floor. Two practice kicks are made at each line before the three kicks for the record are made.

Scoring: The subject receives the number of points indicated on the target area into which the ball is kicked. If the ball is kicked on a line between two areas, the score is that for the area with the larger number. A ball kicked from in front of the restraining floor line counts zero, and another trial is given.

Testing Personnel: One trained assistant to supervise the testing station and to observe, count and record the scores.

ITEM NUMBER IV—THROW-AND-CATCH

Purpose: To measure the fundamental skill of throwing.

Facilities and Equipment: One 8½-inch playground ball (grades 1, 2, 3) and a regulation-sized volleyball (grades 4, 5, 6). An area on the gym wall and floor is marked as follows:

A 3-foot square is placed on a flat wall with one-half inch tape. Its bottom line is 4 feet from the floor. An inner square, 10 inches in from all four sides, is placed on the wall target. Starting 3 feet from the wall, and in line with the wall target, there are placed five 2-foot squares, each one foot behind the other.

Directions: With both feet inside the first square, the subject stands facing the wall target and throws the ball at the wall target; keeping both feet inside the square, he attempts to catch the ball in the air when it rebounds from the wall. The throw should be made with an underhand motion. After two practice trials the subject is given three trials from each of the five squares.

Scoring: Two points for successfully throwing a ball in or on the inner wall target square; two points for successfully catching the rebounding ball in the air while standing in the floor square; one point for successfully throwing a ball in or on the outer wall target square; one point for successfully catching the rebounding ball in the air, on or outside the floor square. The subject's score is the total points scored from all five squares. If the subject steps out of the square while throwing, the throw is nullified and another trial is given.

Testing Personnel: One trained assistant to supervise the testing station and to observe, count, and record the scores.

ITEM NUMBER V—BATTING-TEST

Purpose: To measure the fundamental skill of batting.

Facilities and Equipment: One "batter-up kit" (may be purchased from Tigrett Industries, Jackson, Tennessee). One softball base placed far enough from the "batter-up" so that when the machine is started, the plastic balls in its circle of rotation will pass directly over the base.

Directions: The student, facing the base, stands in a batting position and swings, with a bat, at the ball as it is thrown toward him. Two practice swings are permitted followed by ten trials for the record.

Scoring: One point is scored when the bat makes contact with the ball in such a way as to make the ball complete at least a three-fourths turn in the opposite direction from which it was going. When the bat hits the nylon string, no point is scored.

Testing Personnel: One trained assistant to supervise the testing station and to observe, count and record the scores.

Score Card

JOHNSON FUNDAMENTAL SKILLS TEST
SCORE CARD

Name ————————————————————————
          Last   First   Middle

Grade ————————————Age ————————————

Test Item	Raw Score	Percentile score
Zigzag Tests		
Jump-and-Reach		
Kicking Test		
Throw-and-Catch		
Batting-Test		

Norms

Table 7–5.   Grade 1, Boys and Girls: Percentiles for Kick, Throw-and-Catch, Jump-and-Reach, Zigzag Run, Batting

	Kick (pts.)		Throw-and-Catch (pts.)		Jump-and-Reach (in.)		Zigzag Run (sec.)		Batting (No. of hits)	
Percentile	B	G	B	G	B	G	B	G	B	G
100	34	30	34	29	11-5	10-5	8.0	8.8	6	5
95	28	27	26	23	9-0	8-5	9.2	9.4	5	4
90	27	26	24	21			9.4	9.9	4	3
85	26	25	23	20	8-5	8-0	9.8	10.0		
80			22	19			9.9	10.4	3	
75	25	24	21	18	8-0	7-5	10.0	10.8		
70			20	17	7-5	7-0	10.2	10.9		2
65	24	23	19			6-5	10.4	11.0		
60		22	18	16	7-0		10.6	11.4		
55	23			15		6-0	10.8	11.5		
50			17		6-5		10.9	11.6	2	
45	22	21		14		5-5		11.8		
40			16	13	6-0		11.0			1
35	21		15	12		5-0	11.2			
30	20	20	14	11	5-5		11.4	12.0		
25		19	13	10		4-5	11.6	12.2		
20	19	18	12		5-0	4-0	11.8	12.4	1	
15	18	16	11	9	4-5		12.0	12.6		
10	17	14	10	8	4-0	3-5	12.2	12.8		0
5	14	10	9	5	3-5	3-0	12.8	13.4	0	
0	12	8	6	3	3-0	2-5	13.0	13.6		

Table 7–6. Grade 2, Boys and Girls: Percentiles for Kick, Throw-and-Catch, Jump-and-Reach, Zigzag Run, Batting

Percentile	Kick (pts.)		Throw-and-Catch (pts.)		Jump-and-Reach (in.)		Zigzag Run (sec.)		Batting (No. of hits)	
	B	G	B	G	B	G	B	G	B	G
100	36	35	39	35	12-5	11-0	7.6	7.8	7	6
95	33	33	38	31	10-0	9-5	8.0	8.2	6	5
90	31	31	34	28	9-5	9-0	8.4	8.6	5	4
85	30	30	32	27			8.8	8.8	4	
80	28	29	31	26	9-0	8-5	8.9	9.0		3
75		28	30	25	8-5		9.0	9.4		
70	27	27	29	24		8-0	9.2	9.5	3	
65		26	28	23			9.4	9.6		
60	26		27	22	8-0	7-5	9.5	9.8		2
55		25	26	21			9.6			
50	25	24	25		7-5		9.8	9.9		
45			24	20		7-0				
40	24	23		19			9.9	10.0		
35	23	22	23	18	7-0	6-0		10.2	2	
30	21	20	22	17	6-5		10.0	10.4		1
25	20		21	16	6-0		10.1	10.8		
20	19	19	20	15		5-5	10.2		1	
15	18	18	19	14	5-5	5-0	10.6	11.0		
10	17	16	17	12	5-0	4-5	10.9	11.2		
5	14	14	13	10	4-5	4-0	11.2	11.8	0	0
0	10	12	8	7	4-0	3-5	11.4	12.0		

Table 7–7. Grade 3, Boys and Girls: Percentiles for Kick, Throw-and-Catch, Jump-and-Reach, Zigzag Run, Batting

Percentile	Kick (pts.)		Throw-and-Catch (pts.)		Jump-and-Reach (in.)		Zigzag Run (sec.)		Batting (No. of hits)	
	B	G	B	G	B	G	B	G	B	G
100	40	36	41	38	13-0	12-0	7.4	7.4	8	7
95	37	34	40	34	11-5	10-0	7.8	8.0	7	
90	36	32	39	33	11-0	9-5	8.0	8.2	6	5
85	34	31	38	32	10-0	9-0	8.2	8.4	5	4
80	33	30	37	30			8.4	8.8	4	
75			36	29	9-5	8-5	8.6	8.9		
70	32	29	35	28			8.7	9.1		
65	31	28	34		9-0	8-0	8.8	9.2		3
60	30	27	33	27			9.0	9.3		
55		26		26	8-5			9.4		
50	29	25	32	25		7-5		9.5	3	
45		24	31				9.2	9.6		
40	28		30	24	8-0	7-0	9.3	9.8		2
35	27	23		23			9.4			
30		22	29	22			9.6			
25	26	21		21	7-5	6-5	9.8	10.0	2	
20	25	20	28	20	7-0	6-0	10.0	10.4		1
15	23	19	27	19	6-5		10.2	10.6		
10	22	18	25	18	6-0	5-5	10.4	10.8	1	
5	20	17	21	16	5-0	5-0	10.6	11.0		
0	16	16	17	13	4-5	4-5	10.8	11.2		

Table 7–8.   Grade 4, Boys and Girls: Percentiles for Kick, Throw-and-Catch, Jump-and-Reach, Zigzag Run, Batting

Percentile	Kick (pts.) B	G	Throw-and-Catch (pts.) B	G	Jump-and-Reach (in.) B	G	Zigzag Run (sec.) B	G	Batting (No. of hits) B	G
100	42	39	50	43	15-0	14-0	7.0	7.2	9	7
95	38	37	47	40	13-0	11-0	7.6	7.8	8	
90	37	35	45	39	12-0	10-5	7.8	8.0	7	6
85	36	34	43	38	11-5	10-0	8.0	8.4		
80	35	33	42	37	11-0		8.2	8.6	6	5
75		32	41	36	10-5	9-5	8.4	8.8		
70	34	31	40	35	10-0		8.5	9.0		
65				34		9-0	8.6	9.1	5	4
60	33	30	39				8.7	9.2		
55			38	33	9-5	8-5	8.8	9.4		
50	32	29		32			9.0	9.5		
45	31		37		9-0	8-0	9.1	9.6	4	
40		36	31				9.2	9.7		3
35	30	28	35	30		7-5	9.3	9.8		
30	29	27	34	29	8-5	7-0	9.4	10.0		
25		26	33	28	8-0		9.6	10.2		2
20	28	25	32	27		6-5	9.8	10.4	3	
15	27	24	31	26	7-5	6-0	10.0	10.6		1
10	25	22	30	24	7-0	5-5	10.2	10.8	2	
5	23	20	27	21	6-5	5-0	10.6	11.2	1	
0	19	16	23	16	6-0	4-5	10.8	11.4		

Table 7–9.   Grade 5, Boys and Girls: Percentiles for Kick, Throw-and-Catch, Jump-and-Reach, Zigzag Run, Batting

Percentile	Kick (pts.) B	G	Throw-and-Catch (pts.) B	G	Jump-and-Reach (in.) B	G	Zigzag Run (sec.) B	G	Batting (No. of hits) B	G
100	43	40	57	53	16-0	15-0	6.6	6.8	10	8
95	40	38	54	50	14-0	13-0	7.0	7.2	9	7
90	39	36	52	45	13-0	12-0	7.2	7.4	8	
85	38	35	50	44	12-5		7.3	7.8	7	6
80	37	34	48	43	12-0	11-5	7.4			
75	36	33	47	42		11-0	7.5			5
70	35		46	41	11-5	10-5	7.6	8.0	6	
65		32	45	40	11-0		7.8	8.1		
60	34	31	44		10-5	10-0		8.2		
55				39				8.3		4
50	33		43	38	10-0	9-5	8.0	8.4	5	
45		30	42	37			8.1	8.5		
40	32		41		9-5	9-0	8.2	8.6		
35		29	40	36			8.3	8.8		
30	31	28	39	35	9-0	8-5	9.4	8.9		3
25		27	38	34		8-0	8.5	9.0	4	
20	30	26	37	33	8-5	7-5	8.6	9.2		
15	29	25	36	32	8-0	7-0	8.8	9.4		2
10	28	23	34	31	7-5	6-5	9.0	9.8	3	
5	26	20	33	29	7-0	6-0	9.2	10.0		1
0	23	14	29	24	6-5	5-5	9.4	10.2		

Table 7–10. Grade 6, Boys and Girls: Percentiles for Kick, Throw-and-Catch, Jump-and-Reach, Zigzag Run, Batting

Percentile	Kick (pts.)		Throw-and-Catch (pts.)		Jump-and-Reach (in.)		Zigzag Run (sec.)		Batting (No. of hits)	
	B	G	B	G	B	G	B	G	B	G
100	44	42	59	55	17-5	16-0	6.0	6.6	10	9
95	41	40	56	51	16-0	14-0	6.8	7.0		8
90	40	38	54	49	15-0	13-0	7.0	7.2	9	
85	39	36	53	47	14-0	12-0	7.2	7.4	8	7
80	37	35	52	46	13-5		7.3	7.5		
75		34	51	45	13-0	11-5	7.4	7.6		
70	36		50	44	12-5		7.5	7.7	7	6
65	35	33	49	43	12-0	11-0	7.6	7.8		
60			48				7.8	7.9		
55		32	47	42	11-5	10-5		8.0		5
50	34		46	41		10-0	7.9	8.1	6	
45		31		40	11-0			8.2		
40	33		45				8.0	8.3		
35	32	30	44	39	10-5		8.1	8.4		4
30			43	38		9-5	8.2	8.6	5	
25	31	29	42	37	10-0		8.4	8.8		
20	30	28	41	36		9-0	8.5	9.0		3
15	29	27	40	35	9-5	8-5	8.6	9.2	4	
10	28	25	39	33	9-0	8-0	8.8	9.6		
5	26	20	37	31	8-5	7-0	9.2	10.0	3	2
0	23	15	34	28	8-0	6-5	9.0	10.5		

Morrison Test of Basic Sports Skills for College Women*

Purpose. To measure basic sports skills for purposes of classification and guidance.

Evaluation. Multiple R of .9289 with a standard error .0137.

Level and Sex. College women but could be adapted for high school girls.

Time Allotment and Number of Subjects. A class of 40 students in a one hour period can be tested.

Floor Plan and Space Requirements. A single gymnasium provides ample space. Figure 7–4 shows the floor plan.

Class Organization. The three item battery can best be administered by the station-to-station plan. Since the three items are not strenuous the order of events is not important. However, the test maker recommends this order: running jump and reach, basketball throw for distance, and the obstacle race. The students can be given the carry-type individual score cards when they report and move through the stations either in squads or on an individual basis. Since the running jump and reach is more time consuming, multiple stations can be set up if enough leadership is available.

* Adapted from the following source: Morrison, L. L., A Test of Basic Sports Skills for College Women. Unpublished Thesis, Indiana University, Bloomington, Indiana, 1964.

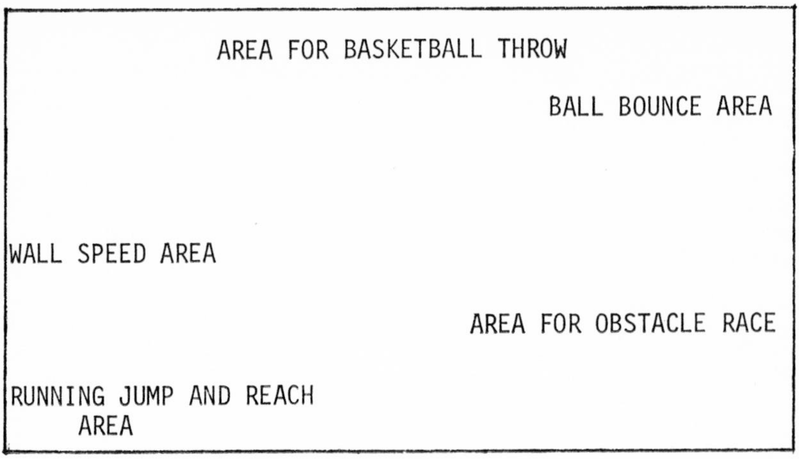

```
┌─────────────────────────────────────────────────────────────┐
│                                                             │
│                  AREA FOR BASKETBALL THROW                  │
│                                                             │
│                       BALL BOUNCE AREA                      │
│                                                             │
│                                                             │
│                                                             │
│  WALL SPEED AREA                                            │
│                                                             │
│                              AREA FOR OBSTACLE RACE         │
│                                                             │
│  RUNNING JUMP AND REACH                                     │
│       AREA                                                  │
└─────────────────────────────────────────────────────────────┘
```

Fig. 7–4.   Floor plan for Morrison test of basic sports skills.

Scoring can be done by squad leaders, a trained assistant at each station or by partners. The five item battery can be administered in similar fashion. The suggested order of testing for the five item battery is as follows: Ball Bounce, Wall Speed, Running Jump and Reach, Basketball Throw for Distance and Obstacle Race.

General Procedure. 1. All three items should be explained and demonstrated at the beginning of the period.

2. The students should report in uniform, including shoes.

3. A warm-up period should precede the actual testing.

4. After the test is given the raw scores can be converted to T-Scores or Weighted Scores and the profile card completed.

Uses. The results of this basic sports skills test may be used to classify students into ability groups. If the student's rank is in the superior group, she could be encouraged to enroll in an advanced class. If the student's rank is in the inferior group, she could be assigned to classes in fundamental movement. If the student's rank places her in the middle three groups, she should be encouraged to elect sports in which she has an interest and some skill already.

The unweighted T-scores are placed on the score card and can be used for the construction of basic sports skills profile.

In addition to sectioning for all classes, scores can also be used as a basis within the class for both competition and instruction (see Chapter 13).

Test Description

ITEM NUMBER I—BALL BOUNCE

Purpose: To measure the ability to bounce a ball on the end of a bat.

Facilities and Equipment: A medium weight softball bat, volleyball. A circle six feet in diameter is drawn on the floor.

Directions: The subject stands in the middle of the circle, holding the bat in the preferred hand, one hand's length from the heavy end of the bat.

The subject tries to bounce the volleyball on the *very top* of the bat continuously for as many as ten bounces. The ball must bounce at least six inches above the bat and the subject must stay within the circle.

Organization: This test is individually administered. Other students to be tested stand around the circle to assist in recovering the ball.

Scoring: The score on each of ten trials stops when: ten bounces have been scored; or, the ball hits the body; or the subject steps on or over the circle line; or, the ball does not bounce six inches from the bat. The final score is the sum of the successful bounces up to ten on each of the ten trials.

Testing Personnel: One trained assistant is needed to supervise the station and to count and record scores.

ITEM NUMBER II—WALL SPEED (Young and Moser)

Purpose: To measure the speed of passing and catching a rebounding ball.

Facilities and Equipment: Basketball for each station, stop watch. A restraining line is marked on the floor six feet from a flat wall surface.

Directions: The tester stands behind the subjects taking the test and times the trials. The subject stands behind the restraining line facing the wall with the ball in her hands. On the signal, "Ready—Go," she throws the ball against the wall and catches it as it rebounds. She continues throwing and catching in this manner until the signal, "Stop." Any type of throw may be used but the subject must throw from behind the restraining line. If the ball goes out of control, the subject must recover it.

Organization: The subjects are in groups of three; one subject takes the test as one watches for foot faults, and one counts the number of times the ball hits the wall. Positions are rotated until each subject has had two trials. As many groups can be tested at one time as wall space permits.

Scoring: The score is the sum of hits recorded in two trials of 30 seconds each. If the subject steps over the restraining line, that hit does not count.

Testing Personnel: One trained test administrator is needed to time the trials.

ITEM NUMBER III—RUNNING JUMP AND REACH

Purpose: To measure the ability to run and jump for height.

Facilities and Equipment: Stall bar bench or stool, jump board, reach scale. A 6-foot long line is marked on the floor 5 feet in front of the jump board.
    The jump board is constructed of wood and masonite or heavy rubber strips. Heavy rubber strips are preferable. Twenty-four graduated strips (numbered from 1–24) of masonite or rubber $\frac{3}{8}$ inch thick and 1 inch wide are suspended by means of small key chains from a board 72 inches long and $5\frac{1}{2}$ inches wide. The shortest strip is 4 inches long and each successive strip is 1 inch longer than the previous strip. Two holes are drilled in each strip $\frac{3}{8}$ inch from the top of the strip and $\frac{1}{4}$ inch in from each edge. Screw eye hooks are secured in pairs to the bottom of the main board so that there is 1 inch leeway at either end of the board. The hooks are $\frac{1}{2}$ inch apart and there is $1\frac{1}{2}$ inches between pairs of hooks. The jump board is attached to a balcony or from the ceiling so the strips will swing freely and so the

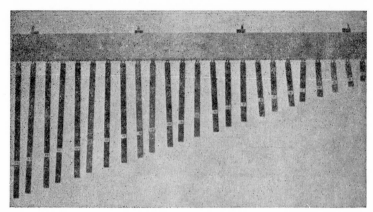

Fig. 7–5.   Jump board for the running jump and reach.

longest strip is within reach of the shortest subject and the shortest strip cannot be reached by the tallest subject.   The board must be level with the floor.   The distance in inches is measured from the longest strip to the floor and a jump chart is constructed.   The chart gives the number of each strip, and the number of inches each strip is from the floor.

The reach scale is drawn on butcher paper and secured to a flat wall surface.   The scale is in $\frac{1}{2}$ inches starting 70 inches from the floor and extending to 90 inches from the floor.

Directions: To secure the reach score, the tester stands on a stool next to the reach scale.   The subject stands facing the scale with her feet flat on the floor.   With both hands she reaches as high as possible and places the palms of the hands against the scale.   The distance from the middle finger of the preferred hand to the nearest $\frac{1}{2}$ inch mark is the reach height.

To secure the jump score the tester stands near the jump board.   The subject stands at any distance behind the starting line opposite the strip she thinks she can run and jump and reach.   She is allowed any number of steps.   If she reaches the chosen strip, she moves to a higher strip and continues in this fashion, until she has failed to reach a strip in two consecutive attempts.

Organization: Individually administered.   The tester records the reach height of all members of a group.   Then she records the number of the highest strip touched by each subject and the height of the strip from the floor.

Scoring: The score is the difference between the reach height and the run and jump height.

Testing Personnel: One trained assistant is needed to supervise and to measure and record scores.

ITEM NUMBER IV—BASKETBALL THROW FOR DISTANCE (Scott)

Purpose: To measure the ability to throw a ball for distance (arm and shoulder girdle strength and coordination).

Facilities and Equipment: Three basketballs, measuring tape, three wooden discs approximately one and one-half inches in diameter.   The throwing area should be about 90 feet long and there should be at least ten feet behind the throwing line. A throwing line is marked on the floor. Beginning ten feet in front of the throwing line, the area is marked off with lines parallel to the throwing line and at five foot intervals. Lines are marked with the amount of distance from the throwing line.

Directions: The tester stands beside the throwing area. The subject stands behind the throwing line and throws the basketball down the throwing area as far as possible. The subject has three trials. The tester should not demonstrate the throw. The tester marks each throw with one of the wooden discs and measures the longest throw to the nearest foot.

Organization: This test is individually administered. Several subjects can be used to recover balls after the balls have bounced.

Scoring: The score is the distance from the throwing line to the spot where the longest throw first touched, measured to the nearest foot. If the subject steps on or across the throwing line that throw is not counted.

Testing Personnel: One trained assistant to mark throws and record scores.

ITEM NUMBER V—OBSTACLE RACE (Scott)

Purpose: To measure a fast start with change of level, running around, changes of direction, and getting under an obstacle.

Facilities and Equipment: Three jump standards, one pole 6½ feet long, stop watch. The obstacle course is set up the same as the Scott Motor Ability Test (see page 180).

Directions: Same as the Scott Motor Ability Test

Organization: Same as the Scott Motor Ability Test

Scoring: Same as the Scott Motor Ability Test

Testing Personnel: Same as the Scott Motor Ability Test

Score Card

BASIC SPORTS SKILLS BATTERY SCORE CARD

Name _____ Class standing_____ Date _____

Campus address _____ PO Box _____ Age_____

Item	Trials										Raw Score	T- Score	Wtd. Score
	1	2	3	4	5	6	7	8	9	10			
1. Ball Bounce (sum of trials)											___	___	___
2. Wall Speed (sum of trials)	1			2							___	___	___
3. Running Jump and Reach (Jump minus Reach)	strip no.		Jump		Reach						___	___	___
4. Basketball Throw for Distance (nearest foot)											___	___	___
5. Obstacle Race (nearest 10th second)											___	___	___

Classification   TOTAL ___

Superior _____ Good _____ Average _____ Poor _____ Inferior _____

Table 7–11.   Scoring Tables for the Three Item Basic Sports Skills Battery
for College Women

Obstacle Race (Weight 1.1)			Running Jump and Reach (Weight 1.0)		Basketball Throw for Distance (Weight 1.1)		
Raw score (10th sec)	T-Score	Wtd. score	Raw score (inches)	T-Score	Raw score (feet)	T-Score	Wtd score
11.7–11.6	100	110	30.5	100	101	100	110
11.9–11.8	99	109			100	99	109
12.1–12.0	98	108	30.0	98	99	98	108
12.3–12.2	97	107			98	97	107
12.5–12.4	96	106	29.5	96	97	96	106
12.7–12.6	95	105	29.0	95	96–95	95	105
12.9–12.8	94	103			94	94	103
13.1–13.0	93	102	28.5	93	93	93	102
13.3–13.2	92	101			92	92	101
13.5–13.4	91	100	28.0	91	91	91	100
13.7–13.6	90	99	27.5	90	90	90	99
13.9–13.8	89	98			89	89	98
14.1–14.0	88	97	27.0	88	88–87	88	97
14.3–14.2	87	96			86	87	96
14.5–14.4	86	95	26.5	86	85	86	95
14.7–14.6	85	94	26.0	85	84	85	94
14.9–14.8	84	92			83	84	92
15.1–15.0	83	91	25.5	83	82	83	91
15.3–15.2	82	90			81	82	90
15.5–15.4	81	89	25.0	81	80	81	89
15.7–15.6	80	88	24.5	80	79–78	80	88
15.9–15.8	79	87			77	79	87
16.0	78	86	24.0	78	76	78	86
16.2–16.1	77	85			75	77	85
16.4–16.3	76	84	23.5	76	74	76	84
16.6–16.5	75	83	23.0	75	73	75	83
16.8–16.7	74	81			72	74	81
17.0–16.9	73	80	22.5	73	71–70	73	80
17.2–17.1	72	79			69	72	79
17.4–17.3	71	78	22.0	71	68	71	78
17.6–17.5	70	77	21.5	70	67	70	77
17.8–17.7	69	76			66	69	76
18.0–17.9	68	75	21.0	68	65	68	75
18.2–18.1	67	74	20.5	67	64	67	74
18.4–18.3	66	73			63–62	66	73
18.6–18.5	65	72	20.0	65	61	65	72
18.8–18.7	64	70			60	64	70
19.0–18.9	63	69	19.5	63	59	63	69
19.2–19.1	62	68	19.0	62	58	62	68
19.4–19.3	61	67			57	61	67
19.6–19.5	60	66	18.5	60	56	60	66
19.8–19.7	59	65			55	59	65
20.0–19.9	58	64	18.0	58	54–53	58	64
20.2–20.1	57	63	17.5	57	52	57	63
20.4–20.3	56	62			51	56	62
20.6–20.5	55	61	17.0	55	50	55	61
20.8–20.7	54	59			49	54	59
20.9	53	58	16.5	53	48	53	58
21.1–21.0	52	57	16.0	52	47	52	57
21.3–21.2	51	56			46–45	51	56

Table 7–11. Scoring Tables for the Three Item Basic Sports Skills Battery for College Women (Continued)

Obstacle Race (Weight 1.1)			Running Jump and Reach (Weight 1.0)		Basketball Throw for Distance (Weight 1.1)		
Raw score (10th sec)	T-Score	Wtd. score	Raw score (inches)	T-Score	Raw score (feet)	T-Score	Wtd. score
21.5–21.4	50	55	15.5	50	44	50	55
21.7–21.6	49	54			43	49	54
21.9–21.8	48	53	15.0	48	42	48	53
22.1–22.0	47	52	14.5	47	41	47	52
22.3–22.2	46	51			40	46	51
22.5–22.4	45	50	14.0	45	39	45	50
22.7–22.6	44	48			38–37	44	48
22.9–22.8	43	47	13.5	43	36	43	47
23.1–23.0	42	46	13.0	42	35	42	46
23.3–23.2	41	45			34	41	45
23.5–23.4	40	44	12.5	40	33	40	44
23.7–23.6	39	43			32	39	43
23.9–23.8	38	42	12.0	38	31	38	42
24.1–24.0	37	41	11.5	37	30	37	41
24.3–24.2	36	40			29–28	36	40
24.5–24.4	35	39	11.0	35	27	35	39
24.7–24.6	34	37	10.5	34	26	34	37
24.9–24.8	33	36			25	33	36
25.1–25.0	32	35	10.0	32	24	32	35
25.3–25.2	31	34			23	31	34
25.5–25.4	30	33	9.5	30	22	30	33
25.7–25.6	29	32	9.0	29	21–20	29	32
25.9–25.8	28	31			19	28	31
26.0	27	30	8.5	27	18	27	30
26.2–26.1	26	29			17	26	29
26.4–26.3	25	28	8.0	25	16	25	28
26.6–26.5	24	26	7.5	24	15	24	26
26.8–26.7	23	25			14	23	25
27.0–26.9	22	24	7.0	22	13–12	22	24
27.2–27.1	21	23			11	21	23
27.4–27.3	20	22	6.5	20	10	20	22
27.6–27.5	19	21	6.0	19	9	19	21
27.8–27.7	18	20			8	18	20
28.0–27.9	17	19	5.5	17	7	17	19
28.2–28.1	16	18			6	16	18
28.4–28.3	15	17	5.0	15	5	15	17
28.6–28.5	14	15	4.5	14	4–3	14	15
28.8–28.7	13	14			2	13	14
29.0–28.9	12	13	4.0	12	1	12	13
29.2–29.1	11	12				11	12
29.4–29.3	10	11	3.5	10		10	11
29.6–29.5	9	10	3.0	9		9	10
29.8–29.7	8	9				8	9
30.0–29.9	7	8	2.5	7		7	8
30.2–30.1	6	7				6	7
30.4–30.3	5	6	2.0	5		5	6
30.6–30.5	4	4	1.5	4		4	4
30.8–30.7	3	3				3	3
30.9	2	2	1.0	2		2	2
31.1–31.2	1	1	.5	1		1	1

Table 7-12. Scoring Tables for the Five Item Basic Sports Skills Battery for College Women

Raw Score (10th sec.)	Obstacle Race (Weight 2.0)		Running Jump and Reach (Weight 1.9)			Wall Speed (Weight 1.5)			Basketball Throw for Distance (Weight 1.6)			Ball Bounce	
	T-Score	Wtd. score	Raw score (inches)	T-Score	Wtd. score	Raw score	T-Score	Wtd. score	Raw score (feet)	T-Score	Wtd. score	Raw score	T-Score
11.7–11.6	100	200	30.5	100	190	96	100	150	101	100	160	87	100
11.9–11.8	99	198				95	99	149	100	99	158	86	99
12.1–12.0	98	196	30.0	98	186	94	98	147	99	98	157	85	98
12.3–12.2	97	194							98	97	155	84	97
12.5–12.4	96	192	29.5	96	182	93	96	144	97	96	154	83	96
12.7–12.6	95	190	29.0	95	181	92	95	143	96–95	95	152	82	95
12.9–12.8	94	188				91	94	141	94	94	150	81	94
13.1–13.0	93	186	28.5	93	177	90	93	140	93	93	149	80–79	93
13.3–13.2	92	184							92	92	147	78	92
13.5–13.4	91	182	28.0	91	173	89	91	137	91	91	146	77	91
13.7–13.6	90	180	27.5	90	171	88	90	135	90	90	144	76	90
13.9–13.8	89	178				87	89	134	89	89	142	75	89
14.1–14.0	88	176	27.0	88	167				88–87	88	141	74	88
14.3–14.2	87	174				86	87	131	86	87	139	73	87
14.5–14.4	86	172	26.5	86	163	85	86	129	85	86	138	72	86
14.7–14.6	85	170	26.0	85	162	84	85	128	84	85	136	71–70	85
14.9–14.8	84	168							83	84	134	69	84
15.1–15.0	83	166	25.5	83	158	83	83	125	82	83	133	68	83
15.3–15.2	82	164				82	82	123	81	82	131	67	82
15.5–15.4	81	162	25.0	81	154	81	81	122	80	81	130	66	81
15.7–15.6	80	160	24.5	80	152				79–78	80	128	65	80
15.9–15.8	79	158				80	79	119	77	79	126	64	79
16.0	78	156	24.0	78	148	79	78	117	76	78	125	63	78
16.2–16.1	77	154				78	77	116	75	77	123	62–61	77
16.4–16.3	76	152	23.5	76	144	77	76	114	74	76	122	60	76
16.6–16.5	75	150	23.0	75	143				73	75	120	59	75
16.8–16.7	74	148				76	74	111	72	74	118	58	74
17.0–16.9	73	146	22.5	73	139	75	73	110	71–70	73	117	57	73
17.2–17.1	72	144				74	72	108	69	72	115	56	72
17.4–17.3	71	142	22.0	71	135				68	71	114	55	71

17.6–17.5	**70**	**142**	**21.5**	70	**133**	**73**	**70**	**105**	**67**	70	112	54	70
17.8–17.7	**69**	**138**				**72**	**69**	**104**	**66**	69	110	53–52	69
18.0–17.9	68	136	21.0	68	129	71	68	102	65	68	109	51	68
18.2–18.1	67	134	20.5	67	125				64	67	107	50	67
18.4–18.3	66	132				70	66	99	63–62	66	106	49	66
18.6–18.5	65	130	20.0	65	124	69	65	98	61	65	104	48	65
18.8–18.7	64	128				68	64	96	60	64	102	47	64
19.0–18.9	63	126	19.5	63	120				59	63	101	46	63
19.2–19.1	62	124	19.0	62	118	67	62	93	58	62	99	45	62
19.4–19.3	61	122				66	61	92	57	61	98	44–43	61
19.6–19.5	60	120	18.5	60	114	65	60	90	56	60	96	42	60
19.8–19.7	59	118							55	59	94	41	59
20.0–19.9	58	116	18.0	58	110	64	58	87	54–53	58	93	40	58
20.2–20.1	57	114	17.5	57	108	63	57	86	52	57	91	39	57
20.4–20.3	56	112				62	56	84	51	56	90	38	56
20.6–20.5	55	110	17.0	55	105	61	55	83	50	55	88	37	55
20.8–20.7	54	108							49	54	86	36	54
20.9	53	106	16.5	53	101	60	53	80	48	53	85	35	53
21.1–21.0	52	104	16.0	52	99	59	52	78	47	52	83	34–33	52
21.3–21.2	51	102				58	51	77	46–45	51	82	32	51
21.5–21.4	50	100	15.5	50	95				44	50	80	31	50
21.7–21.6	49	98				57	49	74	43	49	78	30	49
21.9–21.8	48	96	15.0	48	91	56	48	72	42	48	77	29	48
22.1–22.0	47	94	14.5	47	89	55	47	71	41	47	75	28	47
22.3–22.2	46	92							40	46	74	27	46
22.5–22.4	45	90	14.0	45	86	54	45	68	39	45	72	26	45
22.7–22.6	44	88				53	44	66	38–37	44	70	25–24	44
22.9–22.8	43	86	13.5	43	82	52	43	65	36	43	69	23	43
23.1–23.0	42	84	13.0	42	80				35	42	67	22	42
23.3–23.2	41	82				51	41	62	34	41	66	21	41
23.5–23.4	40	80	12.5	40	76	50	40	60	33	40	64	20	40
23.7–23.6	39	78				49	39	59	32	39	62	19	39
23.9–23.8	38	76	12.0	38	72	48	38	57	31	38	61	18	38
24.1–24.0	37	74	11.5	37	70				30	37	59	17	37
24.3–24.2	36	72				47	36	54	29–28	36	58	16–15	36
24.5–24.4	35	70	11.0	35	67	46	35	53	27	35	56	14	35
24.7–24.6	34	68	10.5	34	65	45	34	51	26	34	54	13	34
24.9–24.8	33	66							25	33	53	12	33

7

Table 7-12. Scoring Tables for the Five Item Basic Sports Skills Battery for College Women (Continued)

Obstacle Race (Weight 2.0)			Running Jump and Reach (Weight 1.9)			Wall Speed (Weight 1.5)			Basketball Throw for Distance (Weight 1.6)			Ball Bounce	
Raw score (10th sec.)	T-Score	Wtd. score	Raw score (inches)	T-Score	Wtd. score	Raw score	T-Score	Wtd. score	Raw score (feet)	T-Score	Wtd. score	Raw score	T-Score
25.1–25.0	32	64	10.0	32	61	44	32	48	24	32	51	11	32
25.3–25.2	31	62				43	31	47	23	31	50	10	31
25.5–25.4	30	60	9.5	30	57	42	30	45	22	30	48	9	30
25.7–25.6	29	58	9.0	29	55				21–20	29	46	8	29
25.9–25.8	28	56				41	28	42	19	28	45	7–6	28
26.0	27	54	8.5	27	51	40	27	41	18	27	43	5	27
26.2–26.1	26	52				39	26	39	17	26	42	4	26
26.4–26.3	25	50	8.0	25	48				16	25	40	3	25
26.6–26.5	24	48	7.5	24	46	38	24	36	15	24	38	2	24
26.8–26.7	23	46				37	23	35	14	23	37	1	23
27.0–26.9	22	44	7.0	22	42	36	22	33	13–12	22	35		
27.2–27.1	21	42							11	21	34		
27.4–27.3	20	40	6.5	20	38	35	20	30	10	20	32		
27.6–27.5	19	38	6.0	19	36	34	19	29	9	19	30		
27.8–27.7	18	36				33	18	27	8	18	29		
28.0–27.9	17	34	5.5	17	32	32	17	26	7	17	27		
28.2–28.1	16	32							6	16	26		
28.4–28.3	15	30	5.0	15	29	31	15	23	5	15	24		
28.6–28.5	14	28	4.5	14	27	30	14	21	4–3	14	22		
28.8–28.7	13	26				29	13	20	2	13	21		
29.0–28.9	12	24	4.0	12	23				1	12	19		
29.2–29.1	11	22				28	11	17					
29.4–29.3	10	20	3.5	10	19	27	10	15					
29.6–29.5	9	18	3.0	9	17	26	9	14					
29.8–29.7	8	16											
30.0–29.9	7	14	2.5	7	13	25	7	11					
30.2–30.1	6	12				24	6	9					
30.4–30.3	5	10	2.0	5	10	23	5	8					
30.6–30.5	4	8	1.5	4	8								
30.8–30.7	3	6				22	3	5					
30.9	2	4	1.0	2	4	21	2	3					
31.1–31.0	1	2	.5	1	2	20	1	2					

Composite Norms

Table 7–13.   Composite Norms for Basic Sports Skills

The norms for the three item battery are:	
Superior	204—above
Good	176—203
Average	146—175
Poor	118—145
Inferior	117—below

The norms for the five item battery are:	
Superior	491—above
Good	431—490
Average	370—430
Poor	310—369
Inferior	309—below

These norms are local in nature. T-Scores
should be developed for the particular school
using the batteries.

Profile Card

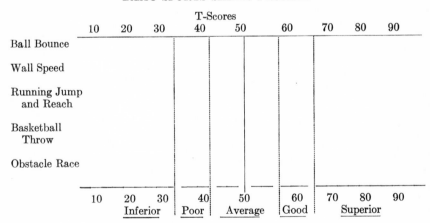

BASIC SPORTS SKILLS PROFILE

Scott Motor Ability Test*
(Battery Number 1 and 2)

Purpose. To measure status in general motor ability.

Evaluation. The three item battery of obstacle run, standing broad jump, and basketball throw has a validity coefficient of .87, while the four item battery which substitutes the 4-second dash and the wall pass for the obstacle run has .91.

Level and Sex. College women, high school girls, and ninth grade boys.[3]

Time Allotment and Number of Subjects. If the proper facilities are available, and if stations are run simultaneously, a class of 35 subjects may be tested in a 45-minute period.

Floor Plan and Space Requirement. When the recommended three items are the only ones being administered, one gym floor can easily accommodate the three stations. The floor plan shown in Figure 7-6 is recommended.

Class Organization. The tests should be administered on a combination station-to-station and squad method of administration. The students should be divided into equal squads, one for each test item. Squad leaders may be assigned to each squad with a squad score card and the leader rotates with his squad from one station to another.

Another way is to issue each student an individual score card, assign him to a squad and permit the squads to rotate as above, except there will be a trained assistant in charge of each test station. In either event, the

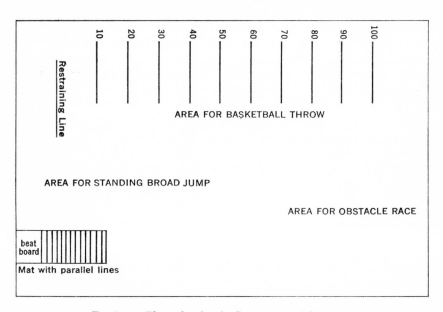

Fig. 7-6.   Floor plan for the Scott motor ability test.

* Scott, M. Gladys, & Esther French: *Measurement and Evaluation in Physical Education.* Dubuque, Iowa, Wm. C. Brown Co. Publishers, 1959. pp 344–363. Adapted by permission of Dr. M. Gladys Scott.

students in each squad may assist the squad leader or the trained assistant with scoring, measuring, and other work.

General Procedure. 1. The broad jump can be administered more effectively if the mat is marked off into lines 2 inches apart.

2. If there is not enough room for the basketball throw indoors, it may be administered outdoors.

3. The general purpose of the tests should be explained first.

4. Both the basketball throw for distance and the 4-second dash might be set up to be run diagonally across the gym if space does not otherwise permit.

5. Several areas may be set up for the wall pass and several students tested at the same time.

6. The test administrator should not give specific instructions on the technique of performing any of these skills.

7. This battery provides meaningful results at any stage of learning but is perhaps more serviceable when administered at the beginning of the junior high school, senior high school, and college.

8. The minimum recommended battery is the obstacle run, basketball throw, and the standing broad jump. The 4-second dash or the wall pass may be substituted for the obstacle race.

9. Composite scores may be computed from these batteries in two ways. The simplified version is to average the T-scores on the three or four items. A second method is through use of the simplified regression equation found from multiple correlation. For the three item test this equation is 2.0 basketball throw $+$ 1.4 broad jump—obstacle race. For the three item battery the equation is .7 basketball throw $+$ 2.0 dash $+$ 1.0 passes $+$ .5 broad jump. In the case of these equations the actual raw scores may be multiplied times these proper weightings. It is perhaps more expedient to use the tables.

Uses. The results of this test may be used to assign students to classes on the basis of general motor skills. This process in itself has many advantages. The results will indicate those students at either end of the scale and special programs can be planned to meet individual needs. Results may be used to identify weaknesses and used diagnostically.

While a motor ability test is not a capacity test, it does give a general estimate of the level of achievement which a student who is just beginning an activity may attain. Many times when motor ability test results are combined with a single valid item from a skill test battery, an adequate basis is available for classification into fairly homogeneous groups for that sport.

Test Description

ITEM NUMBER I—OBSTACLE RACE

Purpose: To measure speed, coordination, and agility.

Facilities and Equipment: A space on the floor of at least 55 by 12 feet is required. In order to complete the course, the following equipment is needed: three jumping standards, one cross bar at least 6 feet, one stop watch, and the course placed on the floor as shown in Figure 7–7.

Procedures: The student starts from a backward-lying position on the floor with his heels at line a. At the starting signal he gets up and runs

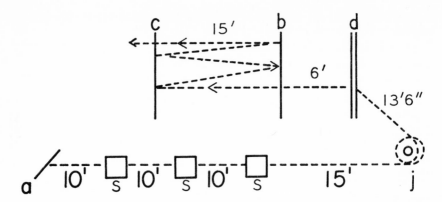

Fig. 7–7.   Floor markings for the Scott obstacle race. *a*, starting line; *b*, line shuttle; *c*, finish line; *d*, cross bar placed 18 inches high; *j*, jump standards; *s* squares on the floor 12 by 18 inches.   Path of runner is shown by dotted line.   The distance from the end of the cross bar to the line of the inner sides of the squares is 4 feet, 4 inches.

toward the jumping standard at point j.   As the student reaches each of the squares on the way, he must step on it with both feet.   On arriving at j he circles it twice and then crawls under the cross bar at d.   He gets up, runs to line c and then shuttles between lines c and b until he arrives at line c for the third time.

Instructions: You lie on your back with your heels touching the starting line.   On the signal "Go!" you get to your feet as rapidly as possible and run to the jumping standard.   On the way you must step on each square with both feet.   You then circle the jumping standard twice and proceed to the cross bar where you crawl under it.   You rise and continue across the first line until you reach the second line on the floor.   You touch this line and then return to the first line.   You then shuttle between these lines until you reach the last line the third time.

Scoring: The final score is the elapsed time to the nearest tenth of a second which is required to run the prescribed course.

Testing Personnel: One instructor or a trained assistant is needed to supervise the testing station and to time and record the scores.

ITEM NUMBER II—BASKETBALL THROW FOR DISTANCE

Purpose: To measure arm and shoulder girdle strength and coordination.

Facilities and Equipment: Several regulation basketballs and an area marked off as shown in Figure 7–6 occupying a space of approximately 20 by 100 feet long.   A throwing or scratch line is placed at one end of the course and parallel lines at intervals of 10 feet.

Procedures: The subject stands behind the throwing line and using any technique of throwing he wishes, he makes the throw down the course.   He must not step on or across the throwing line.   Three consecutive throws are permitted, and the longest throw counts.

Instructions: You may start from any distance behind the throwing line but you may not step on or over the line while throwing. Throw the ball as far as you can and you may use any type throw.

Scoring: The final score is the distance of the best trial measured to the nearest foot.

Testing Personnel: One trained assistant to supervise the testing station and measure the throws. Other assistants are needed to mark the spot where the ball first lands, to record scores, and to chase the balls and return them to the throwing area.

ITEM NUMBER III—BROAD JUMP

Purpose: To measure leg power.

Facilities and Equipment: For outdoor administration a jumping pit with a sunken take-off board 30 inches from the pit may be used. For indoor administration a mat marked at 2-inch intervals and a beat board are recommended.

Procedures: The subject assumes the starting position with feet parallel and the toes slightly curled over the end of the take-off. The jumper may swing the arms and bend the knees in a preliminary movement and then jump forward on the mat.

Instructions: You may crouch before the jump and swing your arms down in a preliminary movement. You must then jump forward as far as possible. You must take off from both feet simultaneously and try not to fall backward on landing.

Scoring: The score is the distance from the take-off board to the closer heel landing or any other part of the body in case that balance is lost. Three trials are permitted and the best one is measured to the nearest inch.

Testing Personnel: One trained assistant to supervise the testing station and measure the event and one assistant to record the score. If mats are used, two other assistants may be needed to stand on the mat to hold it in place.

ITEM NUMBER IV—WALL PASS

Purpose: To measure handling and controlling a ball.

Facilities and Equipment: Regulation basketballs, a flat wall space of at least 8 feet square with a line 9 feet from the wall for a restraining line. One stop watch.

Procedures: The subject stands with his feet behind the restraining line, and passes the ball against the wall as many times as possible in 15 seconds.

Instructions: On the signal to start, you will pass the ball against the wall in any manner you desire and catch it on the return. You keep repeating this act as fast as possible. If you step across the line in making a throw, the hit does not count as a score. If the ball rolls loose between the wall and the line, you may cross the line to retrieve it, but must return to the proper starting position before making the next pass.

Scoring: The final score is the number of times the ball hits the wall in the 15-second time period. If time permits, two or more trials may be used with the best score counting as the final score.

Testing Personnel: One trained assistant to supervise the testing station and operate the stop watch and one assistant to count and record the score.

ITEM NUMBER V—DASH

Purpose: To measure speed of movement.

Facilities and Equipment: A stop watch and whistle and a course marked as follows: a lane of approximately 100 feet long with a minimum width of 4 feet, 10 yards from the starting line this lane should be marked into one-yard zones by placing parallel lines to the starting line. There should be from 30 to 35 such zones. Two or more lanes may be employed.

Procedures: The runner takes any starting position he desires behind the starting line. On the signal to "Go," the runner runs down the lane at top speed until the whistle sounds. The score is the zone she has reached when the whistle sounds at the end of 4 seconds.

Instructions: On the signal to "Go," you run down the lane as fast as you can until you hear the whistle. You should not stop suddenly but slow down gradually to your own pace after the whistle sounds. Your score is the lane zone you have reached at the sound of the whistle.

Scoring: The final score is the distance traveled by the subject in the 4 seconds and is estimated by means of the zones.

Testing Personnel: One trained assistant to supervise the testing station and operate the stop watch, and one assistant to observe the zone and record results. It is possible for one experienced tester to do both the timing and observing.

Score Card

SCORE CARD FOR SCOTT MOTOR ABILITY TEST		
Name_____		
Grade_____ School_____		
Test Event	Raw Score	T—Score
Wall Pass		
Basketball Throw		
Broad Jump		
4—Second Dash		
Obstacle Race		
TOTAL T—SCORE_____ MOTOR ABILITY SCORE (Divide Total T—Score by No. of Events)_____		

Table 7–14. T-Scales for High School Girls

T-Score	Wall Pass (410)*	Basketball Throw (Ft.) (310)*	Broad Jump (In.) (287)*	4 Sec. Dash (Yd.) (398)*	Obstacle Race (Sec.) (374)*	T-Score
80	16	71				80
79			96			79
78						78
77	15	68	94	27		77
76		66			18.5–18.9	76
75		65				75
74		64	92			74
73	14	63				73
72		61				72
71		59	90	26		71
70		55	88		19.0–19.4	70
69	13	54				69
68		52	86	25		68
67		51			19.5–19.9	67
66		50				66
65		49				65
64		48	84	24	20.0–20.4	64
63	12	47				63
62		46	82		20.5–20.9	62
61			80			61
60		45		23		60
59		44	78		21.0–21.4	59
58	11	43				58
57		42	76		21.5–21.9	57
56		41				56
55		40	74	22		55
54					22.0–22.4	54
53		39				53
52	10		72			52
51		37			22.5–22.9	51
50		36		21		50
49		35	70			49
48			68		23.0–23.4	48
47		34	66			47
46	9	33			23.5–23.9	46
45		32	64	20		45
44		31			24.0–24.4	44
43			62			43
42		30			24.5–24.9	42
41	8	29	60	19		41
40		28				40
39			58		25.0–25.4	39
38		27	56			38
37	7		54		25.5–25.9	37
36		26			26.0–26.4	36
35			52	18	26.5–26.9	35

Table 7–14. T-Scales for High School Girls (Continued)

T-Score	Wall Pass (410)*	Basketball Throw (Ft.) (310)*	Broad Jump (In.) (287)*	4 Sec. Dash (Yd.) (398)*	Obstacle Race (Sec.) (374)*	T-Score
34		25	50		27.0–27.4	34
33						33
32		24	47		27.5–27.9	32
31	6	23				31
30			44		28.0–28.4	30
29		22		17	28.5–28.9	29
28					29.0–29.4	28
27		21			29.5–29.9	27
26			40		30.0–30.4	26
25	5	20				25
24				16	30.5–31.9	24
23		19	36		31.5–32.4	23
22				15	32.5–34.9	22
21		16				21
20	4			14	35.0–36.0	20

* Indicates the number of subjects on which the scale is based.

Table 7–15. T-Scales for College Women

T-Score	Basketball Throw	Wall Pass	Broad Jump	Obstacle Race	T-Score
85	75	18	86	17.5–17.9	85
84					84
83	71	17		18.0–18.4	83
82					82
81		16	85		81
80	70	15			80
79	69			18.5–18.9	79
78	68	14	84		78
77	67		83		77
76	66				76
75	65		82	19.0–19.4	75
74	64		81		74
73	62		80		73
72	61	13	79	19.5–19.9	72
71	59				71
70	58		78	20.0–20.4	70
69	57		77		69
68	56		76		68
67	55		75	20.5–20.9	67
66	54	12	74		66
65	52				65
64	51		73	21.0–21.4	64
63	50		72		63
62	48		71	21.5–21.9	62
61	47				61

Table 7–15. T-Scales for College Women (Continued)

T-Score	Basketball Throw	Wall Pass	Broad Jump	Obstacle Race	T-Score
60	46		70		60
59	45	11	69	22.0–22.4	59
58	44		68		58
57	43		67	22.5–22.9	57
56	42				56
55	41		66	23.0–23.4	55
54	40		65		54
53	39		64	23.5–23.9	53
52	38	10	63		52
51	37			24.0–24.4	51
50	36		62		50
49	35		61	24.5–24.9	49
48			60		48
47	34		59	25.0–25.4	47
46	33		58		46
45	32	9	57	25.5–25.9	45
44	31				44
43			56	26.0–26.4	43
42	30		55		42
41			54	26.5–26.9	41
40	29		53	27.0–27.4	40
39	28	8	52		39
38				27.5–27.9	38
37	27		51	28.0–28.4	37
36	26		50		36
35			49	28.5–28.9	35
34	25		48	29.0–29.4	34
33			47	29.5–29.9	33
32		7	46	30.0–30.4	32
31			45	30.5–30.9	31
30	24		44	31.0–31.4	30
29			43	31.5–31.9	29
28	23		42	32.0–32.4	28
27	21		41	32.5–32.9	27
26		6	40	33.0–33.4	26
25	20		39	33.5–33.9	25
24			38	34.0–34.4	24
23		5	37	34.5–34.9	23
22			36		22
21	19			35.0–35.4	21
20					20
19			35	35.5–35.9	19
18					18
17	18	4			17
16					16
15					15
14				43.5–43.9	14
13			30	45.5–45.9	13

Table 7–16. T-Scales for Ninth Grade Boys*

T-Score	Basketball Throw (feet)	Broad Jump (Inches)	Obstacle Race (Seconds)	T-Score
80	117		16.0	80
79			16.1	79
78		104	16.2	78
77	111		16.3	77
76	109	103	16.4	76
75	108	102	16.5	75
74	107	101	16.6	74
73	106		16.7	73
72	104	100	16.8	72
71	102		16.9	71
70	100	99	17.0	70
69	99	98	17.1	69
68	98	97	17.2	68
67	97	96	17.3	67
66	96	95	17.4	66
65	95	94	17.5	65
64	94	93	17.6	64
63	93	92	17.7	63
62	92	91	17.8	62
61	91	90	17.9	61
60	90	89	18.0	60
59	89	88	18.1	59
58	88	87	18.2	58
57	87	86	18.3	57
56	86	85	18.4	56
55	85	84	18.5	55
54	84	83	18.6	54
53	83	82	18.7	53
52	82	81	18.8	52
51	81	80	18.9	51
50	80	79	19.0	50
49	79	78	19.1	49
48	78	77	19.2	48
47	77	76	19.3	47
46	76	75	19.4	46
45	75	74	19.5	45
44	74	73	19.6	44
43	73	72	19.7	43
42	72	71	19.8	42
41	71	70	20.0	41
40	70	69	20.2	40
39	69	68	20.4	39
38	68	67	20.6	38
37	67	66	20.8	37
36	66	65	21.0	36

Table 7–16. T-Scales for Ninth Grade Boys* (Continued)

T-Score	Basketball Throw (feet)	Broad Jump (Inches)	Obstacle Race (Seconds)	T-Score
35	65	64	21.2	35
34	64	63	21.4	34
33	63	62	21.6	33
32	62	61	22.0	32
31	61	60	22.2	31
30	60	59		30
29	59	58		29
28	58	57		28
27	56	56	24.0	27
26	55	55		26
25	54	54		25
24	52	53		24
23	50			23
22	48			22
21	46			21

* Kilday, Kenneth, and Marjorie Latchaw: *Study of Motor Ability in Ninth Grade Boys.* Unpublished studies, Los Angeles, University of California, Los Angeles, 1961. Adapted by permission of Dr. Marjorie Latchaw.

References

1. Barrow, H. M.: *Motor Ability Testing for College Men.* Minneapolis, Burgess Publishing Co., 1957.
2. ———: Test of Motor Ability for College Men. Research Quarterly, *25*, 253–260, October, 1954.
3. Kilday, Kenneth, and Marjorie Latchaw: Study of Motor Ability in Ninth Grade Boys. Unpublished Studies, Los Angeles, University of California, Los Angeles, 1961.
4. Johnson, R. D.: Measurement of Achievement in Fundamental Skills of Elementary School Children. Unpublished Thesis, State University of Iowa, Iowa City, Iowa, 1960.
5. Morrison, L, L.: A Test of Basic Sports Skills for College Women. Unpublished Thesis, Indiana University, Bloomington, Indiana, 1964.
6. Scott, M. Gladys: The Assessment of Motor Ability of College Women Through Objective Tests, Research Quarterly, *10*, 63–83, October, 1939.
7. ———: Motor Ability Tests for College Women, Research Quarterly, *14*, 402–405, December, 1943.
8. Scott, M. Gladys, and Esther French: *Measurement and Evaluation in Physical Education.* Dubuque, Iowa, Wm. C. Brown Co., Publishers, 1959. pp. 344–363.

Additional References

1. Adams, A. R.: A Test Construction Study of Sport-Type Motor Educability for College Men. Doctor's dissertation, Baton Rouge, Louisiana State University, 1954.
2. Barrow, H. M.: All-Around Physical Achievement Test, Unpublished data, Winston-Salem, Wake Forest College, 1960.
3. ———: A Short Screen Test for Motor Ability, The Physical Educator, *14*, 19–20, March, 1957.
4. Brace, David K.: *Measuring Motor Ability,* New York, A. S. Barnes & Co., 1927.
5. Carpenter, Aileen: The Measurement of General Motor Capacity and General Motor Ability in the First Three Grades, Research Quarterly, *13*, 444–465, December, 1942.

6. Cozens, F. W.: *Physical Achievement Scales for Boys in Secondary Schools*. New York, A. S. Barnes & Co., 1936.
7. ———: *The Measurement of General Athletic Ability in College Men*. Eugene, Oregon, University of Oregon Press, 1929.
8. ———: *Achievement Scales in Physical Education Activities for College Men*. Philadelphia, Lea & Febiger, 1936.
9. Greensboro Public Schools: Experimental Testing Project, Physical Education. Greensboro, N. C., 1958.
10. Hatlestad, L. L.: Motor Educability Tests for Women College Students, Research Quarterly, *12*, 10–17, March, 1942.
11. Humiston, Dorothy, A.: A Measurement of Motor Ability in College Women, Research Quarterly, *8*, 181–185, May, 1937.
12. Hunsicker, Paul A., and Henry J. Montoye: *Applied Tests and Measurements in Physical Education*. New York, Prentice-Hall, Inc., 1953.
13. Johnson, K. P.: A Measure of General Sports Skill of College Men. Unpublished doctor's dissertation, Bloomington, Indiana University, 1956.
14. Johnson, G. B.: Physical Skill Test for Sectioning Classes into Homogeneous Units, Research Quarterly, *3*, 128–136, 1932.
15. Knapp, Clyde: Achievement Scales in Six Physical Education Activities for Secondary School Boys, Research Quarterly, *18*, 187, October, 1947.
16. Larson, L. A.: A Factor Analysis of Motor Ability Variables and Tests, with Tests for College Men, Research Quarterly, *12*, 499–517, 1941.
17. Latchaw, Marjorie: Measuring Selected Skills in Fourth, Fifth, and Sixth Grades, Research Quarterly, *25*, 439–449, December, 1954.
18. Latchaw, Marjorie, and Camille Brown: *The Evaluation Process in Health Education, Physical Education and Recreation*. Englewood Cliffs, N.J., Prentice-Hall, Inc., 1962, pp. 84–105.
19. McCloy, C. H.: *The Measurement of Athletic Power*. New York, A. S. Barnes & Co., 1932.
20. ———: An Analytical Study of the Stunt Type Tests as a Measure of Motor Educability, Research Quarterly, *8*, 46–55, 1937.
21. ———: The Measurement of General Motor Capacity and General Motor Ability, Research Quarterly, Supplement, *5*, 46–61, March, 1934.
22. McCloy, C. H., and Norma D. Young: *Tests and Measurements in Health and Physical Education*. New York, Appleton-Century-Crofts, Inc., 1954. pp. 114–126.
23. Metheny, Eleanor: Studies of the Johnson Test as a Test of Motor Educability, Research Quarterly, *9*, 105–114, 1938.
24. Neilson, N. P., F. W. Cozens, and H. J. Cubberly: *Achievement Scales in Physical Education Activities for Secondary School Girls and College Women*. New York, A. S. Barnes & Co., 1937.
25. Neilson, N. P., and F. W. Cozens: *Achievement Scales in Physical Education Activities for Boys and Girls in Elementary and Junior High School*. New York, A. S. Barnes & Co., 1934.
26. Peacock, William H.: *Achievement Scales in Physical Education Activities for Boys and Girls*. University Research Council, Chapel Hill, University of North Carolina.
27. Powell, Elizabeth, and E. C. Howe: Motor Ability Tests for High School Girls, Research Quarterly, *10*, 81–88, December, 1939.
28. Weiss, R. A., and Marjorie Phillips: *Administration of Tests in Physical Education*, St. Louis, C. V. Mosby Co., 1954.
29. Wellesley College Studies in Hygiene and Physical Education, Research Quarterly, Supplement, *9*, 49–53, 1938.

Chapter 8
TESTS OF FITNESS AND ENDURANCE

AAHPER Youth Fitness Test*

Purpose. To measure status and achievement in the physical fitness objective.

Evaluation. A jury of experts in the form of a committee selected the seven items which make up this fitness battery. The Survey Research Center of the University of Michigan selected the schools from which the sample of 8500 boys and girls were drawn. The norms were based on the data from these numbers.

Level and Sex. Boys and girls, grades 5 through 12.

Time Allotment and Number of Subjects. Two testing periods are necessary for the administration of all seven items. During the first period the age, height, and weight can be recorded along with the administration of the pull-up for boys, the flexed-arm hang for girls, the sit-up, the standing broad jump, and the shuttle run. During the second testing period the 50-yard dash, the softball throw for distance, and the 600-yard run-walk can be administered. The aquatic test can be given at a third period whenever time and facilities permit. A class of from 30 to 35 can be tested in the above way in two 45-minute class periods.

Floor Plan and Space Requirement. A basketball court for the indoor items and a football field with track are the ideal space needs.

Class Organization. The tests can be administered on a combination of mass testing with partners and station-to-station. Half of the class can do sit-ups while the other half score. The same method can be applied to the 600-yard run-walk. The other items can be administered and scored by a trained tester at a station. At the beginning of the period each student is supplied with an individual score card. The events for that day of testing are then all explained and demonstrated before testing gets under way.

General Procedure. 1. All pupils should be given a reasonable amount of warm-up before testing begins.
2. When a student's medical status is in question, he should be excused from the test.
3. The norms are based on the Neilson-Cozens Classification Index which uses an exponent system, and a simplified age classification. In this textbook only the age norms are shown.
4. Age for the age classification norms is expressed by the number of birthdays the student has had.

* AAHPER, *Youth Fitness Test Manual*, Washington, D.C.: American Association for Health, Physical Education, and Recreation. (1201 16th Street, N. W., Washington, 6, D.C.) Adapted by permission of the AAHPER.

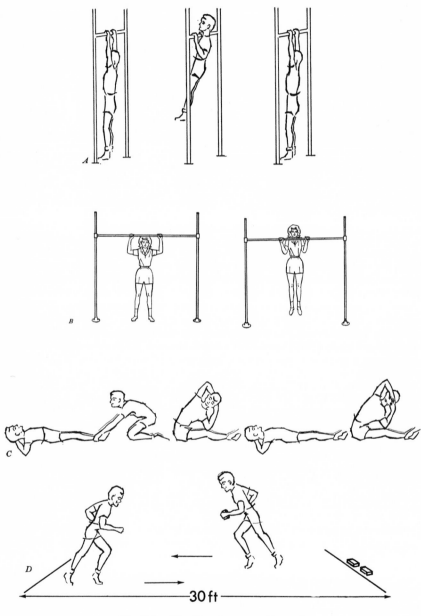

Fig. 8-1. (*Continued on opposite page*)

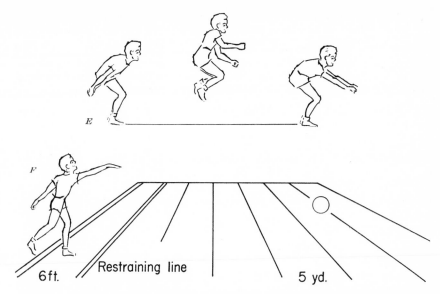

Fig. 8–1. Test items for AAHPER youth fitness test. *A*, Pull-up. *B*, Modified pull-up. *C*, Sit-up. *D*, Shuttle run. *E*, Standing broad jump. *F*, Softball throw for distance.

Uses. The test results may be used to indicate present status in fitness. When there is a re-test, progress may be noted. From such status and achievement records, many other uses are obvious, such as motivation, grading, guidance, and program appraisal. Comparisons may be made between a student's score and those of others in his group or those of others in the schools throughout the country. Two sets of norms have been developed using percentiles in both cases. One set is based on age classification and the other on the Neilson-Cozens Classification Index.

The student's fitness record may be charted on the profile graph shown in Figure 8–2.

Test Description

ITEM NUMBER I—PULL-UP (for boys) (Fig. 8–1 *A*)

Purpose: To measure arm and shoulder strength.

Facilities and Equipment: A metal or wooden bar approximately $1\frac{1}{2}$ inches in diameter and placed at a convenient height should be used. However, for the lower age levels a doorway gym bar can be used. At times it may be necessary to improvise such equipment as a basketball goal support or a ladder.

Procedures: The bar is adjusted to such height that the student can hang free of the floor. The student should grasp the bar with his palms facing away from his body (overhand grasp). The student should then raise his body until his chin is over the bar and then lower it again to the starting position with his arms fully extended.

Instructions: You must not lift your knees or assist your pull-up by kicking. You must return to the hang position with the arms fully straight. You will not be permitted to swing nor snap your way up.

Scoring: One point is scored each time the student completes a pull-up. Part scores do not count and only one trial is permitted unless it is obvious the student did not have a fair chance on his first trial.

Testing Personnel: One trained tester can administer this item, count the scores, and record results.

ITEM NUMBER II—FLEXED-ARM HANG (for girls) (Fig. 8–1 *B*)

Purpose: To measure arm and shoulder strength.

Facilities and Equipment: A metal or wooden bar approximately 1½ inches in diameter and placed at the subject's height should be used. A doorway gym bar adjusted at the desired height in a doorway works very well. If these items are not available, it is necessary to improvise by using some type of pole or pipe across bleachers or ladders. A stop watch is needed.

Procedure: The height of the bar should be adjusted to approximately the standing height of the subject. The student should grasp the bar with an overhand grasp. The subject then raises her body off the floor with the help of assistants to a position where the chin is above the bar. The elbows should be flexed and the chest should be close to the bar. Two spotters, one in front and one in back of the subject, are recommended for assistance in getting to the "hang" position. The subject holds the hang position as long as possible. The stop watch is started as soon as the subject assumes the starting position and is stopped when the chin touches the bar, falls below the bar, or when the subject's head is tilted back to keep the chin above the bar.

Instructions: You grasp the bar with palms facing away from your body and you will be lifted to a position with your chin just above the bar by assistants. You hang in this position as long as possible. It is a violation for your chin to touch the bar, fall below the bar, or for you to tilt your head backward to keep your chin from touching the bar.

Scoring: The score is the elapsed time to the nearest second that the subject maintained the proper hanging position.

Testing Personnel: One trained tester can administer this test and record the score.

ITEM NUMBER III—SIT-UP (Fig. 8–1 *C*)

Purpose: To measure abdominal strength and endurance.

Facilities and Equipment: Mats may be used if they are available; otherwise the floor is satisfactory.

Procedures: The student lies flat on his back with his knees straight and his feet approximately two feet apart. His fingers are interlocked and placed behind his neck. His elbows are flat against the floor or mat. His feet are held by a partner. On the signal to start, the student sits up touching the left elbow to the right knee, returns to the original starting position, sits up again and touches the right elbow to the left knee, and returns. This exercise is repeated, alternating sides. Each time an elbow touches a knee, one point is scored.

Instructions: Your fingers must remain interlocked and in contact with the back of your neck at all times. You may curl up from the starting position but your knees must be straight during the sit-up. However, they may be bent upward when you are touching them with the elbow. When you return to the starting position, your elbows must be flat on the floor or mat.

Scoring: One point is scored for each correct sit-up. The maximum number of sit-ups is: for girls, 50 sit-ups; and for boys, 100 sit-ups.

Testing Personnel: One trained tester can administer this item and count and record the score.

ITEM NUMBER IV—SHUTTLE RUN (Fig. 8–1 *D*)

Purpose: To measure speed and agility.

Facilities and Equipment: Two lines parallel to each other are placed on the floor 30 feet apart. Since the student must overrun both of these lines, it is necessary to have several feet more of floor space at either end. Two blocks of wood, 2 by 2 by 4 inches and a stop watch are needed.

Procedures: The student stands at one of the lines with the two blocks at the other line. On the signal to start, the student runs to the blocks, takes one and returns to the starting line and *places* the block behind that line. He then returns to the second block which he carries across the starting line on his way back. Two students could run at the same time if two timers are available, or if one test administrator has a split-second timer, and of course, if there are two sets of blocks. Two trials are permitted. If the students start first at one line and then at the other, it will not be necessary to return the blocks after each race. Sneakers should be worn or the student may run barefooted.

Instructions: On the signal to "Go" you must run as fast as you can to the next line and pick up a block. You should return the block over the second line where you place it on the floor. Do not throw it. You return for the second block and this time, you may run across the starting line as fast as you can without placing the block on the floor.

Scoring: The score is the elapsed time recorded in seconds and tenths of seconds for the best of two trials.

Testing Personnel: One trained tester can administer this test and time and record the score. If he has a split-second timer, he may have two students running at the same time. If two regular stop watches are available, two timers can be used.

ITEM NUMBER V—STANDING BROAD JUMP (Fig. 8–1 *E*)

Purpose: To measure power.

Facilities and Equipment: Tape measure and a mat, space on the floor, or an outdoor jumping pit.

Procedures: The student stands behind a take-off line with his feet several inches apart. Preliminary to jumping the student dips his knees and swings his arms backward. He then jumps forward by simultaneously extending his knees and swinging his arms forward. Three trials are permitted. Measurement is from the closest heel mark to the take off line. Indoor administration is best accomplished by placing a tape measure on the floor and at right angles to the take-off line and permitting the student to jump along the line. Measurement can then be made by sighting across the tape to the point of the jump. Three trials are permitted.

Instructions: You must take off from both feet simultaneously, jump as far forward as possible, and land on both feet. Try not to fall backward after the landing. You can jump farther by crouching before the jump and swinging your arms.

Scoring: The score is the distance between the take-off line and the nearest point where any part of the student's body touches the floor in feet and inches to the nearest inch. Only the best trial is recorded.

Testing Personnel: One trained tester can administer this item and judge and record the score.

ITEM NUMBER VI—50-YARD DASH

Purpose: To measure speed.

Facilities and Equipment: An area on a track, football field, or playground with a starting line, a 50-yard course, and a finish line. Two stop watches or a split-second timer.

Procedures: After a short warm-up period the student takes his position behind the starting line. Best results are obtained when two students run at the same time for competition. The starter uses the command, "Are you ready?" and "Go!" As he says the latter, he sweeps his arms downward as a signal to the timer. The students run across the finish line. One trial is permitted.

Instructions: You may take any position behind the starting line you wish. On the command, "Go!", you are to run as fast as you can across the finish line. Do not slow up until you are across the finish line. Then, you may slow down gradually.

Scoring: The score is the elapsed time to the nearest tenth of a second between the starting signal and the instant the student crosses the finish line.

Testing Personnel: One starter and two timers are needed to administer this test. If the split-second timer is available, only one timer is needed. The timer can record scores, but testing would be facilitated if he were assisted by a recorder.

ITEM NUMBER VII—SOFTBALL THROW FOR DISTANCE (Fig. 8–1 *F*)

Purpose: To measure arm and shoulder coordination.

Facilities and Equipment: A football field or a comparable place on a playground. The necessary space will depend on the age and sex of the group throwing. Several regulation 12-inch softballs and a measuring tape. Small metal or wooden stakes may be used to mark throws.

Procedures: Two parallel lines 6 feet apart are placed in the throwing area as restraining lines. The throw must be made from within this area. Scoring is facilitated if the field is marked off into additional parallel lines 5 yards apart. The student, using an overhand throw, throws the ball straight down the throwing area. Steps may be taken in making the throw provided the student remains in the 6-foot restraining area. Three trials are permitted and taken in succession. Only the farthest throw is marked by a stake. To facilitate administration the students are asked to stand by their stakes until several students have thrown. Measurement can then be made of several records.

Instructions: You must make your throw from within the space bounded by the two lines. You must throw the ball overhand, and it will help your score to throw as straight as possible. After your last throw, run out and stand by your stake and remain there until you have been scored.

Scoring: The score is the best of the three trials measured to the nearest foot.

Testing Personnel: Two trained assistants are needed to administer this test item. One assistant will judge for fair trials and the second will mark the spot of the throws. These same two assistants can measure the throws and record scores.

ITEM NUMBER VIII—600-YARD RUN-WALK

Purpose: To measure endurance.

Facilities and Equipment: A track or an area within a football field, or a square 50 yards on each side on a playground. Stop watch.

Procedures: Students may run individually or they may run in groups of a dozen or more. When students run in groups, they should be paired into partners and while one student runs, his partner will listen for the timer to call out his partner's time when he crosses the finish line and relay this time to the scorer. The student may interspace his running with periods of walking and should be encouraged to pace himself. When a group is running, the timer can call out times as each student crosses the finish line.

Instructions: You will run three times around this course (one time for a football field) and finish at the line which is clearly marked. You should run as far as you can and then you may have to walk for a short space of time. Try to keep running, however. You must pace yourself by not running too fast at the beginning but keep going at a speed you think you can continue.

Scoring: The score is the elapsed time in minutes and seconds.

Testing Personnel: One trained tester may operate the stop watch and call out the times and one assistant is needed to record the scores.

Score Card

PERSONAL DATA

	Trial 1		Trial 2	
		Exponent		*Exponent*
Age (in months)	_____	_____	_____	_____
Height (in inches)	_____	_____	_____	_____
Weight	_____	_____	_____	_____
Sum of Exponents	_____	_____	_____	_____
Class	_____	_____	_____	_____

	Trial 1		Trial 2	
	Date		Date	
	Score	*Percentile*	*Score*	*Percentile*
Pull-Ups (Boys)	_____	_____	_____	_____
Flexed-Arm Hang (Girls)	_____	_____	_____	_____
Sit-Ups	_____	_____	_____	_____
Shuttle Run	_____	_____	_____	_____
Standing Broad Jump	_____	_____	_____	_____
50-Yard Dash	_____	_____	_____	_____
Softball Throw	_____	_____	_____	_____
600-Yard Run-Walk	_____	_____	_____	_____

PROFILE RECORD

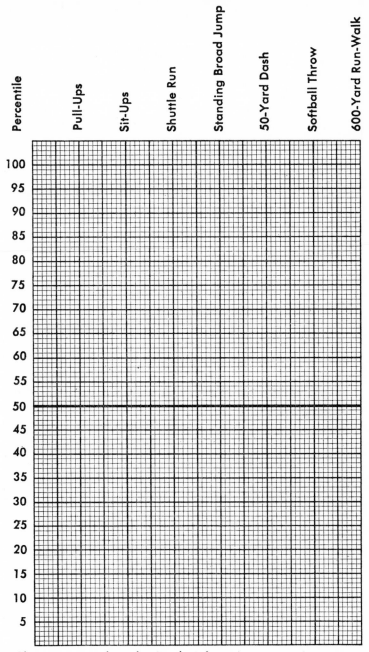

Plot your personal graph using the information on opposite page.
Use a different color for each trial.

Fig. 8–2. Profile for AAHPER youth fitness test.

Table 8-1. Percentile Scores Based on Age for Full-Ups for Boys and Flexed-Arm Hang for Girls

Boys

Age Percentile	10	11	12	13	14	15	16	17	Percentile
100th	16	20	15	24	20	25	25	32	100th
95th	8	8	9	10	12	13	14	16	95th
90th	7	7	7	9	10	11	13	14	90th
85th	6	6	6	8	10	10	12	12	85th
80th	5	5	5	7	8	10	11	12	80th
75th	4	4	5	6	8	9	10	10	75th
70th	4	4	4	5	7	8	10	10	70th
65th	3	3	3	5	6	7	9	10	65th
60th	3	3	3	4	6	7	9	9	60th
55th	3	2	3	4	5	6	8	8	55th
50th	2	2	2	3	5	6	7	8	50th
45th	2	2	2	3	4	5	6	7	45th
40th	1	1	1	2	4	5	6	7	40th
35th	1	1	1	2	3	4	5	6	35th
30th	1	1	1	1	3	4	5	5	30th
25th	0	0	0	1	2	3	4	5	25th
20th	0	0	0	0	2	3	4	4	20th
15th	0	0	0	0	1	2	3	4	15th
10th	0	0	0	0	0	1	2	2	10th
5th	0	0	0	0	0	0	0	1	5th
0	0	0	0	0	0	0	0	0	0

Girls

Age Percentile	10	11	12	13	14	15	16	17	Percentile
100th	66	79	64	80	60	74	74	76	100th
95th	31	35	30	30	30	33	37	31	95th
90th	24	25	23	21	22	22	26	25	90th
85th	21	20	19	18	19	18	19	19	85th
80th	18	17	15	15	16	16	16	16	80th
75th	15	16	13	13	13	14	14	14	75th
70th	13	13	11	12	11	13	12	12	70th
65th	11	11	10	10	10	11	10	11	65th
60th	10	10	8	9	9	10	9	10	60th
55th	9	9	8	8	8	8	8	9	55th
50th	7	8	6	7	7	8	7	8	50th
45th	6	6	6	6	6	6	6	7	45th
40th	6	5	5	5	5	6	5	6	40th
35th	5	4	4	4	4	4	4	4	35th
30th	4	4	3	3	3	3	3	4	30th
25th	3	3	2	2	2	2	2	3	25th
20th	2	2	1	2	1	1	1	2	20th
15th	2	1	0	1	1	0	1	0	15th
10th	1	0	0	0	0	0	0	0	10th
5th	0	0	0	0	0	0	0	0	5th
0	0	0	0	0	0	0	0	0	0

Table 8-2. Percentile Scores Based on Age for Sit-Ups

Boys

Percentile	10	11	12	13	14	15	16	17
100th	100	100	100	100	100	100	100	100
95th	100	100	100	100	100	100	100	100
90th	100	100	100	100	100	100	100	100
85th	100	100	100	100	100	100	100	100
80th	76	89	100	100	100	100	100	100
75th	65	73	93	100	100	100	100	100
70th	57	60	75	99	100	100	100	100
65th	51	55	70	90	99	100	99	99
60th	50	50	59	75	99	99	99	85
55th	49	50	52	70	77	90	85	77
50th	41	46	50	60	70	80	76	70
45th	37	40	49	53	62	70	70	62
40th	34	35	42	50	60	61	63	57
35th	30	31	40	50	52	54	56	51
30th	28	30	35	41	50	50	50	50
25th	25	26	30	38	45	49	50	45
20th	23	23	28	35	40	42	42	40
15th	20	20	25	30	36	39	38	35
10th	15	17	20	25	30	33	34	30
5th	11	12	15	20	24	27	28	23
0	1	0	0	1	6	5	10	8

Girls

Percentile	10	11	12	13	14	15	16	17
100th	50	50	50	50	50	50	50	50
95th	50	50	50	50	50	50	50	50
90th	50	50	50	50	50	50	50	50
85th	50	50	50	50	50	50	50	50
80th	50	50	50	50	49	42	41	45
75th	50	50	50	50	42	39	38	40
70th	50	50	50	45	37	35	34	35
65th	42	40	40	40	35	31	31	32
60th	39	37	39	38	34	30	30	30
55th	33	34	35	35	31	29	28	29
50th	31	30	32	31	30	26	26	27
45th	30	29	30	30	27	25	25	25
40th	26	26	26	27	25	24	24	23
35th	24	25	25	25	23	21	22	21
30th	21	22	22	22	21	20	20	20
25th	20	20	20	20	20	19	18	18
20th	16	19	18	19	18	16	16	16
15th	14	16	16	15	16	14	14	15
10th	11	12	13	12	13	11	11	12
5th	8	10	7	10	10	8	7	9
0	0	0	0	0	0	0	0	0

Table 8-3. Percentile Scores Based on Age for Shuttle Run

	Boys								Percentile	Girls							
Age	10	11	12	13	14	15	16	17		10	11	12	13	14	15	16	17
100th	9.0	9.0	8.5	8.0	8.3	8.0	8.1	8.0	100th	8.5	8.8	9.0	8.3	9.0	8.0	8.3	9.0
95th	10.0	10.0	9.8	9.5	9.3	9.1	9.0	8.9	95th	10.0	10.0	10.0	10.0	10.0	10.0	10.0	10.0
90th	10.2	10.1	10.0	9.8	9.5	9.3	9.1	9.0	90th	10.5	10.2	10.2	10.2	10.3	10.3	10.2	10.3
85th	10.4	10.3	10.0	9.9	9.6	9.4	9.2	9.1	85th	10.8	10.6	10.5	10.5	10.4	10.5	10.4	10.4
80th	10.5	10.4	10.2	10.0	9.8	9.5	9.3	9.2	80th	11.0	10.9	10.8	10.6	10.5	10.7	10.6	10.5
75th	10.7	10.5	10.3	10.1	9.9	9.6	9.5	9.3	75th	11.0	11.0	10.9	10.8	10.6	10.9	10.8	10.6
70th	10.8	10.7	10.5	10.2	9.9	9.7	9.5	9.4	70th	11.1	11.0	11.0	11.0	10.8	11.0	10.9	10.8
65th	10.9	10.8	10.6	10.3	10.0	9.8	9.6	9.5	65th	11.4	11.2	11.2	11.0	10.9	11.0	11.0	11.0
60th	11.0	10.9	10.7	10.4	10.0	9.8	9.7	9.6	60th	11.5	11.4	11.3	11.1	11.0	11.1	11.0	11.0
55th	11.0	11.0	10.9	10.5	10.2	9.9	9.8	9.7	55th	11.8	11.6	11.5	11.3	11.1	11.2	11.2	11.1
50th	11.2	11.1	11.0	10.6	10.2	10.0	9.9	9.8	50th	11.9	11.7	11.6	11.4	11.3	11.3	11.2	11.2
45th	11.4	11.2	11.0	10.8	10.3	10.0	10.0	9.9	45th	12.0	11.8	11.8	11.6	11.4	11.5	11.4	11.4
40th	11.5	11.3	11.1	10.9	10.5	10.1	10.0	10.0	40th	12.0	12.0	11.9	11.8	11.5	11.6	11.5	11.5
35th	11.6	11.4	11.3	11.0	10.5	10.2	10.1	10.0	35th	12.1	12.0	12.0	12.0	11.7	11.8	11.8	11.6
30th	11.8	11.6	11.5	11.1	10.7	10.3	10.2	10.1	30th	12.4	12.1	12.1	12.0	12.0	11.9	12.0	11.8
25th	12.0	11.8	11.6	11.3	10.9	10.5	10.4	10.4	25th	12.6	12.4	12.3	12.2	12.0	12.0	12.0	12.0
20th	12.0	12.0	11.9	11.5	11.0	10.6	10.5	10.6	20th	12.8	12.6	12.5	12.5	12.3	12.3	12.2	12.0
15th	12.2	12.1	12.0	11.8	11.2	10.9	10.8	10.9	15th	13.0	13.0	12.9	13.0	12.6	12.5	12.5	12.3
10th	12.6	12.4	12.4	12.0	11.5	11.1	11.1	11.2	10th	13.1	13.4	13.2	13.3	13.1	13.0	13.0	13.0
5th	13.1	13.0	13.0	12.5	12.0	11.7	11.5	11.7	5th	14.0	14.1	13.9	14.0	13.9	13.5	13.9	13.8
0	15.0	20.0	22.0	16.0	16.0	16.6	16.7	14.0	0	16.6	18.5	19.8	18.5	17.6	16.0	17.6	20.0

Table 8–4. Percentile Scores Based on Age for Standing Broad Jump

Boys

Percentile	10	11	12	13	14	15	16	17	Percentile
100th	6' 8"	10' 0"	7'10"	8' 9"	8'11"	9' 2"	9' 1"	9' 8"	100th
95th	6' 1"	6' 3"	6' 6"	7' 2"	7' 9"	8' 0"	8' 5"	8' 6"	95th
90th	5'10"	6' 0"	6' 4"	6'11"	7' 5"	7' 9"	8' 1"	8' 3"	90th
85th	5' 8"	5'10"	6' 2"	6' 9"	7' 3"	7' 6"	7'11"	8' 1"	85th
80th	5' 7"	5' 9"	6' 1"	6' 7"	7' 0"	7' 6"	7' 9"	8' 0"	80th
75th	5' 6"	5' 7"	6' 0"	6' 5"	6'11"	7' 4"	7' 7"	7'10"	75th
70th	5' 5"	5' 6"	5'11"	6' 3"	6' 9"	7' 2"	7' 6"	7' 8"	70th
65th	5' 4"	5' 6"	5' 9"	6' 1"	6' 8"	7' 1"	7' 5"	7' 7"	65th
60th	5' 2"	5' 4"	5' 8"	6' 0"	6' 7"	7' 0"	7' 4"	7' 6"	60th
55th	5' 1"	5' 3"	5' 7"	5'11"	6' 6"	6'11"	7' 3"	7' 5"	55th
50th	5' 0"	5' 2"	5' 6"	5'10"	6' 4"	6' 9"	7' 1"	7' 3"	50th
45th	5' 0"	5' 1"	5' 5"	5' 9"	6' 3"	6' 8"	7' 0"	7' 2"	45th
40th	4'10"	5' 0"	5' 4"	5' 7"	6' 1"	6' 6"	6'11"	7' 0"	40th
35th	4'10"	4'11"	5' 2"	5' 6"	6' 0"	6' 6"	6' 9"	6'11"	35th
30th	4' 8"	4'10"	5' 1"	5' 5"	5'10"	6' 4"	6' 7"	6'10"	30th
25th	4' 6"	4' 8"	5' 0"	5' 3"	5' 8"	6' 3"	6' 6"	6' 8"	25th
20th	4' 5"	4' 7"	4'10"	5' 2"	5' 6"	6' 1"	6' 4"	6' 6"	20th
15th	4' 4"	4' 5"	4' 8"	5' 0"	5' 4"	5'10"	6' 1"	6' 4"	15th
10th	4' 3"	4' 2"	4' 5"	4' 9"	5' 2"	5' 7"	5'11"	6' 0"	10th
5th	4' 0"	4' 0"	4' 2"	4' 5"	4'11"	5' 4"	5' 6"	5' 8"	5th
0	2'10"	1' 8"	3' 0"	2' 9"	3' 8"	2'10"	2' 2"	3' 7"	0

Girls

Percentile	10	11	12	13	14	15	16	17	Percentile
100th	7' 0"	7'10"	8' 2"	7' 6"	7' 4"	7' 8"	7' 5"	7' 8"	100th
95th	5' 8"	6' 2"	6' 3"	6' 3"	6' 4"	6' 6"	6' 7"	6' 8"	95th
90th	5' 6"	5'10"	6' 0"	6' 0"	6' 2"	6' 3"	6' 4"	6' 4"	90th
85th	5' 4"	5' 8"	5' 9"	5'10"	6' 0"	6' 1"	6' 2"	6' 2"	85th
80th	5' 2"	5' 6"	5' 8"	5' 8"	5'10"	6' 0"	6' 0"	6' 0"	80th
75th	5' 1"	5' 4"	5' 6"	5' 6"	5' 9"	5'10"	5'10"	5'11"	75th
70th	5' 0"	5' 3"	5' 5"	5' 5"	5' 7"	5' 9"	5' 8"	5'10"	70th
65th	5' 0"	5' 2"	5' 4"	5' 4"	5' 6"	5' 7"	5' 7"	5' 9"	65th
60th	4'10"	5' 0"	5' 2"	5' 3"	5' 5"	5' 6"	5' 6"	5' 7"	60th
55th	4' 9"	5' 0"	5' 1"	5' 2"	5' 4"	5' 5"	5' 5"	5' 6"	55th
50th	4' 7"	4'10"	5' 0"	5' 0"	5' 3"	5' 4"	5' 4"	5' 5"	50th
45th	4' 6"	4' 9"	4'11"	5' 0"	5' 1"	5' 3"	5' 3"	5' 3"	45th
40th	4' 5"	4' 8"	4' 9"	4'10"	5' 0"	5' 1"	5' 2"	5' 2"	40th
35th	4' 4"	4' 7"	4' 8"	4' 8"	5' 0"	5' 0"	5' 0"	5' 0"	35th
30th	4' 3"	4' 6"	4' 7"	4' 6"	4' 9"	4'10"	4'11"	5' 0"	30th
25th	4' 2"	4' 4"	4' 5"	4' 6"	4' 8"	4' 8"	4'10"	4'10"	25th
20th	4' 0"	4' 3"	4' 4"	4' 4"	4' 6"	4' 7"	4' 8"	4' 9"	20th
15th	3'11"	4' 1"	4' 2"	4' 2"	4' 3"	4' 6"	4' 6"	4' 7"	15th
10th	3' 9"	3'11"	4' 0"	4' 0"	4' 1"	4' 4"	4' 4"	4' 5"	10th
5th	3' 6"	3' 9"	3' 8"	3' 9"	3'10"	4' 0"	4' 0"	4' 2"	5th
0	2' 8"	2'11"	2'11"	2'11"	3' 0"	2'11"	3' 2"	3' 0"	0

Table 8–5. Percentile Scores Based on Age for 50-Yard Dash

Boys

Percentile	Age 10	11	12	13	14	15	16	17	Percentile
100th	6.0	6.0	6.0	5.8	5.8	5.6	5.6	5.6	100th
95th	7.0	7.0	6.8	6.5	6.3	6.1	6.0	6.0	95th
90th	7.1	7.2	7.0	6.7	6.4	6.2	6.1	6.0	90th
85th	7.4	7.4	7.0	6.9	6.6	6.4	6.2	6.1	85th
80th	7.5	7.5	7.2	7.0	6.7	6.5	6.3	6.2	80th
75th	7.6	7.6	7.3	7.0	6.8	6.5	6.3	6.3	75th
70th	7.8	7.7	7.5	7.1	6.9	6.6	6.4	6.3	70th
65th	8.0	7.8	7.5	7.2	7.0	6.7	6.5	6.4	65th
60th	8.0	7.8	7.6	7.3	7.0	6.7	6.5	6.5	60th
55th	8.1	8.0	7.8	7.4	7.0	6.8	6.6	6.5	55th
50th	8.2	8.0	7.8	7.5	7.1	6.9	6.7	6.6	50th
45th	8.3	8.0	7.9	7.5	7.2	7.0	6.7	6.7	45th
40th	8.5	8.1	8.0	7.6	7.2	7.0	6.8	6.7	40th
35th	8.5	8.3	8.0	7.7	7.3	7.1	6.9	6.8	35th
30th	8.7	8.4	8.2	7.9	7.5	7.1	6.9	6.9	30th
25th	8.8	8.5	8.3	8.0	7.6	7.2	7.0	7.0	25th
20th	9.0	8.7	8.4	8.0	7.8	7.3	7.1	7.0	20th
15th	9.1	9.0	8.6	8.2	8.0	7.5	7.2	7.1	15th
10th	9.5	9.1	8.9	8.4	8.1	7.7	7.5	7.3	10th
5th	10.0	9.5	9.2	8.9	8.6	8.1	7.8	7.7	5th
0	12.0	11.9	12.0	11.1	11.6	12.0	8.6	10.6	0

Girls

Percentile	Age 10	11	12	13	14	15	16	17	Percentile
100th	6.0	6.0	5.9	6.0	6.0	6.4	6.0	6.4	100th
95th	7.0	7.0	7.0	7.0	7.0	7.1	7.0	7.1	95th
90th	7.3	7.4	7.3	7.3	7.2	7.3	7.3	7.3	90th
85th	7.5	7.6	7.5	7.5	7.4	7.5	7.5	7.5	85th
80th	7.7	7.7	7.6	7.6	7.5	7.6	7.5	7.6	80th
75th	7.9	7.9	7.8	7.7	7.6	7.7	7.7	7.8	75th
70th	8.0	8.0	7.9	7.8	7.7	7.8	7.9	7.9	70th
65th	8.1	8.0	8.0	7.9	7.8	7.9	8.0	8.0	65th
60th	8.2	8.1	8.0	8.0	7.9	8.0	8.0	8.0	60th
55th	8.4	8.2	8.1	8.0	8.0	8.0	8.1	8.1	55th
50th	8.5	8.4	8.2	8.1	8.0	8.1	8.3	8.2	50th
45th	8.6	8.5	8.3	8.2	8.2	8.2	8.4	8.3	45th
40th	8.8	8.5	8.4	8.4	8.3	8.3	8.5	8.5	40th
35th	8.9	8.6	8.5	8.5	8.5	8.4	8.6	8.6	35th
30th	9.0	8.8	8.7	8.6	8.6	8.6	8.8	8.8	30th
25th	9.0	9.0	8.9	8.8	8.9	8.8	9.0	9.0	25th
20th	9.2	9.0	9.0	9.0	9.0	9.0	9.0	9.0	20th
15th	9.4	9.2	9.2	9.2	9.2	9.0	9.2	9.1	15th
10th	9.6	9.6	9.5	9.5	9.5	9.5	9.9	9.5	10th
5th	10.0	10.0	10.0	10.2	10.4	10.0	10.5	10.4	5th
0	14.0	13.0	13.0	15.7	16.0	18.0	17.0	12.0	0

Table 8-6. Percentile Scores Based on Age for Softball Throw

Boys

Percentile	10	11	12	13	14	15	16	17
100th	175	205	207	245	246	250	271	291
95th	138	151	165	195	208	221	238	249
90th	127	141	156	183	195	210	222	235
85th	122	136	150	175	187	204	213	226
80th	118	129	145	168	181	198	207	218
75th	114	126	141	163	176	192	201	213
70th	109	121	136	157	172	189	197	207
65th	105	119	133	152	168	184	194	203
60th	102	115	129	147	165	180	189	198
55th	98	113	124	142	160	175	185	195
50th	96	111	120	140	155	171	180	190
45th	93	108	119	135	150	167	175	185
40th	91	105	115	131	146	165	172	180
35th	89	101	112	128	141	160	168	176
30th	84	98	110	125	138	156	165	171
25th	81	94	106	120	133	152	160	163
20th	78	90	103	115	127	147	153	155
15th	73	85	97	110	122	141	147	150
10th	69	78	92	101	112	135	141	141
5th	60	70	76	88	102	123	127	117
0	35	14	25	50	31	60	30	31

Girls

Percentile	10	11	12	13	14	15	16	17
100th	167	141	159	150	156	165	175	183
95th	84	95	103	111	114	120	123	120
90th	76	86	96	102	103	110	113	108
85th	71	81	90	94	100	105	104	102
80th	69	77	85	90	95	100	98	98
75th	65	74	80	86	90	95	92	93
70th	60	71	76	82	87	90	89	90
65th	57	66	74	79	84	87	85	87
60th	54	64	70	75	80	84	81	82
55th	52	62	67	73	78	82	78	80
50th	50	59	64	70	75	78	75	75
45th	48	57	61	68	72	75	74	74
40th	46	55	59	65	70	73	71	71
35th	45	52	57	63	68	69	69	69
30th	42	50	54	60	65	66	66	66
25th	40	46	50	57	61	64	63	62
20th	37	44	48	53	59	60	60	58
15th	34	40	45	49	54	58	55	52
10th	30	37	41	45	50	51	50	48
5th	21	32	37	36	45	45	45	40
0	8	13	20	20	25	12	8	20

Table 8-7. Percentile Scores Based on Age for 600-Yard Run-Walk

Percentile	Boys 10	11	12	13	14	15	16	17	Girls 10	11	12	13	14	15	16	17
100th	1'30"	1'27"	1'31"	1'29"	1'25"	1'26"	1'24"	1'23"	1'42"	1'40"	1'39"	1'40"	1'45"	1'40"	1'50"	1'54"
95th	1'58"	1'59"	1'52"	1'46"	1'37"	1'34"	1'32"	1'31"	2' 5"	2'13"	2'14"	2'12"	2' 9"	2' 9"	2'10"	2'11"
90th	2' 9"	2' 3"	2' 0"	1'50"	1'42"	1'38"	1'35"	1'34"	2'15"	2'19"	2'20"	2'19"	2'18"	2'18"	2'17"	2'22"
85th	2'12"	2' 8"	2' 2"	1'53"	1'46"	1'40"	1'37"	1'36"	2'20"	2'24"	2'24"	2'25"	2'22"	2'23"	2'23"	2'27"
80th	2'15"	2'11"	2' 5"	1'55"	1'48"	1'42"	1'39"	1'38"	2'26"	2'28"	2'27"	2'29"	2'25"	2'26"	2'26"	2'31"
75th	2'18"	2'14"	2' 9"	1'59"	1'51"	1'44"	1'40"	1'40"	2'30"	2'32"	2'31"	2'33"	2'30"	2'28"	2'31"	2'34"
70th	2'20"	2'16"	2'11"	2' 1"	1'53"	1'46"	1'43"	1'42"	2'34"	2'36"	2'35"	2'37"	2'34"	2'34"	2'36"	2'37"
65th	2'23"	2'19"	2'13"	2' 3"	1'55"	1'47"	1'45"	1'44"	2'37"	2'39"	2'39"	2'40"	2'37"	2'36"	2'39"	2'42"
60th	2'26"	2'21"	2'15"	2' 5"	1'57"	1'49"	1'47"	1'45"	2'41"	2'43"	2'42"	2'44"	2'41"	2'40"	2'42"	2'46"
55th	2'30"	2'24"	2'18"	2' 7"	1'59"	1'51"	1'49"	1'48"	2'45"	2'47"	2'45"	2'47"	2'44"	2'43"	2'45"	2'49"
50th	2'33"	2'27"	2'21"	2'10"	2' 1"	1'54"	1'51"	1'50"	2'48"	2'49"	2'49"	2'52"	2'46"	2'46"	2'49"	2'51"
45th	2'36"	2'30"	2'24"	2'12"	2' 3"	1'55"	1'53"	1'52"	2'50"	2'53"	2'55"	2'56"	2'51"	2'49"	2'53"	2'57"
40th	2'40"	2'33"	2'26"	2'15"	2' 5"	1'58"	1'56"	1'54"	2'55"	2'59"	2'58"	3' 0"	2'55"	2'52"	2'56"	3' 0"
35th	2'43"	2'36"	2'30"	2'17"	2' 9"	2' 0"	1'58"	1'57"	2'59"	3' 4"	3' 3"	3' 3"	3' 0"	2'56"	2'59"	3' 5"
30th	2'45"	2'39"	2'34"	2'22"	2'11"	2' 3"	2' 1"	2' 0"	3' 3"	3'10"	3' 7"	3' 9"	3' 6"	3' 0"	3' 1"	3'10"
25th	2'49"	2'42"	2'39"	2'25"	2'14"	2' 7"	2' 5"	2' 4"	3' 8"	3'15"	3'11"	3'15"	3'12"	3' 5"	3' 7"	3'16"
20th	2'55"	2'48"	2'47"	2'30"	2'19"	2'13"	2' 9"	2' 9"	3'13"	3'22"	3'18"	3'20"	3'19"	3'10"	3'12"	3'22"
15th	3' 1"	2'55"	2'57"	2'35"	2'25"	2'20"	2'14"	2'16"	3'18"	3'30"	3'24"	3'30"	3'30"	3'18"	3'19"	3'29"
10th	3' 8"	3' 9"	3' 8"	2'45"	2'33"	2'32"	2'22"	2'26"	3'27"	3'41"	3'40"	3'49"	3'48"	3'28"	3'30"	3'41"
5th	3'23"	3'30"	3'32"	3' 3"	2'47"	2'50"	2'37"	2'40"	3'45"	3'59"	4' 0"	4'11"	4' 8"	3'56"	3'45"	3'56"
0	4'58"	5' 6"	4'55"	5'14"	5'10"	4'10"	4' 9"	4'45"	4'47"	4'53"	5'10"	5'10"	5'50"	5'10"	5'52"	6'40"

Cooper's Aerobics Test*

Purpose. To measure present level of physical fitness.

Level and Sex. Norms are based on men 17 and up and junior high school girls but the test is suitable for all age groups and both sexes.

Time Allotment and Number of Subjects. Any number of subjects may be tested in a thirty minute testing period.

Space Requirement. An outdoor or indoor track. A quarter mile track or a course that is accurately marked for distance.

Class Organization. The class or classes can be tested in mass with everyone running and times checked on a regular cross country score chart with cards numbered consecutively and handed to runners as they cross the finish line or partners can be used to observe each other's time.

General Procedure. 1. All subjects should be given the same instructions.
2. If a student's medical status is in question, he should not run.
3. Any size group may be started with a signal or by blowing a whistle.
4. One timer operating a stop watch can do all the timing and can call out the times as the runners cross the finish line.
5. If the 12-minute run is substituted for the $1\frac{1}{2}$-mile run or the $1\frac{1}{4}$-mile run, the track can be marked into zones and as the 12-minute time is reached, the starter blows his whistle. All runners stop and their distances identified, by means of the zones.

Uses. The results of the test are used to appraise physical condition and determine status. When status is determined, subjects are placed in one of five categories. Cooper has developed a training program for each. The test is not only a good initial test for determining status but can be used as a re-test to measure progress.

Test Description

ONE AND ONE-HALF MILE RUN TEST

Purpose: To measure cardiovascular fitness.

Facilities and Equipment: A quarter mile track is preferable so the runners may complete six laps. If none is available, distance can be measured on a football field, a play field or any open area.

Procedures: The group running can be divided into two sections for testing purposes. Each student works with a partner and while one student is running, the other partner checks laps and marks the time at the finish. The instructor should talk about pace and the time a student should be running at the end of each lap. The students are instructed to listen for the elapsed time to be called out as he passes the finish at the end of each lap. After he has finished the run, the student is instructed to continue walking or jogging for at least a lap in order to regain normal breathing.

Instructions: You should begin to run on the signal "go" and as you cross the finish line following each lap, you should call out the lap number and

* Cooper, Kenneth, *Aerobics:* New York, M. Evans and Company, Inc., 1968. Adapted by permission of Col. Cooper.

then listen for your elapsed time. When you have finished, continue to walk or jog for one more lap but stay on the outside of the track so you will not interfere with late finishers.

Scoring: The partner who is not running listens for his partner's time as he crosses the finish line for the last time. This time is recorded by the instructor after all runners have finished.

Testing Personnel: One trained instructor can administer the test as he serves as timer, calls out times, and records results.

12-MINUTE RUN TEST

The same as above except for:

Facilities and Equipment: Flags are placed around the track at 40-yard intervals.

Procedures: The partner is instructed to count the number of laps which are run within the allotted time. When eleven minutes have elapsed, the instructor calls out the time left to run. At the end of 12 minutes, the instructor blows a blast on his whistle and the runner notes the flag he has just passed.

Scoring: The observing partner gives the runner the number of completed laps he has run. The runner then reports his score in terms of number of laps plus the number of flags passed on the last lap.

Norms

Table 8–8. T-Score Norms for the 12-Minute Test and the $1\frac{1}{4}$-Mile Run Test for Junior High School Girls

	12-Minute Test N = 502 Distance		$1\frac{1}{4}$-Mile Test N = 496 Time
T-Score	Laps	Miles	
84	6 G	1.425	
82	6 F	1.40	
81	6 E	1.375	
79	6 D	1.35	
78	6 C	1.325	
76	6 B	1.30	
74	6 A	1.275	
73	5 J	1.25	8:27–8:40
72			8:41–8:54
71	5 I	1.225	8:55–9:08
70	5 H	1.20	9:09–9:22
69			9:23–9:36
68	5 G	1.175	9:37–9:51
67			9:52–10:05
66	5 F	1.15	10:06–10:19
65	5 E	1.125	10:20–10:33
64			10:34–10:47
63	5 D	1.10	10:48–11:02

Table 8–8   (continued)

T-Score	12-Minute Test N = 502 Distance Laps	Miles	1¼-Mile Test N = 496 Time
62	5 C	1.075	11:03–11:16
61			11:17–11:30
60	5 B	1.05	11:31–11:44
59			11:45–11:58
58	5 A	1.025	11:59–12:12
57	4 J	1.000	12:13–12-27
56			12:28–12:41
55	4 I	.975	12:42–12:55
54	4 H	.95	12:56–13:09
53			13:10–13:23
52	4 G	.925	13:24–13:38
51			13:39–13:52
50	4 F	.90	13:53–14:06
49	4 E	.875	14:07–14:20
48			14:21–14:34
47	4 D	.85	14:35–14:49
46	4 C	.825	14:50–15:03
45			15:04–15:17
44	4 B	.80	15:18–15:31
43			15:32–15:45
42	4 A	.775	15:46–16:00
41	3 J	.75	16:01–16:14
40			16:15–16:28
39	3 I	.725	16:29–16:42
38	3 H	.70	16:43–16:56
37			16:57–17:11
36	3 G	.675	17:12–17:25
35			17:26–17:39
34	3 F	.65	17:40–17:53
33	3 E	.625	17.54–18:07
32			18:08–18:22
31	3 D	.60	18:23–18:36
30	3 C	.575	18:37–18:50
29			18:51–19:04
28	3 B	.55	19:05–19:18
27			19:19–19:33
26	3 A	.525	19:34–19:47
25	2 J	.50	19:48–20:01
24			20:02–20:15
23	2 I	.475	20:16–20:29
22	2 H	.45	20:30–20:44
21			20:45–20:58
20	2 G	.425	20:59–21:12
19			21:13–21:26
18	2 F	.40	
17	2 E	.375	
15	2 D	.35	

* Hielscher, Patricia Ann. The Equivalency of Cooper's 12-Minute Test and a 1¼-Mile Run for Junior High School Girls. Masters Thesis, University of North Carolina at Greensboro, 1970. Used by permission.

8

Table 8–9.   Scoring Table for Twelve Minute Running Test for College
Men and Women*

CATEGORY	MEN (Distance)	WOMEN (Distance)
SUPERIOR	More than 2.25 Miles	More than 1.90 Miles
EXCELLENT	2.00 to 2.24 Miles	1.65 to 1.89 Miles
GOOD	1.75 to 1.99 Miles	1.40 to 1.64 Miles
FAIR	1.50 to 1.74 Miles	1.15 to 1.39 Miles
POOR	1.25 to 1.49 Miles	.90 to 1.14 Miles
VERY POOR	Less than 1.25 Miles	Less than .90 Mile

* Courtesy of Kermit O. Nelson, Ambassador College, Big Sandy, Texas.

Table 8–10.   Scoring Table for the $1\frac{1}{2}$-Mile Run for College Men*

Standard Score	Minutes: Seconds
100	7:09
95	7.29
90	7:50
85	8:10
80	8:31
75	8:51
70	9:12
65	9:32
60	9:53
55	10:13
50	10:34
45	10:54
40	11:15
35	11:35
30	11:56
25	12:16
20	12:37
15	12:57
10	13:18
5	13:38
0	13:59

* Courtesy of Wake Forest University, Department of Physical Education. N –354,
M– 10.34

Table 8–11.   Cooper's Physical Fitness Categories for Men
for the 1½-Mile Run*

AGE (Years)	I—Very Poor	II—Poor	III—Fair	IV—Good	V—Excellent
17–29	16.30 up	14:31 16:30	12:01 14:30	10:16 12:00	10:15 Down
30–34	17:00 up	15:01 17:00	12:31 15:00	10:31 12:30	10:30 Down
35–39	17:30 up	15:31 17:30	13:01 15:30	10:46 13:00	10:45 Down
40–44	18:00 up	16:01 18:00	13:31 16:00	11:01 13:30	11:00. Down
45–49	18:30 up	16:31 18:30	14:01 16:30	11:16 14:00	11:15 Down
50 up	19:00	17:01 19:00	14:31 17:00	11:31 14:30	11:30 Down

* Department of the Air Force. GMT USAF Aerobics: Physical Fitness Program. Air Force Pamphlet. November 1969. Used by permission.

Glover Physical Fitness Items for Primary Grade Children*

Purpose. To measure status in physical fitness type items.

Evaluation. Face validity was used in the selection of the items along with validation by means of the jury technique.

Level and Sex. Boys and girls in the primary grades (ages 6, 7, 8, and 9).

Time Allotment and Number of Subjects. In view of the fact that it is difficult to make use of trained student assistants at the primary level to the extent that it is possible at a higher level, it will probably require two periods to test a class of 35 to 40 pupils.

Floor Plan and Space Requirements. An indoor or outdoor area slightly larger than 40 feet in length is needed. The testing could be set up on a station-to-station basis as shown in Figure 8–3 on the next page.

Class Organization. If leadership is available, the squad method of organizing is the best approach to testing. It can be done on a station-to-station basis for the seal crawl, the standing broad jump, and the shuttle run. The sit-ups can be administered on a mass basis with partners scoring. At this level it may be possible to use other teachers, parents, or high school students as trained assistants to man the other stations.

General Procedures. 1. The children can perform in their school clothes.
2. If possible, they should wear tennis shoes.
3. Score cards can be prepared and distributed in advance.

* Glover, Elizabeth G.: Physical Fitness Test Items for Boys and Girls in the First, Second, and Third Grades, Unpublished Master's Thesis, The Woman's College, University of North Carolina, Greensboro, N.C., 1962. Adapted by permission of the author.

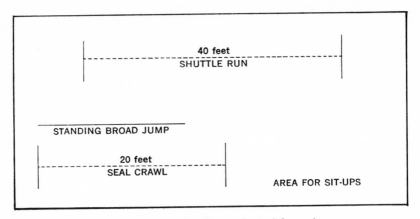

FIG. 8-3.   Floor plan for Glover physical fitness items.

Uses.   The results of these items are useful in determining the status and achievement of primary age children in physical fitness.   When the scores are analyzed, it is possible to detect weaknesses.   Undoubtedly the items have a motivating effect on the individuals.   Weaknesses should be used to plan a better program and should indicate to the teacher there is a job to be done.

Test Description

ITEM NUMBER I—STANDING BROAD JUMP

Purpose: To measure power and leg strength.

Facilities and Equipment: Take-off mark on the floor with chalk or masking tape, tape measure, and chalk.   Mats are optional.

Procedure: See North Carolina Fitness Test.

Instructions: For first grade students the following instructions: "Stand right behind this line.   Are your toes touching the line?   Good!   I want to see how far you can jump.   Let's see if you can be a big frog and jump right over the water!   That time you landed in the water. . . . Let's see if you can jump over the water this time!   Are your feet set?   Good!   One more time, let's see if you can really jump all the way over the water!   Very good!"   For second and third graders the following instructions will suffice: "Stand right behind this line.   Bend your knees and swing your arms, and show me how far you can jump.   Good!   Now try jumping to here (point the yardstick to a distance of 6 inches beyond the last distance jumped).   Very good!   Let's try one more time and see if you can jump to here!   Good!"

Scoring: The measurement is made from the take-off line to the nearest point where any part of the body touches the floor.   Three trials are permitted and the best one is recorded to the nearest inch.

Testing Personnel: One trained assistant to judge, score, and record results.

ITEM NUMBER II—SHUTTLE RACE

Purpose: To measure leg strength, speed, and endurance.

Facilities and Equipment: Two lines on the floor 40 feet apart marked with chalk or masking tape indoors or lime outdoors; two waste paper baskets placed on the floor—one inside and touching the starting line and the other inside and touching the other line 40 feet away; a stop watch.

Procedure: The student stands with his feet behind the starting line. On the signal, "Ready, go," he runs as fast as possible around the two waste paper baskets until he has completed five round trips or a distance of 400 feet. If he becomes tired running, he may walk. The timer should count each trip as the runner completes it.

Instructions: "Stand behind the starting line. Are your feet behind the line? Do you see these two baskets? Good! How fast can you go around *both* of the baskets *five* times? See, I will show you how to make one trip. Up to this basket and back to this basket is one time around both baskets. If you become tired—walk, but show me how fast you can go around the baskets five times. Ready, go!"

Scoring: The score is the elapsed time to the nearest tenth of a second that it takes the student to run or walk around both baskets five times.

Testing Personnel: One trained assistant can administer this test and time and record the scores.

ITEM NUMBER III—SEAL CRAWL (Fig. 8–4)

Purpose: To measure arm and shoulder girdle strength, endurance, and speed.

Facilities and Equipment: A starting line and a finish line 20 feet apart marked with chalk or masking tape; a stop watch.

Procedure: The subject assumes a prone position behind the starting line. He raises and supports his chest and shoulders by placing his hands on the floor and keeping his elbows straight. His finger tips face backward and his wrists forward. The knees should be off the floor and the feet extended so the toes point backward. At the signal, "Go!" the student moves toward and across the finish line by pulling his body with the arms. The exercise will have the appearance of a seal crawl. If the student falls, he should lift his body and continue. It is a foul to touch the floor with the knees or to push with the feet. In case of a foul, the test should be taken again.

Instructions: "Do you know how a seal crawls? Get flat on the floor and hold yourself up with your arms. Good! Now see if you can move your

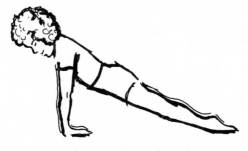

Fig. 8–4.   The seal crawl.

hands and pull yourself with your fingers pointing backward! Don't let your knees touch the floor. Very good! Are your hands behind the line? Show me how quickly you can crawl just like a seal all the way over the tape. Ready. Go!"

Scoring: The score is the elapsed time to the nearest tenth of a second that it takes the student to travel with the seal crawl from the starting line to the finish line. The watch should be stopped when his hand touches the finish line.

Testing Personnel: One trained assistant can administer this test and time and record scores.

ITEM NUMBER IV—SIT-UPS

Purpose: To measure abdominal strength, endurance, and speed.

Facilities and Equipment: A stop watch.

Procedure: The student lies down on his back with his legs bent up and his feet flat on the floor close to his body. His hands should be clasped behind his head. On the signal, "Ready. Go!" the student will sit up, touching his elbows to his knees and go back down to the floor to the starting position. He should do as many sit-ups as possible in 30 seconds and a partner should hold his feet to the floor.

Instructions: "Lie on your back and bend your knees. Good! Put your hands behind your head. Show me how many times you can roll up into a very tiny ball. Ready. Go!"

Scoring: The score is the number of complete sit-ups in the 30-second time period.

Testing Personnel: One leader can administer the test from a central location and the partner who holds the feet can count the scores.

Score Card

GLOVER PHYSICAL FITNESS ITEMS FOR PRIMARY GRADE CHILDREN

Name _____ School _____

Grade _____ Age _____ Sex _____ Date _____

Event	First Test		Second Test	
	Raw Score	Percentile	Raw Score	Percentile
Broad Jump				
Shuttle Race				
Seal Crawl Race				
Sit-Ups				

Norms

Table 8–12. Percentile Norms for Age Six

Percentile	Broad Jump (In.)	Shuttle Race (Sec.)	Seal Crawl Test (Sec.)	Sit-Ups (No.)	Percentile
95	51	41.1	7.0	12	95
90	49	42.8	7.6		90
85	48	43.5	8.1		85
80	47	44	8.7	11	80
75	46	44.5	9.0	10	75
70	45	44.9	9.4	9	70
65		45.4	9.8		65
60	44	45.6	10.1	9	60
55	43	46.0	10.5	8	55
50	42	46.4	10.9		50
45	41	46.7	11.3	7	45
40	40	47.4	11.7	6	40
35		47.9	12.2	5	35
30	39	48.6	12.6	4	30
25	38	49.5	13.1	3	25
20	37	50.5	14.3		20
15	36	51.3	19.0	2	15
10	35	52.3	25.1		10
5	33	54.0	33.1	1	5

Charlotte Public Schools, Charlotte, N.C.   N = 73

Table 8–13. Percentile Norms for Age Seven

Percentiles	Broad Jump (In.)	Shuttle Race (Sec.)	Seal Crawl Test (Sec.)	Sit-Ups (No.)	Percentiles
95	53	41.3	7.6	15	95
90	51	42		14	90
85	50	42.5	8.0	13	85
80	49	43.1	8.8	12	80
75		43.5	9.0		75
70	48	43.8	9.5	11	70
65	46	44.4	10.0		65
60	45	44.8	10.3	10	60
55	44	45.5	10.9	9	55
50	43	46.1	11.1		50
45	42	46.5	11.3		45
40	41	47.0	11.8	8	40
35		47.6	12.6	7	35
30	40	48.4	13.3	6	30
25	39	48.8	15.0	5	25
20	38	49.5	16.7	4	20
15		50.3	19.5	2	15
10	37	50.8	24.2		10
5	34	52.6	39.5	1	5

Charlotte Public Schools, Charlotte, N.C.   N = 83

Table. 8–14. Percentile Norms for Age Eight

Percentiles	Broad Jump (In.)	Shuttle Race (Sec.)	Seal Crawl Test (Sec.)	Sit-Ups (No.)	Percentiles
95	63	39.9	5.9	17	95
90	59	41.1	6.9	15	90
85	58	41.5		14	85
80	57	41.6	7.1	13	80
75	55	42.0	7.4		75
70	54	42.5	7.8		70
65	53	42.8	8.0	12	65
60	51	43.2	8.4		60
55		43.5	8.8	11	55
50	50	43.8	9.2	10	50
45	49	44.2	9.5		45
40	48	44.5	9.9	9	40
35	47	45.0	10.5	8	35
30	46	45.4	10.9	7	30
25	45	45.9	11.5	6	25
20	43	46.5	12.0	5	20
15	42	47.5	13.3	4	15
10	40	48.8	14.9	2	10
5	38	50.0	18.5	1	5

Charlotte Public Schools, Charlotte, N.C.   N = 118

Table 8–15. Percentile Norms for Age Nine

Percentiles	Broad Jump (In.)	Shuttle Race (Sec.)	Seal Crawl Test (Sec.)	Sit-Ups (No.)	Percentiles
95	62	38.5	4.9	18	95
90	59	39.2	5.3	16	90
85	58	39.5	5.8		85
80		40.2	6.3	14	80
75	57	40.9	6.5		75
70	56	41.5	6.9		70
65		41.7	7.3	13	65
60	55	41.9	7.6		60
55	54		8.0		55
50	52	42.0	8.3		50
45	51	42.5	8.7		45
40	50	42.9	9.1	12	40
35	49	43.5	9.5	11	35
30	48	44.1	9.9		30
25	47	45.0	11.0		25
20	46	45.9	12.4	10	20
15	45	46.5	13.4	8	15
10	44	47.0	14.4	6	10
5	43	47.9	16.9	2	5

Charlotte Public Schools, Charlotte, N.C.   N = 50

The Harvard Step Test*

Purpose. To measure general capacity of the body and especially the heart and circulatory system to adapt to and recover from hard work.

Evaluation. The Harvard Step Test has been validated by means of endurance in treadmill running, maximum heart rate per minute, and blood lactate level, and it measures a kind of general endurance.

Level and Sex. This test was originally designed for college men by Brouha, but has been modified and adapted to both sexes from elementary school through college by Brouha and others.[6,10]

Time Allotment and Number of Subjects. If sufficient bench space is available along with enough trained leadership, a class of 30 to 35 can be tested in one period. The 5-minute step test will require approximately 10 minutes to administer to each group.

Floor Plan and Space Requirement. If just one or two students are to be tested at a time, only a small space is needed. However, when one half the class takes the test while the other half observes and records scores, more space is required and the benches should be set up in an orderly fashion so that there will be as little interference as possible. Benches should be arranged in rows and if a wall clock is used, the benches should be placed so the observers can face the clock. (See Fig. 8–5.)

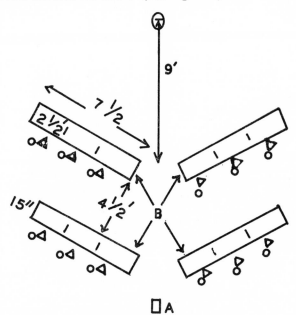

Fig. 8–5. Suggested floor plan for the Harvard step test. *A*, Instructor counting cadence. *B*, Benches. △, Students taking the test. *O*, Students observing and counting pulse. (Weiss, R. A., and Marjorie Phillips, *Administration of Tests in Physical Education.* St. Louis, The C. V. Mosby Co., 1954. Adapted by permission of the publisher and R. A. Weiss.)

* Brouha, Lucien: The Step Test: A Simple Method of Measuring Physical Fitness for Muscular Work in Young Men, Research Quarterly, *14*, 31–36, March, 1942. Adapted by permission of the author.

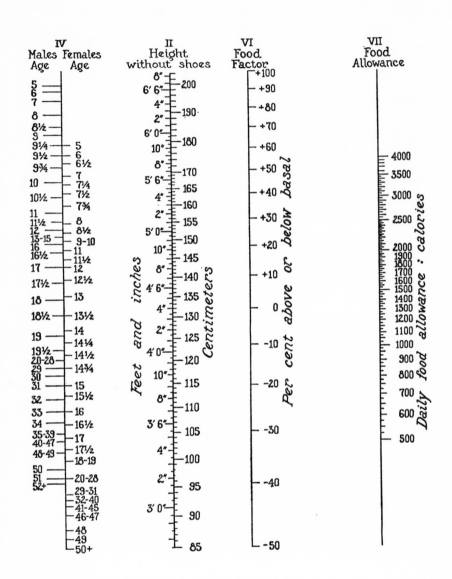

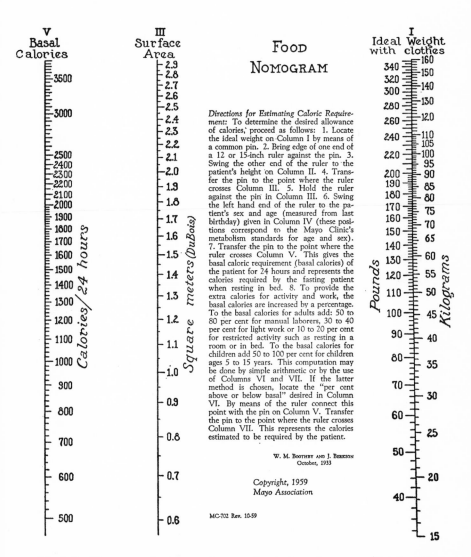

V
Basal Calories

=3500

=3000

=2500
=2400
=2300
=2200
=2100
=2000
1900
1800
1700
1600
1500
1400
1300
1200
1100
1000
900
800
700
600
500

Calories/24 hours

III
Surface Area

2.9
2.8
2.7
2.6
2.5
2.4
2.3
2.2
2.1
2.0
1.9
1.8
1.7
1.6
1.5
1.4
1.3
1.2
1.1
1.0
0.9
0.8
0.7
0.6

Square meters (DuBois)

FOOD

NOMOGRAM

Directions for Estimating Caloric Requirement: To determine the desired allowance of calories, proceed as follows: 1. Locate the ideal weight on Column I by means of a common pin. 2. Bring edge of one end of a 12 or 15-inch ruler against the pin. 3. Swing the other end of the ruler to the patient's height on Column II. 4. Transfer the pin to the point where the ruler crosses Column III. 5. Hold the ruler against the pin in Column III. 6. Swing the left hand end of the ruler to the patient's sex and age (measured from last birthday) given in Column IV (these positions correspond to the Mayo Clinic's metabolism standards for age and sex). 7. Transfer the pin to the point where the ruler crosses Column V. This gives the basal caloric requirement (basal calories) of the patient for 24 hours and represents the calories required by the fasting patient when resting in bed. 8. To provide the extra calories for activity and work, the basal calories are increased by a percentage. To the basal calories for adults add: 50 to 80 per cent for manual laborers, 30 to 40 per cent for light work or 10 to 20 per cent for restricted activity such as resting in a room or in bed. To the basal calories for children add 50 to 100 per cent for children ages 5 to 15 years. This computation may be done by simple arithmetic or by the use of Columns VI and VII. If the latter method is chosen, locate the "per cent above or below basal" desired in Column VI. By means of the ruler connect this point with the pin on Column V. Transfer the pin to the point where the ruler crosses Column VII. This represents the calories estimated to be required by the patient.

W. M. BOOTHBY AND J. BERKSON
October, 1933

Copyright, 1959
Mayo Association

MC-702 Rev. 10-59

I
Ideal Weight with clothes

340
320
300
280
260
240
220
200
190
180
170
160
150
140
130
120
110
100
90
80
70
60
50
40

Pounds

160
150
140
130
120
110
105
100
95
90
85
80
75
70
65
60
55
50
45
40
35
30
25
20
15

Kilograms

Fig. 8–6.   Nomogram chart for use in computing body surface area. (Use the following directions: (1) Locate weight in column I. (2) Locate height in column II. (3) Connect these two points with a ruler. (4) The point on column III which intersects with the ruler gives the body surface area. (Reproduced by permission of the Mayo Association, Rochester, Minnesota.)

Class Organization. The quickest and most economical method of class organization is the mass technique with partners observing and scoring.

General Procedure. 1. Orientation of all students may be done at the same time by the director of testing.

2. If some students must await their turn to be tested, they should remain quietly seated until their testing turn begins.

3. Timing may be done in one of three ways: first, it may be done by each partner if enough stop watches are available; second, it may be done by use of a large wall clock which is placed so that all partners doing the scoring can see it; and third, and perhaps the most economical way, the director of testing himself may do all the timing and calling out the signals.

4. Pulse count may be taken at either the wrist or the carotid artery.

5. The bench height should be gauged to the level and sex of the group.

6. The height and weight should be measured for high school boys and their surface area calculated by means of the nomographic chart. (See Figure 8–6.)

Uses. The results of this test are used to appraise physical condition. Since the test obviously does not measure specifically such factors as strength, muscular endurance, nor cardiovascular endurance, it does measure a general endurance which seems to be necessary for living one's daily normal activities in an effective and efficient manner. Its results may be used to classify individuals into three groups: (*a*) the least fit, (*b*) fit, and (*c*) the most fit. After classification, fitness programs may be designed for each group based on the individual's need.

Test Description

Facilities and Equipment: For college men[2] and for high school boys[7] with a body surface area of at least 1.85 square meters, a 20-inch bench is used. For college women[5] and high school boys with a body surface area of less than 1.85 square meters, an 18-inch bench is employed. For high school girls[3] the bench has been reduced to 16 inches, and for both boys and girls below the age of 12 years,[7] the bench height is 14 inches. The bench should be secured to the floor or be heavy enough not to move around when the subjects are stepping up and down. A stop watch, timer, or wall clock with a large minute hand is needed for timing. A metronome is desirable to help the instructor count the cadence.

Procedures: This is a one-item test which includes step-ups on a bench for a prescribed period of time followed by a count of the pulse rate. The group which is to be tested can be divided into partners by counting off into two's so there will be one observer for each student being tested. Number one's will take the test first while number two's will serve as observers and scorers. The students being tested will face the bench and wait for the signal to start. The director of testing will give the commands as follows: "Ready," "Up," "Two," "Three," "Four," "Up," "Two," "Three," "Four," etc. The signal "Up" should be called out every 2 seconds. On the command of "Up" the testee will step up on the bench with one foot. On the command of "Two" he will step up with the other foot to an erect position. On the command "Three" he will step down with the lead foot, and on the command of "Four" he will step down with the other foot to the original starting position. These four counts make up one complete cycle and the testee will repeat this cycle at the rate of 30 cycles per minute for 5 minutes for college men,[2] 4 minutes for high school boys[7] (age 12 to 18 years) and high school girls[3] and college women,[5] 3 minutes for elementary children (8 to 12 years old), and 2 minutes for children under 8 years.[4] The cadence for these mounts and dismounts is called out by the test director. The subject will continue for the duration of the time limit unless he is forced to drop out sooner due to exhaustion. The testee may change the lead-off foot no more than three times during the time limit. At the end of the exercise period, the test director will give the command, "Stop," "Sit down." The testee should sit down immediately on the bench and remain quiet (Fig. 8–7).

The number two's will locate their partner's pulse so they may be ready to count on the signal. The pulse may be felt at either the wrist or the side of the throat over the carotid artery. The instructor will call out the following signals at the times indicated:

> One minute after exercise he calls, "Start Counting!"
> One and one-half minutes after exercise he calls, "Stop!"
> Two minutes after exercise he calls, "Start Counting!"
> Two and one-half minutes after exercise he calls, "Stop!"
> Three minutes after exercise he calls, "Start Counting!"
> Three and one-half minutes after exercise he calls, "Stop!"

After each counting period the observer will record the number of pulse counts on the score card and when all three counts have been taken, he will find the total count for the three. At this point, number two's will take the test while number one's serve as observers and scorers.

If, during the time limit, a testee fails to finish the test or if he can't keep pace with the cadence and is stopped, his observer should record the actual time he performed.

Instructions: Number one's (the testees) stand in front of your bench. On the signal to begin, you step up on the bench with your lead foot on the count of "Up" and the other foot on the count of "Two." At this point you should have both feet firmly planted on the bench and be standing erect with your legs straight. On the count of "Three" you step down to the rear with the lead foot and on "Four" you should be in the starting position and ready to start the next cycle. You will step up and down keeping pace with the cadence until the instructor calls, "Stop." At this point you will sit down on your bench and remain there until your pulse rate has

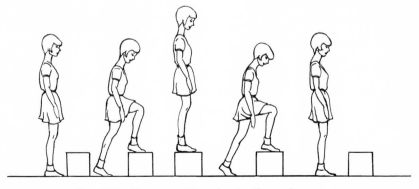

Fig. 8–7.   Various positions for the Harvard step test.

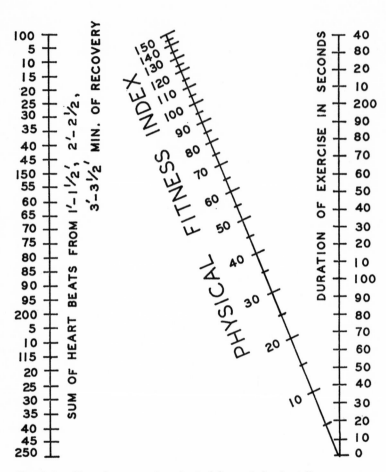

FIG. 8–8. Chart for computing physical fitness index for college women.

been counted three different times. During the exercise period you may change the lead foot in stepping up on the bench not more than three times.

Number two's (observers and scorers) will stand near to your partner but to one side so as not to interfere with his performance. You should observe that your partner is keeping pace with the cadence that is being called out and is coming to an erect position with each step-up. If he is failing to do so for either one or the other or both, you should try to encourage and coach him into the correct procedure. When the time limit is up and the instructor calls, "Stop!" see that your partner sits down on his bench and remains quiet. While you are awaiting a signal from your instructor, locate your partner's pulse. The pulse in the wrist can be found on the palm side of the hand just an inch or so up the radial edge of the wrist from the base of the thumb. When you locate this area, place your first and second finger lightly over the point. Do *not* use the thumb. When the instructor calls out, "Start Counting!" you count the number of pulse beats until he says, "Stop." You record this score on the score card and locate the pulse again and follow instructions until you have counted the pulse rate three times. After you record the third pulse count, sum the scores for a final index.

Scoring: The score is calculated with data from the duration of the exercise in seconds and the sum of the three one-half minute pulse counts. The following *formula* is used.

$$\text{Fitness Index} = \frac{\text{Length of the exercise in seconds} \times 100}{2 \times \text{sum of the pulse counts in the three recovery periods}}$$

However, except for those students who fail to finish the exercise, it is not necessary to use the formula since tables have been computed in order to convert the raw scores to index scores quickly. The scores from the three pulse counts should be summed and referred to the appropriate table. The following tables are available: Table 8–12 for college men,[2] Table 8–13 for high school boys,[7] and Table 8–14 for high school girls.[3] College women[5] scores may be obtained from Figure 8–8.

In order to use the chart shown in Figure 8–8 for scoring college women, the following instructions apply. The scale at the left of the chart carries the sum of the three pulse counts and the scale at the right carries the duration of the exercise in seconds. When a straight edge or ruler is used to connect a student's pulse count for the three periods with the duration of her exercise in seconds, her physical fitness index can be read at the point indicated by the straight edge on the diagonal scale.

College men and women and high school boys may have their scores interpreted according to a classification scheme. The classification chart for college men and women (the same table is used for interpreting women's scores as men's) is shown at the bottom of Table 8–15. The classification for high school boys is shown at the bottom of Table 8–16.

If the student does not continue to exercise for the prescribed period of time, his three pulse counts should be taken from the point when he stopped exercising, and the formula applied. However, for some levels, less exact scoring bases may be used for those students who fail to finish the full time allotment. This makes it unnecessary to break into the routine of counting pulse rate for the drop-outs. This is handled in an arbitrary manner as shown by the following:

For college men		For high school girls	
Duration	*Score*	*Duration*	*Score*
Less than 2 minutes	25	2 minutes	25
		$2\frac{1}{2}$ minutes	30
From 2 to 3 minutes	38	3 minutes	35
From 3 to $3\frac{1}{2}$ minutes	48	$3\frac{1}{2}$ minutes	40
From $3\frac{1}{2}$ to 4 minutes	52	(Those who finish but	45
From 4 to $4\frac{1}{2}$ minutes	55	lag or fail to follow	
From $4\frac{1}{2}$ to 5 minutes	59	instructions)	

For high school boys—all who fail to finish are given a score of 45 and those who finish but lag are given a score of 55.

The average scores for children 12 years of age and under are as follows:

Age	*Average Score*
7 and under	40
7 to 10	57
10 to 12	61

Scores above average may be considered as good and those below average as poor.

Testing Personnel: One instructor can do all the timing and calling the cadence and signals. The counting of scores and the observation of performance can be done by student partners with a minimum of training.

Score Card

HARVARD STEP TEST
SCORING FORM

Name _____ Age _____ Sex _____

Recovery Period	Pulse Count	
$1'–1\frac{1}{2}'$	_____	Index = $\dfrac{\text{Duration of the exercise} \times 100}{2 \times \text{sum of 3 pulse counts}}$
$2'–2\frac{1}{2}'$	_____	$= \dfrac{(\quad) \times 100}{2 \times (\quad)}$
$3'–3\frac{1}{2}'$	_____	$= \dfrac{(\quad)}{(\quad)}$
Sum of 3 pulse counts	_____	Index =
Classification	_____	

(Courtesy of Raymond A. Weiss: *Administration of Tests in Physical Education* by Weiss, R. A., and Phillips, Marjorie. St. Louis, The C. V. Mosby Co., 1954.)

Norms

Table 8–16. Norms for College Men

Pulse	Score	Pulse	Score	Pulse	Score
100	150	129	116	172–173	87
101	149	130	115	174–175	86
102	147	131–132	114	176–177	85
103	146	133	113	178–179	84
104	144	134	112	180–181	83
105	143	135	111	182–184	82
106	142	136	110	185–186	81
107	140	137–138	109	187–188	80
108	139	139	108	189–191	79
109	138	140	107	192–193	78
110	136	141–142	106	194–196	77
111	135	143	105	197–198	76
112	134	144	104	199–201	75
113	133	145–146	103	202–204	74
114	132	147	102	205–206	73
115	130	148–149	101	207–209	72
116	129	150	100	210–212	71
117	128	151–152	99	213–215	70
118	127	153	98	216–218	69
119	126	154–155	97	219–222	68
120	125	156–157	96	223–225	67
121	124	158	95	226–229	66
122	123	159–160	94	230–232	65
123	122	161–162	93	233–236	64
124	121	163	92	237–239	63
125	120	164–165	91	240–243	62
126	119	166–167	90	244–247	61
127	118	168–169	89	248–250	60
128	117	170–171	88		

CLASSIFICATION

Excellent	above 90
Good	80–89
Average	65–79
Below Average	55–64
Poor	Up to 54

Table 8–17. Norms for High School Boys

Pulse	Score	Pulse	Score	Pulse	Score
110	109	140	86	172	70
111	108	141	85	173	70
112	107	142	85	174	69
113	106	143	84	175	69
114	105	144	83	176	68
115	104	145	83	177	68
116	103	146	82	178	67
117	102	147	82	179	67
118	102	148	81	180	67
119	101	149	81	181	66
120	100	150	80	182	66
121	99	151	80	183	66
122	98	152	79	184	65
123	98	153	78	185	65
124	97	154	78	186	65
125	96	155	77	189	64
126	95	156	77	190	63
127	95	158	76	191	63
128	94	160	75	192	63
129	93	161	75	193	62
130	92	162	74	194	62
131	92	163	74	195	61
132	92	164	73	196	61
133	90	165	73	197	61
134	90	166	72	198	60
135	89	167	72	199	60
136	88	168	71	200	60
137	88	169–	71	201	59
138	87	170	71	203	59
139	86	171	70	208	58

CLASSIFICATION

Superior	91 and up
Excellent	81–90
Good	71–80
Fair	61–70
Poor	51–60
Very poor	50 and down

Table 8–18. Norms for High School Girls

Pulse	Score	Pulse	Score	Pulse	Score
105	114	140	86	177	68
106	113	141	85	178	67
107	112	142	85	179	67
108	111	143	84	180	67
109	110	144	83	181	66
110	109	145	82	182	66
111	108	146	82	183	66
112	107	147	82	184	65
113	106	148	81	185	65
114	105	149	81	186	65
115	104	150	80	189	64
116	103	151	80	190	63
117	102	152	79	191	63
118	102	153	78	192	63
119	101	154	78	193	62
120	100	155	77	194	62
121	99	156	77	195	61
122	98	158	76	196	61
123	98	160	75	197	61
124	97	161	75	198	61
125	96	162	74	199	60
126	95	163	74	200	60
127	95	164	73	201	60
128	94	165	73	203	59
129	93	166	72	208	58
130	92	167	72	210	57
131	92	168	71	214	56
132	92	169	71	218	55
133	90	170	71	222	54
134	90	171	70	226	53
135	89	172	70	230	52
136	88	173	70	235	51
137	88	174	69	240	50
138	87	175	69		
139	86	176	68		

New York State Physical Fitness Test*

Purpose. To measure status and progress in physical fitness.

Evaluation. The items were evaluated and selected on the basis of their validity, reliability and ease of administration.

Level and Sex. Boys and girls, grade 4 through grade 12.

Time Allotment and Number of Subjects. A class of 30 pupils will require four or five 45-minute periods for completing the test. This assumes that one teacher will direct the testing and that a separate period will be used for orientation procedures and for posture, and two or three periods for the actual testing of the six other items. If more stations and assistants are used, the time for testing can be materially reduced.

Floor Plan and Space Requirements. Posture—For each posture testing station an area of 5 by 15 feet will be needed.

Accuracy, strength, and agility—Any size gymnasium can be used for the next three test items and a number of testing stations can be set up for each item.

Speed—This testing area will require an area several yards wide and at least 75 yards long and will probably need to be set up for outdoor administration.

Balance and endurance—These areas can be set up in a similar manner at one end or side of the gymnasium. If the mass system of testing is applied, enough stations to test one half the class can be set up.

Class Organization. The test battery can be administered on a combination of the station-to-station and squad methods of class organization. The number of test stations for the various items is always related to the type of item and the availability of leadership.

The posture test can be administered on a station basis and as many stations should be provided as there are trained examiners.

The pull-up, target throw, and side stepping can be administered during one period with the class being divided into squads and a station for each squad, with partners scoring. The 50-yard dash, the squat-stand, and the treadmill can be administered during another class period in the same manner with respect to squads, stations, and scoring.

General Procedure. 1. If more than one item is administered to any pupil during one testing period, the following order of events should be maintained: target throw, push-up or pull-up, side step, 50-yard dash, squat-stand, and treadmill.

2. One period should be devoted to orientation of the students. This would include giving the purpose, explanation of procedures, demonstration of test items, and a practice period for students to practice unfamiliar items, layout of the testing stations, organization of the class, use of the score card, and scoring and recording results.

3. The student may fill out his score card during the orientation period.

4. No student should be given this test battery if his medical status is questionable.

---

* State of New York: *The New York State Physical Fitness Test: A Manual for Teachers of Physical Education.* Albany, Division of Health, Physical Education, and Recreation, New York State Education Department, 1958. Adapted by permission of the State Department of Education.

5. If the results of this test are to be interpreted according to the test norms, the specific directions and procedures for administration must be followed exactly.

Uses. The results of this physical fitness test may be used specifically as follows:

First, such test results provide information for comparison of the student's status in physical fitness with other students of similar sex and grade.

Second, such test results provide information for comparing one component of physical fitness with another for each individual student.

Third, such test results provide information for the comparison of any student's status in either total physical fitness or any component with that of any other student at the local level.

Fourth, such test results provide information for indicating the progress or achievement in any component or for total physical fitness.

In general, the information provided above may be used to motivate the student, to assist in evaluation of the program, to help in planning program and instruction to more nearly meet the individual needs of students, to classify students into homogeneous groups, to grade, and to inform the parents concerning the physical fitness of their children.

Test Description

ITEM NUMBER I—POSTURE TEST

Purpose: To evaluate lateral and anteroposterior posture.

Facilities and Equipment: For each testing station an area 5 by 15 feet in the gym or any convenient place, heavy duty plumb line, a support for the plumb line, masking tape approximately 1 inch in width, and a screen or backdrop. The testing station should be set up as shown in Figure 8–9.

Procedures: The student takes a standing position between the plumb line and the screen with his back toward the plumb line and his feet straddling the line. The examiner assumes his position about ten feet directly to the rear of the student being tested. After the student has been rated for the lateral position, he assumes the anteroposterior position for rating by making a one-quarter turn to the left and stands comfortably and naturally with his left side to the plumb line and his feet at right angles to the floor line and his left ankle bone in line with the plumb bob. The examiner, using the Posture Rating Chart, rates each student by scoring him in each of the 13 segments. Each segment is scored 5, 3, or 1 according to the illustrations and descriptions (see Figure 8–10).

Instructions: Take your position with feet comfortably apart and straddling the end line with your back just in front of the plumb line and facing the screen. Stand comfortably and naturally in a relaxed manner. On the signal "Turn" you are to make a one-quarter turn toward your left with your feet at right angles to the floor line and your left ankle bone in line with the plumb bob. Stand comfortably and naturally in the same manner as before.

Scoring: By making comparisons with Posture Rating Chart, each student is scored from 5, 3, or 1 in each of thirteen segments. These thirteen scores are summed with a possible low of 13 and a high of 65.

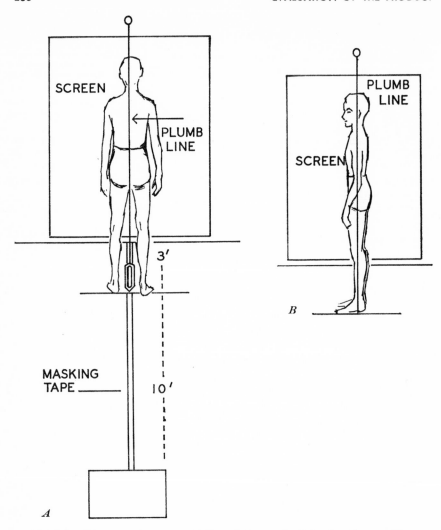

Fig. 8–9. Diagram of posture testing station. *A*, Lateral rating position.
B, Anteroposterior rating position.

Testing Personnel: Posture ratings should be made by the physical education teacher, nurse, or physician, or any other person whose training qualifies him to make such ratings.

ITEM NUMBER II—ACCURACY TEST (TARGET THROW) (Fig. 8–11 *A*)

Purpose: To measure accuracy.

Facilities and Equipment: The following equipment is needed: four or more inseam 12-inch softballs, masking tape 1-inch wide, small box for the balls at the throwing line, and a target. The target with an outside diameter of

2 feet and the center placed 4 feet from the floor can be scribed on a mat hanging from the wall or on some other padded wall surface. Directly in front of the target on the floor a restraining or throwing line is placed with the masking tape. The distance from the target is 30 feet for all girls and for 4, 5, and 6 grade boys. The distance is 35 feet for all boys above the 6th grade.

Procedures: The student takes a position behind the restraining line and uses an overhand throw. He has two series of 10 throws each to hit the target. These series may not be taken in succession.

Instructions: You must stand behind the restraining line and make your throw overhand. It is a foul to step over the line in making the throw.

Scoring: One point is scored each time the ball hits the target and a ball hitting the line is good. Highest possible score is 20.

Testing Personnel: One leader can administer the test while the class is paired into partners and partners can judge the hits, count the score, and record results.

ITEM NUMBER IIIa—STRENGTH TEST (MODIFIED PUSH-UP) (Fig. 8–11 *B*)

Purpose: To measure strength for 4, 5, 6 grade boys and girls.

Facilities and Equipment: The same general area used in the target throw will suffice for the modified push-ups. One large size mat and a stall bar bench 11 by 21 by 14 inches. The bench and mat are placed so the student's feet will touch the wall when he is being tested.

Procedures: The student assumes a front leaning rest position on the bench with his feet flat against the wall and his hands grasping the outer edges of the bench. The body and arms should form a right angle. The student from this position dips down by bending his arms until his chest touches the edge of the bench lightly. He then pushes up to the starting position.

Instructions: You place your feet flat against the wall. Grasp the bench with your hands on the outside edges and assume a straight arm position with your back straight. Let your chest down until it touches the bench by bending your arms, and then push back up to the straight arm position. You may go as fast or slow as you like but you may not rest between push-ups. It is a foul not to go all the way down, or all the way up, and not to keep the body straight at all times. The body must not be arched nor sway forward on the up or down stroke.

Scoring: One point is scored each time a complete push-up is made. No half scores may be counted.

Testing Personnel: One leader is necessary to administer the test while the partners judge the push-ups, count the number, and record the score.

ITEM NUMBER IIIb—STRENGTH TEST (MODIFIED PULL-UP) (Fig. 8–11 *C*)

Purpose: To measure strength for girls grades 7 through 12.

Facilities and Equipment: A large mat and either a horizontal bar or ladder. The bar should be adjusted to a height even with the bottom of girl's breast bone. If a ladder is used, it should be placed at a 45-degree angle.

POSTURE RATING CHART

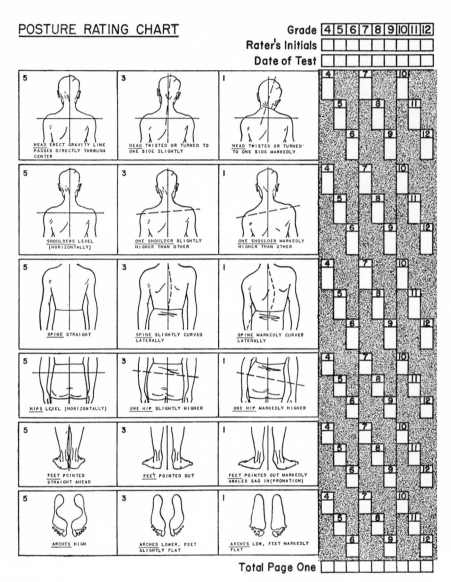

Grade | 4 | 5 | 6 | 7 | 8 | 9 | 10 | 11 | 12

Rater's Initials

Date of Test

Total Page One

Fig. 8–10. (*Continued on opposite page.*)

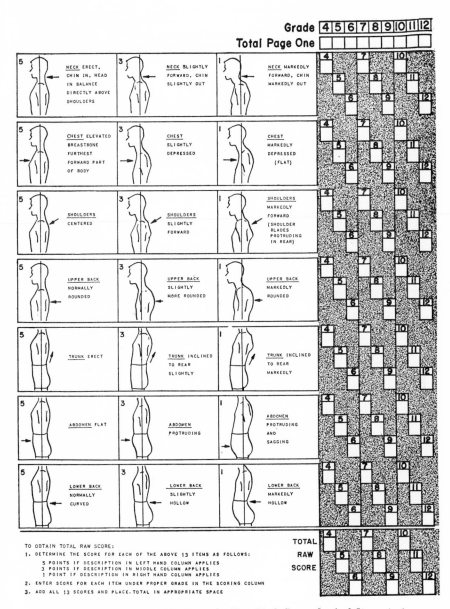

Fig. 8–10. Posture profiles from the New York State physical fitness test.

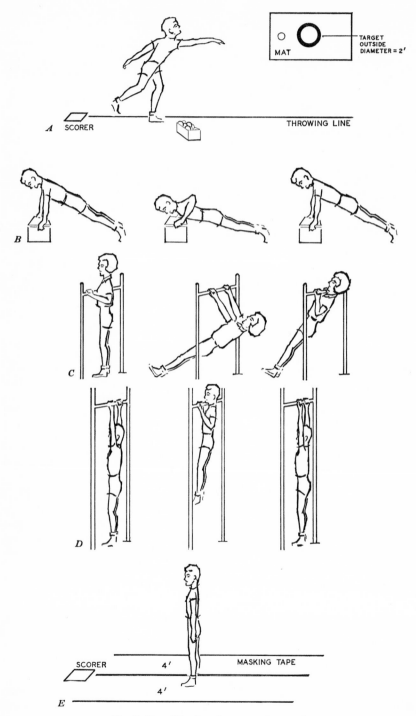

Fig. 8–11. *(Continued on opposite page.)*

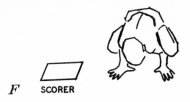

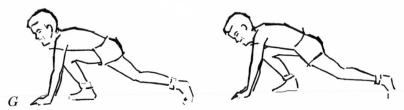

Fig. 8–11. Test items for the New York State physical fitness test. *A*, Target throw. *B*, Modified push-up. *C*, Modified pull-up. *D*, Pull-up. *E*, Side step. *F*, Squat-stand. *G*, Treadmill.

Procedures: The girl should grasp the bar with her palms facing upward and slide her feet under the bar until her body and legs are completely extended with the arms now at an angle of 90 degrees with the chest. The legs and body should comprise a straight line and form an angle of approximately 45 degrees with the floor with the weight of the body resting on the heels. The feet of the student can be braced to prevent slipping by the scorer placing her foot sideways under the insteps. From this position the girl pulls up with her arms until they are completely bent and her chest touches the bar or rung. She then returns to the starting position and repeats as many times as possible.

Instructions: Grasp the bar with your hands facing toward you. You must touch your chest against the bar on the pull-up. You must not let your hips sag or rise during the performance but keep the trunk and legs in a straight line, and you must straighten your arms completely as you lower your body back to the starting position. You may go as fast or slow as you like, but you may not rest between pull-ups.

Scoring: One point is scored for each complete pull-up.

Testing Personnel: One leader is necessary to administer the test while the partners judge the pull-ups, count the number, and record the score.

ITEM NUMBER IIIc—STRENGTH TEST (PULL-UP) (Fig. 8–11 *D*)

Purpose: To measure strength for boys, grades 7 through 12.

Facilities and Equipment: Standard horizontal bar with a mat underneath for protection. The bar should be adjusted so the tallest boy may hang freely.

Procedures: The boy should grasp the bar with his palms facing toward him and from a still hang from full extension of the arms pull himself up by flexing his arms until his chin is level with the bar. He then lowers his body to the starting position with his arms fully extended. This movement is repeated as many times as possible.

Instructions: You must grasp the bar with your palms facing toward you. You must lift your chin level with the bar and go all the way down until your arms are fully extended. You may proceed as fast or slow as you like but you may not rest between pull-ups. You must not lift your knees or assist your pull-up by kicking or swaying the body.

Scoring: One point is scored for each complete pull-up.

Testing Personnel: One leader is necessary to administer the test while partners judge the pull-ups, count the number, and record the score.

ITEM NUMBER IV—AGILITY TEST (SIDE STEP) (Fig. 8–11 *E*)

Purpose: To measure agility.

Facilities and Equipment: Three 5-foot long parallel lines on the floor a distance of 4 feet apart and a stop watch. The lines may be made with 1–inch masking tape.

Procedures: The student assumes a starting position astride the center line with feet parallel to the lines. On the signal to start, the student sidesteps to his left until his left foot has touched the floor beyond the left hand line. This counts another point. He continues to sidestep back and forth in this manner as rapidly as possible in 10 seconds.

Instructions: You must face in the same direction with your feet parallel to the lines throughout the performance. You must not cross your feet at any time and you must not turn or twist the hips or shoulders. You must step beyond the outside lines.

Scoring: One point is scored each time the student crosses one of the three lines in the allotted 10 seconds. The score is the total number of such crossings.

Testing Personnel: One examiner is necessary to operate the stop watch and call out the start and finish of the time interval. Partners can judge the crossings, count the number and record the score. This can be done within each squad or, if there are sufficient stations for the entire class.

ITEM NUMBER V—(SPEED TEST) (50-YARD DASH)

Purpose: To measure speed.

Facilities and Equipment: A hard surface area of at least 75 yards long with sufficient width to permit enough lanes of 3 feet width. There should be one lane for each squad. Stop watch, starting flag, and rubber-soled shoes for all students. The lanes should be marked with a starting and finishing line 50 yards apart.

Procedures: The first student in each squad assumes a standing position behind the starting line. Squad leaders are at the finish and judge the times which are called out by the starter and record the scores. The starter uses the commands, "Take Your Mark! Get Set! Go!"

Directions: Start from a standing position behind the starting line and on the signal "Go!" run as fast as you can across the finish line. Do not slow down until you are across the line and then do not try to stop suddenly.

Scoring: The score is the elapsed time to the nearest half second between the starting line and the finish line.

Testing Personnel: One examiner is needed to administer the test. If there are sufficient stop watches and if the student squad leaders can operate them, the examiner may serve as the starter and permit the squad leaders to time and record scores for their squad members. If there are not sufficient stop watches or if the students are not trained in how to operate and read them, the examiner can act as timer and call out the times as the various runners cross the finish. The squad leaders can observe and record the times. The examiner may select a student to act as starter.

ITEM NUMBER VI—BALANCE TEST (SQUAT-STAND) (Fig. 8-12 *F*)

Purpose: To measure balance.

Facilities and Equipment: Mats and a stop watch or metronome.

Procedures: The student assumes a squat position. He places his hands on the floor close to the mat and just inside his feet with fingers spread and pointing outward toward the mat. His elbows are between his knees and his hands are slightly wider than shoulder width apart. He presses in with his legs at the juncture between the thigh and calf against his elbows. With head up he tips forward and assumes a hand balance with his toes off the floor. This position is held for as long a time as possible without any part of the body touching the floor except the hands.

Instructions: Your score will start to be counted when you assume the balance position with the feet off the floor. You must not touch either foot to the floor or the head to the mat. If you lose your balance before the count of five, you may try a second time and your best score is counted.

Scoring: One point is scored for each second the student remains in a squat-balance position.

Testing Personnel: One examiner is needed to administer the test and operate the stop watch or metronome and squad leaders can judge, count, and score points.

ITEM NUMBER VII—ENDURANCE TEST (TREADMILL) (Fig. 8-11 *G*)

Purpose: To measure endurance.

Facilities and Equipment: Stop watch and a mat.

Procedures: The student assumes a starting position by taking a front leaning rest similar to that for a push-up. From this position one leg is flexed until the knee is between the arms and the thigh is against the chest.

From this position with one leg fully flexed and the other fully extended the test starts. On the command, "Ready, Go!" the student exchanges the positions of his feet as fast as possible. The action of the feet is a jump from one position to the other with both feet. This jump exchange is continued as rapidly as possible for 30 seconds for all girls and 4, 5, 6 grade boys. The time is 1 minute for boys, grades 7 through 12.

Instructions: You must actually jump from one position. Your thigh must touch the chest on each exchange forward and your leg must be straight on the exchange backward. You must not slide your feet on the mat.

Scoring: One point is scored for each exchange of positions.

Testing Personnel: One examiner is needed in the same manner as the squat-stand to operate the stop watch. Judging, counting, and recording of scores can be done by squad leaders.

Score Card

New York State Physical Fitness Test
Pupil Score Card

Name _____
       Last   First   Middle

Grade	_____	
Date	Mo. _____	19 _____
Age	Yrs. _____	Mos. . _____
Height	Ft. _____	In. . _____
Weight	Lbs. _____	
Component	*raw score*	*achievement level*
1. Posture		
2. Accuracy		
3. Strength		
4. Agility		
5. Speed		
6. Balance		
7. Endurance		
Total Physical Fitness	Sum =	

Examiner_____ Date_____

CLASS RECORD SHEET

New York State Physical Fitness Test

The University of the State of New York
The State Education Department
Division of Health, Physical Education and Recreation
Bureau of Physical Education

School...Grade.........................

Date...Class.........................

NAME OF PUPIL	ACHIEVEMENT LEVELS							
	Posture	Accuracy	Strength	Agility	Speed	Balance	Endurance	Total Fitness
1.								
2.								
3.								
4.								
5.								
6.								
7.								
8.								
9.								
10.								
11.								
12.								
13.								
14.								
15.								
16.								
17.								
18.								
19.								
20.								
21.								
22.								
23.								
24.								
25.								
26.								
27.								
28.								
29.								
30.								
Total								

SUMMARY

component	class total	class average
P.		
Ac.		
St.		
Ag.		
Sp.		
B.		
E.		
total fitness		

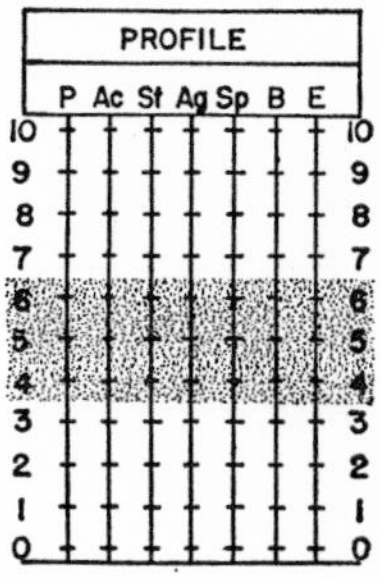

PROFILE

P Ac St Ag Sp B E

10 9 8 7 6 5 4 3 2 1 0

Fig. 8–12.   Class score card for New York State physical fitness test.

TABLE OF ACHIEVEMENT LEVEL NORMS

Table 8-19. Boys—Begin Grade 4

Achievement Level	Percentile Rank	Posture	Accuracy	Strength	Agility	Speed	Balance	Endurance	Total Physical Fitness With Posture	Without Posture	Achievement Level
10	99	—	16–20	44+	20+	0–6.5	36+	76+	53+	46+	10
9	98	65	13–15	36–43	18–19	7.0	21–35	70–75	49–52	43–45	9
8	93	63	11–12	30–35	16–17	7.5	14–20	63–69	46–48	39–42	8
7	84	61	9–10	21–29	15	8.0	8–13	57–62	42–45	36–38	7
6	69	59	7–8	16–20	14	8.5	4–7	51–56	38–41	32–35	6
5	50	57	5–6	11–15	12–13	—	3	44–50	34–37	29–31	5
4	31	53–55	3–4	7–10	11	9.0	2	34–43	30–33	25–28	4
3	16	49–51	2	3–6	10	9.5	1	21–33	26–29	22–24	3
2	7	43–47	1	1–2	8–9	10.0–10.5	0	14–20	22–25	18–21	2
1	2	39–41	0	0	6–7	11.0–11.5	—	8–13	18–21	15–17	1
0	1	13–37	—	—	0–5	12.0+	—	0–7	0–17	0–14	0

Table 8-20. Boys—Begin Grade 5

Achievement Level	Percentile Rank	Posture	Accuracy	Strength	Agility	Speed	Balance	Endurance	Total Physical Fitness With Posture	Without Posture	Achievement Level
10	99	—	18–20	47+	21+	0–6.5	45+	80+	53+	46+	10
9	98	65	15–17	36–46	19–20	7.0	27–44	74–79	49–52	43–45	9
8	93	63	13–14	31–35	17–18	—	16–26	66–73	46–48	39–42	8
7	84	61	11–12	23–30	16	7.5	9–15	60–65	42–45	36–38	7
6	69	59	9–10	16–22	15	8.0	5–8	53–59	38–41	32–35	6
5	50	57	7–8	11–15	13–14	8.5	3–4	46–52	34–37	29–31	5
4	31	53–55	5–6	7–10	12	—	2	35–45	30–33	25–28	4
3	16	49–51	3–4	3–6	11	9.0	1	22–34	26–29	22–24	3
2	7	43–47	2	1–2	9–10	9.5–10.0	0	15–21	22–25	18–21	2
1	2	39–41	1	0	7–8	10.5–11.0	—	8–14	18–21	15–17	1
0	1	13.27	0					0–7	0–17	0–14	0

Table 8-21. Boys—Begin Grade 6

Achievement Level	Percentile Rank	Posture	Accuracy	Strength	Agility	Speed	Balance	Endurance	Total Physical Fitness With Posture	Total Physical Fitness Without Posture	Achievement Level
10	99	—	18-20	48+	23+	0-6.5	61+	82+	53+	46+	10
9	98	65	16-17	37-47	20-22	—	35-60	75-81	49-52	43-45	9
8	93	63	14-15	32-36	18-19	7.0	19-34	69-74	46-48	39-42	8
7	84	61	12-13	24-31	17	7.5	10-18	62-68	42-45	36-38	7
6	69	59	10-11	17-23	16	—	5-9	55-61	38-41	32-35	6
5	50	57	8-9	11-16	14-15	8.0	3-4	48-54	34-37	29-31	5
4	31	53-55	6-7	7-10	13	8.5	2	35-47	30-33	25-28	4
3	16	49-51	4-5	3-6	12	9.0	1	23-34	26-29	22-24	3
2	7	43-47	2-3	1-2	10-11	9.5-10.0	0	15-22	22-25	18-21	2
1	2	39-41	1	0	8-9	10.5-11.0	—	8-14	18-21	15-17	1
0	1	13-37	0	—	0-7	11.5+	—	0-7	0-17	0-14	0

Table 8-22. Boys—Begin Grade 7

Achievement Level	Percentile Rank	Posture	Accuracy	Strength	Agility	Speed	Balance	Endurance	Total Physical Fitness With Posture	Total Physical Fitness Without Posture	Achievement Level
10	99	—	18-20	18+	24+	0-6.0	73+	137+	53+	46+	10
9	98	65	16-17	14-17	21-23	6.5	44-72	126-136	49-52	43-45	9
8	93	63	14-15	11-13	19-20	7.0	23-43	117-125	46-48	39-42	8
7	84	61	12-13	8-10	17-18	—	12-22	105-116	42-45	36-38	7
6	69	59	10-11	5-7	16	7.5	7-11	93-104	38-41	32-35	6
5	50	57	7-9	3-4	15	8.0	4-6	78-92	34-37	29-31	5
4	31	53-55	6	1-2	14	—	2-3	62-77	30-33	25-28	4
3	16	49-51	4-5	0	12-13	8.5	1	47-61	26-29	22-24	3
2	7	43-47	2-3	—	10-11	9.0-9.5	0	36-46	22-25	18-21	2
1	2	39-41	1	—	8-9	10.0-11.0	—	21-35	18-21	15-17	1
0	1	13-37	0	—	0-7	11.5+	—	0-20	0-17	0-14	0

Table 8-23. Boys—Begin Grade 8

Achievement Level	Percentile Rank	Posture	Accuracy	Strength	Agility	Speed	Balance	Endurance	Total Physical Fitness With Posture	Total Physical Fitness Without Posture	Achievement Level
10	99	—	19-20	19+	24+	0-6.0	80+	147+	53+	46+	10
9	98	65	17-18	15-18	21-23	—	56-79	135-146	49-52	43-45	9
8	93	63	15-16	12-14	20	6.5	29-55	125-134	46-48	39-42	8
7	84	61	13-14	9-11	18-19	7.0	16-28	113-124	42-45	36-38	7
6	69	59	11-12	6-8	17	—	9-15	102-112	38-41	32-35	6
5	50	57	9-10	4-5	16	7.5	5-8	89-101	34-37	29-31	5
4	31	53-55	7-8	2-3	15	8.0	3-4	75-88	30-33	25-28	4
3	16	49-51	6	1	13-14	8.5	2	59-74	26-29	22-24	3
2	7	43-47	4-5	0	11-12	9.0	1	40-58	22-25	18-21	2
1	2	39-41	2-3	—	9-10	9.5-10.0	0	25-39	18-21	15-17	1
0	1	13-37	0-1	—	0-8	10.5+	—	0-24	0-17	0-14	0

Table 8-24. Boys—Begin Grade 9

Achievement Level	Percentile Rank	Posture	Accuracy	Strength	Agility	Speed	Balance	Endurance	Total Physical Fitness With Posture	Total Physical Fitness Without Posture	Achievement Level
10	99	—	19-20	19+	25+	0-5.5	84+	149+	53+	46+	10
9	98	65	17-18	16-18	22-24	6.0	63-83	137-148	49-52	43-45	9
8	93	63	16	13-15	21	—	35-62	126-136	46-48	39-42	8
7	84	61	14-15	10-12	19-20	6.5	20-34	116-125	42-45	36-38	7
6	69	59	12-13	8-9	18	7.0	11-19	105-115	38-41	32-35	6
5	50	57	10-11	5-7	16-17	—	6-10	95-104	34-37	29-31	5
4	31	53-55	8-9	3-4	15	7.5	4-5	80-94	30-33	25-28	4
3	16	49-51	6-7	2	13-14	8.0	2-3	64-79	26-29	22-24	3
2	7	43-47	4-5	1	11-12	8.5	1	43-63	22-25	18-21	2
1	2	39-41	2-3	0	9-10	9.0-9.5	0	29-42	18-21	15-17	1
0	1	13-37	0-1	—	0-8	10.0+	—	0-28	0-17	0-14	0

Table 8-25. Boys—Begin Grade 10

Achievement Level	Percentile Rank	Posture	Accuracy	Strength	Agility	Speed	Balance	Endurance	Total Physical Fitness With Posture	Without Posture	Achievement Level
10	99	—	19-20	20+	26+	0-5.5	88+	149+	53+	46+	10
9	98	65	18	17-19	24-25	6.0	67-87	137-148	49-52	43-45	9
8	93	63	17	14-16	22-23	—	43-66	127-136	46-48	39-42	8
7	84	61	15-16	11-13	20-21	6.5	24-42	118-126	42-45	36-38	7
6	69	59	13-14	9-10	19	7.0	14-23	107-117	38-41	32-35	6
5	50	57	11-12	6-8	17-18	—	8-13	97-106	34-37	29-31	5
4	31	53-55	9-10	4-5	16	7.5	5-7	82-96	30-33	25-28	4
3	16	49-51	7-8	3	14-15	8.0	3-4	64-81	26-29	22-24	3
2	7	43-47	5-6	1-2	12-13	8.5	1-2	43-63	22-25	18-21	2
1	2	39-41	3-4	0	10-11	9.0-9.5	0	31-42	18-21	15-17	1
0	1	13-37	0-2	—	0-9	10.0+	—	0-30	0-17	0-14	0

Table 8-26. Boys—Begin Grade 11

Achievement Level	Percentile Rank	Posture	Accuracy	Strength	Agility	Speed	Balance	Endurance	Total Physical Fitness With Posture	Without Posture	Achievement Level
10	99	—	19-20	21+	27+	0-5.5	92+	149+	53+	46+	10
9	98	65	18	18-20	25-26	—	71-91	138-148	49-52	43-45	9
8	93	63	17	15-17	22-24	6.0	51-70	129-137	46-48	39-42	8
7	84	61	16	12-14	21	—	28-50	120-128	42-45	36-38	7
6	69	59	14-15	10-11	20	6.5	17-27	109-119	38-41	32-35	6
5	50	57	12-13	8-9	18-19	7.0	10-16	98-108	34-37	29-31	5
4	31	53-55	10-11	5-7	17	—	5-9	82-97	30-33	25-28	4
3	16	49-51	7-9	4	15-16	7.5	3-4	64-81	26-29	22-24	3
2	7	43-47	5-6	2-3	13-14	8.0	2	43-63	22-25	18-21	2
1	2	39-41	4	1	10-12	8.5-9.5	1	31-42	18-21	15-17	1
0	1	13-37	0-3	0	0-9	10.0+	0	0-30	0-17	0-14	0

Table 8-27. Boys—Begin Grade 12

Achievement Level	Percentile Rank	Posture	Accuracy	Strength	Agility	Speed	Balance	Endurance	Total Physical Fitness With Posture	Total Physical Fitness Without Posture	Achievement Level
10	99	—	20	22+	27+	0-5.5	97+	149+	53+	46+	10
9	98	65	19	18-21	25-26	—	72-96	138-148	49-52	43-45	9
8	93	63	18	15-17	22-24	6.0	53-71	130-137	46-48	39-42	8
7	84	61	16-17	13-14	21	—	31-52	121-129	42-45	36-38	7
6	69	59	14-15	10-12	20	6.5	19-30	110-120	38-41	32-35	6
5	50	57	12-13	9	18-19	—	11-18	98-109	34-37	29-31	5
4	31	53-55	10-11	6-8	17	7.0	6-10	82-97	30-33	25-28	4
3	16	49-51	8-9	4-5	15-16	7.5	3-5	65-81	26-29	22-24	3
2	7	43-47	6-7	2-3	13-14	8.0	2	43-64	22-25	18-21	2
1	2	39-41	5	1	10-12	8.5-9.5	1	31-42	18-21	15-17	1
0	1	13-37	0-4	0	0-9	10.0+	0	0-30	0-17	0-14	0

Table 8-28. Girls—Begin Grade 4

Achievement Level	Percentile Rank	Posture	Accuracy	Strength	Agility	Speed	Balance	Endurance	Total Physical Fitness With Posture	Total Physical Fitness Without Posture	Achievement Level
10	99	—	11-20	44	18+	0-6.5	25+	77+	53+	46+	10
9	98	65	8-10	31-43	17	7.0	14-24	65-76	49-52	43-45	9
8	93	63	6-7	24-30	16	7.5	8-13	59-64	46-48	39-42	8
7	84	61	4-5	17-23	14-15	8.0	5-7	54-58	42-45	36-38	7
6	69	59	3	11-16	13	8.5	3-4	49-53	38-41	32-35	6
5	50	57	2	7-10	12	9.0	2	41-48	34-37	29-31	5
4	31	53-55	1	3-6	11	9.5	1	32-40	30-33	25-28	4
3	16	49-51	0	1-2	9-10	10.0	0	24-31	26-29	22-24	3
2	7	43-47	—	0	7-8	10.5-11.0	—	16-23	22-25	18-21	2
1	2	39-41	—	—	5-6	11.5-12.0	—	9-15	18-21	15-17	1
0	1	13-37	—	—	0-4	12.5+	—	0-8	0-17	0-14	0

Table 8-29. Girls—Begin Grade 5

Achievement Level	Percentile Rank	Posture	Accuracy	Strength	Agility	Speed	Balance	Endurance	Total Physical Fitness With Posture	Total Physical Fitness Without Posture	Achievement Level
10	99	—	13-20	48+	21+	0 6.5	35+	77+	53+	46+	10
9	98	65	10-12	31-47	19-20	7.0	17-34	69-76	49-52	43-45	9
8	93	63	8-9	23-30	17-18	7.5	11-16	64-68	46-48	39-42	8
7	84	61	6-7	16-22	15-16	8.0	6-10	58-63	42-45	36-38	7
6	69	59	4-5	10-15	14	8.5	4-5	52-57	38-41	32-35	6
5	50	57	2-3	6-9	13	9.0	2-3	44-51	34-37	29-31	5
4	31	53-55	1	3-5	12	9.5	1	36-43	30-33	25-28	4
3	16	49-51	0	1-2	10-11	10.0	0	27-35	26-29	22-24	3
2	7	43-47	—	0	8-9	10.5-11.0	—	18-26	22-25	18-21	2
1	2	39-41	—	—	5-7	11.5-12.0	—	11-17	18-21	15-17	1
0	1	13-37	—	—	0-4	12.5+	—	0-10	0-17	0-14	0

Table 8-30. Girls—Begin Grade 6

Achievement Level	Percentile Rank	Posture	Accuracy	Strength	Agility	Speed	Balance	Endurance	Total Physical Fitness With Posture	Total Physical Fitness Without Posture	Achievement Level
10	99	—	15-20	50+	21+	0-6.5	41+	79+	53+	46+	10
9	98	65	12-14	31-49	19-20	7.0	21-40	72-78	49-52	43-45	9
8	93	63	9-11	23-30	18	7.5	13-20	67-71	46-48	39-42	8
7	84	61	7-8	16-22	16-17	—	6-12	61-66	42-45	36-38	7
6	69	59	5-6	10-15	15	8.0	4-5	54-60	38-41	32-35	6
5	50	57	3-4	5-9	14	8.5	2-3	46-53	34-37	29-31	5
4	31	53-55	2	2-4	12-13	9.0	1	39-45	30-33	25-28	4
3	16	49-51	1	1	11	9.5	0	29-38	26-29	22-24	3
2	7	43-47	0	0	9-10	10.0-10.5	—	20-28	22-25	18-21	2
1	2	39-41	—	—	7-8	11.0-11.5	—	12-19	18-21	15-17	1
0	1	13-37	—	—	0-6	12.0+	—	0-11	0-17	0-14	0

Table 8-31. Girls—Begin Grade 7

Achievement Level	Percentile Rank	Posture	Accuracy	Strength	Agility	Speed	Balance	Endurance	Total Physical Fitness With Posture	Total Physical Fitness Without Posture	Achievement Level
10	99	—	16–20	75+	21+	0–6.5	49+	81+	53+	46+	10
9	98	65	13–15	58–74	19–20	7.0	24–48	73–80	49–52	43–45	9
8	93	63	10–12	49–57	18	—	14–23	67–72	46–48	39–42	8
7	84	61	8–9	38–48	16–17	7.5	7–13	61–66	42–45	36–38	7
6	69	59	6–7	25–37	15	8.0	4–6	54–60	38–41	32–35	6
5	50	57	4–5	17–24	14	8.5	3	46–53	34–37	29–31	5
4	31	53–55	2–3	12–16	13	9.0	2	39–45	30–33	25–28	4
3	16	49–51	1	7–11	11–12	9.5	1	31–38	26–29	22–24	3
2	7	43–47	0	4–6	9–10	10.0	0	22–30	22–25	18–21	2
1	2	39–41	—	2–3	7–8	10.5–11.0	—	13–21	18–21	15–17	1
0	1	13–37	—	0–1	0–6	11.5+	—	0–12	0–17	0–15	0

Table 8-32. Girls—Begin Grade 8

Achievement Level	Percentile Rank	Posture	Accuracy	Strength	Agility	Speed	Balance	Endurance	Total Physical Fitness With Posture	Total Physical Fitness Without Posture	Achievement Level
10	99	—	17–20	73+	21+	0–6.0	55+	81+	53+	46+	10
9	98	65	14–16	57–72	20	6.5	25–54	73–80	49–52	43–45	9
8	93	63	11–13	50–56	18–19	7.0	14–24	66–72	46–48	39–42	8
7	84	61	9–10	37–49	17	7.5	7–13	61–65	42–45	36–38	7
6	69	59	7–8	23–36	16	—	4–6	54–60	38–41	32–35	6
5	50	57	5–6	17–24	15	8.0	3	47–53	34–37	29–31	5
4	31	53–55	3–4	12–16	14	8.5	2	40–46	30–33	25–28	4
3	16	49–51	2	7–11	12–13	9.0	1	32–39	26–29	22–24	3
2	7	43–47	1	4–6	10–11	9.5	0	23–31	22–25	18–21	2
1	2	39–41	0	2–3	8–9	10.0–10.5	—	15–22	18–21	15–17	1
0	1	13–37	—	0–1	0–7	11.0+	—	0–14	0–17	0–14	0

Table 8–33. Girls—Begin Grade 9

Achievement Level	Percentile Rank	Posture	Accuracy	Strength	Agility	Speed	Balance	Endurance	Total Physical Fitness With Posture	Without Posture	Achievement Level
10	99	—	18–20	71+	22+	0–6.0	56+	79+	53+	46+	10
9	98	65	15–17	57–70	20–21	6.5	28–55	71–78	49–52	43–45	9
8	93	63	12–14	51–56	19	7.0	14–27	65–70	46–48	39–42	8
7	84	61	9–11	37–50	17–18	7.5	7–13	59–64	42–45	36–38	7
6	69	59	7–8	27–36	16	—	5–6	53–58	38–41	38–35	6
5	50	57	5–6	19–26	15	8.0	3–4	47–52	34–37	29–31	5
4	31	53–55	4	13–18	14	8.5	2	39–46	30–33	25–28	4
3	16	49–51	2–3	8–12	12–13	9.0	1	31–38	26–29	22–24	3
2	7	43–47	1	4–7	10–11	9.5	0	22–30	22–25	18–21	2
1	2	39–41	0	2–3	8–9	10.0–10.5	—	14–21	18–21	15–17	1
0	1	13–37	—	0–1	0–7	11.0+	—	0–13	0–17	0–14	0

Table 8–34. Girls—Begin Grade 10

Achievement Level	Percentile Rank	Posture	Accuracy	Strength	Agility	Speed	Balance	Endurance	Total Physical Fitness With Posture	Without Posture	Achievement Level
10	99	—	18–20	71+	23+	0–6.0	58+	75+	53+	46+	10
9	98	65	15–17	57–70	21–22	6.5	30–57	69–74	49–52	43–45	9
8	93	63	12–14	51–56	19–20	7.0	15–29	64–68	46–48	39–42	8
7	84	61	10–11	37–50	18	7.5	8–14	58–63	42–45	36–38	7
6	69	59	8–9	28–36	16–17	—	5–7	52–57	38–41	32–35	6
5	50	57	6–7	20–27	15	8.0	3–4	46–51	34–37	29–31	5
4	31	53–55	5	14–19	14	8.5	2	39–45	30–33	25–28	4
3	16	49–51	3–4	9–13	13	9.0	1	30–38	26–29	22–24	3
2	7	43–47	2	4–8	11–12	9.5	0	23–29	22–25	18–21	2
1	2	39–41	1	2–3	9–10	10.0–10.5	—	13–22	18–21	15–17	1
0	1	13–37	0	0–1	0–8	11.0+	—	0–12	0–17	0–14	0

Table 8-35. Girls—Begin Grade 11

Achievement Level	Percentile Rank	Posture	Accuracy	Strength	Agility	Speed	Balance	Endurance	Total Physical Fitness With Posture	Total Physical Fitness Without Posture	Achievement Level
10	99	—	18-20	70+	24+	0-6.0	59+	75+	53+	46+	10
9	98	65	15-17	57-69	21-23	6.5	31-58	70-74	49-52	43-45	9
8	93	63	12-14	49-56	19-20	7.0	16-30	64-69	46-48	39-42	8
7	84	61	10-11	37-48	18	7.5	9-15	58-63	42-45	36-38	7
6	69	59	8-9	27-36	16-17	—	5-8	52-57	38-41	32-35	6
5	50	57	7	20-26	15	8.0	3-4	46-51	34-37	29-31	5
4	31	53-55	5-6	13-19	14	8.5	2	39-45	30-33	25-28	4
3	16	49-51	3-4	8-12	13	9.0	1	31-38	26-29	22-24	3
2	7	43-47	2	4-7	11-12	9.5	0	24-30	22-25	18-21	2
1	2	39-41	1	1-3	9-10	10.0-10.5	—	14-23	18-21	15-17	1
0	1	13-37	0	0	0-8	11.0+	—	0-13	0-17	0-14	0

Table 8-36. Girls—Begin Grade 12

Achievement Level	Percentile Rank	Posture	Accuracy	Strength	Agility	Speed	Balance	Endurance	Total Physical Fitness With Posture	Total Physical Fitness Without Posture	Achievement Level
10	99	—	18-20	67+	24+	0-6.0	60+	76+	53+	46+	10
9	98	65	16-17	56-66	21-23	6.5	32-59	71-75	49-52	43-45	9
8	93	63	13-15	46-55	19-20	7.0	16-31	64-70	46-48	39-42	8
7	84	61	11-12	36-45	18	7.5	9-15	58-63	42-45	36-38	7
6	69	59	9-10	26-35	16-17	—	5-8	52-57	38-41	32-35	6
5	50	57	7-8	19-25	15	8.0	3-4	46-51	34-37	29-31	5
4	31	53-55	5-6	12-18	14	8.5	2	40-45	30-33	25-28	4
3	16	49-51	3-4	7-11	13	9.0	1	32-39	26-29	22-24	3
2	7	43-47	2	3-6	12	9.5	0	25-31	22-25	18-21	2
1	2	39-41	1	1-2	10-11	10.0-10.5	—	15-24	18-21	15-17	1
0	1	13-37	0	0	0-9	11.0+	—	0-14	0-17	0-14	0

North Carolina Fitness Test*

Purpose. To measure achievement in the physical fitness objective.

Evaluation. Items were selected through the jury technique on the basis of criteria established by a Fitness Committee.

Level and Sex. Boys and girls age 9 through 18.

Time Allotment and Number of Subjects. A class of 30 to 35 pupils can be tested in a 45-minute class period.

Floor Plan and Space Requirement

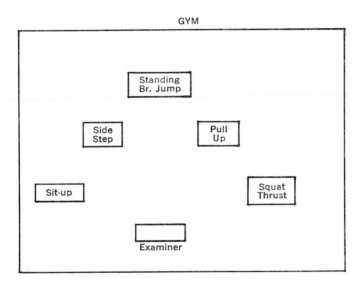

Fig. 8–13. Floor plan for North Carolina fitness test.

Class Organization. The tests should be administered on a combination of the station-to-station and squad method of administration. The class should be divided into five squads which will rotate from one station to another until all squads have visited all five stations.

At the beginning of the period all students are supplied with an individual score card. All five test items are explained and demonstrated to the entire class. The squads then go to the stations assigned. Score cards are collected by the student assistant at the last station where the student is tested.

General Procedure. 1. The five testing stations should be arranged in the order of the rotation mentioned in 2 below.

2. The following sequence should be maintained for rotation: Sit-Ups, Side-Stepping, Broad Jump, Pull-Ups, and Squat Thrusts. One squad should start at each station and from that starting position should continue in the order just listed. For example, a squad starting with the Side-

* State of North Carolina. *North Carolina Fitness Test.* Raleigh, Department of Public Instruction, North Carolina, 1961. Adapted by permission of the State Department of Public Instruction.

Stepping will move to Broad Jump, Pull-Ups, Squat Thrust, and Sit-Ups. This sequence is planned so that a student will not be using the same muscle groups in succession.

3. Student leaders should be trained to administer the tests and score them at each station.

4. The instructor can serve as the director of the entire testing program. He can operate the watch from a central position and give the starting and stopping signals for all stations at the same time. Each station may use its own watch, but this method would require two trained assistants at each station—one to time and one to score.

5. Since the Standing Broad Jump is not operated on a 30-second time limit, its administration may be speeded up by having two stations.

Uses. The results of this test may be used for measuring status and progress in fitness. Specifically, such results have always been good for motivation purposes and frequently used as a basis for partial marks in the physical education class. Students may be classified into homogeneous groups on the basis of fitness.

When all scores from a class or a school are analyzed, certain weaknesses may be revealed. These knowledges might lead to a change in program or methodology.

One of the most graphic uses of this test is the profile chart shown on the obverse side of the score card. It is used to plot the performance of the student. This provides a graphic illustration of the student's performance and indicates strengths and weaknesses. Also, by plotting two administrations of the same test to the same student, it is possible to have a graph of the change in status. Thus, the profile becomes a means of showing graphically both status and progress.

This test has been revised and is in the process of being re-normed. Interested persons may write the authors or the State Department of Public Instruction in North Carolina.

Test Description

ITEM NUMBER I—SIT-UPS (Fig. 8–14 *A*)

Purpose: To measure abdominal strength, endurance, and speed.

Facilities and Equipment: If enough mats are available, they should be used; otherwise, the floor is satisfactory. Watch with a second hand, or a stop watch.

Procedures: The student lies on his back with his fingers clasped behind his neck and elbows touching the floor, his knees bent, and his feet flat on the floor pulled in close to his body. His feet are held securely by a partner. He sits up, turning the trunk to the left, touching the right elbow to the left knee, returns to the starting position, then sits up, touching the left elbow to the right knee. The exercise is repeated as the subject alternates sides.

Instructions: You must return to the starting position with the elbows touching the floor. Your fingers must remain in contact behind the neck throughout the exercise. You may not rest between sit-ups, and you must touch the knee with the opposite elbow. Do as many sit-ups as you can in 30 seconds.

Scoring: A sit-up is scored each time an elbow touches a knee. The score is the number of correct sit-ups performed in 30 seconds.

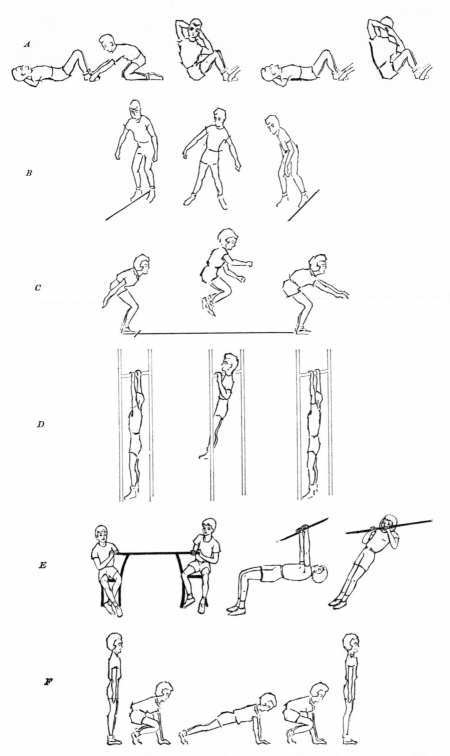

Fig. 8-14.   Test items for the North Carolina fitness test.   *A*, Sit-ups.   *B*, Side-stepping.   *C*, Standing broad jump.   *D*, Pull-ups.   *E*, Modified pull-ups.   *F*, Squat thrust.

251

Testing Personnel: One leader can administer the entire test from a central position and this item can be scored by one scorer who might be a squad leader or a trained assistant.

ITEM NUMBER II—SIDE-STEPPING (Fig. 8–14 *B*)

Purpose: To measure agility, endurance, and speed.

Facilities and Equipment: Two lines on the floor 10 feet apart. Watch with a second hand or a stop watch.

Procedures: The subject assumes a starting position with one foot touching a side line. On the signal to start he moves sideward with a side-step leading with the foot nearest the line he is approaching and repeats this step until his foot has touched or gone beyond the line. He then moves to the other side line in the same manner.

Instructions: You must face in the same direction throughout the exercise. You must reach the line and you must never cross your feet at any time.

Scoring: One point is scored each time the subject touches a side line. The final score is the number of one-way trips completed in 30 seconds.

Testing Personnel: One trained student assistant to count the score and record it.

ITEM NUMBER III—STANDING BROAD JUMP (Fig. 8–15 *C*)

Purpose: To measure power.

Facilities and Equipment: Mats are desirable if they are marked off at intervals. Otherwise, the floor can be used with a take-off mark and tape measure.

Procedures: The subject should stand with his feet several inches apart and with his toes just back of the take-off mark. He may swing his arms and bend his knees in making the jump forward. Both feet should leave the floor at the same time.

Instructions: You should crouch before the take-off and swing your arms down in a preliminary movement. As the jump is made, you should throw your arms up and out. Jump from both feet and try not to fall backwards on landing.

Scoring: The measurement is made from the take-off line to the nearest point where any part of the body touches the floor. Three trials are permitted and the best one is estimated to the nearest inch.

Testing Personnel: One trained student assistant to score and record results.

ITEM NUMBER IV—PULL-UPS (for boys age 12 through 17) (Fig. 8–14 *D*)

Purpose: To measure arm and shoulder girdle strength, endurance, and speed.

Facilities and Equipment: A bar approximately 1 inch in diameter secured to prevent rotation should be used. Preferably the bar should be adjustable to various heights. Watch with a second hand or a stop watch.

Procedures: The subject starts by grasping the bar with the palms of the hands turned away from the face and extending the body in a hanging position with the feet off the floor. Using his arms he raises his body until his chin touches the bar and then lowers it to the starting position.

Instructions: You must not swing your body to aid in chinning. You must not lift your knees or kick to aid in the action of chinning, and the chin must be a continuous movement without a snap. You must lower your body until the arms are fully extended, and you must not rest between pull-ups.

Scoring: One point is scored for each correct pull-up in the 30-second time period. A correct pull-up requires raising the body until the chin touches the bar and returns to the starting position.

Testing Personnel: One trained student assistant to count and record the score.

ITEM NUMBER V—MODIFIED PULL-UPS (for all girls and boys age 9 through 11) (Fig. 8–14 *E*)

Purpose: To measure arm and shoulder girdle strength, endurance, and speed.

Facilities and Equipment: Two chairs of equal height with a minimum height of 30 inches support a bar 1 inch in diameter and 4 feet long. A student sits in each chair and holds the bar on the chair to prevent it from sliding or rotating. Watch with a second hand or a stop watch.

Procedure: The student should grasp the bar with his palms away from the face and position his body under the bar with his feet flat on the floor directly under the knees so that the area between the *knees and the head comprises a straight line.* The arms are extended to form a 90-degree angle with the chest. From this position the subject pulls up with the arms until they are completely bent and then lowers to the full extension of the arms.

Instructions: You are not permitted to rest between pull-ups. Your feet must be kept under the knees at all times and your body must be kept straight between the knees and the head. You must flex your arms until your chest or chin touches the bar and your arms must be fully extended between pull-ups.

Scoring: The score is the number of correct pull-ups performed in 30 seconds.

Testing Personnel: One trained student assistant to appoint students to hold the bar. This assistant also can count and record the score.

ITEM NUMBER VI—SQUAT THRUST (for boys and girls age 9 through 17) (Fig. 8–14 *F*)

Purpose: To measure endurance, agility, and speed.

Facilities and Equipment: Watch with a second hand or a stop watch.

Procedures: The subject starts in a standing position. (1) He goes to a full squat position placing both hands on the floor about shoulder width apart in front of his feet; (2) He thrusts both legs backward to a front leaning rest position with the body resting on both hands and the toes and approximately straight from his shoulders to his feet; (3) He returns to the full squat position; (4) Then he stands erect.

Instructions: You must reach the full squat position before your legs are thrust backward. Your back should be kept straight in this front leaning rest position. You must come to an upright position with the body in a straight line at the hips. You cannot rest between any of these movements.

Scoring: The score is the number of complete repetitions correctly executed in 30 seconds.

Testing Personnel: One trained student assistant to count the score and record results.

Score Card

NORTH CAROLINA FITNESS TEST SCORE CARD

Name_____Age____ Height____ Weight____
　　　(Last)　　　　　　(First)

School_____ Grade_____ Sex_____

Test Item	First Test		Second Test	
	Date:		Date:	
	Raw Score	Percentile	Raw Score	Percentile
Sit-Ups (number in 30 seconds)				
Side-Stepping (number in 30 seconds)				
Standing Broad Jump (number of inches)				
Pull-Ups (number in 30 seconds)				
Squat Thrusts (number in 30 seconds)				

This score card may be reproduced on 5″ by 8″ cards

Profile

PROFILE CHART FOR NORTH CAROLINA FITNESS TEST

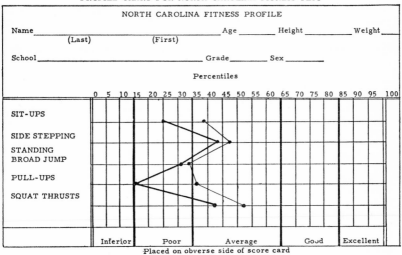

Fig. 8–15.   Profile for North Carolina Fitness Test.

References

1. AAHPER: *Youth Fitness Test Manual*, Washington, D.C. AAHPER, 1961 (Revised).
2. Brouha, L.: The Step Test: A Simple Method of Measuring Physical Fitness for Muscular Work in Young Men. Research Quarterly, *14*, 31–36, March, 1943.
3. Brouha, L., and J. R. Gallagher: A Functional Fitness Test for High School Girls. Journal of Health & Physical Education, *14*, 517, December, 1943.
4. Brouha, L., and Ball, M. V.: *Canadian Red Cross Society's School Meal Study.* Toronto, University of Toronto Press, 1952, pp. 55–56.
5. Clarke, H. L.: A Functional Physical Fitness Test for College Women. Journal of Health & Physical Education, *14*, 517, September, 1943.
6. Cooper, Kenneth. *Aerobics:* New York, M. Evans and Company, Inc., 1968.
7. Gallagher, J. R., and L. Brouha: A Simple Method of Testing the Physical Fitness of Boys. Research Quarterly, *14*, 23–30, March, 1943.
8. Glover, Elizabeth Gay: Physical Fitness Test Items for Boys and Girls in the First, Second, and Third Grades, Unpublished Master's Thesis. The Woman's College of the University of North Carolina, Greensboro, N. C., 1962.
9. Hielscher, Patricia Ann. The Equivalency of Cooper's 12-Minute Test and a $1\frac{1}{4}$-Mile Run for Junior High School Girls. Unpublished Master's Thesis. The University of North Carolina at Greensboro, Greensboro, N.C., 1970.
10. State of New York: The New York State Physical Fitness Test: A Manual for Teachers of Physical Education. Albany, Division of Health, Physical Education, and Recreation, New York State Education Department, 1958.
11. State of North Carolina: North Carolina Fitness Test. Raleigh, Department of Public Instruction, North Carolina, 1961.
12. United States Air Force. *GMT USAF Aerobics:* Physical Fitness Program. Washington, D.C., 1969.

Additional References

1. AAU: Junior Physical Fitness Standards (For boys and girls). The Amateur Athletic Union, 233 Broadway, New York.
2. Anhalt, Carol J.: A Reliable and Valid Motor Fitness Test Battery for Upper Elementary School Girls. Unpublished Master's Thesis, University of Oregon, Eugene, Oregon, 1958.
3. Baltimore Public Schools: Physical Fitness Test, Physical Education Bulletin, Vol. 17, No. 3, Baltimore, Division of Physical Education, Department of Education, 1963.
4. Bookwalter, K. W., and C. W. Bookwalter: A Measure of Motor Fitness for College Men, Bulletin of the School of Education. Bureau of Cooperative Research and Field Services, Indiana University, Vol. 19, March, 1943.
5. Bookwalter, K. W.: Further Studies of Indiana University Motor Fitness Index, Bulletin of School of Education. Bureau of Cooperative Research and Field Services, Indiana University, Vol. 19, September, 1943.
6. ————: Test Manual for Indiana Motor Fitness Indices for High School and College Men, Research Quarterly, 14, 356–365, December, 1943.
7. Cureton, Thomas K.: Physical Fitness Appraisal and Guidance. St. Louis, The C. V. Mosby Co., 1947, Chapter 13.
8. Cureton, T. K., Lyle Welser, and W. J. Huffman: A Short Screen Test for Predicting Motor Fitness. Research Quarterly, 16, 106–119, May, 1945.
9. Franklin, C. C., and N. G. Lehsten: Indiana Physical Fitness Test for Elementary Level (Grades 4–8), The Physical Educator, 5, 38–45, May, 1948.
10. Ismail, A. S., and C. C. Cowell: Purdue Motor Fitness Test Batteries and a Development Profile for Pre-Adolescent Boys. Research Quarterly, 33, 553–558, December, 1962.
11. Kirchner, Glenn: Elementary School Physical Fitness Test. Cheney, Washington, Washington Association for Health, Physical Education, and Recreation, 1959.
12. Kraus, Hans, and Ruth P. Hirschland: Minimum Muscular Fitness Tests in School Children. Research Quarterly, 25, 178–188, May, 1954.
13. McClane, John P.: A Motor Fitness Test for High School Boys. Unpublished Master's Thesis, State College of Washington, Pullman, Washington, 1958.
14. NSWA Committee (Eleanor Metheny, Chairman): Physical Performance Levels for High School Girls. Journal of Health & Physical Education, 16, 32–35, June, 1945.
15. O'Connor, M. E., and Thomas K. Cureton: Motor Fitness Tests for High School Girls. Research Quarterly, 16, 302–314, December, 1945.
16. Phillips, B. E. The JCR Test. Research Quarterly, 18, 12–29, March, 1947.
17. President's Council on Youth Fitness: Youth Physical Fitness: Suggested Elements of a School-Centered Program. Washington, D.C., U.S. Government Printing Office, 1961. pp. 19–26, 44–55.
18. Scott, M. Gladys, and Marjorie Wilson: Physical Efficiency Tests for College Women. Research Quarterly, 19, 62–69, May, 1948.
19. State of California: California Physical Performance Test. Sacramento, State Department of Education, California, 1958.
20. State of Indiana: High School Physical Education Course of Study. Bulletin No. 222, Department of Public Instruction, Indiana, 1958, pp. 170–177.
21. State of Minnesota: The Minnesota Physical Efficiency Test, A Guide for Instruction in Physical Education. Curriculum Bulletin, No. 11, St. Paul, State Department of Education, 1950, pp. 42–48.
22. State of Oregon: Motor Fitness Tests for Oregon Schools. Salem, State Department of Education, Oregon, 1962.
23. Tuttle, W. W.: The Use of the Pulse-Ratio Test for Rating Physical Efficiency. Research Quarterly, 2, 5–8, May, 1931.
24. United States Navy: Physical Fitness Manual for the U. S. Navy. Bureau of Naval Personnel, Training Division, Chapter 4, 1943.
25. WAC Department: WAC Physical Fitness Rating. Washington, D.C., U.S. Government Printing Office, 1944.
26. Woodall, Ann Wescott: The Construction and Standardization of a Cardiovascular Test for Girls. Unpublished Master's Thesis, Woman's College of the University of North Carolina, Greensboro, N.C., 1959.

Chapter 9
TESTS OF SPECIFIC SPORTS SKILLS

BADMINTON
French Short Serve Test*

Purpose. To measure ability to serve accurately and low.

Evaluation. A validity coefficient of .66 was reported using a criterion of tournament rankings. The reliability was .96. The reliability will not hold up well for beginning players. A rating of the serve might be a better measure of serving skill for beginning players. This test is appropriate for intermediate players.

Level and Sex. May be used for boys and girls who have developed a degree of skill in the Short Serve.

Time Allotment and Number of Subjects. The test is time consuming unless areas can be marked and prepared for taking the test off to the side of the regulation courts. If several courts can be marked, the testing goes faster. Both the right and left courts on the same side of the net can be marked. Two take the test at the same time. One to the right court and one to the left.

Floor Plan and Space Requirements. A regulation badminton court can be used unless the needed portions of a court can be measured off in the side line areas of the gymnasium floor. This usually requires more preparations than will seem feasible.

Class Organization. Some can take the serve test while others are taking the volleying test. This test will be slower, however, so several stations will expedite the administration.

General Procedures. 1. Provide new or good shuttlecocks. Each player should be allotted at least 6 shuttlecocks.
2. The rope should be easily visible so the scorer can judge the flight of the shuttlecock between it and the net.
3. Some practice sessions prior to the testing day should be permitted.
4. If the left court is used, 10 serves should be from the right court, and 10 from the left. A group of 4 students could be on a court at one time: 2 taking the test and 2 scoring.

Uses. To increase awareness that the short serve must be low.
To use as a self-testing device for motivation.

Test Description

Purpose: To measure accuracy of the short, low serve.

* Scott, M. Gladys, Aileen Carpenter, Esther French, and Louise Kuhl: Achievement Examinations in Badminton, Research Quarterly, *12*, 242–253, May, 1941. Used by permission of the AAHPER.

Facilities and Equipment: Badminton court, rope, shuttlecocks, racket, and floor markings. The circular lines are 1½ inches wide and the width of them is included in the amount of each radius. The use of different colors for the circles will make scoring more accurate.

Procedure: The player stands in the regulation right court for serving and serves 20 times into the opposite right service court for the doubles game. The shuttlecock must go under the rope placed 20 inches above the net and parallel to it and must otherwise be a legal serve. The serves should be taken in groups of at least 5 and preferably 10 if there is a sufficient number of shuttlecocks.

Instructions: "Stand in the service court wherever you would like. Serve low and short to the opposite right service court for the doubles game and try to place the shuttlecock in the areas counting the most values. The serve must go under the rope and must be a legal serve. You will have 20 trials and your score is the total score for the 20 serves. Jane will score the serves for you and then she will take her turn while you score for her."

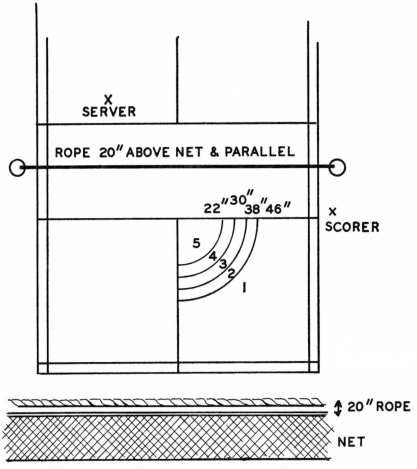

Fig. 9–1. Specifications for the short serve test.

Norms

Table 9–1. Norms for the French Short-Serve Test

T-Score	Short* Serve[1]	Short Serve[2]	T-Score
80	68	86	80
75	66	79	75
70	59	73	70
65	53	66	65
60	44	59	60
55	37	52	55
50	29	46	50
45	22	39	45
40	13	32	40
35	8	26	35
30	4	19	30
25	1	12	25
20		6	20

[1] Based on the performance of 385 college women after a 25-lesson beginning course in badminton.

[2] Based on the performance of 46 college women after a 30-lesson beginning course in badminton.

* Norms from *Measurement and Evaluation in Physical Education*. Dubuque, Iowa: Wm. C. Brown Publishers, 1959, pp. 156–157. Used by permission of M. Gladys Scott and Esther French.

Scoring: Score each serve by the numerical value of the area in which it first lands. Shuttlecocks which land on a line will score the higher value. Serves which fail to go between the rope and net, which are out of the bounds of the right service court for doubles, and which are not executed legally, will score zero. The final score is the total of the values made on 20 serves.

Testing Personnel: A scorer who stands on the target side of the net out of the way of the flight of the shuttlecock.

French Clear Test*

Purpose. To measure ability to use the clear shot.

Evaluation. French originally developed this test on 29 major students at the University of Iowa. The reliability, using the Spearman-Brown Prophecy Formula, was .96. The validity coefficient was .60 using tournament rankings as the criterion. This item is recommended for use with a service measure and a footwork measure to ascertain overall playing ability.

Level and Sex. For secondary and college students.

* French, Esther and Evelyn Stalter: Study of Skill Tests in Badminton for College Women, Research Quarterly, *20*, 257–272, October, 1949. Used by permission of the AAHPER.

Time Allotment and Number of Students. One or two students can be
tested on each badminton court. If several testing areas can be used,
and if the class members can help with testing assignments, the test
probably can be given to a class of 20 in 2 class periods.

Floor Plan, Space Requirements, and Equipment. A badminton court, a
rope, rackets, and shuttlecocks will be needed for each testing station.

Stretch a rope across the court 14 feet from the net and parallel to it at a
height of 8 feet from the floor on the same side as the target area.

Mark a line 1½ inches wide 2 feet nearer the net than the rear service line
and parallel to it. On the same side of the net mark a line 2 feet farther
from the net than the rear service line (singles) and parallel to it. Measure
from the exact center of the line. Extend lines from one outer alley line to
the other outer line. The lines of the target should be marked in different
colors to increase accuracy in scoring.

Class Organization. Groups of 4 can be tested by using one to hit, one to
record, and two to retrieve the shuttlecocks. The instructor or an advanced player should be the server. For advanced classes, the students
can serve for each other.

Uses. To measure improvement.
To develop distance in the clear shot.
To use as a partial grade.
To use with other badminton tests to measure overall playing ability.

Test Procedures and Instructions. The player to be tested shall stand
anywhere behind the short service line on the court opposite the target
and receive twenty shuttles (consecutively or divided into two groups of
ten), which he will try to send, by means of a clear stroke, above the rope
so that the shuttle lands on the target. The shuttles shall be served to the
player by an experienced player, standing anywhere behind the short
service line on the same side as the target, who must serve the shuttle with

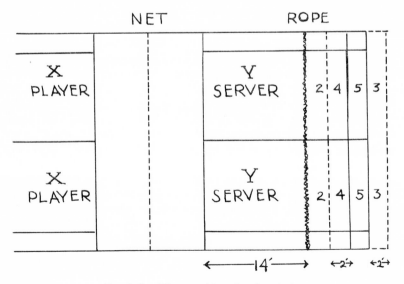

FIG. 9–2.   Floor markings for clear test.

enough force that it will carry beyond the short service line opposite the target. Only shuttles played by the player being tested shall count as trials. A trial which is carried or slung shall be repeated. Two practice trials shall be given. The instructor shall demonstrate a clear stroke using good form.

Scoring. The server shall act as scorer and shall call out the score of each of the 20 trials to the recorder. Two players can be tested at one time on a regulation badminton court if two servers are available. The target area would include the entire court for each player. The area between the two rear lines of the regulation court counts 5 points, the space just behind it counts 3 points, and the space just in front of the two rear lines of the regulation court counts 4 points. Any shuttle going over the net but failing to reach the target counts zero. Shuttles landing on a line shall be given the value of the higher area. Score each shuttle in accordance with the area in which the tip portion of the shuttle first hits. Record all 20 trials. The score shall be the total value of the 20 trials.

Miller Wall Volley Test*

Purpose. To measure ability to use the clear shot in badminton.

Evaluation. Miller made an accumulative record of the number of times each stroke was used in the Ninth Annual U.S. Amateur Badminton Championship. For both men's and women's singles events, the clear was used most often and drop shots were second. Once she had decided on the clear as the stroke to use for the development of a test, she then made a cinematographic study of the clear shot. It was essential to know the minimum height that an ideal-driven clear would cross the net and still go over an average sized opponent's head when the racket was extended into the air. This information set the wall line at $7\frac{1}{2}$ feet and the restraining line at 10 feet. The specifications call for an outdoor shuttlecock with a sponge end. Many students of less than championship level skill are unable to hit the shuttlecock the 10 foot distance using an indoor shuttlecock. Miller[30] adapted the original Miller test by changing the restraining line to 8 feet and used it successfully with junior and senior high school girls. The reliability was .83 for three trials. Miller developed the original test using 100 college girls of all ranges of ability. The reliability was .94 on a total of three trials in a test-retest situation. The validity was based on a continuous round robin tournament using 20 players. Altogether 380 games were played. The validity coefficient was .83.

Level and Sex. Developed for college men and women. Appropriate for secondary school students, especially if the restraining line is placed at 8 feet from the wall.

Time Allotment and Number of Students. This can be given easily in one class period.

Floor Plan and Space Requirements. Wall—a 1 inch line is extended across the wall $7\frac{1}{2}$ feet from the floor and parallel to it. The width of the wall space should be at least 10 feet and the height preferably 15 feet or higher.

Floor—A straight line 10 feet from the wall is extended the length of the wall distance and parallel to the wall.

* Miller, Frances A.: A Badminton Wall Volley Test, Research Quarterly, *22*, 208–213, May, 1951. Used by permission of the AAHPER.

Class Organization. Partners or doubles foursomes can be spaced at testing stations around the wall. One scores, one takes the test, and a rotation plan is used so some rest is possible between trials. In this way, several can be tested at the same time.

General Procedures. A 1-minute practice should be given before the first trial but not between trials. A short rest period should be allowed between trials.

Due to the fact that a subject encounters difficulty when trying to look at the line on the floor along with watching the shuttlecock, it is suggested that a chalk line 3 inches back from the 10-foot line be added, and the subject told to stay behind that line if possible. This allows the foot to slide as much as 3 inches without penalizing the person being tested. Also the scorer should say "Back" whenever the subject consistently goes over the line. Any stroke may be used to keep the shuttlecock in play. A "carried bird" or a double hit is counted as good if the hit eventually goes on or over the 7½-foot wall line.

Uses. A grading device, a practice device, a diagnostic tool, a measure of achievement, a device for adding interest and variety to teaching, and a classification test.

Test Instructions. On the signal, "Ready, Go," the subject serves the shuttlecock in a legal manner against the wall from behind the 10-foot floor line. The serve puts the shuttlecock in a position to be rallied with a clear on each rebound. If the serve hits on or above the 7½-foot wall line, that hit counts as one point and each following rebound hit, made on or above the 7½-foot wall line when the subject is behind the 10-foot floor line, counts as one point. The hit is not counted if any part of the foot goes over the 10-foot restraining line. The hit is not counted if the shuttlecock goes below the 7½-foot wall line. However, either in the case of the foot going over the restraining line or the shuttlecock going below the wall line, the subject is permitted to keep the shuttlecock in play. The subject may step in front of the restraining line to keep the shuttlecock in play, but hits failing to follow the specifications do not count. The shuttlecock may be stopped at any time and restarted with a legal service from behind the 10-foot floor line. If the shuttlecock is missed or falls to the floor, the subject picks up the same shuttlecock as quickly as possible, gets behind the restraining line, and puts the shuttlecock into play with a legal service.

Scoring. An accumulative number of hits made within 30 seconds is the score for each individual trial. Three 30-second trials are given. The score consists of the sum of three trials.

Lucey Badminton Rating Scale*

Purpose. To judge degree of proficiency in badminton.

Procedure. The rating sheet is structured to accommodate both players in a singles game. The instructor can rate the players or classmates can rate depending on how it will be used. The scale covers 14 aspects of the game. A student could get a score as high as 70 points.

* Lucey, Mildred A.: A Study of the Components of Wrist Action as They Relate to Speed of Learning and the Degree of Proficiency Attained in Badminton, Ph.D., New York University, 1952. Used by permission of the author.

The Scale

| Judge _____ | Date _____ |
| Student _____ | Student _____ |

Items

1 2 3 4 5			1 2 3 4 5
	Clear Shot—	high, deep, used at needed times	
	Smash Shot—	steep, powerful, good placement	
	Net Shot—	close to net, not too deep, uses full width of court	
	Drop Shot—	drops close to net, deceptive	
	Drive Shot—	flat and not too high above net, uses it to run opponent	
	Low Serve—	close to net, quick, accurate, varies spot, does not telegraph	
	Driven Serve—	executes well, uses strategically	
	High Serve—	high, deep, deceptive, does not telegraph, varies spot	
	Grip—	loose, though firm, not tense, changes appropriately for backhand	
	Body Control—	complete freedom of action, not caught off balance easily, moves body	
	Footwork—	good balance, not flatfooted, starts toward shuttle correctly, gets back to base	
	Judgment—	sizes up court situations quickly, plays appropriate shots	
	Deception—	ability to deceive opponent by making proper feints	
	Wrist Control—	full use of wrist in controlling and alternating direction of strokes, clean follow through without slipping	

Score 1 if shot is very poorly executed according to standards listed above or if never attempts shot.
Score 2 if shot is poorly executed.
Score 3 if shot is fairly executed.
Score 4 if shot is well executed.
Score 5 if shot is excellently executed.

Additional Badminton References

Davis, Phyllis R.: The Development of a Combined Short and Long Badminton Service Skill Test, MSPE, University of Tennessee, Knoxville, 1968.

Greiner, Marilyn R.: Construction of a Short Serve Test for Beginning Badminton Players, MSPE, University of Wisconsin, Madison, 1964.

Hicks, Joanna V.: The Construction and Evaluation of a Battery of Five Badminton Skill Tests, Ph. D., Texas Woman's University, Denton, 1967.

Johnson, Rose Marie: Determination of the Validity and Reliability of the Badminton Placement Test, MSPE, University of Oregon, Eugene, 1967.

Kowert, Eugene A.: Construction of a Badminton Ability Test Battery for Men, MAPE, University of Iowa, Iowa City, 1968.

Lockhart, Aileene, and Frances A. McPherson: Development of a Test of Badminton Playing Ability, Research Quarterly, *20*, 402–405, December, 1949.

McDonald, E. Dawn: The Development of a Skill Test for the Badminton High Clear, MS in Ed., Southern Illinois University, Carbondale, 1968.

Washington, Jean: Construction of a Wall Test for the Badminton Short Serve, and the Effect of Wall Practice on Court Performance, MSPE, North Texas State University, Denton, 1968.

BASKETBALL—BOYS

Johnson Basketball Test*

Purpose. To measure the basic skills of shooting, throwing, and dribbling in boys' basketball.

Evaluation. The test is the result of work with 19 tests to determine the best ones to measure basketball playing ability. The reliability coefficients ranged from .73 to .93 and the validity coefficients reported were .84 and .88.

Level and Sex. The test is designed for use with high school boys.

Time Allotment and Number of Subjects. The 3-item battery is not unduly time consuming if the station method of class organization is used. Not more than 2 class periods should be required to complete the test.

Floor Plan and Space Requirement. A regulation basketball court and a wall area are needed.

Class Organization. The station plan can be used if assistants are trained. The throw for accuracy causes a bottleneck. Prepare more than 1 target or have 2 students alternate throwing at the same target. The two 30-second items could be timed by a central timer. Assistants would be needed at the test stations to give directions and score.

General Procedures. The three raw scores for the three test items can be added to obtain a battery score.

Uses. To measure improvement from the beginning to the end of a unit in basketball.

To be a partial basis for grading a basketball unit.

* From the unpublished thesis by L. W. Johnson: Objective Tests in Basketball for High School Boys, State University of Iowa, in H. Harrison Clarke, *Application of Measurement to Health and Physical Education,* © 1959 by Prentice-Hall, Inc., Englewood Cliffs, N. J. Used by permission of the publisher.

Test Description

ITEM NUMBER I—FIELD GOAL SPEED TEST

Purpose: To measure ability to make successive field goals under the stress of time.

Facilities and Equipment: basketball goal, basketball, stop watch.

Procedures: The student throws as many baskets as possible in any style from any distance starting close under the basket.

Instructions: "Stand close under the basket in any position you wish and make as many baskets as you can in 30 seconds.   Ready, Go!"

Scoring: One 30-second trial is given.   One point is scored for every basket made.

Testing Personnel: One person to score and time.

ITEM NUMBER II—BASKETBALL THROW FOR ACCURACY

Purpose: To measure the strength of the shoulders and the ability to throw accurately with consistency.

Facilities and Equipment: A target area, a space of about 50 feet, a basketball.

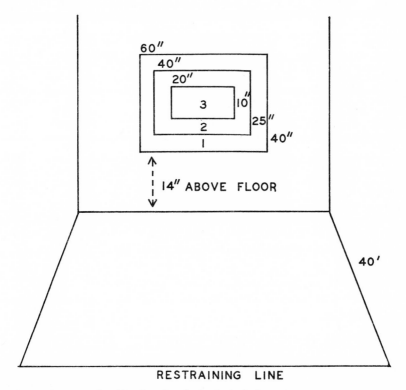

Fig. 9–3.   Specifications for the basketball throw for accuracy test.

Procedure: The student stands behind a line 40 feet from the target and throws either a baseball or hook pass to the target for 10 trials. Jacobson[20] used a 35-foot restraining line for the 7th grade boys and a 42-foot restraining line for the 8th and 9th grade boys.

Instructions: "Please stand behind this restraining line and throw the basketball to the target area. You will have 10 trials. Try to make as many points as possible."

Scoring: Score 3 points for every ball hitting in the center of the target or on the inner line. Score 2 points for balls landing in the middle rectangle and line. Score 1 point for balls landing in the outer rectangle or on the line. A total of 30 points is possible.

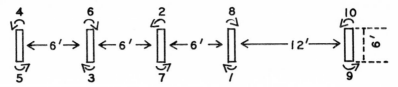

Fig. 9–4. Specifications for the dribble test.

Norms

Table 9–2. Norms for the Johnson Basketball Test* for Junior High School Boys

T-Score	Throw for Accuracy†			Field Goal Speed Test			Dribble Test			T-Score
	7th Grade	8th Grade	9th Grade	7th Grade	8th Grade	9th Grade	7th Grade	8th Grade	9th Grade	
85	25	23	25	14	19	22	24	26	26	85
80	23	21	23	13	18	21	23	25	26	80
75	21	19	20	12	16	19	22	24	25	75
70	19	16	18	10	14	17	21	23	24	70
65	16	14	16	9	13	15	20	22	22	65
60	14	12	14	7	11	12	19	20	21	60
55	11	10	11	6	9	10	18	19	20	55
50	9	8	9	5	7	8	17	18	19	50
45	7	5	7	4	6	6	16	17	18	45
40	4	3	4	2	4	4	15	16	17	40
35	2	1	2	1	2	2	14	15	16	35
30							13	14	15	30
25							12	13	14	25
20							11	12	13	20
15							10	11	12	15

* Norms used by permission of Theodore Vernon Jacobson and located in An Evaluation of Performance in Certain Physical Ability Tests Administered to Selected Secondary School Boys, M. S. in Physical Education, U. of Washington, Seattle, 1960.

† 35-foot restraining line for 7th grade boys, 42-foot restraining line for 8th and 9th grade boys.

Table 9–3.   Grade Ranges for the Johnson Basketball Ability Test*

Event	Grade	(Based on the Raw Scores) 7th Grade	8th Grade	9th Grade
Basketball Throw	A	18 & over	16 & over	18 & over
(In points)	B	13–17	11–15	13–17
	C	7–12	6–10	7–12
	D	1–6	1–5	1–6
	E	0	0	0
	A	10 & over	14 & over	16 & over
Basketball Shooting	B	7–9	10–13	12–15
(Baskets made)	C	4–6	6–9	7–11
	D	1–3	2–5	2–6
	E	0	1 & under	1 & under
	A	21 & over	23 & over	24 & over
Basketball Dribbling	B	19–20	20–22	21–23
(In points)	C	16–18	18–19	18–20
	D	14–15	15–17	16–17
	E	13 & under	14 & under	15 & under
	A	46 & over	48 & over	53 & over
Total Test	B	37–45	39–47	43–52
(Total points)	C	27–36	29–38	32–42
	D	18–26	20–28	22–31
	E	17 & under	19 & under	21 & under

* Used by permission of Theodore Vernon Jacobson.

Score Card

```
                    JOHNSON BASKETBALL TEST
        Name_____ Grade_____ Date_____
                                  Raw Score        T-Score
        1. Field Goal Speed Test
             (points)           _____     _____
        2. Basketball Throw for Accuracy
             (points)           _____  _____
                                _____  _____
                                _____  _____
                                _____  _____
                                _____  _____

                     Total      _____     _____
        3. Dribble (points)     _____     _____

                                           Average
                  Total Points  _____  T-Score_____
```

Testing Personnel: One assistant to score the test. Students waiting for their turns can help keep the ball available to the thrower.

ITEM NUMBER III—DRIBBLE

Purpose: To measure ball handling ability and agility of the player.

Facilities and Equipment: An area at least 40 feet in length is needed to set up the test. Sawhorses used as supports for Table Tennis tables or chairs or hurdles can be used as the obstacles. A ball and a stop watch.

Procedures: The test is started from behind a line which is 6 feet long and 12 feet from the first obstacle. The student dribbles the ball in "figure 8" fashion around the obstacles for 30 seconds. He continues with a second trip if time is remaining when he returns to the starting line.

Instructions: "Stand behind this line and on the signal, 'Ready, Go!', dribble in and out the obstacles in a figure 8 pattern passing as many areas as possible in 30 seconds."

Scoring: Score 1 point for every area passed; that is, 1 point every time the student passes the end of a hurdle or sawhorse.

Testing Personnel: One assistant to score and time.

Pimpa Modification of Bunn Basketball Test*

Purpose. To measure basketball ability of boys and men.

Evaluation. Pimpa reduced the 6-item Bunn test to two items. The original items included alternate lay-up, wall bounce, penny cup, dribble maze, stop and pivot, and dribble shot. Pimpa retained the alternate lay-up test and the penny cup test and found a relationship of .879 between these two items and the 6-item Bunn battery for unskilled players and a coefficient of .947 for skilled players.

Level and Sex. Pimpa used 100 men students at Springfield College; 50 skilled and 50 unskilled. The test seems appropriate for junior and senior high school age boys.

Time Allotment and Number of Students. An average size class can take the two items in one period if sufficient testing stations and stop watches are available.

Floor Plan and Space Requirements. A basketball court is needed. Both the basket areas and open space areas can be used.

Class Organization. The squad plan seems most feasible. Several stations of the Penny Cup test will be needed. The number of stations will be determined by the number of stop watches available. The Alternate Lay-up test can be given with a sweep hand wrist watch but a stop watch will be needed for the Penny Cup test.

Uses. To classify students for instruction and for competition.

* Pimpa, Udom: A Study to Determine the Relationship Between Bunn's Basketball Skill Test and the Writer's Modified Version of that Test, MSPE, Springfield College, Springfield, Massachusetts, 1968.

Test Description

ITEM NUMBER I—ALTERNATE LAY-UP

Purpose: To see how fast the student can make ten alternating lay-up shots.

Facilities and Equipment: Basketball goal, basketball, stop watch or sweep hand wrist watch.

Procedures and Instructions: "The purpose of this test is to see how fast you can make ten alternating lay-up shots. I will start the watch on the signal, 'Go' and I will stop the watch when you make the tenth basket. You may start on either side of the basket, but you will alternate each shot even though you lose control of the ball and it rolls away. You cannot go on until you have made a basket on one side."

Scoring: The score is the amount of time required to make ten alternating lay-up shots.

Testing Personnel: The instructor gives directions, demonstrates, and lets the students practice a few shots. A timer is needed for each testing station.

ITEM NUMBER II—PENNY CUP TEST

Purpose: To measure the agility and reaction time of boys.

Facilities and Equipment: Three tin cups and several pennies are needed for each testing area, stop watch, red, white, and blue paint or tape to put on the cups.

Procedures: The student stands on the starting line with his back to the cups; he has a penny in his hand. On the signal "Go," he turns and runs toward the cups. As he crosses the signal line, he is given a direction signal by the teacher; he continues to the cup indicated by the teacher and places the penny in that cup. The signal is one of three words: "red," "white," or "blue." The time that elapses between the starting signal and the sound of the penny striking in the cup is measured with a stop watch. The process is repeated four times. The score is the sum of times required in the four repetitions.

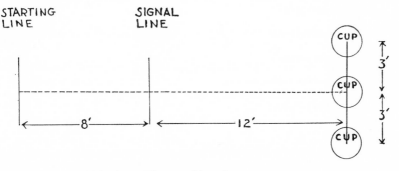

Fig. 9–5. Floor markings for penny cup test.

Instructions: "Watch me! I stand on this line with a penny in my hand. Notice that my back is toward the cups and I am in a crouched position. At the signal 'Go,' I turn and start toward the cups; as I cross the signal line, I hear the signal 'red,' and so I continue to the red cup and put the penny in it. If, as I crossed the signal line, I had heard the signal 'blue,' I would have gone to the blue cup. I want you to do the same thing, but do it as quickly as you can. The watch will start with the signal 'Go,' and will stop at the sound of the penny entering the cup. The watch will continue to run until the penny is in the cup. You will not be timed while you are returning to the starting line. You will repeat the test 4 times."

Testing Personnel: One test administrator at each testing station to time the student and to signal the cup color in random order.

Walter Basketball Evaluation Chart*

SCHOOL ————————————————   DATE——————————, 19——

PLAYER————————————— AGE—— HEIGHT—————— WEIGHT——————

	EXCELLENT	GOOD	AVERAGE	FAIR	POOR
	All-Conference Level	Varsity Level	Junior Varsity Level	Sophomore Level	Intramural Level
Speed					
Quickness					
Agility					
Jumping Ability					
Dribbling Skill					
Passing Skill					
Ball Handling Skill					
Foul Shooting Skill					
Side Shooting Skill					
Front Shooting Skill					
Close-in Shooting Skill					
Overall Skill Ability					
Overall Team Contribution					

* Walter, Ronald J.: A Comparison Between Two Selected Evaluative Techniques for Measuring Basketball Skill, M.S. Ed., Western Illinois University, Macomb, 1968. Used by permission of the author.

BASKETBALL—GIRLS
Leilich Basketball Test*

Purpose. To measure achievement in basketball skills.

Evaluation. The battery resulted from a factor analysis study covering all the basketball tests available. The four factors were identified as basketball motor ability, speed, ball handling for accuracy and speed in passing, and ball handling for accuracy in goal throwing.

Level and Sex. This battery was designed for college women and is appropriate for secondary school girls also.

Time Allotment and Number of Subjects. The three-item battery can be completed in 2 class periods. It might be done in only one if sufficient test stations and assistants are used for the size of the class.

Floor Plan and Space Requirements. A basketball court with wall space is needed. The test administration will be greatly expedited if 6 goals are available, since two of the three items in the battery make use of the goal.

Class Organization. The station method will facilitate testing. The 2 tests which require 30 seconds, the half-minute shooting, and the push-pass, could be administered by a central timer if the test stations are adjacent. The other goal could be used for the Bounce and Shoot test. Multiple stations can be used depending on the number of baskets available.

General Procedures. 1. Rest periods should be planned between each trial for each of the tests.
2. The circular target may need to be lowered and the distance to the restraining line shortened when giving the test to younger students.

Uses. To detect weaknesses in basic skills.
To include in unit grades.
To measure achievement.

Test Description

ITEM NUMBER I—BOUNCE AND SHOOT

Purpose: To measure agility and ball handling ability involving speed and accuracy of shooting.

Facilities and Equipment: 2 basketballs, a regulation basketball goal, stop watch, 2 chairs.

Procedures: The student starts from behind the 18-foot mark on the B side of the basket. When the signal is given, she picks up the ball from the chair, bounces, shoots, rebounds, and passes the ball back to the receiver who is standing behind the B chair. She then runs to the chair on the A side, picks up the ball, bounces, shoots, rebounds, and throws the ball to the receiver standing behind the A chair. This pattern is followed until ten shots have been made alternately from the B and A areas. The bounce must start from behind the 18-foot line. The timer starts the watch on signal and stops it when the student has caught the ball on rebound after making the 10th shot for the basket.

---

* Leilich, Avis: The Primary Components of Selected Basketball Tests for College Women, Unpublished doctoral dissertation, Indiana University, Bloomington, 1952. Used by permission of the author.

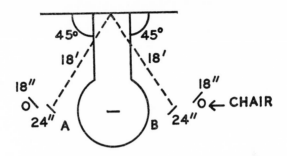

Fig. 9–6.   Specifications for the bounce and shoot test.

Instructions: "Stand behind this line which is 18 feet from the end line When 'Go!' signal is given, pick up the ball from the chair, bounce it once shoot for the basket, rebound, and pass the ball back to Sally who will be standing behind the chair.   Run immediately to get the ball in the chair on the left side of the basket and repeat the procedure.   You will do this, alternating sides, until you have made 10 shots for the basket and rebounded the ball.   You must start the bounce from behind the line, you may bounce only once, and you may not travel with the ball.   Your time and your baskets will count in the score."

Scoring: Time is recorded from the "Go" signal until the student has rebounded the ball following the 10th attempt for a basket.   Two scores are obtained.   One for accuracy and one for speed.   The accuracy score comprises two points for every basket, one point for hitting the rim but missing the basket, and no points for missing the rim and the basket.   The speed score is the total number of seconds required to complete the test.   One second is added to the score for every foul.   The best of 3 trials is recorded.

Testing Personnel: 2 pass receivers, 1 to time, and 1 additional to score and to notify the timer when the 9th shot is being made so the timer will be alert to stop the watch on the 10th rebound.

ITEM NUMBER II—HALF-MINUTE SHOOTING

Purpose: To measure accuracy of shooting.

Facilities and Equipment: Basketball, regulation goal, and a stop watch.

Procedures: The student stands near the basket holding a ball and shoots continuously for thirty seconds.   Any position is permissible and any type shot.

Instructions: "Stand near the basket, wherever you like, holding the ball. On the signal, 'Ready, Go!', shoot for the basket and make as many goals as possible in 30 seconds.   You may use any type shot you like.   You will have 2 trials and your better one will count."

Scoring: The score is the number of baskets made in 30 seconds. The basket counts if the ball has left the hands of the player when the 30 seconds is up. Two trials are given and the better one is the final score.

Testing Personnel: A timer who can also score.

ITEM NUMBER III—PUSH-PASS

Purpose: To measure the speed and accuracy of passing.

Facilities and Equipment: A target area, a basketball, and a stop watch.

Procedures: The student stands behind a 10-foot restraining line facing a target placed on the wall. She uses a two-hand chest pass to throw to the target for 30 seconds. The student must have both feet behind the restraining line when she passes but she may go forward of it to retrieve the ball.

Instructions: "Stand behind this line and pass to the target using a push-pass. You will be timed for 30 seconds and should try to accumulate as many points as possible during this time. The better of two trials will count. Ready, Go!"

Scoring: The score is the total points made in 30 seconds. A ball which lands on a circle is scored by the value of the inside circle. A ball which lands outside the circle counts no points. Two trials are given, the better one counting.

Testing Personnel: 1 person to time, 1 to call the point values, and 1 to record them after each pass. The passes will be so fast that the addition of points will be difficult for the spotter. They can be added more accurately after someone has recorded them.

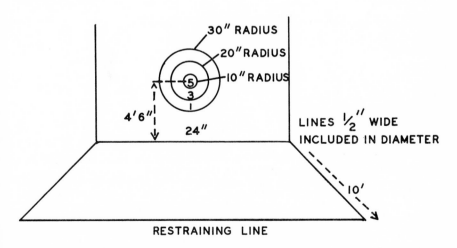

Fig. 9–7. Specifications for the push-pass test.

Score Card

LEILICH BASKETBALL TEST

Name_____ Grade_____ Date_____

	Raw Scores		T-Scores
	Time	Points	
Bounce and Shoot	____	____	
	____	____	
	____	____	____ ____
Half-Minute Shooting	____		
	____		____
Push-Pass	____		
	____		____

Norms

Table 9–4.   Norms for Leilich Basketball Test*

T-Score	½-Minute Shooting	½-Minute Shooting	Bounce and Shoot Accuracy	Speed	Push-Pass	T-Score
80	20	15			137	80
75	18	14		41	130	75
70	16	12		46	123	70
65	14	9	19	52	117	65
60	13	8	17	58	110	60
55	11	6	15	64	103	55
50	9	5	13	70	96	50
45	7	4	11	76	90	45
40	6		9	82	83	40
35	4	3	7	88	76	35
30	2	2	5	94	70	30
25	1		3	100	63	25
20		1	1	106	56	20

* Norms by Miller, Wilma K.:   Achievement Levels in Basketball Skills for Women Physical Education Majors, Research Quarterly, *25*, 450–455, December, 1954, except for 2nd column of norms for ½-Minute Shooting which are located in *Measurement and Evaluation in Physical Education* by M. Gladys Scott and Esther French, Dubuque, Iowa, Wm. C. Brown Publishers, 1959, pages 160–161. The norms by Miller used by permission of the AAHPER and the norms by Scott and French based on the performance of high school girls and used by permission of M. Gladys Scott and Esther French.

Table 9–5. Norms for Leilich Basketball Test for College Major Students*

Percentile	½-Minute Shooting	Bounce and Shoot		Push-Pass	Percentile
		Speed	Accuracy		
100	18	50	20	125	100
95	14	56		115	95
90	13	58	17	110	90
85	12	60		108	85
80			16	105	80
75	11	61		104	75
70		63	15	103	70
65	10	64		101	65
60		66	14	100	60
55	9	67		99	55
50		68	13	97	50
45	8	70		95	45
40		71	12	94	40
35	7	72	11	92	35
30		74	10	91	30
25	6	76		89	25
20		79	9	86	20
15	5	81	8	83	15
10	4	86	6	79	10
5	3	89	4	73	5
1	1			44	1

* Norms by Wilma K. Miller and used by permission of the AAHPER.

Table 9–6. Classification of Raw Scores on Leilich Test*

Classification	½-Minute Shoot	B & S Speed	B & S Accuracy	Push-Pass
Superior	16 & above	47 & below	21 & above	122 & above
Good	12–15	48–61	16–20	106–121
Average	7–11	62–77	10–15	89–105
Fair	3–6	78–91	6–9	72–88
Poor	2 & below	92 & above	5 & below	71 & below
	N 1812	N 1645	N 1645	N 1646
	M 9.11	M 69.69	M 12.95	M 96.66
	SD 3.50	SD 12.00	SD 4.12	SD 13.47

* Norms based on college major students. Prepared by Wilma K. Miller and used by permission of the AAHPER.

Cunningham Basketball Test*

Purpose. To measure the basketball playing ability of high school girls.

Evaluation. Cunningham used Incidence Charts to identify the fundamental skills in basketball. Passing ranked first, then dribbling, rebounding, shooting, pivoting, and intercepting in that order. She began with 7 items and finished with a 3-item battery which had a multiple correlation of .69 using the sum of 4 judges' ratings as the validity criterion. She used 108 high school girls to develop the battery. The judges' ratings intercorrelated with coefficients ranging from .88 to .91.

	Reliability	*Validity*
Run and Pass	.71	.46
Dribbling	.89	.46
Modified Edgren	.94	.60

The intercorrelations for the 3-item battery were as follow:

Run and Pass—Dribbling	.30
Run and Pass—Modified Edgren	.33
Dribbling—Modified Edgren	.39

The multiple correlation for the 3-item battery was .69 and .71 for the 7-item battery. The weighted formula is 1.8 Run and Pass + 1.0 Dribbling + 3.3 Modified Edgren. The norms reported seemed to be from raw scores and not from weighted scores.

The Modified Edgren test was located in the literature. The other items were developed by Cunningham within the high school situation.

Cunningham recommends the 3-item battery but suggests that the addition of a shooting item would make the total measure more representative of the important skills of the game and might make the battery more meaningful to the students.

Level and Sex. High school girls.

Time Allotment and Number of Students. Two class periods will be needed to administer the battery to a regular class because of the nature of the items and the endurance factor in one item.

Floor Plan and Space Requirements. A basketball court and unobstructed wall space will be required.

Class Organization. The squad plan should be used with several stations of each test item.

General Procedures. Use a central timer for the two 30-second items. Allow practice time. If time permits, administer 4 instead of 3 trials on each item. Give 2 trials on 2 different days.

Uses. To aid in classification.
For student motivation.
For grading.
For practice devices.
Cunningham states, however, that these items should not be used to provide the sole measurement for such purposes.

* Cunningham, Phyllis: Measuring Basketball Playing Ability of High School Girls, Ph.D., University of Iowa, Iowa City, 1964. Used by permission of the author.

Test Description

ITEM NUMBER I—RUN AND PASS

Purpose: To assess running ability, including both speed and endurance.

Equipment: Two regulation basketballs, two chairs with a shallow box (6 inches depth) fastened to the seat, a ball in each box.

Markings: Center line in the gymnasium. A line 4 feet long, 15 feet from each end of the gymnasium. A chair with box attached is placed opposite each of the 4 foot lines, chairs facing the same side wall.

Procedure: The player starts behind one of the 4-foot lines. On signal, *Ready, Go!* she runs forward to the opposite chair, picks up the ball, throws it to the end wall, catches the ball and places it back in the box. If the ball bounces out she must pick it up and put it back into the box. She runs to the opposite chair, repeats, and continues running and passing for 90

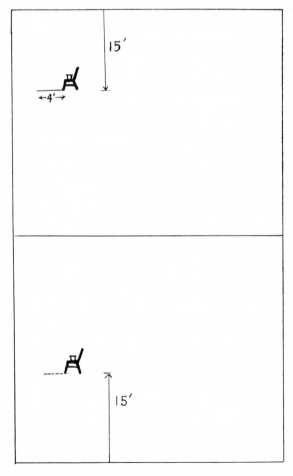

Fig. 9–8. Markings for run and pass test.

seconds. The timer calls the time every 15 seconds ("15 . . . 30 . . . 60 . . . 75 . . .") and blows the whistle after 90 seconds. The player stops where she is when the whistle blows and remains there until the scorer announces the score. One trial is given. The test is explained and demonstrated but no practice is allowed. This is a strenuous test. Tell students to go as fast as they can but to try to pace themselves, listening for the time announcements.

Scoring: The score is the number of times the ball is placed back in the box after running, throwing and catching, plus $\frac{1}{4}$ point for crossing the center line, $\frac{1}{2}$ point for having the ball in the hands before the throw, and $\frac{3}{4}$ point if the ball has been thrown but not returned to the box when time is up.

Testing Personnel: A central timer can be used. The instructor should explain and demonstrate the test. The students can score for each other at each station.

ITEM NUMBER II—DRIBBLE

Purpose: To assess body control and dribbling ability.

Equipment: Official basketball, stop watch.

Markings: A flat unobstructed wall space at least 16 feet long and 7 feet high fronted by floor space about 10 feet deep. Four 12-inch radius circles placed as follows: (All measurements are center to center.) Circle I 4 feet from the wall, II 3 feet to the right of I and 7 feet from wall, III 6 feet to the right of II and 7 feet from the wall, IV 3 feet to the right of III and 4 feet from the wall.

Procedure: An extra player stands in circle II facing circle IV; another player stands in circle III facing circle I. The player taking the test stands in Circle I with basketball in hands. On signal *Ready, Go!* she dribbles between the two players standing in the circles, around the player in circle

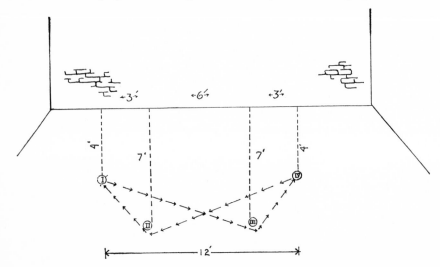

Fig. 9–9. Markings for dribble test.

III and into circle IV, passes to the wall, catches the ball and dribbles back going between the two players, around the player in circle II and into circle I. She throws to the wall, catches and repeats the entire sequence as rapidly as possible, moving until the whistle blows at the end of 30 seconds. Three trials are given.

The player must not travel with the ball. The pass and catch are not counted as a score if the player travels anytime between the start in circle I or IV and the throw in circle IV or I.

After explanation and demonstration, each girl takes one complete practice trial.

Scoring: The score on each trial is the number of times the ball is caught after being passed to the wall (without traveling on the dribble), plus one half point for being even with the player standing in the far circle when the whistle blows. The player's score is the total of three trials.

ITEM NUMBER III—MODIFIED EDGREN BALL HANDLING

Purpose: To assess ball handling and change of direction abilities.

Equipment: Properly inflated basketball, stop watch.

Markings: A flat unobstructed wall space at least 15 feet long and 7 feet high and a floor space in front of it 15 feet long and 10 feet deep.

A line on the floor parallel to the wall and 7½ feet from it. Two parallel lines on the wall, lines 4 feet long, 3 feet apart (width of lines included in 3 feet), starting 18 inches above floor. Two lines on the floor, each line 15 inches to the outside of one of the lines on the wall (5½ feet apart, lines included) so that they are perpendicular to the line parallel to the wall.

I on floor = starting zone for first and other odd-numbered throws
I on the wall = target for odd-numbered throws
II on floor = starting zone for second and other even-numbered throws
II on wall = target for even-numbered throws

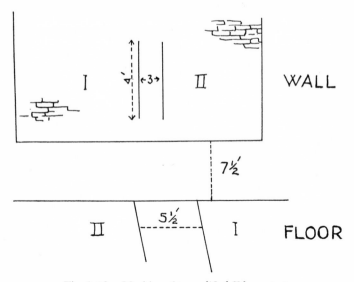

Fig. 9–10. Markings for modified Edgren test.

Procedure: The player stands in area I with basketball in hands. On signal *Ready, Go!* she throws the ball to area I on the wall, runs to corner II or beyond so that she catches the ball on the rebound. She repeats from II throwing to II on the wall, and continues throwing alternately to I and II as rapidly as possible until the whistle blows at the end of 30 seconds. Three trials are given. Allow each girl one complete practice trial. The player must stay behind the $7\frac{1}{2}$-foot line at all times, and the throws must be made while in the proper area. The ball may not hit in the 3-foot neutral zone on the wall. The player may use any type of pass, and any type of pivot or turn; she is not penalized for traveling. The ball may bounce on the floor one or more times before being caught.

Scoring: The score on each trial is the number of successful hits made in the proper wall area (without line violations being made in the recovery) before time is called. The player's score is the total for three trials.

Testing Personnel: A central timer can be used for the Modified Edgren Ball Handling item and the Dribbling item. Students can score for each other. The items should be described to the entire group and then the students should disburse to the testing stations.

Score Card

Cunningham Basketball Test

Name_____ Grade_____ Date_____

Offensive Player_____ Defensive Player_____

Run and Pass (Total of 2 trials)

    1._____   2._____   Total_____   T-Score_____

Dribbling (Total of 3 trials)

    1._____   2._____   3._____   Total_____   T-Score_____

Modified Edgren Ball Handling
   (Total of 3 trials)

    1._____   2._____   3._____   Total_____   T-Score____

                                       Total T-Score_____

                                   Average T-Score_____

Norms

Table 9–7.   T-Scale Norms—Cunningham Basketball Test

T-Score	Run and Pass N = 132	Dribbling N = 137	Modified Edgren N = 131	T-Score
75	111	77	61	75
70	109	75	58	70
65	105	70	52	65
60	100	65	48	60
55	96	60	45	55
50	92	54	43	50
45	88	50	40	45
40	84	42	35	40
35	82	36	32	35
30	78	30	27	30
25	73	18	23	25

Based on the performance of high school girls.

Additional Basketball References

Barrow, H. M.: Basketball Skill Test, The Physical Educator, *16*, 26–27, March, 1959.

Brace, David K.: Consultant, *Skills Test Manual—Basketball for Boys*, Washington, D.C.: AAHPER, 1966.

———: Consultant, *Skills Test Manual—Basketball for Girls*, Washington, D.C.: AAHPER, 1966.

Bonner, Donald A.: A Comparative Study of the Ability of High School Basketball Players to Perform Basic Skills at Three Stages of the Season, Master's Thesis, North Carolina College, Durham, 1963.

Edgren, H. D.: An Experiment in the Testing of Ability and Progress in Basketball, Research Quarterly, *3*, 159, March, 1932.

Elbel, E. R., and Forrest C. Allen: Evaluating Team and Individual Performance in Basketball, Research Quarterly, *5*, 538–555, October, 1941.

Gilbert, Raymond R.: A Study of Selected Variables in Predicting Basketball Players, MSPE, Springfield College, Springfield, Massachusetts, 1968.

Jones, Edith: A Study of Knowledge and Playing Ability in Basketball for High School Girls, Unpublished Master's Thesis, State University of Iowa, Iowa City, 1941.

Kay, H. Kenner: A Statistical Analysis of the Profile Technique for the Evaluation of Competitive Basketball Performance, MA, University of Alberta, Edmonton, Alberta, Canada, 1966.

Knox, Robert D.: Basketball Ability Test, Scholastic Coach, *17*, 45, March, 1947

Lehsten, Nelson: A Measure of Basketball Skills in High School Boys, The Physical Educator, *5*, 103–109, December, 1948.

Loose, W. A. Robert, Jr.: A Study to Determine the Validity of the Knox Basketball Test, M.S. in Physical Education, Washington State University, Pullman, 1961.

Matthews, Leslie E.: A Battery of Basketball Skills Test for High School Boys, MSPE, University of Oregon, Eugene, 1963.

Mortimer, Elizabeth M.: Basketball Shooting, Research Quarterly, *22*, 234–243, May, 1951.

Peters, Gerald V.: The Reliability and Validity of Selected Shooting Tests in Basketball, MAPE, University of Michigan, Ann Arbor, 1964.

Plinke, John F.: The Development of Basketball Physical Skill Potential Test Batteries by Height Categories, P. E. D., Indiana University, Bloomington, 1966.

Schwartz, Helen: Achievement Tests in Girls Basketball at the Senior High School Level, Research Quarterly, *8*, 143–156, March, 1937.

Stroup, Francis: Relationship Between Measurement of Field of Motion Perception and Basketball Ability in College Men, Research Quarterly, *28*, 72–76, March, 1950.

Stubbs, Helen C.: An Explanatory Study of Girls Basketball Relative to the Measurement of Ball Handling Ability, MSPE, University of Tennessee, Knoxville, 1968.

Thornes, Ann B.: An Analysis of a Basketball Shooting Test and Its Relation to Other Basketball Skill Tests, MSPE, University of Wisconsin, Madison, 1963.

Voltmer, E. F., and Ted Watts: A Rating Scale for Player Performance in Basketball, Journal of Health and Physical Education, *2*, 94–95, February, 1947.

Wilbur, Carol D.: Construction of a Simple Skills Test, *Basketball Guide—1959–60*. Washington, D.C.: AAHPER, 1959, pp. 30–33.

Young, Genevieve, and Helen Moser: A Short Battery of Tests to Measure Playing Ability in Women's Basketball, Research Quarterly, *5*, 3–23, May, 1934.

FENCING

Cooper Fencing Rating Scale*

5—Superior. The fencer almost always displays proper form. She shows good balance in performing the actions. Her movements are quick and sharp with little waste motion.

4—Excellent. The fencer usually displays proper form. Her movements and balance are above average.

3—Average. The fencer displays the proper form more than half of the time. Her movements and balance are good.

2—Fair The fencer sometimes displays the proper form. Her movements are awkward and she tends to have an excess of wasted motion.

1—Poor. The fencer rarely displays proper form. Her balance is poor and there is a great deal of wasted motion. She displays little knowledge of the fundamentals of fencing.

Additional Fencing References

Bower, Muriel G.: A Test of General Fencing Ability, Unpublished Master's Thesis, University of Southern California, Los Angeles, 1961.

Schutz, Helen J.: Construction of an Achievement Scale in Fencing for Women, Unpublished Master's Thesis, University of Washington, Seattle, 1940.

Wyrick, Waneen: A Comparison of the Effectiveness of Two Methods of Teaching Beginning Fencing to College Women, Unpublished Master's Thesis, The Woman's College of the University of North Carolina, Greensboro, 1958.

FIELD HOCKEY

Schmithals-French Achievement Tests in Field Hockey†

Purpose. To aid in the classification of students for instructional purposes.

Evaluation. The total battery includes 6 items:
1. Goal shooting left.
2. Dribble, dodge, circular tackle, and drive.

---

* Cooper, Cynthia K.: The Development of a Fencing Skill Test for Measuring Achievement of Beginning Collegiate Women Fencers in Using the Advance, Beat, and Lunge, MS in Ed., Western Illinois University, Macomb, 1968. Used by permission of the author.

† Schmithals, Margaret, and Esther French: Achievement Tests in Field Hockey for College Women, Research Quarterly, *11*, 84–92, October, 1940. Used by permission of the AAHPER.

3. Fielding and drive.
4. Drive for distance.
5. Combined goal shooting.
6. Push pass.

Only the second item is included here because it proved to be the best single measure. The goal shooting left and the fielding and drive test were the best combination for a 2-item battery.

The validity with subjective ratings as criterion was .44 and the reliability was .92.

Level and Sex. This test was developed using college women as subjects. It has been widely used for secondary school girls.

Time Allotment and Number of Subjects. The test is time consuming because each player must have 6 trials. Each trial, however, is not long— 30 seconds. Several test stations might be arranged off to the side of the hockey field.

Floor Plan and Space Requirements. A field space of 50 by 20 feet is needed for each station.

Class Organization. The squad method works well because the girls will need to rest between trials.

General Procedures. 1. Arrange test stations to the side of the field so testing can proceed while play is scheduled.
2. Keep testing stations set up as practice stations.
3. Do not administer indoors.

Uses. To classify students at the first of the unit.
To measure progress.
To use as a practice drill.
To use as only one phase of the total grade.

Test Description

Purpose: To measure ability to control the ball for a combination of fundamental hockey skills.

Facilities and Equipment: Hockey sticks, ball, 2 obstacles, stop watch.

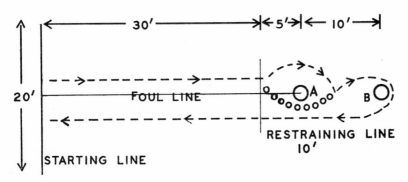

Fig. 9–11. Specifications for the dribble, dodge, circular tackle, and drive test.

Procedures: The player begins by standing behind the starting line to her left of the foul line. She is holding a hockey stick and a ball is on the starting line anywhere to the left of the foul line. She dribbles to the restraining line, keeping the ball to the left of the foul line, sends the ball to the right of the standard while she goes to the left, regains control of the ball and dribbles it around the second standard going to the right. She then drives the ball back around the starting line and may follow it up to hit it again if more distance is needed.

Instructions: "Stand behind the starting line to the left of the foul line and be ready to start dribbling the ball on the signal, 'Ready, Go!' Dribble to the restraining line, keeping the ball from crossing the foul line—keep to the left of it. You then dodge to the left of the first obstacle while sending the ball to the right of it. Regain control of the ball and dribble it around the second obstacle to the right like performing a circular tackle. Once around far enough to get a good drive, drive the ball across the starting line. You may follow the ball to give it additional hits if necessary. Both you and the ball must stay to the left of the foul line on the dribble, you and the ball must go opposite ways around the first obstacle, and you must dribble to the right around the second obstacle and then refrain from making 'sticks' when you drive the ball across the starting line. You will have six timed trials which will be averaged for your final score."

Scoring: Time is taken from the "Go" signal until the ball crosses the starting line. Six trials are recorded and then averaged for the final score.

Testing Personnel: A timer.

Score Card

```
┌─────────────────────────────────────────────────────────────────────┐
│            NAME_____                           │
│            CLASS_____                          │
│            DATE _____                          │
│                    Dribble, Dodge, Circular Tackle, Drive Test        │
│                            1. _____                              │
│                            2. _____                              │
│                            3. _____                              │
│                            4. _____                              │
│                            5. _____                              │
│                            6. _____                              │
│            Total               _____                            │
│            Average             _____                            │
│            T-Score             _____                            │
└─────────────────────────────────────────────────────────────────────┘
```

Norms

The condition of the field and the skill of the players will vary greatly so the preparation of local norms is recommended. Scott and French[41] report a mean T-score of 14 seconds based on the performance of 310 college women. See the norms given with the Friedel Test based on the performance of 68 high school girls.

Friedel Field Hockey Test*

Purpose. To measure ball control and maneuverability of the player to adjust to a moving ball.

Evaluation. Reliability r = .90 on trials from the left.
                  = .77 on trials from the right.
        Validity   r = .87 using the Schmithals-French test of dribble, dodge, circular tackle, and drive as the criterion.

A group of 68 high school girls was used as the study group.

Level and Sex. Designed for high school girls.

Time Allotment and Number of Subjects. The administration is time consuming because each student has 20 trials. Multiple stations would expedite the administration element. Testing concurrently with game play is recommended.

Floor Plan and Space Requirements. A field space 30 by 15 yards is needed for each testing station.

Class Organization. Several test stations should be available. Practice trials should be permitted during the lessons prior to the test. Rest periods should be permitted between trials.

General Procedures. 1. Practice with several students on the speed and direction of the roll-in so they can help administer the test and so that part of the test will be as standardized as possible.

2. Do not have a student take all 20 trials on one day.

Uses. To classify students.

To measure progress in game-like skills.

To provide a self-testing situation which will motivate practice.

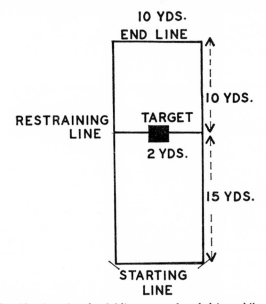

Fig. 9–12. Specifications for the fielding, control and drive while moving test.

* Friedel, Jean Elizabeth: The Development of a Field Hockey Skill Test for High School Girls, Unpublished Master's Thesis, Illinois State University, Normal, 1956. Used by permission of the author.

Test Description

Purpose: To measure ability to control the ball in a variety of game-like situations.

Facilities and Equipment: Hockey sticks, ball, stop watch. The target should be 2 yards in length and 1 yard in width and should be placed in the center of the restraining line. The diagonal lines from which the balls are rolled are 1 yard in length.

Procedures: The player stands behind the starting line and, on the signal, runs forward to control a ball which has been rolled in either from the right or left corner. The ball should be aimed toward the target area, and if not accurate, it should be rolled in again. The player should have the ball in control by the time she passes the restraining line. She dribbles to the end line, turns around and drives the ball back to the starting line A follow up drive may be needed The return drive must stay within the 10-yard lane for the trial to count

Instructions: "Stand behind the starting line holding your hockey stick. On the signal, 'Ready, Go!' run toward the target area to receive the ball which will be rolled in to you from the left (or right) side. Have it in control, dribbling as you pass the restraining line on the way to the end line. Once at the end, turn around and drive the ball back to the starting line, keeping it within the lane. You may follow the ball to drive again if needed. If the roll-in is not accurate, the trial will be repeated. You will have 10 trials from the left and 10 from the right. The total time for the 20 trials will be your score."

Scoring: Time each trial from the "Go" signal until the ball crosses the starting line on the return trip. Total the number of seconds for all 20 trials.

Testing Personnel: Timer. Trained assistants to roll in the ball. Speed and accuracy of the roll-in should be fairly consistent for every trial and for every student, as this will influence the performance of the student taking the test.

Score Card

FRIEDEL FIELD HOCKEY TEST

NAME_____ DATE_____

GRADE_____ CLASS_____

Right		*Left*	
1	_____	1	_____
2	_____	2	_____
3	_____	3	_____
4	_____	4	_____
5	_____	5	_____
6	_____	6	_____
7	_____	7	_____
8	_____	8	_____
9	_____	9	_____
10	_____	10	_____

Sub-Total _____   Sub-Total _____

Final Total _____   T-Score _____

Norms

Table 9–8. Norms for Field Hockey Test*

T-Score	Friedel Test (Total seconds in 20 trials)	Schmithals-French Test (Average seconds in 6 trials)	T-Score
80	193		80
75	209	11.0	75
70	224	12.3	70
65	239	13.6	65
60	255	14.9	60
55	270	16.2	55
50	285	17.5	50
45	301	18.8	45
40	316	20.1	40
35	331	21.4	35
30	347	22.6	30
25	361	23.9	25
20	376		20

* Based on the performance of 68 high school girls.

Strait's Field Hockey Rating Scale*

EXCELLENT—5 points

1. stick work is superior
2. footwork is consistently controlled
3. ball control is excellent
4. passes are well timed and accurate
5. very rarely fouls
6. positions herself well
7. cuts to receive passes
8. takes advantage of nearly all opportunities

GOOD—4 points

1. shows ability to make proper use of the stick
2. feet are used to good advantage most of the time
3. ball is usually under control
4. passes are well timed and accurate
5. fouls rarely
6. positions herself well most of the time
7. is able to see opportunities and take advantage of them
8. cuts to receive passes

* Strait, C. Jane: The Construction and Evaluation of a Field Hockey Skills Test. Unpublished Master's Thesis, Smith College, Northampton, Mass., 1960. Used by permission of the author.

AVERAGE—3 points

1. drives and fielding are good, but lacks fine control of the ball for consistent dodges and tackles
2. full use is not made of the feet
3. when in possession of the ball, occasionally loses it because of poor control
4. some passes are good, but others are not well timed or accurate
5. fouls moderately often
6. is not sure as to where her position should be many times
7. misses some available opportunities
8. does not consistently cut for passes

LOW—2 points

1. drives are not strong
2. when fielding, often misses the ball
3. rarely tries dodges
4. tackles unsuccessfully
5. feet are sometimes in the way
6. has small degree of ball control
7. passes are poorly timed and not accurate
8. fouls fairly often
9. lacks good positioning
10. usually fails to take advantage of opportunities
11. is slow in getting to the ball

POOR—1 point

1. lacks general control of the stick
2. feet are in the way
3. ball is rarely under control
4. passes are poorly timed and are not well directed
5. fouls often
6. appears not to realize the benefits of good positioning
7. rarely takes advantage of opportunities
8. usually does not move to meet the ball
9. lacks body control, in general

Additional Field Hockey References

Illner, Julee A.: The Construction and Validation of a Skill Test for the Drive in Field Hockey, M.S. in Ed., Southern Illinois University, Carbondale, 1968.

Stewart, Harriet E.: A Test for Measuring Field Hockey Skill of College Women, P.E.D., Indiana University, Bloomington, 1965.

FOOTBALL AND TOUCH FOOTBALL
Borleske Touch Football Test*

Purpose. To measure the basic skills in touch football for classifying students into competitive groups and for a partial basis of grading.

Evaluation. The 3-item battery correlated .88 with the objective criterion of composite scores. Judgments were also used on the performance of each student.

Level and Sex. This test battery was originally designed for college men. It has been used widely and adapted slightly for use with secondary school boys.

Time Allotment and Number of Subjects. The original battery contains 5 items, but 3 are considered a valid measure of touch football performance. The reduction in the size of the battery shortens the time requirement. The nature of any distance item requires more time and more organization for efficient test administration. Two class lessons would be needed to give the 3-item battery to a class of boys.

Floor Plan and Space Requirement. Use both ends of the football field for 2 stations of each item if enough equipment is available and if several classes must be accommodated.

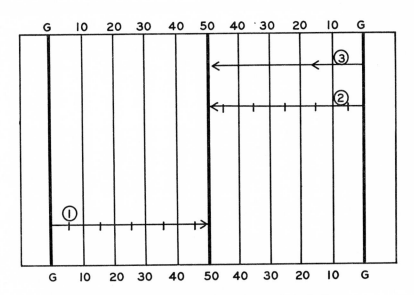

Fig. 9–13. Field plan for the Borleske touch football test.
(1) Punt for distance. (2) Pass for distance. (3) Sprint.

* Borleske, Stanley E.: A Study of Achievement of College Men in Touch Football, Unpublished Master's Thesis, University of California, Berkeley, 1936. Reported by Cozens, Frederick W., Ninth Annual Report of the Committee on Curriculum Research of the College Physical Education Association, Research Quarterly, *8*, 73–78, May, 1937. Used by permission of the AAHPER.

Class Organization. The 50-yard sprint will take less time to administer. One instructor or student leader could administer this item and then divide the class between the other two stations. Two stations of each of the distance items would speed the administration considerably. An individual score card should be taken by each student to the test station. Borleske suggests that the students take the tests in partners—1 performing and 1 recording the score.

General Procedures. 1. Borleske suggests that the pass for distance and the punt for distance be preceded by a pass from center to the performer. This practice was *not* used in the norms presented.

2. The plan of organization should be explained to the students.

3. The assistants should be trained prior to the testing period.

Test Description

ITEM NUMBER I—FORWARD PASS FOR DISTANCE

Purpose: To measure the ability to pass far and straight.

Facilities and Equipment: A football field should be marked every 5 yards. Several footballs will speed the administration.

Procedures: One minute of warm-up is permitted. The player receives the pass from the center and passes. Three trials are given and the best one counts. If the pass from center is not good, another one is made.

NOTE: The test was not administered with the pass from center for the norms reported.

Instructions: "Stand here to receive a pass from the center and then pass the ball as far and as straight as you can. You will have three trials and the best one will score. Be sure you have allowed enough space behind the line to get off your pass without going over the line."

Scoring: The distance is measured to the nearest yard and the best of 3 trials is recorded.

Testing Personnel: One to give instructions and administer the test. One or two in the field to spot the distance and retrieve the footballs.

ITEM NUMBER II—PUNT FOR DISTANCE

Purpose: To measure ability to punt for distance.

Facilities and Equipment: A football field marked every 5 yards. Several footballs.

Procedures: The kicker stands behind a line 7 yards behind the center, receives the pass from center, and within 2 seconds, punts the ball. A warm-up period of 1 minute is permitted.

NOTE: The test was not administered with the snap from center for the norms presented.

Instructions: "Stand behind this line and receive the ball on the snap from center. If the snap is not good, it will be repeated. Within 2 seconds, you must get the ball away, punting it as far and as straight as you can. The best of 3 trials will be recorded."

Scoring: The distance is estimated to the nearest yard measuring from the 5-yard markers.   The best of 3 punts is recorded.

Testing Personnel: 1 test administrator, 1 spotter, and several ball retrievers.

ITEM NUMBER III—RUNNING—STRAIGHT-AWAY, SPEED, OR SPRINT

Purpose: To measure ability to make a fast take-off after receiving the ball and to run for 50 yards.

Facilities and Equipment: A 50-yard area marked from 5 yards back of center, a football, and a stop watch.

Procedures: The student, in a backfield stance (three-point stance), receives the pass from center who is 5 yards away, and immediately runs 50 yards carrying the ball.

Instructions: "Start 5 yards behind the center in a three-point stance.   He will snap the ball to you.   Receive it and carry it for 50 yards running as fast as possible.   If the snap is bad, it will be repeated.   You will have only one trial.   Time will be taken from the second you receive the ball until you cross the 50-yard line."

Scoring: Time one trial from the instant the player receives the ball from center until he has crossed the 50-yard mark.

Testing Personnel: A timer, center, and recorder.

Score Card

BORLESKE TOUCH FOOTBALL TEST

Name_____ Grade_____ Date_____

T-Score

1. Pass for Distance   Best of 3   _____   _____
                        (yards)

2. Punt for Distance   Best of 3   _____   _____
                        (yards)

3. 50-yd. Sprint   (seconds)   _____   _____

Norms

Table 9–9.   Norms for the Borleske Touch Football Test for Junior High School Boys*

T-Score	Pass for Distance			Punt for Distance			Run for Speed			T-Score
	7th Grade	8th Grade	9th Grade	7th Grade	8th Grade	9th Grade	7th Grade	8th Grade	9th Grade	
85	41	48	53	38	43	47				85
80	39	45	50	36	40	44	6.3	5.8	5.7	80
75	36	41	46	33	37	41	6.7	6.2	6.0	75
70	34	38	43	31	34	38	7.0	6.6	6.3	70
65	31	35	39	28	31	34	7.3	7.0	6.7	65
60	28	32	36	26	28	32	7.7	7.4	7.0	60
55	25	29	33	23	25	28	8.0	7.7	7.3	55
50	23	26	29	20	22	25	8.3	8.1	7.6	50
45	20	23	26	18	19	22	8.6	8.5	7.9	45
40	18	20	23	16	16	19	9.0	8.9	8.3	40
35	15	17	19	13	13	16	9.3	9.2	8.6	35
30	13	14	16	11	10	13	9.6	9.6	8.9	30
25	10	10	13	8	7	10	10.0	10.0	9.2	25
20	8	8	10	6		7	10.3	10.4	9.5	20
15	5	6					10.6	10.7	9.9	15

* Norms used by permission of Theodore Vernon Jacobson and located in An Evaluation of Performance in Certain Physical Ability Tests Administered to Selected Secondary School Boys, Unpublished Master's Thesis, University of Washington, Seattle, 1960.

Table 9–10. Grade Ranges for the Borleske Touch Football Test*

Event	Grade	7th Grade	8th Grade	9th Grade
Pass for Distance (Measured in yards)	A[a]	33 & over	38 & over	42 & over
	B	27–32	30–37	34–41
	C	21–26	23–29	26–33
	D	15–20	15–22	18–25
	E	14 & under	14 & under	17 & under
Punt for Distance (Measured in yards)	A	30 & over	34 & over	37 & over
	B	24–29	26–33	30–36
	C	18–23	19–25	22–29
	D	12–17	12–18	15–21
	E	11 & under	11 & under	14 & under
Running Speed (Measured in seconds)	A	7.1 & under	6.7 & under	6.4 & under
	B	7.2–7.8	6.8–7.6	6.5–7.1
	C	7.9–8.7	7.7–8.5	7.2–7.9
	D	8.8–9.5	8.6–9.4	8.0–8.7
	E	9.6 & over	9.5 & over	8.8 & over
Total Test (Measured in T-scores)	A	195 & over	193 & over	195 & over
	B	166–194	165–192	165–194
	C	137–165	137–164	136–164
	D	108–136	108–136	106–135
	E	107 & under	107 & under	105 & under

Legend

Seventh Grade Pass for Distance

M = 23.5   S.D = 5.14

(GRADING ON THE 5 S.D. RANGE)

[a]A = 1.8 S.D. and up
B = .6 S.D. to 1.8 S.D.
C = −.6 S.D. to + .6 S.D.
D = −1.8 S.D. to −.6 S.D.
E = below −1.8 S.D.

A = 23.5 + 1.8 S.D. (5.14) and up = *33 yards and up*
B = 23.5 + .6 S.D. (5.14) to 33 yards = 23.5 + 3.02 (or 26.52) to 27 or *27 to 32 yards*
C = (23.5 − 3.02) to 27 = 20.48 to 27 or *21 to 26 yards*
D = (23.5 − 9.05) to 21 = 18.47 to 21 or *15 to 20 yards*
E = (23.5 − 9.05) or below 14.45 or *14 yards and under*

* Used by permission of Theodore Vernon Jacobson

Wallrof Rating Scale for Defensive Linemen*

Purpose. To provide coaches a yardstick for evaluating their players and to provide incentive for the players.

Evaluation. Wallrof used the judgment of coaches to identify the desirable and undesirable characteristics of defensive performance. These characteristics provided the basis for developing the rating scale. A scale for Defensive Linebackers and Backs was developed also.

Procedures. The coaches study game motion pictures to evaluate their players after each football game. They develop a profile graph for each player which represents his performance for the season.

The Scale

I. A Five Point Score for a Defensive Lineman

A grade of five is awarded when a defensive lineman makes an outstanding play; a play that is above and beyond the expected. Also the following would make five points possible:

1. The aggressiveness of the defensive player caused a fumble and a team recovery.
2. He scored a safety by tackling an offensive ball carrier in his end zone.
3. The defensive player intercepted a pass and scored.
4. He blocked a try for point after touchdown.
5. He blocked a punt and scored.
6. He picked up a fumble and scored.

II. A Four Point Score for a Defensive Lineman

A grade of four is given when a defensive lineman does a good job with his assignment:

1. He shows aggressiveness and aids in stopping the offensive threat.
2. His mental alertness helps him to adapt rapidly to the offensive play.
3. He shows quickness of initial movement.
4. He keys and diagnoses the offensive play.
5. With agility, he escapes from the blocker and makes a tackle.
6. He takes the proper pursuit of the ball.

III. A Three Point Score for a Defensive Player

A grade of three is given when the average job is done and the defensive player is still effective.

1. His aggressiveness and mental alertness are such that he is still effective.
2. His initial movement and his ability to key and diagnose show a passable performance.
3. His agility and escape from the blocker are mediocre.
4. He makes the tackle but with imperfections.
5. His pursuit is fair.
6. His stance and alignment are passable.

IV. A Two Point Score for a Defensive Lineman

A grade of two is given when a poor defensive play is made.

1. He shows poor reaction to the offensive move and a lack of agility.

* Wallrof, Paul J.: Methods for Rating Defensive Proficiency of High School Football Players, MSPE, University of Washington, Seattle, 1965. Used by permission of the author.

      2. He fails to move on the ball.
      3. He fails to make the tackle.
      4. He is blocked.
      5. His pursuit of the ball is inferior.
      6. His alignment and lateral movement are defective.
      7. His stance is faulty.
 V. A One Point Score for a Defensive Lineman
      A grade of one is given for an inferior defensive performance.
      1. The defensive lineman allows a score or allows the opponent to make a long gain.
      2. He quits.
      3. He shows no courage.
      4. His lack of aggressiveness gives the offensive team the advantage.
      5. He is blocked out of the play and makes no effort to recover.
      6. He is responsible for a penalty which gives the opponent a definite advantage.

SAMPLE DEFENSIVE PLAYER RECORDING CHART

Player: 2   Game: Cleveland versus Roosevelt

Total Plays Graded: 17   Total Score: 39   Game Average: 2.2

Number	Away	Toward	Grade	Remarks
1	X		2	Poor pursuit
2	X		3	Keep head up on tackle
3		Pass	3	Fair rush
4		X	3	React quicker
5	X		2	Poor pursuit angle
6		Pass	2	Get hands up
7	X		1	No pursuit
8		Pass	3	Get hands up
9		Pass	3	Keep outside containment
10	X		1	No pursuit, did not read or diagnose
11	X		2	Pursuit angle poor
12		Pass	3	Get hands up
13		X	2	Poor reaction
14		X	2	Took yourself out of the play
15		Pass	3	Get hands up sooner
16		X	1	No reaction, no pursuit, nothing!
17		Pass	3	Need to rush with outside leverage

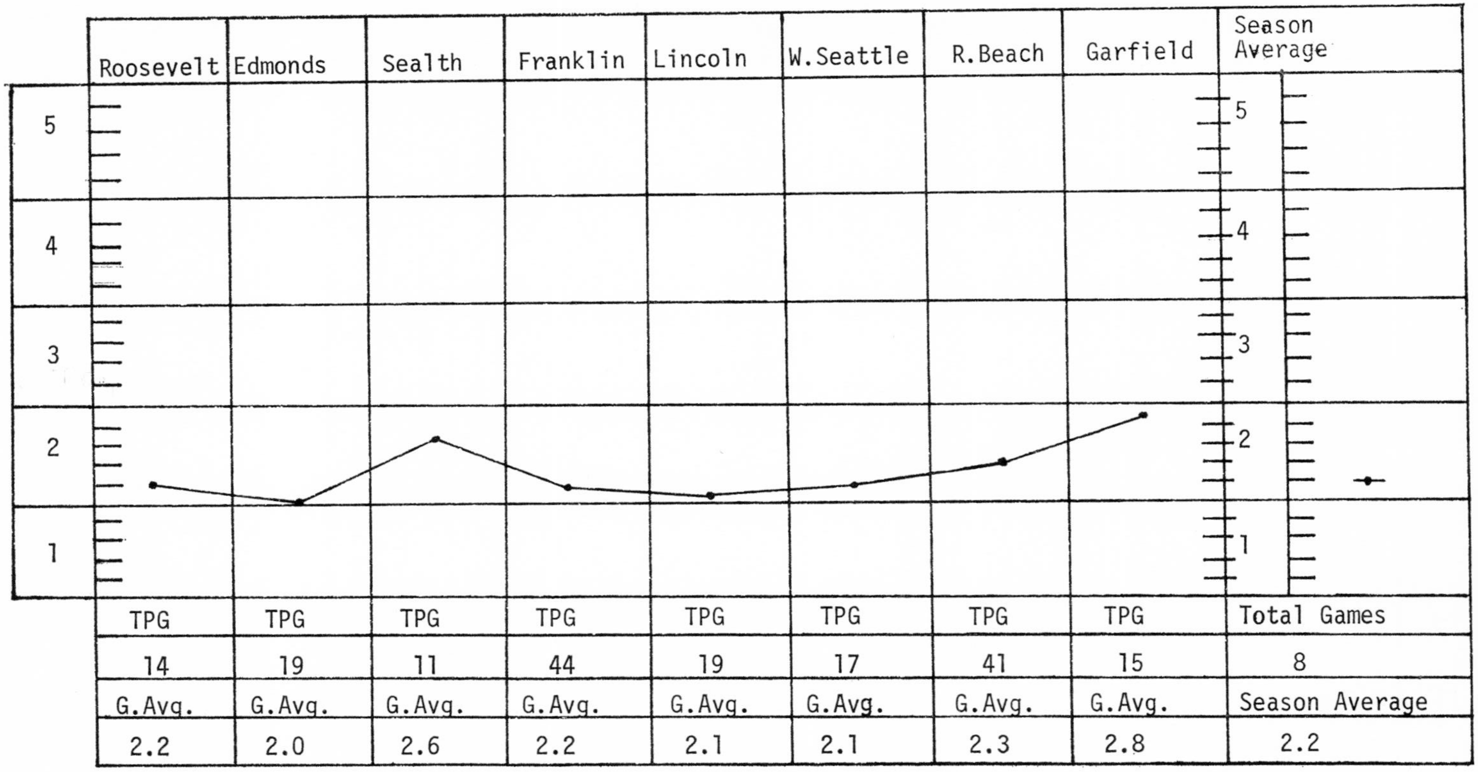

Fig. 9–14. Defensive profile graph for player No. 1

TPG = Total Plays Graded   G.Avg. = Game Average

Additional Football References

Brace, David K., Consultant: *Skills Test Manual—Football*, Washington, D.C.: AAHPER, Revised Edition, 1966.

Brace, David K.: Validity of Football Achievement Tests as Measures of Learning and as a Partial Basis for the Selection of Players, Research Quarterly, *14*, 372, December, 1943.

Cowell, C. C., and A. H. Ismail: Validity of a Football Rating Scale and Its Relationship to Social Integration and Academic Ability, Research Quarterly, *32*, 461–467, December, 1961.

Lee, Robert Charles: A Battery of Tests to Predict Football Potential, MSPE, University of Utah, Salt Lake City, 1965.

See the Football Play Ability and Attitude Rating Scale in Chapter 12, page 451.

GOLF

Vanderhoof Golf Test*

Purpose. To measure golfing ability.

Evaluation. Two criteria were used for validity purposes—one was a subjective rating and one was scores from playing 6 holes of golf. The rating proved to be more satisfactory and the validity coefficients reported made use of the ratings as the criterion.

	Reliability	Validity
Drive Test	.90	.71
5-Iron Test	.84	.66

The Drive Test proved to be the best single indicator of playing ability as judged by ratings. The Multiple R including the Drive Test and the 5-Iron Test was .78.

Level and Sex. The test was developed for college women who had received 15 lessons of group instruction in golf.

Time Allotment and Number of Subjects. The test is time consuming unless the administration can proceed while others are occupied elsewhere. Multiple stations would enhance the efficient use of time.

Floor Plan and Space Requirements. An indoor gymnasium space is recommended. The test area requires a space of at least 74 by 13 feet for each station. Gymnasium space is also recommended so there will be no low overhead ceiling to obstruct the flight of the ball.

Class Organization. If a gymnasium floor is used, several stations can be arranged side by side using one long rope to go the length of the floor. If available space permits only one station, the class members should rotate to the testing station in small groups.

General Procedures. 1. Practice with cocoa mats should be a usual procedure for the class members.

2. The use of a permanent tee for the Drive Test will stabilize the height of the ball for each golfer and will save time from replacing the tee after each stroke. A 3-legged plastic tee was used by Vanderhoof and sewed to the mat with elastic thread.

* Vanderhoof, Ellen R.: Beginning Golf Achievement Tests, Master's Thesis, State University of Iowa, Iowa City, 1956. Used by permission of the author.

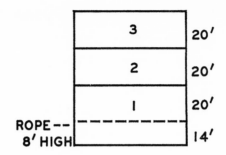

Fig. 9–15.   Specifications for the drive and #5 iron
approach shot tests.

Uses.   To use as a practice device.
To measure improvement.
To use as a partial basis for grading.
To analyze the pattern of the scoring to detect possible consistent errors.

Test Description

ITEM NUMBER I—DRIVE TEST

Purpose: To measure ability to use a full swing with a wood.

Facilities and Equipment: Mat with a permanent tee, #2 wood, plastic
practice balls, 2 standards, 1 rope about 20 feet in length, and a ten pin.
The ten pin or some other obstacle is placed in the distance behind the
testing area to serve as a target for the golfer.

Procedures: The golfer takes several practice swings, hits 2 or 3 practice
balls as a warm-up, and then drives 15 plastic balls. Each must go under
the rope to score but must be in the air when it passes directly under the
rope. Two topped balls in succession count as only 1 trial.

Instructions: "Stand at the cocoa mat with a #2 Wood and take some practice swings and hit 2 or 3 of these plastic practice balls. Then drive 15
times aiming for the ten pin in the distance. The ball must go under the
rope on the fly and land in the areas marked on the floor to score."

Scoring: Score each ball by the value of the area in which it lands if it went
under the rope above the floor. Total the score for 15 trials. Count only
1 trial for 2 balls in a row which are topped. See the score card to note a
method of recording each drive by the number of the drive within the
15 trials.

Testing Personnel: A scorer.

ITEM NUMBER II—#5 IRON APPROACH SHOT

   This test is administered exactly as the Drive Test except that no tee is
used.

Score Card

```
                        GOLF  TEST
Name_____ Class_____ Date_____
      Drive Test                    5-Iron Test
```

9		4	5		
	7		13	3 x <u>6</u> = 18	
		6			
	14	3	11	2 x <u>4</u> = 8	
			10		
	1	2	12	1 x <u>4</u> = 4	
		15			
	8			Total <u>30</u>	

T-Score <u>57</u>

5-Iron Test:
3 x ___
2 x ___
1 x ___
Total___

T-Score____

The score card shows the *number* of each trial, 1–15, and its location. This particular golfer consistently hit to the right side of the target. Once detection of directional errors is made, corrections can be suggested.

Norms

Table 9–11. Norms for the Vanderhoof Drive Test*

T-Score	(Total of 15 trials) Raw Score
75	45
70	41
65	38
60	33
55	28
50	24
45	19
40	13
35	9
30	7
25	4

* Based on the performance of 110 college women after 15 lessons of golf.

Reece 5-Iron Test*

Purpose. To measure ability to hit a regulation golf ball with a five iron.

Evaluation. Reece used 120 beginning women students and 25 women intermediate students to compare an indoor and outdoor golf test using the 5 iron.

The reliability for the beginners was .87 and .88 for the intermediates. The scores ranged from 12 to 131 on the outdoor test. It correlated .45 with the indoor test for beginning golf students and .56 with intermediate golf students. Reece concluded that the 2 tests could not be interchanged and that possibly the loft as measured by the indoor test and the distance as measured by the outdoor test did not have a close relationship.

Level and Sex. Designed for college women. Appropriate for secondary school girls as well. The idea of the test is appropriate for men but the dimensions of the scoring area would have to be changed.

Time Allotment and Number of Students. Half a class can be tested at a time using partners to score. The number of balls available and the size of the golf range will dictate the number who can be tested at one time.

Space Requirements. A hitting area approximately 20–30 yards by 100 yards should safely accommodate a class of 20 students.

Class Organization. Assign partners for testing. One scores while the other completes the test including practice hits, practice swings, and 20 trials. The partners then change places.

Uses. To use as a practice device.
To use as a partial basis for grading.
To assess improvement.

Test Description—5-Iron Test

Equipment: One half the number of five irons as the size of the class. 23 regulation golf balls for each student, score cards and pencils.

Field Markings: The hitting line is the line behind which students must stand to take test. It is designated by white flags. The target lines are 20 yards, 40 yards, and 60 yards from the hitting line. They are marked by green flags, red flags, and yellow flags respectively.

Directions: "This test is intended to measure your ability to hit a regulation golf ball with the five iron. These scores will serve as a basis for part of your skill grade, so do as well as you can.

"Decide who is going to hit first, you or your partner. You will be allowed three practice hits before any scoring begins, and you may take a *single* practice swing between trials if you desire. During the test you will hit 20 trials in succession, then change places with your partner and score 20 trials for her. Be careful that you do not step in front of the hitting line and that you do not interfere with others who are hitting.

"The score is determined by where the ball first lands, not by where it finally comes to rest. The ball must go as high as your head to score beyond the 20 yard marker."

* Reece, Patsy Anne: A Comparison of the Scores Made on an Outdoor and the Scores Made on an Indoor Golf Test by College Women, M.S., University of Colorado, Boulder, 1960. Used by permission of the author.

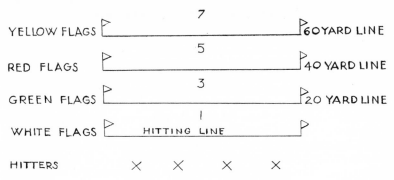

Fig. 9–16.   Diagram of target area.

Scoring: The scorer should stand about ten feet behind the person taking the test in a position where she can see well.   She must watch closely to see if the ball rises higher than the head of the person who is hitting, and to see in which area it first touches the ground.   All trials are scored according to where the ball lands, not according to where it rolls.   The following procedures should be followed for recording the scores:

1. Place the number of the trial on the target diagram of the score card in the area corresponding to the score the trial should receive.   Use con-
2. secutive numbers, *i.e.* 1, 2, 3, etc. up to 20.
   When the girl for whom you are scoring has completed 20 trials, write the number of hits made in each scoring area on the blank beside the scoring area.
3. Multiply the number of hits in each area by the point value for that area and add the total score.   Have your partner double check her own score card to make sure the total is correct.

Testing Personnel: One instructor will explain the test procedures and scoring plan.   Partners will score for each other.

Score Card

OUTDOOR GOLF SKILL TEST

60	Yellow	_____	× 7 =	_____	
40	Red	_____	× 5 =	_____	
20	Green	_____	× 3 =	_____	
0			× 1 =	_____	

Balls beyond 20 yards, but
not higher than head   _____   _____
                                                                  Name

Balls missed or which do   _____
not pass 20 yard line   _____   Class
                                                                  _____
                                                                  Date
                          Total _____   _____
                                                                  Scorer

Vanderhoof Rating Scale for Golf*

5. Good   Consistent, relaxed, well-coordinated swing and follow
                     through. Good stance and grip. Good timing with
                     entire swing in approximately the same plane.
4. Above Average   Consistent, coordinated swing and follow through.
                     Good stance, grip and timing. Minor errors in plane
                     of swing and use of wrists.
3. Average.   Fair form for stance, grip, swing, and follow through.
                     Fair coordination and timing. Fairly consistent.
2. Below Average   Fair form for stance, grip and swing. Poor timing and
                     coordination. Inconsistent.
1. Poor   Generally poor form for stance, grip and swing. Tense
                     and inconsistent.

Additional Golf References

Bowen, Robert T.: Putting Errors of Beginning Golfers Using Different Points of Aim,
    Research Quarterly, *39*, 31–35, March, 1968.
Clevett, Melvin A.: An Experiment in Teaching Methods in Golf, Research Quarterly
    2, 104–106, December, 1931.
Cochrane, June Fleurette: The Construction of an Indoor Golf Skills Test as a Measure
    of Golfing Ability. Unpublished Master's Thesis, University of Minnesota, Minne-
    apolis, 1960.
McKee, Mary Ellen: A Test for the Full-Swinging Shot in Golf, Research Quarterly,
    21, 40–46, March, 1950.
Watts, Harriet: Construction and Evaluation of a Target on Testing the Approach
    Shot in Golf. Unpublished Master's Thesis, University of Wisconsin, Madison,
    1942.
West, Charlotte, and JoAnne Thorpe: Construction and Validation of an Eight-Iron
    Approach Test, Research Quarterly, *39*, 1115–1120, December, 1968.

* Vanderhoof, Ellen, R.: Beginning Golf Achievement Tests. Master's Thesis,
State University of Iowa. Iowa City, 1956. Used by permission of the author.

GYMNASTICS AND TUMBLING

Scale for Judging Quality of Performance in Stunts and Tumbling*

Criteria for judging the quality of performance:
Relaxation
Control of the body
Technique
Accuracy
Timing or rhythm
Approach
Finish

10 —Excellent	A finished performance. Body relaxed and completely controlled. Proper technique applied. Accuracy obtained. Correct timing or rhythm. Excellent approach and finish.
7–9—Good	Above average, but not a finished performance. Lack of excellence in one or two details.
4–6—Average	Fair performance. Activity accomplished, but as a whole, shows a lack of finish in most details.
1–3—Poor	Activity barely accomplished. Lack of control. Deficient technique used.
0 —Failed	Activity not accomplished.

Harris Tumbling and Apparatus Proficiency Test†

Purpose. To measure proficiency in tumbling and apparatus.

Evaluation. Harris started with a battery of 22 items which he narrowed to 6. His work was accomplished using men students at the University of North Dakota. The test-retest reliability was satisfactory and the 6-item battery discriminated well between high, medium, and low skill levels as judged by raters.

* Bonnie and Donnie Cotteral: *The Teaching of Stunts and Tumbling,* Copyright 1936 The Ronald Press. Used by permission of the publisher.
† Harris, J. Patrick: A Design for a Proposed Skill Proficiency Test in Tumbling and Apparatus for Male Physical Education Majors at the University of North Dakota. MS in Ed., University of North Dakota, Grand Forks, 1966. Used by permission of the University of North Dakota and the author.

The Test

Name:	Judge:	Class:	Date:

Directions: Circle the number which indicates the performers score in areas of form
and execution respectively. Leave the totals until all testing has been
completed.

Tumbling

  1. Forward roll to head stand.

form: 1 2
execution: 1 2 3 4 5   Total ____

Parallel Bars

  2. Back uprise, shoulder balance, front roll.

form: 1 2
execution: 1 2 3 4 5   Total ____

  3. Shoulder kip from arm support,
     swing, front dismount.

form: 1 2
execution: 1 2 3 4 5 6   Total ____

Horizontal Bar

  4. Cast to kip up.

form: 1 2
execution: 1 2 3 4 5 6   Total ____

  5. Front pull-over, cast,
     back hip circle.

form: 1 2
execution: 1 2 3 4 5   Total ____

Trampoline

  6. Back, front, seat, feet.

form: 1 2
execution: 1 2 3 4 5   Total ____

Total Points ____

Scoring. There is a possible score of 44 points. The total point value was
divided into form points and execution points to help lessen the possibility
of scoring confusion with regard to beauty of performance as compared to
beauty of the performer. For example, a student could receive maximum
execution points and a zero score for form. However, the form score should
in no way influence the performer's execution points.

Additional Gymnastics References

Bowers, Carolyn O.: Gymnastics Skill Test for Beginning to Low Intermediate Girls
and Women, M.A. in P.E., Ohio State University, Columbus, 1965.
Landers, Daniel M.: A Comparison of Two Gymnastics Judging Methods, MSPE,
University of Illinois, Urbana, 1965.
Schwarzkoph, Robert J. The Iowa-Brace Test as a Measuring Instrument for Predicting
Gymnastics Ability, MSPE, University of Washington, Seattle, 1962.

HANDBALL

Handball Test*

Purpose. To measure status and progress in the acquisition of handball skills.

Evaluation. This test was developed using the average score per game obtained in a partial round robin tournament as the criterion. A multiple r of .802 was obtained between the criterion and the 3 test items of service accuracy, total wall volley, and back-wall volley. These results were de-

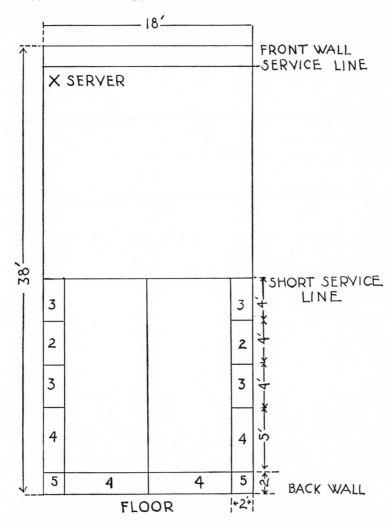

Fig. 9–17. Court markings for service placement test.

* Pennington, G. Gary, James A. P. Day, John N. Drowatzky, and John F. Hansan: A Measure of Handball Ability, Research Quarterly, *38*, 247–253, May, 1967. Used by permission of the AAHPER.

11

rived from the performance of 37 male undergraduates at the University
of Oregon. The multiple r was .791 for the two-item battery of service
placement and total wall volley.

Test Description

ITEM NUMBER I—SERVICE PLACEMENT TEST

The court is divided into areas that are assigned numerical values.
Serving in a regulation manner, the student attempts to place the service
into the area having the highest numerical value. Each student is given
10 trials.

ITEM NUMBER II—TOTAL WALL VOLLEY

A. Thirty-second wall volley with dominant hand. The student stands
   at the center of the court behind the short service line, drops the ball
   to the floor and strokes it against the front wall repeatedly for 30
   seconds. He is permitted to step ahead of the line for one return,
   but the next must be played behind the line. If he violates this rule
   or loses control, he must recover the ball and begin a new series in
   the same way. The score is the number of times the ball is stroked
   against the front wall in 30 seconds.
B. Thirty-second wall volley with nondominant hand. This test is
   administered in the same way but the subject may not strike the ball
   with his dominant hand.

The score for this item is the sum of wall hits for items A and B.

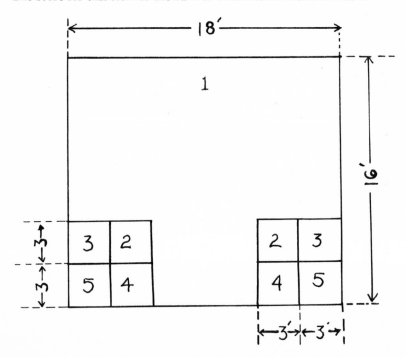

Fig. 9–18.   Court markings for wall placement test.

ITEM NUMBER III—BACK-WALL PLACEMENT TEST

The front wall is divided into different areas with assigned numerical values. The subject throws the ball high and hard against the front wall, and, after it hits the floor and rebounds off the back wall, he attempts to stroke it into the high scoring areas of the front wall. The student is allowed five trials with the right hand off the right back wall and five trials with the left hand off the left back wall.

Scoring: The following weighted formula was given by the authors for computing the final score:

Handball ability = 1.37 (Service Placement) + 2.27 (Total Wall
Volley) + 1.59 (Back-Wall Placement) + .29.

The suggested score card shows an application of the formula using average performance.

HANDBALL TEST

Name: Class: Date:

1. Service Placement Test

3	4
0	3
2	0
0	0
5	3

Total   20   × 1.37   27.40

2. Total Wall Volley Score

Dominant Hand   8
Nondominant Hand   6   Total   14   × 2.27   31.78

3. Back-Wall Placement Test

Rt Hand   Lt Hand
Rt Back Wall Lt Back Wall

2	3
0	0
0	2
1	2
0	0

Total   10   × 1.59   15.90

Constant   .29

T-Score:_____   Final Weighted Score   75.37

Additional Handball References

Cornish, Clayton: A Study of Measurement of Ability in Handball, Research Quarterly, *20*, 215–222, May, 1949.

Griffith, Malcolm Anstett: An Objective Method of Evaluatiing Ability in Handball Singles, Unpublished Master's Thesis, Ohio State University, Columbus, 1960.

McCachren, James R.: A Study of the University of Florida Handball Skill Test, Master's Thesis, University of North Carolina at Chapel Hill, 1949.

Montoye, H. J., and Brotzman, J.: An investigation of the validity of using the results of a doubles tournament as a measure of handball ability. Research Quarterly, *22*, 214–218, 1951.

LACROSSE
Hodges Lacrosse Rating Scale*

Purpose. To judge performance of basic lacrosse skills.

Evaluation. The scale was designed originally as a criterion measure for developing skills tests in lacrosse. It considers eight basic areas of lacrosse skill and distinguishes five levels of performance for each.

The Rating Scale:

Name:	Judge:	Class:	Date:

Skills:

Cradling
E. Smooth, well-timed, ball under control.
G. Fairly smooth, ball under control.
A. Movements not absolutely synchronized, but maintains possession of the ball.
F. Characterized by jerky movements.
P. Does not cradle.

Picking Up
E. Accomplished with ease and full control.
G. Is successful, but does not gain full control immediately.
A. Experiences difficulty, but eventually is successful.
F. Does not gain control; pushes the ball along the ground.
P. Completely misses the ball.

Catching
E. Accomplished with ease and full control.
G. Is successful but does not gain full control immediately.
A. Has difficulty controlling the ball.
F. Ball hits the stick but bounces off.
P. Completely misses the ball.

Passing
E. Pass is accurate and well-timed.
G. Pass is accurate but not well-timed.
A. Gets free to make pass, but pass is not accurate.
F. Tries to make pass when marked too closely; passes just to get rid of the ball.
P. Drops the ball or makes a poor pass.

Evading Opponents
E. Dodges, pivots, or otherwise evades opponents with ease and control.
G. Evades opponent fairly effectively.
A. Is checked in the evading attempt, but maintains possession of the ball.

* Hodges, Carolyn V.: Construction of an Objective Knowledge Test and Skills Tests in Lacrosse for College Women, MSPE, University of North Carolina at Greensboro, 1967. The scoring procedures have been adapted and the scale is used by permission of the author.

F. Attempts to evade opponent, but loses the ball.
P. Does not attempt to evade opponent.

Shifting from Offense to Defense
E. Shifts immediately when opponent gets ball; constantly checks and challenges opponent.
G. Shifts quickly from offense to defense.
A. Shifts, but not soon enough.
F. Is very slow in shifting.
P. Does not shift at all when the opponent gets the ball.

Field Positioning
E. Effectively makes spaces for self or teammate.
G. Is fairly effective in making spaces.
A. Tries to make spaces, but cuts in wrong direction.
F. Crowds teammate who has the ball.
P. Stands in one place; does not cut to make spaces.

Body Control
E. Has excellent body control; rarely fouls.
G. Has body control; seldom fouls.
A. Has body control; fouls infrequently.
F. Usually has body control; fouls occasionally.
P. Lacks body control; fouls often.

Scoring: E. = Excellent = 5 points
          G. = Good   = 4 points
          A. = Average = 3 points
          F. = Fair   = 2 points
          P. = Poor   = 1 point
A player can score a maximum of 40 points or a minimum of 8 points.
A score card could be arranged to rate individually or by teams

Additional Lacrosse References

Lutze, Margaret C.: Achievement Tests in Beginning Lacrosse for Women, MAPE, University of Iowa, Iowa City, 1963.
Wilke, Barbara J.: Achievement Tests for Selected Lacross Skills of College Women, M. Ed., University of North Carolina at Greensboro, 1967.

SOCCER AND SPEEDBALL

Warner Test of Soccer Skills*

Purpose. To measure the fundamental skills of soccer. To arouse interest in learning fundamental skills. To measure improvement during the sports season. To help select a varsity team.

Evaluation. The test items were evaluated by soccer coaches who rated

* Warner, Glenn F. H.: Warner Soccer Test, Newsletter of the National Soccer Coaches Association of America, *6*, 13–22, December, 1950. Used by permission of the author.

them according to their importance and the degree of difficulty to learn.
A 7-item battery was suggested:
1. Kicking for distance, right foot
2. Kicking for distance, left foot
3. Corner kicking for accuracy
4. Heading for accuracy
5. Throw-ins for distance
6. Penalty kicking for accuracy
7. Dribbling for time
Only 3 items will be presented here: Nos. 1, 2, and 7.

Level and Sex. Designed for junior and senior high school boys and for high school varsity soccer players.

Time Allotment and Number of Subjects. The test can be administered to an average size class in one period if well organized.

Floor Plan and Space Requirements. Outdoor field space is required.

Class Organization. One squad can take the test while the others scrimmage. One item could be given each day.

General Procedures. 1. Leather soccer balls should be used.
2. The test should not be given on a rainy or windy day.
3. Tennis shoes should be worn.

Uses. To help with grading procedures.
To increase interest in the activity by reporting scores quickly.
To help the beginner see that skill with both feet should be developed

Test Description

ITEM NUMBER I—KICKING FOR DISTANCE, RIGHT FOOT

Purpose: To measure kicking ability for distance with a degree of accuracy using the right foot.

Facilities and Equipment: Soccer balls and field markings.

Procedures: The player runs to kick a stationary ball. The ball must stay within a lane which is 25 yards wide. The distance the ball advances in the air is measured. Three trials are given.

Instructions: "Take a running start and kick this ball with your right foot as far as you can down this marked-off lane. It will be measured at the first bounce. You will have three trials and the best one will count."

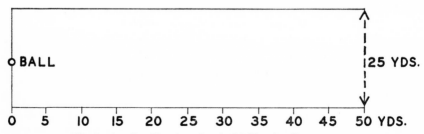

Fig. 9-19. Specifications for the kicking for distance test.

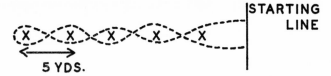

Fig. 9–20. Specifications for the dribbling for time test.

Scoring: Measure the distance of the kick to the first bounce. Record the best of 3 kicks measured to the nearest yard.

Testing Personnel: Classmates can be used to retrieve and spot the balls. The squad leader or instructor should record the score.

ITEM NUMBER II—KICKING FOR DISTANCE, LEFT FOOT

This test is administered exactly like Item No. I except that the left foot is used for the kicking foot.

ITEM NUMBER III—DRIBBLING FOR TIME

Purpose: To measure ability to control the ball with the feet.

Facilities and Equipment: 5 objects, soccer ball, stop watch.

Procedures: The student dribbles the soccer ball in and out among the objects and is timed for the course of the trip.

Instructions: "On the signal, 'Ready, Go!' dribble the ball to the right and left of the five objects, around the end one, and back in the same manner, and cross the starting line. You will be timed and will be given 3 trials to get your best time."

Scoring: Three trials are timed and the best one is recorded.

Testing Personnel: Timer and recorder.

Score Card

WARNER SOCCER TEST				
Name_____ Date _____				
Class Period_____ Grade_____				
	1st Testing	*Standard Score*	*2nd Testing*	*Standard Score*
Right foot, Kick for Distance	_____	_____	_____	_____
Left foot, Kick for Distance	_____	_____	_____	_____
Dribble for Time	_____	_____	_____	_____

Norms

Table 9–12.   Norms for Warner Soccer Test*

Standard Score	Kicking for Distance Right Foot (yards)			Kicking for Distance Left Foot (yards)			Dribbling (seconds)			Standard Score
	12–13 yrs.	14–15 yrs.	16–17 yrs.	12–13 yrs.	14–15 yrs.	16–17 yrs.	12–13 yrs.	14–15 yrs.	16–17 yrs.	
95	42	52	54			47				95
90	39	49	52	39	44	44				90
85	37	46	49	36	42	41	12			85
80	35	43	47	31	39	39	15		12	80
75	33	40	44	29	36	36	19	14	15	75
70	31	38	41	26	34	33	22	17	18	70
65	28	35	39	24	31	31	25	21	21	65
60	26	32	36	22	26	28	29	24	24	60
55	24	29	33	19	23	25	33	28	27	55
50	22	26	31	17	20	23	36	31	30	50
45	19	23	28	15	18	20	40	34	32	45
40	17	21	25	12	15	18	43	38	35	40
35	15	18	23	10	12	15	47	41	38	35
30	13	15	20	8	10	12	50	45	41	30
25	11	12	17	5	7	10	54	48	44	25
20	8	9	15	3	4	7	57	51	47	20
15	6	7	12	1	1	4	61	55	50	15
10	4	4	9			2	64	58	53	10
5	2	1	7				68	62	55	5

* Based on the performance of 319 high school boys.

Mitchell Modification of the McDonald Soccer Skill Test*

Purpose.   To measure soccer playing ability at the upper elementary level.

Evaluation.   The original McDonald test was validated by correlating subjective ratings with the performance of varsity and freshman soccer players. The coefficient was .85 for the combined group.[28]   Mitchell has adapted the test to make it more suitable for 5th and 6th grade boys. The target area is smaller, the restraining line is closer, and the floor area is enclosed with classmates to keep the ball in the testing area.

Johnson[21] has developed still another modification of the McDonald test which specifies a target area 24 × 8 feet, a restraining line 15 feet back, three 30-second trials, starting the test with the ball in the hands, and the use of spare balls when the test ball goes out of control.

* Mitchell, J. Reid: The Modification of the McDonald Soccer Skill Test for Upper Elementary School Boys, M.S., University of Oregon, Eugene, 1963. Used by permission of the author.

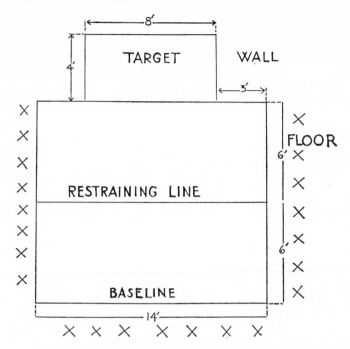

Fig. 9–21.   Specifications for the Mitchell soccer test.

Level and Sex.   This version of the McDonald Soccer test is designed for 5th and 6th grade boys and seems appropriate, as well, for upper elementary school girls and junior high school boys and girls.

Time Allotment.   The test can be taken in about 1 minute per student. If several testing stations are available, a class can be tested in one class period.

Floor Plan and Space Requirements.

Class Organization.   The squad plan should be used.   One student takes the test while the squad members stand back a pace or two from the boundary lines to stop any ball that comes over the line.

General Procedure.   1. A retrial is given if a ball is mishandled by a retriever resulting in undue delay for the kicker.
2. A practice trial is recommended.
3. The 3 trials are given consecutively.

Uses.   To use as a practice device.
To measure improvement.
To measure achievement in the basic skills of soccer.

Test Description

Facilities and Equipment: A wall area about 20 × 10 feet fronted by a floor area about 20 × 20 feet is necessary, soccer balls, stop watch.

Norms

Table 9–13.   T-Scale for the Total Score of Three Trials on the Mitchell Modification of McDonald Soccer Test*

T-Score	*Test Score*
75	55
70	51
65	46
60	41
55	37
50	32
45	28
40	25
35	21
30	17
25	14

*Based on the performance of 192 5th and 6th grade boys.

Procedures: The ball is set on the restraining line and the subject stands back of the ball, ready to kick on the command, "Go." He continues to kick as many times as possible any way he desires, with either foot, by immediately kicking the ball or blocking and steadying it, soccer-style, before re-kicking. Use of the hands at any time is prohibited and discounts the score by one point for each infraction.

Three 20-second trials are taken consecutively.

Scoring: A student's score is determined by the number of times within the twenty second time limit that he successfully propels the ball against the wall. The ball may be directed by the foot, leg, knee or other part of the body, except the hands or arms, to the area marked as the target or on the lines thereof. The subject must stand and maintain a balanced position back of the restraining line. If he touches the ground on the other side of this line during the kicking motion or follow through, or kicks from a position in advance of the line, that kick does not count toward his score. A ball that does not rebound to the restraining line can be retrieved by the kicker and dribbled back out over the line or kicked against the wall hard enough to rebound out where he can start again. In this latter case of retrieving, the illegal kick would not score. Use of the hands at any time to steady or retrieve the ball discounts the score by one point for each infraction.

Testing Personnel: One test administrator can explain the procedures and serve as the central timer. The students can score for one another.

Smith Kick-Up to Self Test*

Purpose. To measure the ability to convert a ground ball to an aerial ball.

Evaluation. This test correlated .54 with a criterion of subjective ratings and had a reliability coefficient of .90 for a group of college women.

* Smith, Gwen: Speedball Skill Tests for College Women, Unpublished study, Illinois State University, Normal, 1947. Used by permission of the author.

Level and Sex. This test was designed for college women but is appropriate for junior and senior high school boys and girls.

Time Allotment and Number of Subjects. It will take approximately 4 minutes for each student plus 1 minute of rest time between each of the 6 trials. Use of the rotation plan will save time.

Floor Plan and Space Requirements. Some wall space and adjoining floor space is required.

Class Organization. Plan for several stations and use a central timer.

General Procedures. 1. Be sure a rest period is taken between each trial. 2. Be sure the scorers know how to judge a legal kick-up. 3. Combine this test with various ones of the soccer tests to make a battery of tests appropriate to speedball.

Uses. To measure a skill unique and fundamental to speedball. To motivate learning a new skill. To use as a partial basis for a speedball grade.

Test Description

Purpose: To measure ability to convert a ball to an aerial ball successively and quickly.

Facilities and Equipment: Soccer ball, stop watch, wall and floor space.

Procedures: The student stands behind a 7-foot restraining line, tosses the ball against the wall and executes a kick-up to self when it rebounds. This pattern is repeated for 30 seconds. The student may go in front of the line to recover the ball with his hands, but he must be behind the line when he makes the next throw. A toss against the wall of about 2 to 3 feet seems best.

Instructions: "Stand behind this 7-foot line, holding the soccer ball. On the signal, 'Ready, Go!' throw the ball against the wall and perform a kick-up to self when it rebounds. Continue as fast as possible to perform during a 30-second period. You need to do as many kick-ups as possible in that time. If the ball gets out of control, retrieve it with your hands and return to the line to make the next throw."

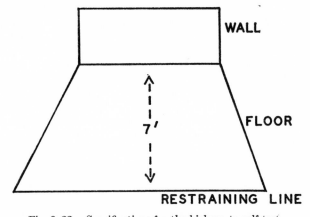

Fig. 9–22. Specifications for the kick-up to self test.

Scoring: Score each legal kick-up accomplished during the 30-second trial. Total all the kick-ups for 6 trials.

Testing Personnel: A timer and a scorer.

Additional References for Soccer-Type Sports

Bontz, Jean: An Experiment in the Construction of a Test for Measuring Ability in Some of the Fundamental Skills Used by Fifth and Sixth Grade Children in Soccer, Unpublished Master's Thesis, State University of Iowa, Iowa City, 1942.

Buchanan, Ruth E.: A Study of Achievement Tests in Speedball for High School Girls, Unpublished Master's Thesis, State University of Iowa, Iowa City, 1942.

Crew, Vernon N.: A Skill Test Battery for Use in Service Program Soccer Classes at the University Level, MSPE, University of Oregon, Eugene, 1968.

MacKenzie, John: The Evaluation of a Battery of Soccer Skill Tests as an Aid to Classification of General Soccer Ability, MSPE, University of Massachusetts, Amherst, 1968.

McDonald, Lloyd C.: The Construction of a Kicking Skill Test as an Index to General Soccer Ability, Unpublished Master's Thesis, Springfield College, Springfield, Mass., 1951.

Schaufele, Evelyn F.: The Establishment of Objective Tests for Girls of the Ninth and Tenth Grades to Determine Soccer Ability, Unpublished Master's Thesis, State University of Iowa, Iowa City, 1940.

Stephyns, Opal Ruff: Achievement Tests in Speed-A-Way for High School Girls, MSPE, Illinois State University, Normal, 1965.

Streck, Bonnie: An Analysis of the McDonald Soccer Skill Test as Applied to Junior High School Girls, MSPE, Fort Hays State College, Fort Hays, Kansas, 1961.

Whitney, Alethea Helen, and Grace Chapin: Soccer Skill Testing for Girls, *Soccer-Speedball Guide—1946–48*. Washington, D.C.: NSWA of AAHPER, 1946, pp. 19–24.

SOFTBALL

Fringer Softball Battery*

Purpose. To measure the important aspects of softball in a manner which would be meaningful to students and economical in time, space, and equipment.

Evaluation.

	Reliability	*Validity*
3-item Battery:		
Fly Balls	.87	.76
Fielding Grounders, Agility, Speed, and Accuracy	.72	.70
Softball Throw for Distance	.90	.72
Criterion:		
Repeated Throw	.87	

The 3-item battery had a multiple correlation of .83 with the criterion. The 2-item battery of the 1st two tests had a multiple R of .80.

The Repeated Throws test correlated well with the Distance Throw so could be substituted if an all indoor battery is needed.

* Fringer, Margaret Neal: A Battery of Softball Skill Tests for Senior High School Girls, Unpublished Master's Thesis, University of Michigan, Ann Arbor, 1961. Used by permission of the author.

Level and Sex. The battery was designed for high school girls. The items are appropriate for boys but the norms included here are not.

Time Allotment and Number of Subjects. Fielding Grounders, Agility, Speed, and Accuracy Test requires 2 minutes per person plus rest periods between trials. The Softball Throw for Distance Test requires 1½ minutes per person. The Fly Balls Test requires 1½ minutes per person plus rest periods between trials. The Repeated Throws test requires 4 minutes per person plus rest time between trials.

Floor Plan and Space Requirements. If the 2-item battery of Fielding Grounders and Fly Balls is used, only indoor floor and wall space is required. If the 3-item battery is used, which includes the Softball Throw for Distance, outdoor space is needed also. This may be a factor in helping the teacher decide which battery is most appropriate to her situation.

Class Organization. Stations can be used if the students are trained to assist with the test administration.

General Procedures. Warm-up exercises are suggested.

Rest periods can be scheduled if the students rotate after each trial except on the Throw for Distance.

Uses. To help students and teachers note progress over the season.

To determine which skills need particular attention in the future.

To remove false judgment of a person's playing ability.

Test Description

ITEM NUMBER I—FLY BALL TEST

Purpose: To measure the ability to catch fly balls and throw quickly.

Facilities and Equipment: Several good softballs, stop watch, unobstructed wall space.

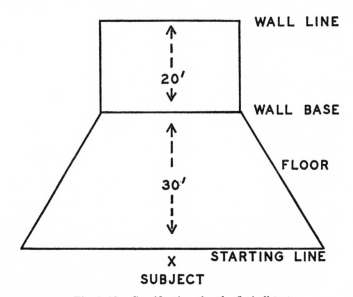

Fig. 9–23. Specifications for the fly ball test.

Procedures: The player stands behind a 30-foot restraining line to start. She throws the ball against the wall above a line 20 feet from the floor. After the first throw she may retrieve from anywhere on the floor and throw from anywhere using either an overarm or sidearm throw. Three 30-second trials are given with rest periods between.

Instructions: "Stand behind this line holding a softball. On the signal, 'Ready, Go!' throw the ball against the wall so it will hit above the 20-foot mark. Once you have thrown the first time, you may move anywhere to catch and throw the ball. Using either overarm or sidearm throws, see how many fly balls you can catch in 30 seconds. Balls which are fumbled or which bounce before the catch will not count. The total number of catches made in all three trials will be your final score."

Scoring: Count the number of catches made. The ball must hit the wall above the 20-foot mark. An overarm or sidearm throw must be used. Balls which are fumbled or are caught on the bounce do not count. The total number of catches made in 3 trials is recorded for the final score.

Testing Personnel: 1 timer and 1 scorer. If well trained, 1 person can perform both duties.

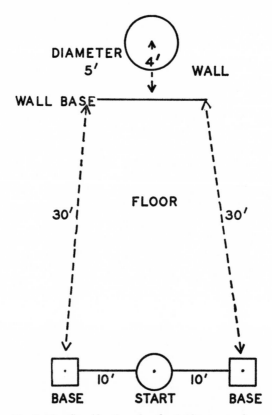

Fig. 9–24. Specifications for the fielding grounders, agility, speed and accuracy test.

ITEM NUMBER II—FIELDING GROUNDERS, AGILITY, SPEED AND ACCURACY TEST

Purpose: To measure the ability to field grounders, to run quickly to a base, and to throw quickly to a target with accuracy.

Facilities and Equipment: A floor space approximately 30 by 40 feet with a wall space approximately 20 by 20 feet. Balls and a stop watch.

Procedures: The test is started at a mark 30 feet from the wall midway between the two bases. The student alternates throws from each base to the target, retrieving the ball after each throw and proceeding to the appropriate base. She makes as many target hits as possible in 45 seconds. A rest period is taken between 2 trials. A retrial is permitted only if the ball hits another person.

Instructions: "Stand midway between the 2 bases with a softball in hand. On the signal, 'Ready, Go!' run to a base and, while your foot is on it, throw the ball to the target on the wall. Retrieve the ball, run to the opposite base and throw to the target from it. You must be touching the base when you throw and the throw must hit in or on the target circle to score. You will have 45 seconds to make as many target hits as possible."

Scoring: One point is scored for every target hit. The player must alternate bases to make the throws and must be touching the base when the throw is made. The final score is the total number of target hits in 2 trials.

Testing Personnel: 1 scorer, 1 timer, and a classmate at each base to check for foot faults.

ITEM NUMBER III—SOFTBALL THROW FOR DISTANCE

Purpose: To measure ability to throw long distances with some degree of accuracy.

Facilities and Equipment: Several softballs, markers to place in the field.

Procedures: The student is allowed to take one step into a throw for distance and must release the ball before stepping over the restraining

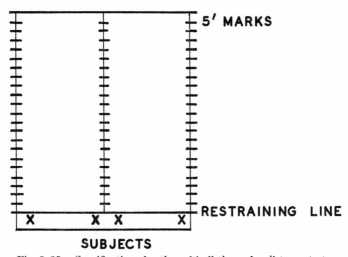

Fig. 9–25. Specifications for the softball throw for distance test.

line. Three successive throws are made and the best one counts. A warm-up of 20 jumping jacks is recommended.

Instructions: "Stand behind this line and allow yourself enough room to take one step into your throw without stepping over the line. You will throw 3 times and the longest throw will be recorded."

Scoring: Measure each throw to the nearest foot and record the best of 3 trials.

Testing Personnel: Spotters who call out the distance, ball retrievers, a scorer who explains the test.

Score Card

FRINGER SOFTBALL TEST

Name_____ Section_____ Squad_____

Grade_____1st Test Date_____ 2nd Test Date_____

	First Testing			Second Testing		
Test	*Trials*	*Score*	*T-Score*	*Trials*	*Score*	*T-Score*
Fielding	1	___		1	___	
Grounders,	2	___		2	___	
Agility, Speed,						
and Accuracy	Total	___	___	Total	___	___
Fly Balls	1	___		1	___	
	2	___		2	___	
	3	___		3	___	
	Total	___	___	Total	___	___
Distance Throw	Best	___	___	Best	___	___

Norms

Table 9–14. Norms for Fringer Softball Battery for High School Girls

T-Score	Fielding Grounders — Total of 2 trials	Fly Balls — Total of 3 trials	Distance Throw — Best trial	T-Score
75	25	31	150	75
70	24	30	115	70
65	21	28	105	65
60	18	25	95	60
55	15	21	83	55
50	12	17	71	50
45	10	11	61	45
40	7	7	55	40
35	5	2	47	35
30	2		41	30
25			37	25

Softball Repeated Throws*

Purpose. To measure softball playing ability similar to what the softball throw for distance measures. The two tests relate highly. This one can be administered indoors in a short period of time.

Evaluation. Reliability has been reported to be around .94 for college women, .84 for junior high school girls, and .87 for senior high school girls.

Level and Sex. This test is appropriate for use with junior and senior high school boys and girls.

Time Allotment and Number of Subjects. An entire class can take this test in 15 to 20 minutes if there is enough wall space for several stations. Six trials are required. Three would be sufficient during any one period.

Floor Plan and Space Requirements. An unobstructed indoor floor and wall space is needed for each station.

Class Organization. Arrange the class in squads for several to be tested at a time if enough space is available for several test stations. This also permits rest between trials as the students take turns.

General Procedures. The 6 trials can be administered by giving 3 trials for 2 days to reduce soreness and fatigue.

Uses. To combine with a subjective rating of batting for grading overall playing ability.

To check periodically during the unit to show progress.

To strengthen the shoulder girdle.

Test Description

Purpose: To measure ball handling skills of throwing and catching with a degree of speed.

Facilities and Equipment: A wall space about 15 feet high and 10 feet wide, balls, stop watch.

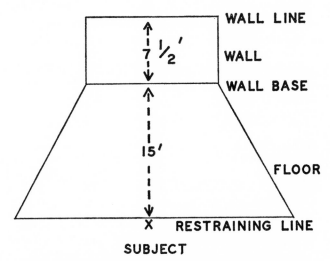

Fig. 9-26. Specifications for the repeated throws test.

* Located in Scott, M. Gladys, and Esther French: *Measurement and Evaluation in Physical Education.* Dubuque, Iowa: Wm. C. Brown Publishers, 1959. pp. 199-202. Used by permission of the authors.

Procedures: The student stands behind the 15-foot restraining line and throws the ball repeatedly at the wall above the $7\frac{1}{2}$-foot mark. Only one ball may be used during the test. The student may go ahead of the line to recover a ball but must be behind it for the throw to count. A 2-minute rest period between each of the 6 trials is recommended.

Instructions: "Stand behind this line to start and be sure you are behind it each time you throw the ball to the wall. Continue throwing and catching for 30 seconds. The ball must hit above the $7\frac{1}{2}$-foot mark on the wall. You will have 6 trials in all and they will be totaled, so do your very best on each trial."

Score Card

		REPEATED THROWS TEST		
Name_____		Date_____		
Class_____		Period_____		
Repeated Throws	*1st Testing*	*T-Score*	*2nd Testing*	*T-Score*
Trials:				
1	_____		_____	
2	_____		_____	
3	_____		_____	
4	_____		_____	
5	_____		_____	
6	_____		_____	
Total	_____ _____		_____ _____	

Norms

Table 9–15. Norms on Repeated Throws

T-Score	Scott, College Women	Fringer, High School Girls	T-Score
75	120	123	75
70	114	111	70
65	103	105	65
60	92	95	60
55	84	87	55
50	76	79	50
45	70	71	45
40	65	67	40
35	61	63	35
30	54	53	30
25	52	47	25

Total of 6 trials.

Scoring: Score 1 point for every hit against the wall which lands on or above the 7½-foot mark and which is released from behind the 15-foot line. The final score is the total number of hits for all 6 trials.

Testing Personnel: A central timer can signal for several stations. A scorer is needed at each station.

Check List for Rating Softball Batting Skills*

Student's Name _____ Date_____

Rated By_____ Score_____

Directions: First check student's performance as good, fair, or poor on each item and then check deviations noted. Determine the student's score by assigning 1 point for poor, 2 for fair, and 3 for good, and totaling points.

	Rating	*Deviations from Standard Performance*
1. Grip	____Good	____Hands too far apart
	____Fair	____Wrong hand on top
	____Poor	____Hands too far from end of bat
2. Preliminary Stance	____Good	____Stands too near the plate
	____Fair	____Stands too far from plate
	____Poor	____Stands too far forward toward pitcher
		____Stands too far backward toward catcher
		____Feet not parallel to line from pitcher to catcher
		____Rests bat on shoulder
		____Shoulders not horizontal
3. Stride or Footwork	____Good	____Fails to step forward
	____Fair	____Fails to transfer weight
	____Poor	____Lifts back foot from ground before swing
4. Pivot or Body Twist	____Good	____Fails to "wind up"
	____Fair	____Fails to follow-through with body
	____Poor	____Has less than 90° pivot
5. Arm Movement or Swing	____Good	____Arms held too close to body
	____Fair	____Rear elbow held too high
	____Poor	____Bat not held approximately parallel to ground
		____Not enough wrist motion used
		____Wrists not uncocked forcefully enough
6. General (Eyes on ball, judgment of pitches, and the like)	____Good	____Body movements jerky
	____Fair	____Tries too hard; "presses"
	____Poor	____Fails to look at center of ball
		____Poor judgment of pitches
		____Appears to lack confidence
		____Bat used not suitable

* Reprinted from *Teachers Guide to Physical Education for Girls in High School.* Compiled by Genevie Dexter, California State Department of Education, Sacramento, 1957, p. 315. Used by permission of the Department.

NOTE: The skills tests presented for softball fail to measure batting ability. The various batting tests available either use a pitcher, which is not desirable because of the partial dependence on the skill of the pitcher, or a batting tee which eliminates the approaching ball. As a supplement to the skills tests, this rating form for softball batting is included.

Additional Softball References

Brace, David K., Consultant: *Skills Test Manual—Softball for Boys*, Washington, D.C.: AAHPER, 1966.

————: *Skills Test Manual—Softball for Girls*, Washington, D.C.: AAHPER, 1966.

Everett, Peter W.: The Prediction of Baseball Ability, Research Quarterly, *23*, 15–19, March, 1952.

Fox, Margaret G., and Olive G. Young: A Test of Softball Batting Ability, Research Quarterly, *25*, 26–27, March, 1954.

Hooks, G. Eugene: Prediction of Baseball Ability Through An Analysis of Measures of Strength and Structure, Research Quarterly, *30*, 38–43, March, 1959.

Kehtel, Carmen H.: The Development of a Test to Measure the Ability of a Softball Player to Field a Ground Ball and Successfully Throw It at a Target, Unpublished Master's Thesis, University of Colorado, Boulder, 1958.

Kelson, Robert E.: Baseball Classification Plan for Boys, Research Quarterly, *24*, 304–309, October, 1953.

Thomas, Jesselene: Skill Tests, *Softball-Volley Ball Guide—1947–49*. Washington, D.C.: NSWA of the AAHPER, 1947, pp. 33–39.

SWIMMING

Rosentsweig Revision of the Fox Swimming Power Test*

Purpose. To evaluate five basic swimming strokes on form and power.

Evaluation. Rosentsweig revised the Fox test by changing the starting procedures, by adding a form rating, and by testing 5 strokes. He used 184 college women for the analysis. The reliability coefficients are computed on 2 trials. The form rating was correlated with the better of the power scores, not as a validity measure, but to show the relationship of the two components.

	Reliability	*Judge's Ratings*
Front Crawl	.89	.72
Side Crawl	.91	.81
Elementary Back Stroke	.96	.83
Back Crawl	.91	.63
Breast Stroke	.95	.74

Time Allotment and Number of Students. The students can help each other with starting procedures and power scoring but an instructor will need to rate the form, probably. This means individual testing which would be time consuming. The various strokes could be tested at different times toward the end of the unit.

Test Description

Procedures: The pool deck is marked off in 1-foot intervals beginning 8 feet from the shallow end to designate the starting line.

The test is started by having a student stand to the side of the swimmer being tested and use forearms as a cradle, holding the legs of the swimmer to the surface of the water. The student sculls or floats in the appropriate

* Rosentswieg, Joel: A Revision of the Power Swimming Test, Research Quarterly, *39*, 818–819, October, 1968. Used by permission of the AAHPER.

position with her shoulders parallel to the starting line. All measurements are taken at the shoulders. When the student is ready she swims away from the helper by using an arm stroke first. If a kick is made prior to the arm stroke, the trial is immediately stopped. Twelve arm strokes or six cycles are allowed depending upon the stroke. Two trials are allowed and the better distance accepted as the score.

A subjective rating of the swimmer's form is made at the same time the factor is being measured. A 5-point scale is used for the rating. Form and distance are evaluated at the same time and both scores are considered in the final grade.

Burris Speed-Stroke Test of the Crawl*

Purpose. To measure crawl stroking ability.

Evaluation. Five tests of crawl stroking ability were administered to 69 college men and women. The scores were converted to T-scores and added to get a composite criterion. Reliabilities were computed on a test-retest basis.

	Reliability	*Validity*	*Objectivity*
Men	.910	.887	.999
Women	.902	.864	.999

Chapman[5] compared three methods of measuring stroke proficiency:
1. Number of strokes constant, time and distance vary.
2. Time constant, number of strokes and distance vary.
3. Distance constant, time and number of strokes vary.

The third method proved most satisfactory. This supports the method used by Burris: 25-yard distance was constant and the time and number of strokes varied with the swimmer.

Level and Sex. Appropriate for men and women swimmers at the inter- mediate level or above. Norms would need to be adjusted for boys and girls but the test is appropriate.

Instructions. "This is a test of your crawl stroking ability. Swim as fast as you can, at the same time using as few strokes as possible. This means you will have to get as much power as you can from your kick and from your arm pull. Use the regular crawl stroke with the flutter kick and with rhythmic breathing on every second or third stroke (Demonstrate). Start in the deep water with one hand grasping the gutter, and with your feet vertical in the water and away from the wall. When I say, 'Ready-Go!', begin swimming without pushing off from the wall. Do not start until I say, 'Go', and do not stop until you have touched the wall."

Scoring. 1. *Speed.* On the signal, "Go," the watch is started. The watch stops when any part of the student's body touches the wall at the twenty-five yard distance. Time is recorded to the nearest tenth of a second.

* Burris, Barbara J.: A Study of the Speed-Stroke Test of Crawl Stroking Ability and Its Relationship to Other Selected Tests of Crawl Stroking Ability, M. Ed., Temple University, Philadelphia, 1964. Used by permission of the author.

Table 9-16. Scoring Table for Men for 25 Yards of Speed-Stroke Test of the Crawl

Seconds

Seconds	10	11	12	13	14	15	16	17	18	19	20	21	22	23	24	25	26	27	28	29	30	31	32	33	34
T-Scores	90	85	80	75	70	65	61	58	55	52	50	47	45	42	40	38	36	35	33	31	29	28	27	26	25

DIRECTIONS

Place the corner of the score sheet in the angle between the two sets of conversion scores. Round the time score to the nearest second and look for the appropriate number along the top row of figures marked seconds. Immediately below the score in seconds is the T-score equivalent of that score. Look up the raw score in strokes in the left hand column marked strokes. Just to the right of the stroke score is the T-score equivalent for strokes. Add the T-score for strokes to the T-score for seconds for the combined speed-stroke score.

Strokes / T-Score

Strokes	T-Score
10	92
11	89
12	85
13	83
14	80
15	77
16	75
17	72
18	70
19	68
20	66
21	64
22	62
23	60
24	58
25	56
26	54
27	52
28	50
29	48
30	46
31	44
32	42
33	40
34	38
35	36
36	34
37	32
38	31
39	30
40	28
41	27
42	25

Table 9–17. Scoring Table for Women for 25 Yards of Speed-Stroke Test of the Crawl

Seconds	16	17	18	19	20	21	22	23	24	25	26	27	28	29	30	31	32	33	34	35	36	37	38	39	40	41
T-Scores	91	85	80	75	70	66	62	58	55	53	51	49	48	46	44	43	42	40	39	38	36	34	33	31	30	27

Strokes	T-Score
14	89
15	85
16	82
17	80
18	78
19	75
20	73
21	71
22	68
23	66
24	64
25	62
26	60
27	57
28	55
29	53
30	51
31	49
32	47
33	45
34	44
35	42
36	41
37	40
38	39
39	37
40	36
41	35
42	34
43	33
44	31
45	30
46	28
47	26
48	25

DIRECTIONS

Place the corner of the score sheet in the angle between the two sets of conversion scores. Round the time score to the nearest second and look for the appropriate number along the top row of figures marked seconds. Immediately below the score in seconds is the T-score equivalent of that score. Look up the raw score in strokes in the left hand column marked strokes. Just to the right of the stroke score is the T-score equivalent for strokes. Add the T-score for strokes to the T-score for seconds for the combined speed-stroke score.

2. *Stroke.* Each time either hand enters the water for a pull, one stroke is counted. The touch to the wall is counted as a stroke if part of the arm pull has occurred. The first stroke is counted when the hand that had been touching the wall on the start enters the water for the first time.

Scoring Tables. Norms were developed on 89 men and 143 women swimmers at Temple University. Local norms will need to be developed. The format of the scoring table is worthy of note. Since the speed-stroke scores represent 2 T-scores combined, the average score is 100 instead of 50.

Additional Swimming References

Arrasmith, Jean L.: Swimming Classification Test for College Women, Ph.D., University of Oregon, Eugene, 1967.

Bennett, La Verne Means: A Test of Diving for Use in Beginning Classes, Research Quarterly, *13*, 109–115, March, 1942.

Durrant, Sue M.: An Analytical Method of Rating Synchronized Swimming Stunts, Research Quarterly, *35*, 126–134, May, 1964.

Fox, Margaret G.: Swimming Power Test, Research Quarterly, *28*, 233–238, October, 1957.

Hewitt, Jack E.: Achievement Scale Scores for High School Swimmers, Research Quarterly, *20*, 170–179, May, 1949.

———: Achievement Scale Scores for War Time Swimming, Research Quarterly, *14*, 391, December, 1943.

———: Swimming Achievement Scales for College Men, Research Quarterly, *19*, 282, December, 1948.

Kilby, Emelia-Louise Jepson: An Objective Method of Evaluating Three Swimming Strokes, Ph.D., University of Washington, Seattle, 1956.

Munt, Marilynn R.: Development of an Objective Test to Measure the Efficiency of the Front Crawl for College Women, MA, University of Michigan, Ann Arbor, 1964.

Wilson, Marcia Ruth: A Relationship Between General Motor Ability and Objective Measures of Achievement in Swimming at the Intermediate Level for College Women, Unpublished Master's Thesis, The Woman's College of the University of North Carolina, Greensboro, 1962.

TABLE TENNIS
Mott-Lockhart Table Tennis Test*

Purpose. To measure skill in table tennis.

Evaluation. A reliability of .98 is reported along with a validity coefficient of .81 using as a criterion subjective ratings of performance during tournament games.

Level and Sex. The test was developed using college women, but it is appropriate for secondary school boys and girls.

Time Allotment and Number of Subjects. A class can be tested in a period if multiple testing stations are available.

Floor Plan and Space Requirements. A hinged table tennis table needs to be arranged so half of the table can lean against a wall or post and so it will be perpendicular to the half in its regular position.

*Mott, Jane A., and Aileene Lockhart: Table Tennis Backboard Test, Journal of Health and Physical Education, *17*, 550–552, November, 1946. Used by permission of the AAHPER.

Class Organization. Provide several testing stations if possible. Arrange the students in squads at each testing station. Use one central timer.

General Procedures. 1. Arrange some practice in the days preceding the testing.

2. Arrange for the players to rotate so at least a little rest is provided between trials.

3. Thumb tack the little box which holds the extra balls to the right side of the table.

4. Provide one practice trial immediately preceding the official test.

Uses. To use as a practice drill.
To motivate.
To indicate achievement.
To classify tournament players.

Test Description

BACKBOARD TEST

Purpose: To measure ability to rally a table tennis ball against an upright surface.

Facilities and Equipment: A table tennis table which can be divided in the middle and half of it placed perpendicularly on the other half, or boards which are of table quality which can be placed upright on the table, or wall space against which the tables can be placed, balls, paddle, stop watch, and a small cardboard box to hold the balls and thumbtacks.

Procedures: The player rallies the ball against the upright surface. The ball must hit above the 6-inch net line and it must bounce at least once on the table surface before being returned. The ball is put into play by bouncing it on the table and then stroking it. The extra balls in the little box attached to the side of the table are used whenever the ball goes out of control. The player may not place his hands on the table.

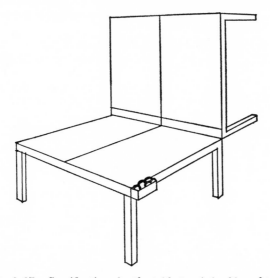

Fig. 9–27. Specifications for the table tennis backboard test.

Instructions: "Stand at the end of the table holding a paddle and a ball. On the signal, 'Ready, Go!' bounce the ball against the table and stroke it against the upright portion of the table. Rally for 30 seconds accumulating as many hits as possible. The ball must bounce at least once before you play it, it must hit above the net line, and you may not use your free hand on the table during the stroking. You will have three 30-second trials and the best one will score."

Scoring: Count 1 point for each ball hitting above the 6-inch net line which has been stroked after a bounce with no help from the free hand on the table. The final score is the best of three 30-second trials.

Testing Personnel: A scorer and a timer.

Score Card

```
                          TABLE TENNIS TEST
  Squad No._____ Class_____ Period_____ Date_____

                    Trial        Trial        Trial
       Name          #1           #2           #3          T-Score

  1. _____  _____   _____    _____    _____
  2. _____  _____   _____    _____    _____
     .
     .
     .
  8. _____  _____   _____    _____    _____
```

Norms

Table 9–18.   Norms for the Mott-Lockhart Table Tennis Test*

T-Score	Raw Score
75	59
70	54
65	49
60	46
55	43
50	39
45	33
40	29
35	25
30	21
25	17

* Based on the performance of 162 college women.

TENNIS
Scott-French Revision of the Dyer Wallboard Test*

Purpose. To measure ability to rally with forehand and backhand drives.

Evaluation. Validity r was .61 with a criterion of subjective ratings.

One reliability r was reported as .80 computed on the performance of college women.

The Revised Dyer backboard test which is reported in the 1938 *Research Quarterly* calls for a restraining line of 5 feet. The present revision which is reported in Scott and French[41] specifies a restraining line of 27½ feet to encourage better form. An even farther restraining line is suggested for more advanced players in order to give them the opportunity to use the full strength of their drives.

Level and Sex. This test is suitable for boys and girls of all ages. Care should be taken to apply appropriate norms for each group.

Time Allotment and Number of Subjects. An entire class can be tested in one class period.

Floor Plan and Space Requirements. A wall space at least 10 feet in height and 20 feet in width is needed for each station. Court or floor space to a depth of at least 35 feet is needed.

Class Organization. Squads will work since several students can be used to keep the ball supply adequate and since rest periods between trials are desirable. A regular gym floor can usually accommodate at least 4 test stations and perhaps 6, depending on the amount of free wall space.

General Procedures. 1. The racket with the extra balls on it should be placed in the same location at each station so the supply of balls will be standardized. The balls should not be handed to the player.

2. The racket should be on the restraining line but toward the end of it and should be to the left of a right handed player as he faces the wall.

3. The students can pool their balls to have an adequate number at each station.

4. The students should be sure to stay out of the way of the player being tested.

Uses. To classify students for instructional groups.
To classify students for competition.
To measure achievement.
To use as a partial grade in a tennis unit.
Note: The rally test should be supplemented with a service placement test or a service rating to get a better over-all skill grade of tennis playing ability.

Test Description

ITEM NUMBER I—BACKBOARD TEST

Purpose: To measure ability to rally the ball using forehand and backhand drives.

*Scott, M. Gladys, and Esther French: *Measurement and Evaluation in Physical Education.* Dubuque, Iowa: Wm. C. Brown Company, Publishers, 1959, pp. 222–225. Used by permission of the authors.

Facilities and Equipment: Two rackets, 10 to 12 balls, wall and floor space, the net line should be 3 inches in width and should be included in the 3-foot distance.

Procedures: The player stands behind the restraining line holding a racket and 2 balls. The ball is put into play by bouncing it and stroking it against the wall. The rally continues for 30 seconds, using any stroke desired. If the ball gets out of control, another one is started in the same manner in which the test was started. Balls hit short of the restraining line or which land below the 3-foot mark do not score but sometimes help to keep the rally going. After the initial bounce to start the rally, the ball may be hit on the volley or after any number of bounces. The player should get 2 more tennis balls from the racket face whenever they are needed to keep the rally going.

Instructions: "Stand behind the restraining line holding your racket and two balls. On the signal, 'Ready, Go!' bounce a ball and drive it against the wall. Continue to rally the ball for 30 seconds getting as many hits as possible. Get additional balls from the racket face if the two you have go out of control. To score you must be standing behind this line when you stroke the ball and it must hit above the 3-foot line. It is permissible to go ahead of the line to keep the rally going but balls hit from this area do not score. You may hit the ball on the volley or after any number of bounces. Your score will be the total number of hits you make in three 30-second trials."

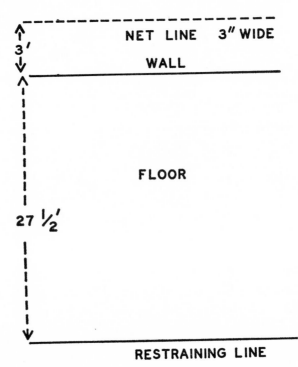

Fig. 9–28. Specifications for the tennis backboard test.

Scoring: Three 30-second trials are given. The score is the total hits for all 3 trials. A legal hit must land above the 3-foot line on the wall and must be contacted from behind the 27½-foot restraining line.

Testing Personnel: One to time, one to score, and several to retrieve the balls which go astray and to place them on the face of the extra racket.

Score Card

```
                      TENNIS TESTS
         Name_____  Date_____

         Class_____  Grade_____

         Wallboard Test: 1. _____     Serve Rating:

                        2. _____      _____

                        3. _____

                   Total _____

                 T-Score _____
```

Norms

Table 9–19.   Norms for Scott-French Revision of Dyer Wallboard Test*

T-Score	Total of 3 trials Wallboard
80	34
75	31
70	29
65	25
60	22
55	18
50	15
45	13
40	11
35	9
30	6
25	3
20	1

* Based on 583 college students. Norms by Scott, M. Gladys, and Esther French, *Measurement and Evaluation in Physical Education.* Dubuque, Iowa: Wm. C. Brown Publishers, 1959, p. 224. Used by permission of the authors.

Broer-Miller Forehand-Backhand Drive Test*

Purpose. To measure ability to place drives in the back court.

Evaluation. Broer and Miller developed this test in conjunction with a tennis knowledge test. The skill test was evaluated using 27 college women of intermediate skill and 32 college women of beginning level skill. They were attempting to develop a test that would do away with the necessity of tossing or hitting the ball to the student being tested. The reliability coefficients were .80 for both beginning and intermediate groups using the split-halves method with the Spearman-Brown Prophecy Formula. Validity was established using subjective ratings as the criterion. Two judges were used with the intermediate group and 3 with the beginning group. Their average ratings correlated .85 for the intermediate level and .61 for the beginning students.

Level and Sex. Developed for college women. Appropriate for secondary and college students.

Time Allotment and Number of Students. Thirty students can be tested in one hour using 1 recorder.

Floor Plan, Space Requirements, Facilities and Equipment. One regulation tennis court, tennis racket, rope, 15–20 balls in good condition, score cards and pencils will be needed. Two lines are drawn across the court 10 feet inside the service line and 9 feet outside the service line and parallel to it. Two lines are drawn across the court 5 feet and 10 feet respectively outside the baseline and parallel to it. Numbers are placed in the center of each area to indicate its scoring value. A rope is stretched 4 feet above the top of the net.

Uses. To serve as a classification device.
To help determine grades.

Test Description. The player taking the test stands behind the baseline, bounces the ball to herself, hits the ball and attempts to place it in the back 9 feet of the opposite court. Each player is allowed fourteen trials on the forehand and fourteen trials on the backhand. In order to score the values designated, balls must go between the top of the net and the rope. Balls

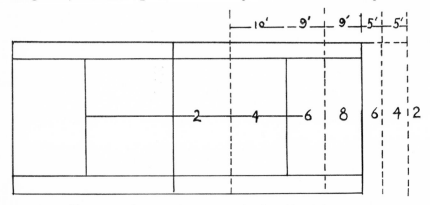

Fig. 9–29.   Court markings for forehand-backhand drive test.

* Broer, Marian R. and Donna Mae Miller: Achievement Tests for Beginning and Intermediate Tennis, Research Quarterly, *21*, 303–321, October, 1950. Used by permission of the AAHPER.

which go over the rope score one-half the value of that area in which they land. If the player misses the ball in attempting to strike it, it is considered a trial. Let balls are taken over.

Scoring. Each ball hit between the net and rope is scored 2-4-6-8-6-4-2, depending upon the area in which it lands. Each ball going over the rope is scored one-half the value of the area in which it lands. The total score equals the sum of fourteen balls on the forehand and fourteen balls on the backhand.

Wisconsin Wall Test for Serve*

Purpose. To measure the effectiveness of the serve as reflected by force and height.

Evaluation. The Serve Test is reported to be reliable and to be valid logically.[12] The time scores had a reliability of .978 using 20 trials on 2 days determined by the Analysis of Variance statistic. Using only 10 trials on one day, the reliability of the velocity score was .942. The final score combining speed and placement values had a reliability of .957 using 20 trials on 2 days and .912 using 10 trials on 1 day. The test also validated well with subjective ratings.

The Wisconsin Wall Test for Serve correlated .62 with tournament rankings in 9 tennis classes, 229 students, at Memphis State University.[13]

Level and Sex. Developed for college women. Appropriate for secondary and college students.

Time Allotment and Number of Students. The test can be administered to a class in one class period if all preliminary preparations have been made.

Markings and Space Requirements. The wall target is $42\frac{1}{2}$ feet away from the serving line. The wall is marked off in 1-foot intervals from the floor to the height of 12 feet. The 3-foot line, designating the height of the net, should be a thicker line. No limit is set on the width of the target.

The test can be administered either indoor or outdoor using a wall or a fence.

Class Organization. The students can score for one another. A person well trained in the use of the stop watch should time the velocity of each serve. Groups of 5 or 6 students could be placed at each testing station: 1 to take the test, 1 to time and note the placement area, 1 to record time and placement, 1 to retrieve, and 1 or 2 to wait their turns in the rotation order.

Uses. To measure improvement in service ability.
To measure achievement in service ability.
To use as a partial basis for a grade.
To diagnose individual needs.

Test Instructions. You will serve at the wall target from this line $42\frac{1}{2}$ feet from the wall. You will serve 10 times. Your point of aim is area 4 on the wall, just above the thick line marking the net height. We will repeat all serves that do not reach the wall before hitting the floor. You will hold 2 balls in your tossing hand for each serve. You may have 3 practice serves and then we will begin. The area where the ball lands will

* Edwards, Janet: A Study of Three Measures of the Tennis Serve, MSPE, University of Wisconsin, Madison, 1965. Used by permission of the Department of Physical Education for Women of the University of Wisconsin and the author.

be recorded and the time it takes the ball to travel from the racket to the target will be recorded. These values will be converted into point values so they can be combined to determine an overall score for the serve test.

Scoring. The scorer-timer stands to the left and approximately 6 feet behind each server in order to note the wall area number and the time for each serve. This information is reported to a recorder. The score is the total number of point values for Velocity and Vertical Placement which are made with 10 serves. The velocity measures for the total of 10 trials should be added and then converted to the point values from Table 9–20.[13] The placement conversions will need to be made from Table 9–20 for each of the 10 serves and then added.

Note. Hulbert[19] used these same conversion values to apply to a forehand drive test. The wall markings and the 42½-foot restraining line are identical to the service test. The player puts the ball into play with a self-toss and uses 10 trials. Content validity is claimed and a reliability of .78 for 10 trials on one day, using the Analysis of Variance statistic, is reported.

Table 9–20. Wisconsin Wall Conversion Tables

Vertical Placement		*Velocity**	
Wall Area	*Point Values*	*Time*	*Point Values*
11′	1	4.00	300
10′	2	4.25	290
9′	4	4.50	280
8′	6	4.75	270
7′	7	5.00	260
6′	8	5.25	250
5′	9	5.50	240
4′ Net	10	5.75	230
3′	6	6.00	220
2′	4	6.25	210
1′	2	6.50	200
		6.75	190
		7.00	180
		7.25	170
		7.50	160
		7.75	150
		8.00	140
		8.25	130
		8.50	120
		8.75	110
		9.00	100
		9.50	90
		10.00	80
		10.50	70
		11.00	60
		11.50	50
		12.00	40
		12.50	30
		13.00	20
		13.50	10
		13.51+	0

* Velocity Scores treated in terms of 10 serves, not in terms of individual serves, as suggested by Farrow, Andrea C.: Skill and Knowledge Proficiencies for Selected Activities in the Required Program at Memphis State University, Ed.D., University of North Carolina at Greensboro, 1971, and used by permission of the author.

Additional Tennis References

Cobane, Edith: Test for the Service, *Tennis and Badminton Guide—June 1962–June 1964*. Washington, D.C.: AAHPER, pp. 46–47.

Cotten, Doyice J., and Jane Nixon: A Comparison of Two Methods of Teaching the Tennis Serve, Research Quarterly, *39*, 929–931, December, 1968.

DiGennaro, Joseph: Construction of Forehand Drive, Backhand Drive, and Serve Tennis Tests, Research Quarterly, *40*, 496–501, October, 1969.

Dyer, Joanna Thayer: Revision of Backboard Test of Tennis Ability, Research Quarterly, *9*, 25–31, March, 1938.

Fonger, Sandra J.: The Development of a Reliable, Objective, and Practical Tennis Serve Test for College Women, MAPE, University of Michigan, Ann Arbor, 1963.

Hewitt, Jack E.: Classification Tests in Tennis, Research Quarterly, *39*, 552–555, October, 1968.

———: Hewitt's Tennis Achievement Test, Research Quarterly, *37*, 231–240, May, 1966.

———: Revision of the Dyer Backboard Tennis Test, Research Quarterly, *36*, 153–157, May, 1965.

Hubbell, Nancy C.: A Battery of Tennis Skill Tests for College Women, Unpublished Master's Thesis, Texas Woman's University, Denton, 1960.

Johnson, Joan: Tennis Serve of Advanced Women Players, Research Quarterly, *28*, 123–131, May, 1957.

Jones, Skirley K.: A Measure of Tennis Serving Ability, MSPE University of California, Los Angles, 1967.

Kemp, Joann, and Marilyn F. Vincent: Kemp-Vincent Rally Test of Tennis Skill, Research Quarterly, *39*, 1000–1004, December, 1968.

Malinak, Nina R.: The Construction of an Objective Measure of Accuracy in the Performance of the Tennis Serve, Unpublished Master's Thesis, University of Illinois, Urbana, 1961.

Ronning, Hilding Earl: Wall Tests for Evaluating Tennis Ability, Unpublished Master's Thesis, Washington State University, Pullman, 1959.

Timmer, Karen L.: A Tennis Skill Test to Determine Accuracy in Playing Ability, MSPE, Springfield College, Springfield, Massachusetts, 1965.

VOLLEYBALL

Rules changes often require changes in skills tests. The one hit rule in the girls' game has caused some changes but the new attack, offensive type volleyball game reflects a change in strategy which has influenced volleyball skills tests even more. The serve is fast and low, the pass or set is high and accurate, and the spike is decisive. The repeated volley tests are described with many variations. The restraining line varies from 3 to 5 to 7 feet, to no restraining line at all, or one only to start the test. The length of trials varies from 15 seconds to 1 minute and the number of trials from 1 to 10. The horizontal wall line ranges from $7\frac{1}{2}$ to 11 feet in height.

Modified Brady Volleyball Test*

Purpose. To indicate overall volleyball playing ability.

Evaluation: Kronqvist and Brumbach revised the Brady test, which had been developed for college men, to fit secondary school boys. Seventy-one 10th and 11th grade boys in West Vancouver, British Columbia were

---

* Kronqvist, Roger A., and Wayne B. Brumbach: A Modification of the Brady Volleyball Skill Test for High School Boys, Research Quarterly, *39*, 116–120, March, 1968. Used by permission of the AAHPER.

12

involved. Three judges used the rating scale suggested by Laveaga[24] to form the validity criterion. Their intercorrelations were .776, .804, and .903. The validity coefficient was .767 and the reliability, established by the test-retest method, was .817.

Level and Sex. Secondary school boys.

Time Allotment and Number of Students. An average size physical education class can be tested within one period if several testing stations are marked on the gymnasium wall.

Uses. To aid in determining grades.
As a screening device for grouping students.
As a motivation for individual practice.

Test Description

Markings: A target area is a 5-foot line on the wall, 11 feet from the floor. From both ends of this line, lines extend toward the ceiling for at least 4 feet. There are no restraining lines on the floor.

Equipment: Volleyballs, stop watch, score cards and pencils.

Instructions:
1. You will receive three trials of 20 seconds' duration.
2. To start, you will throw the ball against the wall within the rebound area on the command, "Ready, Go."
3. When the ball returns to you, begin to volley.
4. Continue until given the command "Stop."
5. If you lose control of the ball or if it touches the floor, you must retrieve the ball, then throw it against the wall as when you started the test.
6. One point is scored for each successful volley (not necessarily consecutive volleys).
7. The time between each trial will be approximately 30 seconds, the length of time it takes the next subject to perform the trial.
8. The scorer will count aloud, so the tester will know whether or not the volleys are acceptable.
9. In order for a volley to be counted, the ball must be clearly hit. When, in the opinion of the scorer, the ball visibly comes to rest at contact, the volley shall not be counted.

Scoring: The score is the number of legal volleys executed in three 20-second trials.

Testing Personnel: The instructor can explain and demonstrate the test and serve as the central timer. The students can score for each other.

High Wall Volley Test*

Purpose. To measure volleyball playing ability.

Evaluation. The rule change to the single hit game for girls and women has made the higher volley important for passing. The developers of this test hoped to incorporate the following factors:
1. minimize, but not eliminate, the height factor

* Cunningham, Phyllis and Joan Garrison: High Wall Volley Test for Women's Volleyball, Research Quarterly, *39*, 486–490, October, 1968. Used by permission of the AAHPER.

2. eliminate a restraining line
3. require the student to use footwork
4. require accurate placement
5. require the use of a high volley.

One hundred and eleven college women were used in the analysis. Judges' ratings intercorrelated .89, .83, and .87 and were totaled to serve as the validity criterion. The new test correlated .72 with the criterion and had a reliability coefficient of .87 correlating trial one with trial two.

Level and Sex. Developed for college women and appropriate for secondary school girls.

Time Allotment and Number of Students. An average sized class can be tested easily within one class period if there are several test stations marked on the wall.

Facilities and Equipment. Leather volleyballs, stop watch, score cards, and pencils.

Floor Plan and Space Requirements. A flat, unobstructed wall space 9 feet wide and 15 feet high is needed for each test station. A target area is 10 feet from the floor. A horizontal line is drawn 3 feet long with 3-foot vertical lines extending upward at right angles to the horizontal line.

Test Description. The test consists of two 30-second trials. The player stands anywhere in front of the target. With the signal, "ready, go" she uses any type of toss or hit to send the ball into the target area on or above the 10-foot line and on or between the two vertical lines or their extensions. When the ball returns, she volleys it repeatedly into the target area. Only one contact of the ball is allowed on each volley.

If the player loses control of the ball, she recovers it and starts again as before. She may not use the sequence, "toss, volley, catch: toss, volley, catch" but must make an attempt to perform a repeated volley. Following the first trial the player rests while the other members of her group (6 to 8 players) take their first trials. A second trial is given as before.

Scoring. One point is scored each time the ball hits in the target area or on the line bounding it following a legal volley of a ball rebounding from the wall. The toss or hit to start the ball does not count. If the player loses control of the ball, scoring continues with the next legal hit. The better score of the two trials is recorded.

Petry Volleyball Serve Test*

Purpose. To measure volleyball serving ability using underhand, side-arm, and overhand serves.

Evaluation. Petry identified three factors crucial to a good serve:
1. getting the ball over the net.
2. placing the ball.
3. hitting the ball low.

She used 118 10th, 11th, and 12th grade girls to develop the serve test.

	Reliabilities
10 underhand trials	.65
10 sidearm trials	.54
10 overhand trials	.78
total 30 trials	.818

* Petry, Kathryn: Evaluation of a Volleyball Serve Test, MAPE, Los Angeles State College, Los Angeles, 1967. Used by permission of the author.

The validity was determined by judging the difference in performance of top and bottom groups. The mean difference was significant so discriminatory validity was established. Petry believed the use of three types of serves would provide a better classification tool.

Level and Sex. For use with secondary school girls. Appropriate for boys as well.

Uses. To classify students.
To use as a partial grade.
To use as a self-testing device for motivation.

Test Description

Equipment and Facilities: Volleyballs, score cards and pencils, rope and a regulation volleyball court.

Floor Markings: Four lines parallel to the net, 6 feet apart and with the first line 6 feet from the net, divide the court into 5 equal areas, 6 by 30

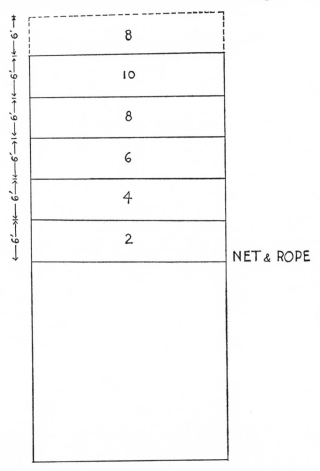

Fig. 9–30. Court markings for serve test.

feet. An additional area is bounded by a line parallel to and 6 feet behind the service line and extensions of the side lines.

A rope is stretched 3 feet above the regulation net and parallel to it.

Procedures: A rotation plan is utilized whereby each girl attempts ten underhand serves and then goes to the end of the line while the remaining girls on the team attempt ten. The second time around she attempts ten sidearm, and the third and final time she serves, she attempts ten overhand serves. This rotation plan is employed to offset fatigue and discomfort.

Instructions and Scoring: The student stands anywhere behind the endline within the service area. She serves ten consecutive times in the required manner, that is underhand, sidearm, and overhand, attempting to hit the ball so that it travels over the net and under the rope. The score is determined by the placement of the ball on the court. In order to obtain full credit, the ball must travel over the net and under the 3-foot rope. If the ball goes over the rope, only one-half credit is received. If the student steps over the endline, hits the ball into the net, or serves the ball in any other illegal manner, the trial is recorded as a zero. The score is the sum of the 30 trials.

Testing Personnel: The students can administer this test for themselves after the instructor has explained it.

Additional Volleyball References

Blackman, Claudia J.: The Development of a Volleyball Test for the Spike, MS in Ed., Southern Illinois University, Carbondale, 1968.

Brady, G. F.: Preliminary Investigation of Volleyball Playing Ability, Research Quarterly, *16*, 14–17, March, 1945.

Camp, Billie Ann: The Reliability and Validity of a Single-Hit Repeated Volleys Test in Volleyball and the Relationship of Height to Performance on the Test, MSPE, University of Colorado, Boulder, 1963.

Chaney, Dawn S.: The Development of a Test of Volleyball Ability for College Women, MA in PE, Texas Woman's University, Denton, 1966.

Clifton, Marguerite: Single Hit Volley Test for Women's Volleyball, Research Quarterly, *33*, 208–211, May, 1962.

Crogan, Corrinne: A Simple Volleyball Classification Test for High School Girls, The Physical Educator, *4*, 34–37, October, 1943.

Jackson, Patricia: A Rating Scale for Discriminating Relative Performance of Skilled Female Volleyball Players, MAPE, University of Alberta, Edmonton, Alberta, Canada, 1967.

Johnson, Judith A.: The Development of a Volleyball Skill Test for High School Girls, MSPE, Illinois State University, Normal, 1967.

Jones, Richard N.: The Development of a Volleyball Skills Test for Adult Males, MSPE, Springfield College, Springfield, Massachusetts, 1964.

Kissler, Adrian A.: The Validity and Reliability of the Sandefur Volleyball Spiking Test, MAPE, California State College, Long Beach, 1968.

Ladner, Jane: Volleyball Wall Volley Skill Test, Southern District Proceedings of the AAHPER, Biloxi, Mississippi, 1954.

Lamp, Nancy A.: Volleyball Skills for Junior High School Students as a Function of Physical Size and Maturity, Research Quarterly, *25*, 189, May, 1954.

Liba, Marie R., and Marilyn R. Stauff: A Test for the Volleyball Pass, Research Quarterly, *34*, 56–63, March, 1963.

Lopez, Delfina: Serve Test, *Volleyball Guide—1957–59*, DGWS of the AAHPER, 1957, pp. 29–30.

Michalski, Rosalie Ann: Construction of an Objective Skill Test for the Underhand Volleyball Serve, MAPE, University of Iowa, Iowa City, 1963.

Mohr, Dorothy R., and Martha V. Haverstick: Repeated Volleys Test for Women's Volleyball, Research Quarterly, *26*, 179, May, 1955.

Russell, Naomi, and Elizabeth Lange: Achievement Tests in Volleyball for Junior High School Girls, Research Quarterly, *11*, 33–41, December, 1940.

Ryan, Mary Frances: A Study of Tests for the Volleyball Serve, M.S., University of Wisconsin, Madison, 1969.

Shaw, John H.: A Preliminary Investigation of a Volleyball Skill Test, MSPE, University of Tennessee, Knoxville, 1967.

Shay, Clayton, Consultant: *Skills Test Manual—Volleyball for Boys and Girls*, Washington, D.C.: AAHPER, 1969.

Shavely, Marie: Volleyball Skill Tests for Girls, *Selected Volleyball Articles*. Washington, D.C.: DGWS of the AAHPER, 1960, pp. 77–78.

Suttinger, Joan: A Proposed Predictive Index of Volleyball Playing Ability for College Women, Unpublished study, University of California, Los Angeles, May, 1957.

West, Charlotte: A Comparative Study Between Height and Wall Volley Test Scores as Related to Volleyball Playing Ability of Girls and Women, Unpublished Master's Thesis, The Woman's College of the University of North Carolina, Greensboro, June, 1957.

WRESTLING
Sickels Amateur Wrestling Ability Rating Form*

Purpose. To measure wrestling ability.

Evaluation. This scale was formulated on the basis of the performance of 129 high school boys who participated in interscholastic competition and in physical education classes.

The Rating Form:

AMATEUR WRESTLING ABILITY RATING FORM

Name_____ Weight Class_____ Date _____

Rating Scale: 7—Superior;   6—Excellent;   5—Good;
                     4—Average;   3—Poor;   2—Very Poor;
                     1—Ineffective

I. WRESTLING ON FEET   A. Balance   1 2 3 4 5 6 7
                          B. Timing and Speed   1 2 3 4 5 6 7
                          C. Strategy   1 2 3 4 5 6 7
                          D. Aggressiveness   1 2 3 4 5 6 7

II. WRESTLING ON MAT
   1. Top Position   A. Balance   1 2 3 4 5 6 7
                          B. Timing and Speed   1 2 3 4 5 6 7
                          C. Wrestling Skills   1 2 3 4 5 6 7

   2. Bottom Position   A. Balance   1 2 3 4 5 6 7
                          B. Timing and Speed   1 2 3 4 5 6 7
                          C. Wrestling Skills   1 2 3 4 5 6 7

TOTAL POINTS _____

Scoring: The scores range from a maximum of 70 points to a minimum of 10 points.

* Sickels, William Loyd: A Rating Test for Amateur Wrestling Ability, MSPE, San Jose State College, San Jose, California, 1967. Used by permission of the author.

Additional Wrestling References

Case, Robert L.: An Evaluation of the Improvement of Wrestling Skills and Competence, MSPE, University of Illinois, Urbana, 1964.

Sources of Tests for Sports Not Included in This Book

Archery

Hyde, Edith I.: An Achievement Scale in Archery, Research Quarterly, *8*, 109, May, 1937.

Bohn, Robert W.: An Achievement Test in Archery, MSPE, University of Wisconsin, Madison, 1962.

Brace, David K., Consultant: *Skills Test Manual—Archery for Boys and Girls*, Washington, D.C.: AAHPER, 1967.

Bowling

Johnson, Norma Jean: Tests of Achievement in Bowling for Beginning Girl Bowlers, MSPE, University of Colorado, Boulder, 1962.

Martin, Joan L.: A Way to Measure Bowling Success, Research Quarterly, *31*, 113–116, March, 1960.

Martin, Joan and Jack Keogh: Bowling Norms for College Students in Elective Physical Education Classes, Research Quarterly, *35*, 325–327, October, 1964.

Olson, Janice and Marie R. Liba: A Device for Evaluating Spot Bowling Ability, Research Quarterly, *38*, 193–201, May, 1967.

Phillips, Marjorie, and Dean Summers: Bowling Norms and Learning Curves for College Women, Research Quarterly, *21*, 377–385, December, 1950.

Ice Sports

Brown, Harriet M.: The Game of Ice Hockey, Journal of Health and Physical Education, *6*, 28–30, January, 1935.

Hacke, Roland E.: An Achievement Test in Ice Hockey, MSPE, University of Massachusetts, Amherst, 1967.

Leaming, Thomas W.: A Measure of Endurance of Young Speed Skaters, Unpublished Master's Thesis, University of Illinois, Urbana, 1959.

Merrifield, H. H., and Gerald A. Walford: Battery of Ice Hockey Skill Tests, Research Quarterly, *40*, 146–152, March, 1969.

Moore, Kathleen Fitzgerald: An Objective Evaluation System for Judging Free Skating Routines, MAPE, Michigan State University, East Lansing, 1967.

Recknagel, Dorothy: A Test for Beginners in Figure Skating, Journal of Health and Physical Education, *16*, 91, February, 1945.

Rogers, Marilyn Helen: Construction of Objectively Scored Skill Tests for Beginning Skiers, Unpublished Master's Thesis, University of Colorado, Boulder, 1960.

Rhythms and Dance

Ashton, Dudley: A Gross Motor Rhythm Test, Research Quarterly, *24*, 253–260, October, 1953.

Benton, Rachel J.: The Measurement of Capacities for Learning Dance Movement Techniques, Research Quarterly, *15*, 137, May, 1944.

Blake, Patricia A.: Relationship Between Audio Perceptual Rhythm and Skill in Square Dance, Research Quarterly, *31*, 229–231, May, 1960.

Briggs, Ruth A.: The Development of an Instrument for Assessment of Motoric Rhythmic Performance, MAPE, University of Missouri, Columbia, 1968.

Coppock, Doris E.: Development of an Objective Measure of Rhythmic Motor Response, Research Quarterly, *39*, 915–921, December, 1968.

Dvorak, Sandra E.: A Subjective Evaluation of Fundamental Locomotor Movement in Modern Dance Using a Five-Point Scale, MSPE, South Dakota State University, Brookings, 1967.

Frial, Paula Isabel S.: Prediction of Modern Dance Ability Through Kinesthetic Tests, Ph.D., University of Iowa, Iowa City, 1965.

Imel, Elizabeth Carmen: Construction of an Objective Motor Rhythm Skill Test, MAPE, University of Iowa, Iowa City, 1963.
Lang, Lucile M.: The Development of a Test of Rhythmic Response at the Elementary Level, M.Ed., University of Texas, Austin, 1966.
Waglow, I. F.: An Experiment in Social Dance Testing, Research Quarterly, *24*, 97, March, 1953.
Withers, Maida Rust: Measuring Creativity of Modern Dancers, Unpublished Master's Thesis, University of Utah, Salt Lake City, 1960.

References

1. Borleske, Stanley E.: A Study of Achievement of College Men in Touch Football, Unpublished Master's Thesis, University of California, Berkeley, 1936. Reported by Cozens, Frederick W., Ninth Annual Report of the Committee on Curriculum Research of the College Physical Education Association, Research Quarterly, *8*, 73–78, May, 1937.
2. Brady, G. F.: Preliminary Investigations of Volleyball Playing Ability, Research Quarterly, *16*, 14–17, March, 1945.
3. Broer, Marian R., and Donna Mae Miller: Achievement Tests for Beginning and Intermediate Tennis, Research Quarterly, *21*, 303–321, October, 1950.
4. Burris, Barbara J.: A Study of the Speed-Stroke Test of Crawl Stroking Ability and Its Relationship to Other Selected Tests of Crawl Stroking Ability, M. Ed., Temple University, Philadelphia, 1964.
5. Chapman, Peggy: A Comparison of Three Methods of Measuring Swimming Stroke Proficiency, MSPE, University of Wisconsin, Madison, 1965.
6. Clarke, H. Harrison: *Application of Measurement to Health and Physical Education*, 4th Ed., Englewood Cliffs, N.J., Prentice-Hall, Inc., 1967.
7. Cooper, Cynthia K.: The Development of a Fencing Skill Test for Measuring Achievement of Beginning Collegiate Women Fencers in Using the Advance, Beat, and Lunge, MS in Ed., Western Illinois University, Macomb, 1968.
8. Cotteral, Bonnie, and Donnie Cotteral: *The Teaching of Stunts and Tumbling.* New York, A. S. Barnes & Co., 1936.
9. Cunningham, Phyllis: Measuring Basketball Playing Ability of High School Girls, Ph.D., University of Iowa, Iowa City, 1964.
10. Cunningham, Phyllis and Joan Garrison: High Wall Volley Test for Women's Volleyball, Research Quarterly, *39*, 486–490, October, 1968.
11. Dexter, Genevie, Compiler: *Teachers Guide to Physical Education for Girls in High School.* Sacramento, California State Department of Education, 1957.
12. Edwards, Janet: A Study of Three Measures of the Tennis Serve, MSPE, University of Wisconsin, Madison, 1965.
13. Farrow, Andrea C.: Skill and Knowledge Proficiencies for Selected Activities in the Required Program at Memphis State University, Ed. D., University of North Carolina at Greensboro, 1971.
14. French, Esther and Evelyn Stalter: Study of Skill Tests in Badminton for College Women, Research Quarterly, *20*, 257–272, October, 1949.
15. Friedel, Jean Elizabeth: The Development of a Field Hockey Skill Test for High School Girls, Unpublished Master's Thesis, Illinois State University, Normal, 1956.
16. Fringer, Margaret Neal: A Battery of Softball Skill Tests for Senior High School Girls, Unpublished Master's Thesis, University of Michigan, Ann Arbor, 1961.
17. Harris, J. Patrick: A Design for a Proposed Skill Proficiency Test in Tumbling and Apparatus for Male Physical Education Majors at the University of North Dakota, M.S. in Ed., University of North Dakota, Grand Forks, 1966.
18. Hodges, Carolyn V.: Construction of an Objective Knowledge Test and Skills Tests in Lacrosse for College Women, MSPE, University of North Carolina at Greensboro, 1967.
19. Hulbert, Bonita A.: A Study of Tests for the Forehand Drive in Tennis, MSPE, University of Wisconsin, Madison, 1966.

20. Jacobson, Theodore Vernon: An Evaluation of Performance in Certain Physical Ability Tests Administered to Selected Secondary School Boys, Unpublished Master's Thesis, University of Washington, Seattle, 1960.
21. Johnson, Joseph Robert: The Development of a Single-Item Test as a Measure of Soccer Skill. M.P.E., University of British Columbia, Vancouver, British Columbia, Canada, 1963.
22. Johnson, L. W.: Objective Basketball Test for High School Boys, Unpublished Master's Thesis, State University of Iowa, Iowa City, 1934.
23. Kronqvist, Roger A. and Wayne B. Brumbach: A Modification of the Brady Volleyball Skill Test for High School Boys, Research Quarterly, *39*, 116–120, March, 1968.
24. Laveaga, R. C.: *Volleyball*, 2nd Ed., New York: Ronald Press Co., 1960.
25. Leilich, Avis: The Primary Components of Selected Basketball Tests for College Women, Unpublished doctoral dissertation, Indiana University, Bloomington, 1952.
26. Lockhart, Aileene, and Frances A. McPherson: Development of a Test of Badminton Playing Ability, Research Quarterly, *20*, 402–405, December, 1949.
27. Lucey, Mildred A.: A Study of the Components of Wrist Action as They Relate to Speed of Learning and the Degree of Proficiency Attained in Badminton, Ph.D., New York University, 1952.
28. McDonald, Lloyd G.: The Construction of a Kicking Skill Test as an Index of General Soccer Ability, Master's Thesis, Springfield College, Springfield, Massachusetts, 1951.
29. Miller, Frances A.: A Badminton Wall Volley Test, Research Quarterly, *22*, 208–213, May, 1951.
30. Miller, Susan Elizabeth: The Relative Effectiveness of High School Badminton Instruction when Given in Two Short Units and One Continuous Unit Involving the Same Total Time, Master's Thesis, University of Washington, Seattle, 1964.
31. Miller, Wilma K.: Achievement Levels in Basketball Skills for Women Physical Education Majors, Research Quarterly, *25*, 450–455, December, 1954.
32. Mitchell, J. Reid: The Modification of the McDonald Soccer Skill Test for Upper Elementary School Boys, M. S., University of Oregon, Eugene, 1963.
33. Mott, Jane A., and Aileene Lockhart: Table Tennis Backboard Test, Journal of Health and Physical Education, *17*, 550–552, November, 1946.
34. Pennington, G. Gary, James A. P. Day, John N. Drowatzky, and John F. Hansan: A Measure of Handball Ability, Research Quarterly, *38*, 247–253, May, 1967.
35. Petry, Kathryn: Evaluation of a Volleyball Serve Test, MAPE, Los Angeles State College, Los Angeles, California, 1967.
36. Pimpa, Udom: A Study to Determine the Relationship Between Bunn's Basketball Skill Test and the Writer's Modified Version of that Test, MSPE, Springfield College, Springfield, Massachusetts, 1968.
37. Reece, Patsy Ann: A Comparison of the Scores Made on an Outdoor and the Scores Made on an Indoor Golf Test for College Women, M.S., University of Colorado, Boulder, 1960.
38. Rosentswieg, Joel: A Revision of the Power Swimming Test, Research Quarterly, *39*, 818–819, October, 1968.
39. Schmithals, Margaret, and Esther French: Achievement Tests in Field Hockey for College Women, Research Quarterly, *11*, 84–92, October, 1940.
40. Scott, M. Gladys, Aileen Carpenter, Esther French, and Louise Kuhl: Achievement Examinations in Badminton, Research Quarterly, *12*, 242–253, May, 1941.
41. Scott, M. Gladys, and Esther French: *Measurement and Evaluation in Physical Physical Education*. Dubuque, Iowa: Wm. C. Brown Publishers, 1959.
42. Sickels, William Loyd: A Rating Test for Amateur Wrestling Ability, MSPE, San Jose State College, San Jose, California, 1967.
43. Smith, Gwen: Speedball Skill Tests for College Women, Unpublished study, Illinois State University, Normal, 1957.
44. Strait, C. Jane: The Construction and Evaluation of a Field Hockey Skills Test, Unpublished Master's Thesis, Smith College, Northampton, Mass., 1960.
45. Vanderhoof, Ellen R.: Beginning Golf Achievement Tests, Unpublished Master's Thesis, State University of Iowa, Iowa City, 1956.

46. Wallrof, Paul J.: Methods for Rating Defensive Proficiency of High School Football Players, MSPE, University of Washington, Seattle, 1965.
47. Walter, Ronald J.: A Comparison Between Two Selected Evaluative Techniques for Measuring Basketball Skills, MS in Ed., Western Illinois University, Macomb, 1968.
48. Warner, Glenn F. H.: Warner Soccer Test, Newsletter of the National Soccer Coaches Association of America, *6*, 13–22, December, 1950.

Chapter 10
OTHER PSYCHOMOTOR TESTS

Meredith Physical Growth Record*

Purpose. To provide interesting and helpful information regarding the status and progress of physical growth for boys and girls.

Evaluation. The four charts are the result of computation of average weight and height of various age levels of large numbers of boys and girls.

Level and Sex. For boys and girls age 4 through 18 years of age.

Time Allotment and Number of Subjects. Since the only data required for applying the Physical Growth Chart are age, weight, and height, these factors can be obtained from any size group at any time. One instructor making height and weight measurements can handle as many as 75 students in one 45-minute period. If more than one station is set up for both height and weight measurements, the time for administration can be materially reduced.

Floor Plan and Space Requirements. Since students are weighed and measured for height with their clothes on, measuring stations may be set up at any convenient place either in the locker room, or in the gymnasium or classroom.

Class Organization. The most practical method of class organization is the squad method. While one squad is being measured, the others can carry on their regular class program.

General Procedures

1. If a standard set of beam-type platform scales with measuring rod is available, both height and weight may be obtained at the same time.

2. Scales should be checked for balance and adjusted before each examination period.

3. The students should remove shoes and sweaters or coats before measurement is taken.

4. For height measurement the student should stand straight and tall, his heels should be in contact with the floor and almost together but not quite touching, his arms should hang naturally at his side, and his head should face straight forward.

5. When girls are measured for height, the instructor should see that there are no obstructions to prevent contact with the top of the head such as combs, braids, etc.

* National Education Association and American Medical Association, Physical Growth Records for Boys and Physical Growth Records for Girls, using data prepared by Howard V. Meredith, State University of Iowa. Adapted by permission of the Joint Committee on Health Problems in Education of the National Education Association and the American Medical Association. (Information and charts may be obtained from the AMA, 535 N. Dearborn St., Chicago, Illinois or the NEA, 1201 Sixteenth St., N.W., Washington, D.C.)

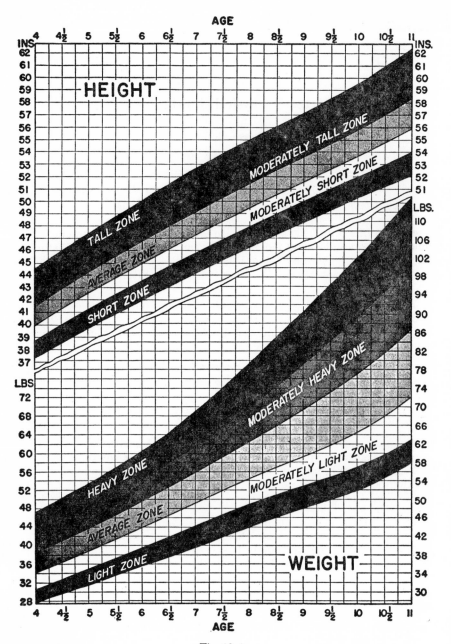

Fig. 10-1.

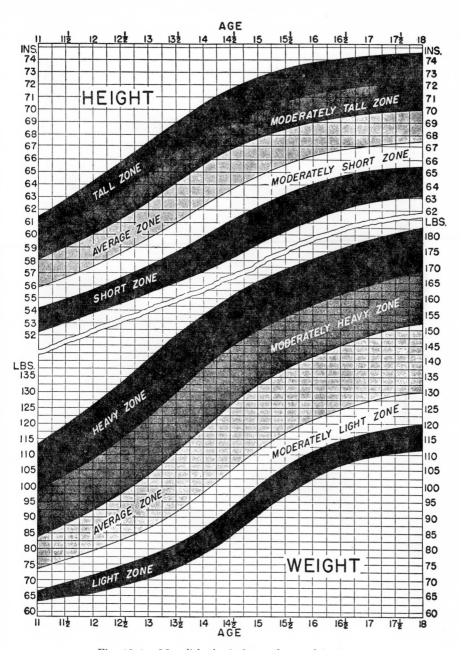

Fig. 10–1. Meredith physical growth record for boys.

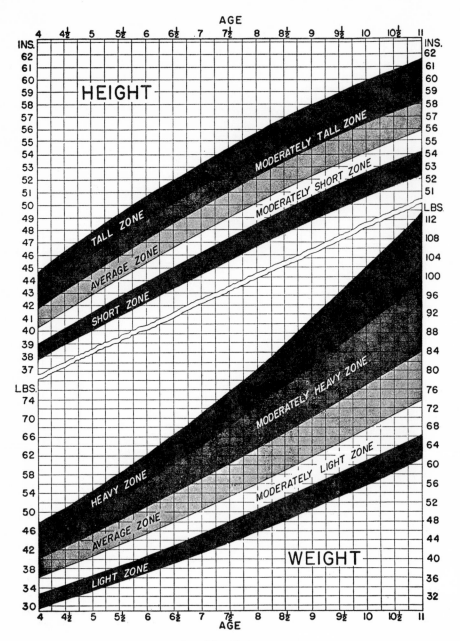

Fig. 10–2.

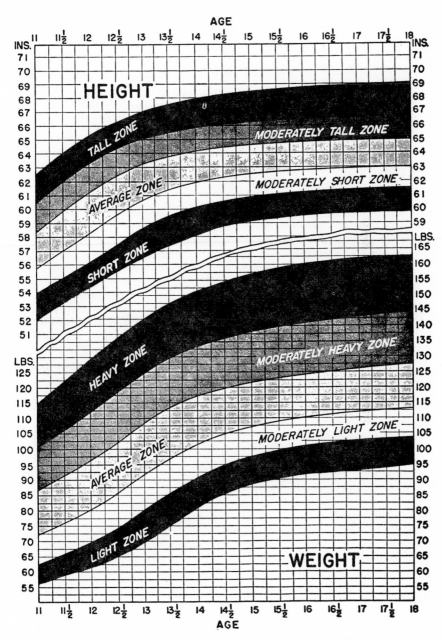

Fig. 10–2.   Meredith physical growth records for girls.

6. Two separate measurements should be taken on each student.

7. Weight should be determined to the nearest one-half pound and height to the nearest one-fourth inch.

8. If no measuring rod is available, the next most expedient method is to take the measurement with the student's back against a smooth wall. A measuring tape may be fastened in place directly on the wall. A wood headpiece with two faces at right angles is used to obtain the exact height measurement. One face of the makeshift headpiece is placed against the wall and the other is brought down on top of the student's head. The height measurement is read from the intersection of this gadget and the tape measure.

Uses. If height and weight measurements do not fall in corresponding zones or if successive measurements result in a jump from one zone to another, the discrepancy may be regarded as an indication of poor health and referral should be made to a physician.

Test Description. The Physical Growth Records are charts for interpreting the height and weight of boys and girls age 4 to 18. There is a separate chart for each sex. Each has five weight-age channels or zones and five height-age. The weight-age zones are at the bottom of the chart and the channels are indicated in various shades to distinguish them from each other. They are listed as light, moderately light, average, moderately heavy, and heavy. The height-age zones are near the top and the channels are listed as short, moderately short, average, moderately tall, and tall. Height and weight horizontal lines run across the width of the charts. Age is indicated by vertical lines with each line representing 3 months of advancement. See Figure 10–1 for boys and Figure 10–2 for girls.

Directions for Use. 1. Height and weight measurements are obtained as recommended.

2. To plot height for each student, first locate his age along the top of the chart. Next locate his height in inches along the upper left hand margin. If these two lines are followed, it will be found that they intersect at some point within one of the five height zones. At this point a dot should be placed and the height written in above it.

3. To plot weight for each student, first locate his age along the bottom of the chart. Then locate his weight in pounds along the lower left hand margin. Where the age and weight lines intersect, a dot is placed and the weight measurements written in. This point will fall within one of the five weight zones.

4. To plot progress for height and weight, successive measurements are made at different times for the various ages of the same individual, thus making a succession of dots. These dots may be connected by drawing lines between them and forming a curve of progress.

Interpretation

1. Interpreting Status
   a. The measurement figures written by each plotted dot provide a description of each student's actual height and weight at the various ages which measurements have been made.
   b. The channel in which the student's height and weight dots for a particular age are located indicates that student's standing in relation to others of the same age.

    c. Whenever a student's height and weight dots do not fall in similar
zones (for example, tall-heavy, moderately tall-moderately heavy,
average-average, moderately short-moderately light, and short-light),
the lack of similarity may be indicative of stockiness or slenderness
and/or it may indicate some health failure. Such dissimilarity calls
for referral to proper medical authorities.
2. Interpreting Progress
    a. The difference between a student's height (or weight) at different
ages indicates the amount of change that has occurred between
measurements.
    b. The relation of a student's height and weight curve to the curve on
the respective charts indicates whether or not he is growing satisfactorily. A normally growing student's curve for height should run
parallel with his height zone on the chart. If, however, the student's
height curve falls off toward a lower zone, his growth warrants
medical investigation.
    c. Although weight growth is frequently less regular than height, if the
student's weight curve shows a downward dip or remains level, he
has lost weight in the first instance and has failed to gain in the second.
In either event he should be referred to a physician. Allowance must
be made, however, in the case of older students for individual differences in the time at which the adolescent "spurt" occurs. This
"spurt" will vary and as long as the student is continuing steady
growth at his childhood rate, his growth should not be judged
"unsatisfactory." This "spurt" may occur as early as 9 years in
girls and 11 in boys but will probably be two or three years later in
the average.

The Wetzel Grid*

Purpose. To measure the physical growth and development of boys and
girls throughout school life.

Evaluation. The earliest applications of the Wetzel Grid were made
during the depression of 1937. Even in those first studies there was 94
per cent agreement when Wetzel Grid results were compared with physicians' estimates of disturbances in growth and nutrition over a population
sample of some 2,000 Ohio children ranging from kindergarten to senior
high school pupils. The Grid, however, has also been based on long-term
data accumulated during the past 25 years on about $4\frac{1}{2}$ million children
from all parts of the world.

Level and Sex. Two different Grids are in use: the Baby Grid is employed
for young infants (both boys and girls) from birth to three years of age.
Apart from its value as a record of pre-school growth, the Baby Grid has no
immediate application in the school program. The second form is sometimes known as the "Big" or "regular" Grid and it is this form to which
the following description applies. It can be used for both sexes, ages 5 to 18.

---

* Wetzel, Norman C.: Grid for Evaluating Fitness. NEA Services, Cleveland, Ohio,
1948. Adapted by permission of the author and the NEA Services. (Further information and grid records may be obtained from the NEA Services, Inc., 1200 W. 3rd St.,
Cleveland, Ohio.)

Time Allotment and Number of Subjects. The only data required to use the Wetzel Grid for judging the growth and physical condition of school children are Age, Weight, and Height. Any convenient number of children can be "gridded" at any time. One instructor taking weight and height measurements can usually handle 75 students in one 45-minute period, and, with the help of an assistant, can also complete plotting the results with little or no extra time. If more than one set of scales (equipped with measuring rods) are available, several stations should be used so that measurement time can be reduced to a minimum. If both sexes are to be measured at the same time, the students may dress in their gym uniforms or even in street clothing. Choice of clothing and measuring technique must be consistent throughout successive measurement periods. For elementary age children, the most expedient place to take measurements is the class room. Measurements without clothing can be made in available locker room space. The most efficient method of class organization is to divide the class into "squads." While one squad is being measured, the others can carry on regular class-work.

General Procedure. 1. A separate Grid should be employed for every student in order to assure that the full power of the Grid is completely utilized to display each child's individual growth characteristics.

2. Maximum value of the Grid will be obtained when it is made a part of the official cumulative school record.

3. As indicated above, any preferred routine for measuring weight and height may be employed so long as this is consistently done.

4. In practice, annual or semi-annual measurements will suffice. Less frequent measurements are to be avoided. On the other hand, *more* frequent measurements are indicated when Grid trends indicate deviation from the normal pattern.

5. A medical examination form, suitable as a permanent school health record, appears on the reverse side of each Grid.

Uses. The Wetzel Grid has many uses:

1. Perhaps its most valuable use is the early detection of abnormal trends in physical growth and development. One example of an abnormal trend is that seen when a child is becoming more obese. Another even more common example is the typical Grid picture formed by the curves of on-coming malnutrition which clearly reveal loss of physique, *i.e.*, with a trend toward a more slender body build and a *slowdown* in the rate of advance.

2. Since sub-standard progress is readily evident in a Grid record, students may be screened out and given further examination.

3. Grid ratings may be used as "classifiers" and have been utilized as criteria for separating students into homogeneous groups for competition in sports and games.

4. Parents, teachers, as well as students, readily learn what various points or positions and trends on a Grid signify since it furnishes a graphic picture of body build and body size and changes therein. As a result, they will easily distinguish "good" from "poor" records and both of these from what is ordinarily regarded as "normal" status and progress.

5. One of the important uses of the Grid is that it measures and identifies a student's individual body type or build. A reliable estimate and indication of body build is obtained when a child's height and weight are plotted in the Grid channel system since each of the seven main channels represents a quite familiar body type ranging from stocky at the left through medium

at the center to linear and extreme slender types at the right. Incidentally, it will be noted that physique is independent of age, contrary to implications of various other methods.

6. The total Grid record with its several results is especially well adapted for counseling and child guidance since parents, teachers, nurses, health and physical education personnel all have the advantage of gaining a common understanding of a given problem from the visual Grid trends.

7. Grid records provide an objective basis for prognosis. In addition to summarizing progress to date, established Grid trends give a dependable indication of what kind of physical and growth progress may be expected to follow under similar conditions of home and school life.

Test Description. The Wetzel Grid is a three-color precision chart shown in Figure 10–3. The Grid consists of three panels:

1. *Grid Panel.* This field is marked by a vertical weight scale graduated both in pounds (shown on the outside of the scale) and in kilograms (on the inside) and by horizontal height scales (top and bottom) graduated in centimeters and inches. The distinctive feature of this panel is a set of 9 adjacent, parallel physique channels running obliquely from SW to NE. A set of short parallel lines cross the channels (NW to SE) at regular intervals to give the panel a football gridiron effect. Hence, the name Grid. The short parallels, numbered 0, 10, 20, ... 180, with half-way distances between them indicated by dashed parallels, are known as *isodevelopmental level lines.* The individual channels, representing different body types, are designated as follows: A_4 at the extreme left represents the potentially obese type; A_3 and A_2 are the channels typical of the familar stocky athletic, and more particularly, football builds. In the center are the channels for those of medium build, A_1, M, and B_1. Beyond these are channels B_2, B_3, where children of extreme linear or slender form are found. The *purpose of the channels* is to afford a ready means of measuring and identifying a child's body physique (type); the *purpose of the isodevelopmental level lines,* however, is to measure the *body size.* Increase in size occurs as a child moves from one level to the next. This one-level distance is normally accomplished in one month's time. Hence, according to the Grid standards, all children, no matter of which body shape or size, and regardless of race or sex, should proceed up-channel one level per month on the average. Failure to do this is cause for investigation. As previously mentioned, observations at 6-month intervals to test whether a child has gained 6 levels during that interval are quite practical and valuable.

2. *Auxodrome Panel.* To the right of center is the Auxodrome Panel through which 5 standard age schedules of development are seen to run in a NE direction. The solid curves are advanced, average and late schedules for boys; the dashed branches represent the corresponding girls' standards of level for age. These standards range from the highly advanced 2 per cent to the highly retarded 98 per cent Auxodrome. The purpose of these Auxodromes is to provide a nearby standard of comparison according to which a child's own Auxodrome, when plotted in terms of attained level and chronological age, may be judged from two standpoints: first, in terms of the *speed* of growth, that is, the increment between any two successive observations (which should closely approximate one level per month) and secondly, to permit a child to be classified—*relative to the general population* —as "advanced," "average" or "retarded." The co-ordinates in this panel are *level* (vertical scale) and *age* (horizontal axis) in years. A child's own Auxodrome is thus produced when successively attained levels—as

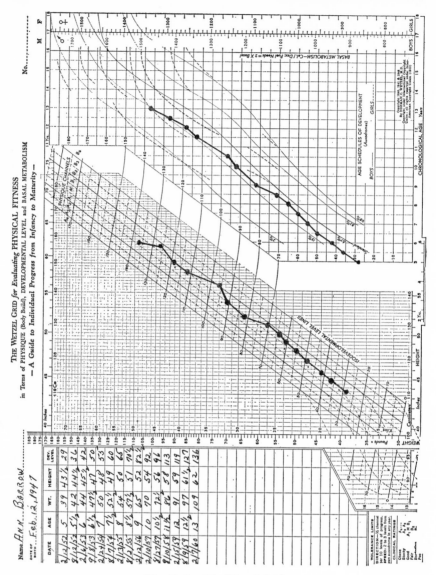

Fig. 10-3. The Wetzel Grid.

listed in column 5 of the tabular entry form at the extreme left—are plotted against corresponding ages. Percentile graduation of these Auxodromic standards has the usual significance, namely, that 2 per cent of children, for instance, will be found on or ahead of this upper standard; that about 15 per cent of all boys and girls will be on or ahead of the second highest Auxodrome and, finally, that only about 2 per cent of children will be found below the 98 per cent Auxodrome. The 67 per cent standard, it may be noted, is taken as the demarcation curve separating "advanced" from comparatively "retarded" children. In brief, the unique advantage of the

Auxodrome panel and its standards is that estimates of growth "speed" in *levels per month* can be readily and directly made independently of any influence such as age, sex, physique, or body size.

3. *Metabolism Panel.* This panel is used less frequently than the other two. It deals with basal heat production caloric requirement per day and the growth and activity total requirement of calories daily.

Directions for Use. 1. Height and weight measurements, along with the corresponding date and age, should be entered in the appropriate column of the data table on the left side of each Grid for each examination.

2. Weight should be plotted as read from the vertical weight scale at the left, against the child's height as read from either the lower or the upper horizontal height scale. Weight and height may be measured in either metric or avoirdupois units. A nurse, teacher, counselor, or even a student can be trained to plot out Grid records. The intersection of the weight and height lines will make the point at which a given height and weight should be plotted and this point, in all but exceptional cases, will be found to lie within the channel system. In fact, it should lie within one of the 9 individual physique channels and will indicate the child's body build (physique). On occasion a point will fall exactly on a channel border, *e.g.*, A_1 A_2, or again, on the B_3 B_4 boundary. Each plotted point will also fall on a Grid level, *e.g.*, level 139 or, again, on level 52 which represents and measures body size.

3. The child's level should be read from the diagonal scale along the left hand border of the channel system and recorded in column 5 of the data table. Then, each level value should be plotted (in the Auxodrome panel) against the corresponding age, utilizing the vertical level scale and the horizontal age scale to do so. Successive points in the Auxodrome panel, connected as before by line segments, produce the child's own Auxodrome. Interpretation of the Auxodrome has been described in paragraph 2 under *Test Description.*

4. It is advisable to repeat steps 1, 2, and 3 at least twice a year for ordinary routine follow-up. Unsatisfactory Grid trends, however, call for more frequent checkups, perhaps quarterly or even as often as monthly in some cases. Successive points should be connected with line segments. Best results are obtained, however, when the segments do not touch the points, but rather leave a bit of white space surrounding the plotted observation.

General Remarks. Interpretation of Grid record from the standpoint of routine school work is quite simple and may be undertaken by school personnel for certain purposes without presuming to encroach upon medical or health responsibilities. What should be kept in mind is that physical growth, although it is a natural process, cannot be counted upon under the stresses of life to proceed at all times in a thoroughly acceptable fashion. Actually, student growth consists of two kinds, good growth and poor growth. It is highly unlikely that any youngster ever proceeds from kindergarten through college without at least some minor growth disturbance. The danger is that too many so-called minor disturbances ultimately become aggravated and amplified into unacceptable growth quality. The fundamental purpose of the Grid is to aid the teacher, nurse, or parent in detecting as early as possible those mild deviations from a normal pattern which, when unattended, result in growth failure. Fundamental to success in education is the development of a sound body and this cannot be accomplished when growth proceeds in an unacceptable manner. In fact, a child who does not have the strength to develop his physique as nature calls for, cannot, under any hypothesis, be expected to achieve his full educational capacity.

With these simple tenets in mind it is readily understood why systematic, periodic follow-up on child growth should be routinely insisted upon. It is necessary in modern education if for no other reason than to avoid those inevitable losses that are incurred when under-par children attempt to match the academic achievement of their physically healthy and up-to-par classmates. The signs of early, simple growth failure are few and are often found when looked for in routine growth trends as revealed by the Grid. Deviation to the extent of one-half channel per 10 levels of advancement, if continued, will eventually result in undesirable loss of physique. During such periods it is quite common that the rate of gain is reduced below the normal of 12 levels per year; many such youngsters, in fact, slow down to the point of gaining no more than a half level per month. A second, and at present, an enlarging group of children are manifesting the signs of obesity, namely, an exceedingly high slope toward A_4, and beyond, which is usually accompanied by an undesirably high rate of developmental advance; speed of growth in such instances may increase to $1\frac{1}{2}$ and even 2 levels per month.

On the other hand, children who remain in their established channels faithfully and who also average 12 levels per year can be considered to be without serious growth disturbance no matter which channel they are in. Similar remarks apply to the need for adhering to a given age schedule or Auxodrome from which they should not deviate by more than about 2 levels per year and even such a deficit should be made up as soon as possible in order to assure that each individual child can attain his full upper growth capacity before puberty may have prematurely closed the door. The value of the Grid from this standpoint, not only to physical education particularly, but also to the entire school curriculum in general, is obvious.

Iowa Posture Test*

Purpose. To measure posture in a sitting, walking, standing, and exercising position.

Evaluation. No validities are available.

Level and Sex. This instrument was originally devised to measure the posture of girls at the college level. However, like most posture tests, it can be adapted to any age and sex level, grade one through college.

Time Allotment and Number of Subjects. Since each student must be observed and rated in a number of positions for a number of situations, it would require one entire period for a class of from 20 to 25.

Floor Plan and Space Requirement. An area on the floor large enough to place 10 or 12 chairs which are set two feet apart with sufficient room in front of this row of chairs for an examiner's station and an area for the student to walk and perform. Figure 10–4 shows a suggested floor plan for administration of all test parts.

---

* Courtesy of Scott, M. Gladys and Esther French: *Measurement and Evaluation in Physical Education*, William C. Brown Company Publishers, Dubuque, 1959 and Frost, Loraine, *Posture and Body Mechanics*, University of Iowa Extension Bulletin, State University of Iowa, Iowa City, 1944.

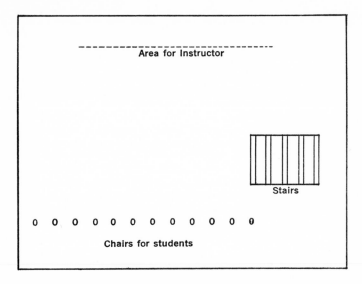

Fig. 10–4. Floor plan for Iowa posture test.

Class Organization. The best method of class organization is the squad method. The squad members should be seated in the chairs in the same order that names appear on the score sheet shown in Figure 10–5.

General Procedure. 1. Ratings can be made more satisfactorily if students are dressed in bathing suits or leotards.

2. Students should be barefooted.

3. Orientation may be given to each squad just prior to testing, or to the entire class a day or two before testing is begun.

4. No more than 10 or 12 students should be tested at one time.

5. The criteria of good standing posture applies equally well to posture during most movements.

Uses. This test is entirely too subjective to be used as a grading device where accurate measurements are necessary for postural deviations. However, by using acceptable criteria of various body segments and by making ratings while the student is carrying on some of his normal daily activities, the ratings can be used as an excellent motivating device. The student's knowledge of posture can be increased and his attitude toward maintenance of good habits and correction of faults can be improved.

Test Description

ITEM NUMBER I—FOOT MECHANICS

Purpose: To check the pronation and direction of the foot.

Facilities and Equipment: Score sheet for each squad. See floor plan for test arrangement.

Procedure: Examiner stands several feet to the side of the row of chairs where the students are sitting. Each student walks out to the instructor and back to his chair as the instructor observes for pronation and foot alignment. *CRITERIA USED:* (1) the heel cord in the rear should be straight and not turned in at the ankle level; (2) the feet should be parallel with no toeing out; (3) there should be no bulge or marked prominence of the inner ankle bone.

Instructions: Rise from your chair, walk naturally toward the examiner, turn, walk back to your seat and be seated.

Scoring: The following scores are given: No pronation –3; some pronation –2; marked pronation –1.   Normal toeing out –3; moderate toeing out –2; and marked toeing out –1.

Testing Personnel: Ratings should be made by the physical education instructor or some other trained examiner.

ITEM NUMBER II—STANDING

Purpose: To evaluate alignment of body segments in a standing position.

Procedure: The students stand at the side of their chairs as the examiner observes body alignment and records scores as he moves down the row of chairs.   *CRITERIA USED:* The head, neck, trunk and legs should be situated one above the other in a straight line with the head and neck erect, the chest up, lower abdomen flat, and the entire body at ease and balanced.   The three curves in the spine should be normal, which means a moderate amount of curve.

Instructions: Rise and stand beside your chair in a balanced, natural position.

Scoring: Correct alignment—3; slightly general deviation or moderate deviation of one part—2; marked general deviation—1.

ITEM NUMBER III—WALKING

Purpose: To measure alignment and the smoothness of action of the body segments in a walking position.

Procedure: Half of the students who are sitting should be examined at one time.   They can rise and walk around the chairs two or three times while the examiner observes and records results.   *CRITERIA USED:* The same as for standing posture.   The important thing is to observe if there has been any change from the standing position.

Instructions: Rise and walk around the row of chairs keeping 5 or 6 feet between you and the person just ahead.

Scoring: Same as for the standing position.

ITEM NUMBER IV—SITTING

Purpose: To measure the posture mechanics of sitting, rising, and being seated in a chair.

Procedure: Each student is examined in turn in a sitting position first, then as he rises from the chair, and again as he sits down. *CRITERIA USED:* Sitting position—head erect, chest high, shoulders back, abdomen flat with the spine curves moderately curved. The upper trunk is balanced over the hips and the hips should be well back in the chair. *Rising and being seated*—one foot should be slightly under the chair and the other out, hips under the body with the body slightly bent, the arms relaxed and the body without stiffness.

Instructions: You are to sit easily and relaxed in your chair until told to arise. You then walk forward for six or seven steps, turn around, walk back to your chair, and be seated.

Scoring: For each of three categories the scoring is as follows: correct position—3; some degree of deviation—2; marked deviation—1.

ITEM NUMBER V—STOOPING

Purpose: To measure the mechanics of posture while the body is in a stooping position.

Procedure: The students in turn walk to a specific point, stoop, pick up an object from the floor and walk to another point and place it on the floor again. *CRITERIA USED:* One foot should be slightly ahead of the other, feet and hips under the body, knees bent and some bend at the hips with a slight rounding of the back. The arms should be relaxed and there should be a smooth, balanced movement of the entire body.

Instructions: You are to walk easily toward the object on the floor. Stop when it is slightly ahead and outside your front foot. Stoop and pick up the object. Walk forward six steps and replace the object on the floor.

Scoring: Good position—3; Fair position—2; Poor position—1.

ITEM NUMBER VI—WALKING UP AND DOWN STAIRS

Purpose: To measure the mechanics of posture in movement on the stairs.

Facilities and Equipment: A specially designed stairs should be constructed with 8 to 10 steps on each side so the students may pass up and down the steps in a continuous line.

Procedure: The students are observed and rated as they ascend and descend the stairs. *CRITERIA USED:* In *ascending* the same criteria as described in standing and walking are true for the various body segments. The body weight should be slightly forward and from the ankles. There should be no sideward sway of the hips. In *descending* the same criteria apply and there should be a controlled lowering of the weight to the front foot and there should be no bobbing.

Instructions: You are to walk up the flight of steps on one side and down the other. Do not hurry, but try to walk in a relaxed manner.

Scoring: Ascending   Good—3; Fair—2; Poor—1
         Descending Good—3; Fair—2; Poor—1

Score Card

Name	Foot Mechanics		Standing	Walking	Sitting		Stooping	Stairs		Total Score*
	Absence of Pronation	Toe Str. Ahead	Alignment	Alignment, Smoothness	Natural Position	Rising, Being Seated		Up	Down	

Scoring: 3—good   2—fair   1—poor

* A total of 27 points would be perfect. Score, however, cannot be considered as entirely significant. Weighting of separate items was attempted, but abandoned due to the wide variety of opinion on the part of experts.

Fig. 10-5.   Score sheet for Iowa posture test.

New York State Posture Test

One of the most recently devised posture tests and perhaps one of the simplest to administer is the New York State Posture Test. This test is described in detail in Chapter 8, page 229 as a part of the New York State Physical Fitness Test. The Posture Rating Chart is shown in Figure 8–10 and the testing station and the method of using it are shown in Figure 8–9. This method is a simple inspection-type measurement with the subjective approach but objectified by means of the pictured standards shown on the rating chart. Posture is observed as shown in Figure 8–9 and, with the aid of the Posture Rating Chart shown in Figure 8–10, posture ratings are made. The rater compares the student being rated with the 13 drawings on the posture chart representing the various segments of the body. Each of the body segments is scored as 1—3— or 5 with a possible range of 13 to 65 in total score. These scores are converted to percentile ranks and finally to Achievement Levels.

Sensory Motor Awareness Survey*

Purpose. To appraise perceptual-motor awareness.

Evaluation. No validities have been furnished.

Level and Sex. Boys and girls age 4 and 5. It may be adapted for older age groups.

Time Allotment and Number of Subjects. For a class of 25 to 30 students two testing periods of at least 45 minutes would be necessary.

Floor Plan and Space Requirements. A small gym or even a playroom would provide sufficient space.

Class Organization. Testing must be administered on an individual basis.

General Procedures. Since testing is on an individual basis and done by the instructor for all children to insure greater reliability, an assistant is needed to keep order and facilitate administration.

Uses. While no norms have been established to date, the results can be used to identify those with perceptual motor problems.

Test Description and Score Card

SENSORY MOTOR AWARENESS SURVEY FOR 4 AND 5 YEAR OLDS

Date of Test_____

Name_____ Sex_____ Birth_____ Center_____

Body Image. $\frac{1}{2}$ point for each correct part; 9 points possible.

_____ 1. Ask the child to touch the following body parts:

head _____	ankles _____	ears _____	stomach _____
toes _____	nose _____	legs _____	chin _____
eyes _____	feet _____	mouth _____	waist _____
wrists _____	chest _____	fingers _____	shoulders _____
back _____	elbows _____		

---

* Braley, William T.: Sensorimotor Skills Program. Dayton, Ohio, Early Childhood Education Program, Dayton Public Schools, 1970. Used by permission of William T. Braley.

Space and Directions. $\frac{1}{2}$ point for each correct direction; 5 points possible.

_____ 2. Ask the child to point to the following directions:

front___   back___   up___   down___   beside you___

Place two blocks on a table about one inch apart. Ask the child to point:

under___   over___   to the top___   to the bottom___ between___

Balance. Score 2 points if accomplished.

_____ 3. Have the child stand on tiptoes, on both feet, with eyes open for eight seconds.

Balance and Laterality. Score 2 points for each foot; 4 points possible.

_____ 4. Have the child stand on one foot, eyes closed, for 5 seconds. Alternate feet.

Laterality. Score 2 points if the child keeps his feet together and does not lead off with one foot.

_____ 5. Have the child jump forward on two feet.

Rhythm and Neuromuscular Control. Score 2 points for each foot if accomplished six times; 4 points possible.

_____ 6. Have the child hop on one foot. Hop in place.

Rhythm and Neuromuscular control. Score 2 points.

_____ 7. Have the child skip forward. Child must be able to sustain this motion around the room or for approximately 30 feet.

Integregation of Right and Left Sides of the Body. Score 2 points if cross patterning is evident, for each.

_____ 8. Have the child creep forward.

_____ 9. Have the child creep backwards.

Eye-Foot Coordination. Score 2 points if done the length of tape or mark.

_____ 10. Use an eight-foot tape or chalk mark on the floor. The child walks in a cross-over step the length of the tape or mark.

Fine Muscle Control. Score 2 points if paper is completely crumpled.
Score 1 point if paper is partially cumpled.
Score 0 points if child needs assistance or changes hands.

_____ 11. Using a half sheet of newspaper, the child picks up the paper with one hand and puts the other hand behind his back. He then attempts to crumple the paper in his hand. He may not use his other hand, the table, or his body for assistance.

Form Perception. Score 1 point for each correct match.

_____ 12. Using a piece of paper with 2-inch circles, squares and triangles, ask the child to point to two objects that are the same.

Form Perception. Score 1 point if circle is identified correctly.
Score 2 points if the triangle and square are identified correctly.

_____ 13. Ask the child to identify by saying, "Point to the circle."
_____   "Point to the square."
_____   "Point to the triangle."

Hearing Discrimination. Score 1 point if the child taps correctly each time.

_____ 14. Ask the child to turn his back to you. Tap the table with a stick three times. Ask the child to turn around and tap the stick the same way.

_____ Ask the child to turn his back to you. Tap the table again with the stick (two quick taps, pause, then two more quick taps). Have the child turn back to you and tap out the rhythm.

Eye-Hand Coordination. Score one point for each successful completion.

_____ 15. A board is used with three holes in it. The holes are $\frac{3}{4}$, $\frac{5}{8}$, and $\frac{1}{2}$ inches in diameter. The child is asked to put his finger through the holes without touching the sides.

References

1. Braley, William T.: Sensorimotor Skills Program: Dayton, Ohio. Unpublished Research Study, Dayton Public Schools, 1970.
2. Frost, Loraine: Posture and Body Mechanics. University of Iowa Extension Bulletin, Iowa City, State University of Iowa, 1955.
3. Meredith, Howard V.: Interpreting Growth: Ways to Use Height and Weight Measures of School Children, Saskatchewan Recreation, Fall, 1947. (Further information and charts may be obtained from the American Medical Association, 535 N. Dearborn Street, Chicago, Illinois, and National Education Association, 1201 Sixteenth Street, N.W., Washington 6, D.C.)
4. Meredith, Howard V.: A Physical Growth Record for Use in Elementary and High Schools, American Journal of Public Health, *39*, 378–385, July, 1949.
5. National Education Association and American Medical Association, Physical Growth Records for Boys and Physical Growth Records for Girls. Joint Committee on Health Problems in Education of the National Education Association and the American Medical Association, using data prepared by Howard V. Meredith, State University of Iowa.
6. Scott, M. Gladys, and Esther French: *Measurement and Evaluation in Physical Education.* Dubuque, Iowa: Wm. C. Brown Co. Publishers, 1959, pp. 227–229.
7. State of New York, The New York State Physical Fitness Test: A Manual for Teachers of Physical Education. Albany, Division of Health, Physical Education, and Recreation, New York State Education Department, 1958.
8. Wetzel, Norman C.: The Treatment of Growth Failure in Children. Cleveland, NEA Services, Inc., 1948. (Further information and grid records may be obtained from NEA Services, Inc., 1200 West Third Street, Cleveland 13, Ohio.)
9. Wetzel, Norman C.: The Simultaneous Screening and Assessment of School Children, Journal of Health, Physical Education, and Recreation, *13*, 200–205, December, 1942.
10. Wetzel, Norman C.: Grid for Evaluating Physical Fitness. NEA Services, Cleveland, Ohio, 1948.

Additional References

1. Bancroft, Jessie H.: *The Posture of School Children.* New York, The Macmillan Co., 1913, pp. 197–203.
2. Barrow, H. M., Marjorie Crisp, and J. W. Long: *Physical Education Syllabus,* 3rd Ed., Minneapolis, Burgess Publishing Co., 1961, (Appendix).
3. Billig, H. E., and Evelyn Loewendahl: A Dynamic Concept of Posture Screening at the Elementary Level, The Physical Educator, *11*, 9–10, March, 1954.
4. Blesh, T. E., C. R. Meyers, and O. W. Kiphuth: Photometric Photography in Posture Evaluation of Yale University Freshmen. New Haven, Yale University Clerical Bureau, 1954.
5. Brownell, C. L.: A Scale for Measuring the Anterior-posterior Posture of Ninth Grade Boys. Teachers College Contribution to Education, No. 325, New York; Bureau of Publications, Teachers College, Columbia University, 1928.

6. Franzen, Raymond, and George Palmer: The ACH Index of Nutritional Status. New York, American Child Health Association, 1934.
7. Fishman, H. R.: One-minute Posture Picture, Journal of Health, Physical Education, and Recreation, *29*, 72, January, 1958.
8. Klein, Armin, and Leah C. Thomas: Posture Exercises. Washington, D.C., U. S. Department of Labor, Children's Bureau, Publication No. 165, United States Government Printing Office, 33 pp. 1937.
9. Kraus, Hans, and W. Weber: Evaluation of Posture Based on Structural and Functional Measurements, Physiotherapy Review, *25*, 267, November-December, 1945.
10. Lowman, C. L., and C. H. Young: *Postural Fitness*, Philadelphia, Lea & Febiger, 1960.
11. MacEwan, C. G., and E. C. Howe: An Objective Method of Grading Posture, Research Quarterly, *3*, 144–147, October, 1932.
12. Manley, Helen: Good Posture for Boys and Girls, The Physical Educator, *6*, 14, May, 1949.
13. Massey, W. W.: A Critical Study of Objective Methods for Measuring Anterior-Posterior Posture with a Simplified Technique, Research Quarterly, *14*, 3–10, March, 1943.
14. Matthews, D. K.: *Measurement in Physical Education*, Philadelphia, W. B. Saunders Co., 1963, pp. 255–258.
15. Pryor, Helen B.: *Width-Weight Tables*. Stanford University, California, Stanford University Press, 1940.
16. Shaw, Virginia: Washington State College Screening Test (Posture). Unpublished data, Washington State College, Pullman, Washington, 1957
17. Sheldon, W. H.: *Atlas of Men*. New York, Harper & Brothers, 1954.
18. Sheldon, W. H., S. S. Stevens, and W. B. Tucker: *The Varieties of Human Physique*. New York, Harper & Brothers, 1940.

Chapter 11
THE MEASUREMENT OF KNOWLEDGES
AND UNDERSTANDINGS

The measurement of knowledges and understandings has become justified as the fuller definition of physical education has evolved. No longer is physical development enough. The meanings behind the performance are now considered a vital part of the total program. The background "how's" and "why's" enhance the performance and consequently justify the teaching and the assessments of knowledges and understandings. If they are important to the physically educated person, then they must be a part of the instructional program and so a phase of the measurement program. Students are no longer expected to accept at face value anything the teacher decides to present. The deeper meanings, the explanations, the causes, and the possible results are explained as well. This richness and fullness of content should be reflected in the measurement program.

Tests of knowledge imply an involvement with facts, while tests requiring an understanding demand an application of the facts and thus a deeper meaning. Written tests in physical education should measure both knowledges and understandings. The more of the latter that can be included in the test, the more difficult it is to construct; but also, the more valuable it is as an instrument designed to give a true picture of the grasp the student has of the subject.

USES

Written tests, or "paper and pencil" tests, serve several uses. Most prevalent is the one of *assessing achievement*. At the completion of a unit, the students are tested to see how much information and meaning they have assimilated. The grade made on the test usually becomes a part of the over-all grade for the unit. A unit test should follow the unit plan in its points of emphasis and its general content. If 50 per cent of the unit was spent on skill techniques, then 50 per cent of the questions should investigate the knowledge and understanding about the execution of the techniques. In more advanced units, more time frequently will be spent on strategy and this emphasis should be reflected in the content of the test.

Tests can be learning experiences. Too often there is little or no follow-up of final unit tests resulting in the loss of fine learning opportunities. The teacher may have the students check the papers immediately with a discussion to follow. A check of the number of students missing each question may give the teacher direction for a follow-up discussion of the test during the next class period. False information and misconceptions can be clarified if the students have the opportunity to study their incorrect answers along with the correct ones. Knowledge of the correct information is the ultimate objective even if it has to be learned after the test.

Tests also serve as *motivational devices*. Unit tests are motivational if the students realize the uses to be made of the final results. They should know the weighting of the test in the over-all grade, the type of test, and the content areas. Plans should be made to go over the test papers to discuss questions and misunderstandings. Such follow-up discussions are helpful to the instructor when test revisions are made. If the test and its results are used in meaningful ways, the students are motivated to learn.

Once or twice during a unit a short test could be given to stimulate the students to keep up with the content of the unit. Short tests on scoring in tennis, on positions and marking in speedball, or on terminology in golf are some examples of this application. This serves a diagnostic purpose as well as a motivational one and tends to keep the students "on their toes." This type of test usually covers only one aspect of the content of the activity and consequently plays a small part in the over-all unit grade.

Whether for grading, for encouraging, for learning, for detecting weak areas, or whatever, it is well for the teacher to remember that knowledge tests help to complete the total measurement program. Skill achievements are not enough, just as information about strategy, techniques, and rules alone is inadequate. The physical educator is teaching the total person and must be concerned with mental as well as physical and social accomplishments.

TYPES OF TESTS

Standardized Tests are considered those which have been scientifically constructed and which *may* be accompanied by norms. The validity and reliability of standardized tests have been established. The norms are of questionable value except for gross comparisons because each must be computed in light of a particular unit of a certain length with a specific content presented to a certain age group. These factors vary so greatly that norms for knowledge tests are seldom appropriate. Standardized tests are carefully developed and usually can be made available. Very few knowledge tests in physical education are available commercially but this is one area in which measurement progress will undoubtedly be made. Standardized tests have several characteristics:

1. They provide valid and reliable measures.
2. They show what content and degree of difficulty can be expected for certain groups.
3. They provide good tests when teacher-made ones cannot be well constructed.
4. They provide tests for a great variety of activities.
5. They serve as examples for format and content balance.
6. They are in print somewhere for distribution.   Not all tests in print, however, have been standardized.   The sample tests in college activities handbooks, courses of study, and state syllabi usually are not standardized.

Teacher-Made Tests are more prevalent and are the work of teachers for their local purposes.   They also have certain characteristics:

1. They fit the unit for which they are planned in content and difficulty.
2. They may or may not be scientifically constructed, depending on whether or not the teacher has ascertained their reliability and validity. The fact that a test has not been analyzed does not mean that it has no validity.   If the test coincides with the unit of instruction it automatically has curricular validity.
3. They may or may not be accompanied by local norms depending on whether or not the instructor has collected the scores year after year and prepared norms.
4. They usually are prepared quickly and, consequently, probably not so well constructed as standardized tests.
5. They generally are not available to others.   They are used only locally.

Essay Tests call for a written answer which involves the organization of information to be presented in logical paragraph form.   Essay questions are usually general and test the ability of the student to write the material to be covered.   Essay tests have several characteristics:

1. They usually involve only five or six questions and thus a limited sample of the subject content.
2. They may be constructed quickly.
3. They are difficult to grade objectively and reliably.
4. They usually require more time to answer than objective tests.
5. They may test general explanations, interpretations, and problem-solving concepts which may be difficult to measure in isolated questions of an objective test.
6. They test ability to compose in prose which may *not* be one of the purposes of the test.
7. They are usually good for creative and exploratory testing.
8. They are more efficient for small scale testing.
9. They favor the verbally inclined student.[8]
10. They promote good study habits.[8]

Objective Tests require a brief response of recall or recognition and generally are concerned with smaller pieces of information. They have certain characteristics:

13

1. Good objective tests are difficult and time-consuming to prepare.
2. They may be quickly, efficiently, and objectively graded.
3. They can be validated and revised.
4. They are reliable.[8]
5. They may test for several types of information such as rules, strategy, techniques, terminology, and history of any activity.
6. They lend themselves to follow-up lessons to correct errors and misconceptions.
7. They too frequently measure only superficial and trivial facts.
8. They should rank the students rather accurately according to their understanding and knowledge of the activity.
9. They encourage guessing.[8]
10. They usually cover an extensive amount of the subject content.
11. They eliminate bluffing.[8]
12. They clearly define the task to be done.

Some critics state that objective tests examine only superficial information. If well constructed, however, an objective test can be a challenging mental exercise which measures insights, understandings, interpretations, and judgments. Too frequently, objective tests are prepared quickly and contain questions on rules almost exclusively. Such tests are criticized justifiably and hopefully are being used less frequently in measurement programs. The trend is for the physical education teacher to prepare objective knowledge tests carefully and to continue to analyze and revise them into refined standardized measurement tools worthy of confidence.

SAMPLE TESTS
9th-Grade Wrestling Test*

Purpose. To measure knowledge and understanding of wrestling.

Evaluation. This test has been administered to 9th-grade boys and has been treated by item analysis. Some of the revisions are incorporated in this edition of the test.

Time Allotment. This test can be taken within one class period.

Class Organization. Each student should be supplied with a copy of the test and an answer sheet.

General Procedures. 1. Explain the use of the answer sheet.
2. Provide opportunity for the students to ask questions about the procedures to follow.
3. Motivate the students to do their own work.

Uses. The result of the test may be used as part of the unit grade. It can be used as a follow-up lesson to re-emphasize and clarify some of the questions which the students will have.

---

* Used by permission of Mr. Milton E. Reece, Physical Education Instructor, Greensboro College, Greensboro, North Carolina.

The Test (with correct answers indicated)

DIRECTIONS: Please do not write on the question sheet. Write your name, the date, and the name of the test on the answer sheet.

TRUE-FALSE: Use the first 2 columns on the answer sheet, using number one for true, number two for false. Make an X in the column that best describes the statement.

T   1. Wrestling is a contest of skill, conditioning, weight, and leverage.
F   2. Professional wrestling and junior high wrestling are similar.
T   3. Wrestlers should wear wrestling helmets to protect their ears.
F   4. The Irish made wrestling their national sport.
T   5. The knees cannot be behind the opponent's feet or in front of his knees or touching the opponent, in the top position.
F   6. The referee's standing position is used at the start of the second and third periods.
F   7. The on-guard position is the same as the lock-up.
F   8. The man in the bottom position is in the position of advantage.
F   9. The top position is taken on the opponent's right side.
F   10. The referee's position on the mat is used at the start of the first period.
T   11. Greek and Roman athletes wrestled at the early Olympics in the Coliseum.
T   12. Try to keep your opponent tied up to force him to waste his energy.
T   13. The choice of position for second and third periods is determined by the toss of a coin in tournaments and alternated between teams in a dual meet.
T   14. At the start of a match, the referee should check both contestants to see that no harmful jewelry or unnecessary bandages are worn.
F   15. The worst position in wrestling is on the knees.
T   16. Wrestling is the oldest of all sports.
T   17. Sitting back on the heels in the bottom position prevents the opponent from getting leverage with the ankle.
F   18. If you are either behind or even on points at the start of the second period and if you have the choice, you should take the top position.
T   19. Wrestling has developed as a sport in every civilized country in the world.
F   20. The lock-up position requires the wrestlers to stand straight up.

MULTIPLE-CHOICE: Choose the correct answer and make an X in the proper column on the answer sheet. (1 to 4.)

21. The half nelson should not be put on when the opponent is

1. standing.
2. on his stomach.
3. sitting.
*4. kneeling.

22. A body slam with one knee on the mat counts

*1. no points.
2. 1 point.
3. 2 points.
4. 3 points.

23. A draw awards each team

1. 1 point.
*2. 2 points.
3. 3 points.
4. 5 points.

24. A counter to a pinning combination is

1. a whizzer.
2. a leg roll.
*3. an arm across the chest.
4. a heel pick up.

25. Junior high school wrestling matches consist of 3 periods of

   *1. 1 minute.
   2. 2 minutes.
   3. 3 minutes.
   4. 4 minutes.

26. A take down is

   1. a half nelson.
   *2. a single leg dive.
   3. a sit out.
   4. an elbow roll.

27. A and B lock-up in the first period and A forces B off the mat. A is awarded

   *1. no points.
   2. 1 point.
   3. 2 points.
   4. 3 points.

28. Which is *not* an illegal hold?

   1. locked hands on the mat.
   *2. locked hands in the standing position.
   3. hammer lock above the right angle.
   4. strangle hold.

29. Which one is *not* an escape?

   1. elbow roll.
   2. step over.
   3. sit out.
   *4. shot put.

30. A decision awards the winner's team

   1. 1 point.
   2. 2 points.
   *3. 3 points.
   4. 5 points.

31. A switch is countered with

   1. an elbow roll.
   2. a power switch.
   3. a shot put.
   *4. a reswitch.

32. What is it called when both shoulders are touching the mat for two seconds?

   1. near fall.
   2. predicament.
   *3. fall.
   4. take down.

33. A second take down by a wrestler counts

   1. no points.
   *2. 1 point.
   3. 2 points.
   4. 3 points.

34. The position of advantage is taken by being

   *1. astraddle your opponent and behind.
   2. astraddle your opponent and in front.
   3. on your knees to the left of your opponent.
   4. on your knees to the right of your opponent.

35. A fall or pin awards the winner's team

   1. 1 point.
   2. 2 points.
   3. 3 points.
   *4. 5 points.

36. In the 6-step switch, the sit-out and reach is the

   1. second step.
   2. third step.
   *3. fourth step.
   4. fifth step.

37. A reversal is a

   *1. switch
   2. tackle.
   3. half nelson.
   3. full nelson.

38. An illegal hold is counted *for* the offended and counts

   1. no points.
   *2. 1 point.
   3. 2 points.
   4. 3 points.

39. On a near fall, one shoulder must be touching the mat and the other within
    1. 1 inch from the mat.
    2. 2 inches from the mat.
    3. 3 inches from the mat.
    *4. 4 inches from the mat.

40. The counter to the shot put is the
    1. lock up.
    2. on guard.
    *3. standing switch.
    4. stall.

41. A breakdown hold is
    1. a whizzer.
    2. an elbow roll.
    3. a double arm bar.
    *4. a tight gut and far ankle.

42. The counter to the tackle is the
    1. sit out.
    *2. shoot the hands inside the crotch.
    3. fake sit out.
    4. standing switch.

43. An escape counts
    1. no points.
    *2. 1 point.
    3. 2 points.
    4. 3 points.

44. A reversal counts
    1. no points.
    2. 1 point.
    *3. 2 points.
    4. 3 points.

45. Which one is *not* a pinning combination?
    1. crotch and half nelson.
    2. chicken wing and half nelson.
    *3. full nelson.
    4. ¾ nelson.

46. The first take down by a wrestler counts
    1. no points.
    2. 1 point.
    *3. 2 points.
    4. 3 points.

47. Which one is *not* an escape?
    1. stand up.
    2. switch.
    *3. arm break down.
    4. fake sit out and turn in.

48. A near fall occurs when both shoulders are on the mat for one second and counts
    1. no points.
    2. 1 point.
    3. 2 points.
    *4. 3 points.

49. A control hold is a
    1. fireman's carry.
    *2. far arm and near ankle.
    3. forward roll.
    4. whizzer.

50. Which one is a legal hold?
    1. pressure scissors.
    2. full nelson.
    3. double arm bar.
    *4. tight gut.

GOLF KNOWLEDGE TEST*
Table of Specifications

Elective Golf: Junior and Senior High School Girls
30 40-minute Lessons
For right handed players

Objectives:	A	B	C
The learner is able to:	Identify specific facts and general principles	Apply knowledges: how to interpret cause and effect, and how to analyze	Recognize favorable social attitudes

* Used by permission of Miss Florence Malizola, Physical Education Instructor, New Trier West High School, Northfield, Illinois.

CONTENT AREA	Objectives			Total no. of items	%
	A	B	C		
1. Rules	10	1		11	22%
2. Etiquette	1		3	4	8%
3. Techniques and Skills	6	10		16	32%
4. Strategy and Tactics		4		4	8%
5. Terminology	7	1		8	16%
6. History and Equipment	5			5	10%
7. Safety	2			2	4%
TOTAL no. of items	31	16	3	50	100%
Percentage	62%	32%	6%		100%

TRUE-FALSE: If the statement is true, place an X in column a. If the statement is false, place an X in column b.

F
1–A*   1. The golfer counts only the strokes in which he makes contact with the ball.

F
6–A   2. The length of the shaft increases as the number of an iron gets higher.

T
1–A   3. The left hand controls the club throughout the swing.

F
1–A   4. A golf course consists of twenty holes.

F
3–B   5. The player should feel that he is using the palm of his left hand to slap a flat surface when swinging the club.

T
1–A   6. There is an allowance of two putts in determining par.

T
5–A   7. The face is that part of the club head which strikes the ball.

F
6–A   8. Of the three woods numbered 1, 2, 3, the driver has the most slant to the club face.

T
5–A   9. The stance refers to the position of the player's feet when addressing the ball.

T
7–A   10. The player farthest from the hole should play first even though he may have to take several strokes before another person plays.

T
6–A   11. The larger the number of the iron club, the heavier and shorter the club and the more loft to its face.

* Key to objectives and content areas.

T   12. The speed and weight of the club head coming accurately into
3–B   contact with the ball is responsible for making the ball go far and
straight rather than sheer strength.

T   13. Courtesy demands that one remain quiet when another person is
2–C   hitting the ball.

F   14. It is all right to leave holes in the ground which you have made
2–C   while playing a shot because they add to the hazards of the course.

T   15. The left hand is placed closer to the top end of grip than the
3–B   right hand.

MULTIPLE CHOICE: Indicate your choice of the one best answer to each
question by making an (X) in the proper space on
the answer sheet.

16.   Which grip is used most widely in putting?
3–A *a.* Overlapping.
     b. Interlocking.
     c. Ten-finger grip
   d. Reverse overlapping

17.   Which practice will cause a slice?
5–B *a.* Hitting too far under the ball.
     b. Hitting above center.
     c. Hitting from inside out.
   d. Hitting from outside in.

18.   Which statement best describes match play?
5–A *a.* Hole-by-hole competition.
     b. Stroke competition.
     c. Players paired according to ability.
     d. Players paired according to draw.

19.   Players A and B are both on the green. Player A is "away" but
1–A player B's ball is directly between A and the cup. What is the correct
procedure?
   a. Player A should ask player B to remove his ball, mark its position and then player A should putt.
    b. Player B should putt first since his ball lies on the line of direction
for A.
    c. Player B must putt first according to the rule since his ball is the
closer one.
    d. Player A must ask B if he will observe the rules of etiquette and
putt first.

20.   Historians credit the origin of golf to which country?
6–A *a.* United States
   b. Holland or the Low Countries
     c. England
     d. Scotland

21. In which instance might one employ a closed stance?
3–A *a*. Short pitch and run shots.
     b. Longer pitch and run shots.
    *c. Driving and long approach shots.
     d. Pitch shots.

22. What procedure should a player follow who has just hit out of a
2–C sand trap?
     a. Leave the trap by the same route he entered.
     b. Refill the hole made by the "explosion" shot
     c. Leave the trap by the shortest route.
    *d. Refill all holes left by the club and feet.

23. You see that the green slopes downward from you and slightly to the
4–B right. What is the best tactic for lining up the putt?
     a. Aim directly at the hole and hit the ball harder than usual to
          overcome the effect of gravity.
    *b. Aim to the left of the hole and let gravity operate.
     c. Aim at the hole but follow through to the left.
     d. Aim to the right of the hole and let gravity operate.

24. Where should the ball be placed in relation to the body on an ap-
3–A proach shot?
    *a. Off the right heel.
     b. Off the left heel.
     c. Slightly to the right of center
     d. In the center of the stance.

25. Which statement best describes the downswing with irons?
3–B *a. The ball is contacted first and then the turf for loft.
     b. The ball is hit on the upswing to insure loft.
     c. The turf is contacted first, then the ball for loft.
     d. The club head hits through the ball, the turf is never contacted.

26. What is the basis for computing par for a hole?
1–A *a. The yardage of the hole.
     b. The difficulty of the hole.
     c. The yardage and difficulty of the hole.
     d. The average score of players on that hole.

27. Figure out the number of strokes a golfer has so far in the following
1–B hole of play. He begins by driving the ball out-of-bounds. He tees
     another ball and hits it. From the fairway he shoots the ball into the
     rough and loses it. He then drops a ball at the spot and hits it
     successfully.
     a. 4
     b. 5
    *c. 6
     d. 7

28. What is a provisional ball?

5–A *a.* An old ball used as a substitute for a "good" ball in a hazardous situation.
  b. A practice shot from the first tee.
  *c. A second ball hit from the tee to save time in case the first ball is out-of-bounds.
  d. A new ball used to replace a lost ball.

29. What would you do to get less distance with a certain iron?

3–B **a.* Decrease the length of the backswing.
  b. Decrease the speed of the club head.
  c. Decrease the power of the swing.
  d. Decrease the length of the follow-through.

30. Which action starts the downswing of the club?

3–B *a.* Uncocking of wrists.
  b. Rotating the hip.
  c. Rotating the shoulder.
  *d. Shifting the weight.

31. What is the basic difference between the pitch and pitch-and-run
5–A shots?

  *a. The amount of roll and time the ball is in the air.
  b. The club selection.
  c. The length of the swing.
  d. The stance and ball placement.

32. What should the player do if greater force is desired?

3–B *a.* Use more wrist action.
  *b. Use longer backswing.
  c. Use firmer wrists at impact.
  d. Use a longer follow-through.

33. Which is a correct statement?

1–A *a.* Birdie is 1 over par, eagle is 2 under par, bogey is 1 under par.
  b. Bogey is 1 under par, birdie is 2 under par, ace is 1 over par.
  c. Eagle is 1 under par, birdie is 2 under par, ace is 1 over par.
  *d. Birdie is 1 under par, eagle is 2 under par, bogey is 1 over par.

34. Which statement describes a hook?

5–A *a.* Ball with clockwise spin traveling straight—then curving to the right.
  *b. Ball with counterclockwise spin traveling straight—then curving to the left.
  c. Ball with clockwise spin traveling straight—then curving to the left.
  d. Ball with counterclockwise spin—then curving to the right.

35. What happens when the ball is out-of-bounds?

1–A *a.* Play it as it lies with no penalty.
  b. Drop a ball over the shoulder on to the fairway and play it from there with no penalty.
  *c. Take it to the place from which it was hit and play it again with a one stroke penalty.
  d. Drop a ball over the shoulder with one penalty stroke.

36.   What is the procedure to follow when your ball lands in a water
1–A   hazard?
    a. Play another ball from the place of the last shot.
    **b*. Drop a ball and add a 1 stroke penalty.
    c. Drop a ball and add a 2 stroke penalty.
    d. Drop a ball without penalty.

37.   Where should the ball be addressed when driving from the tee?
3–A   *a*. Off the right heel.
    **b*. Off the left heel.
    c. Slightly to the right of center.
    d. In the center of the stance.

38.   Why does the player farthest from the hole play first?
7–A   *a*. It is a rule of the game.
    b. It is a convenience.
    **c*. It is safer.
    d. It speeds up the game.

39.   Which iron will give the greatest accuracy of placement and why?
6–A   *a*. #5 iron; distance and roll.
    **b*. #9 iron; more height and less roll.
    c. #7 iron; less height and more roll.
    d. #2 iron; least amount of height and roll.

40.   What is the axis around which the club is swung?
3–A   *a*. Head.
    b. Shoulders.
    c. Hips.
    **d*. Spine.

41.   Your ball is resting just off the apron of the green which slopes down-
4–B   ward toward the cup. What club would you use to hit the ball on
      to the green?
    a. #2 iron
    b. #5 iron
    **c*. #9 iron
    d. #7 iron

42.   What is the *primary* function of the backswing?
3–B   *a*. To get the club head in motion.
    **b*. To position the club to hit the ball.
    c. To establish the arc of the swing.
    d. To ensure a rhythmical swing.

43.   Which statement best describes a correct follow-through?
3–B   *a*. It is stopped when the hands reach shoulder height.
    b. It is stopped when the handle points toward the hole.
    **c*. It is determined by the momentum of the club head.
    d. It continues until the club is over the left shoulder.

44.   Which is an example of an obstacle on the fairway?
5–A   *a*. Dog-leg.
    b. Rough.
    c. Divot.
    **d*. Bunker.

45.   What is the proper procedure when a ball lands in casual water?

1–A   *a.* Remove ball from the water, drop it behind the water, and count a stroke.
      b. Remove the ball and place it in front of the water and count a stroke.
      **c.* Remove the ball, drop it behind the water and do *not* count a stroke.
      d. Play the ball from where it landed.

46.   What is the effect of top spin on the ball when it drops to the ground?

3–B   **a.* Increased forward roll.
      b. No effect.
      c. Decreases the amount of roll.
      d. Makes the ball bounce forward.

47.   A short hole, 125 yards long, has a raised green surrounded by traps.

4–B   What club would you use from the tee and why?
      a. #3 wood for less distance than a driver.
      b. #1 wood for distance.
      **c.* #5 iron for distance.
      d. #7 iron for more lift.

48.   Your ball is in a good lie on the fairway 175 yards from the green.

4–B   There is a creek that runs across the fairway about 50 yards away. What club would you use and why?
      **a.* #2 wood to cover the distance.
      b. #2 iron to raise the ball as well as gain the greatest distance.
      c. #5 iron to raise the ball over the creek and gain some distance.
      d. #7 iron to get the ball over the creek.

49.   What is the accepted practice when you think you have lost your

1–A   ball?
      a. Look until you find it and then continue play.
      b. Immediately wave the group following to play through.
      **c.* Wave the group following you to play through after you have looked for the ball 5 minutes.
      d. Play a provisional ball.

50.   Which player has the honor on the next tee when the hole completed

2–A   was tied?
      **a.* The player winning the preceding hole.
      b. The player with the higher total score.
      c. The player with the lower total score.
      d. The player with the lower handicap.

The Construction of Objective Knowledge Tests

The measurement of knowledges and understandings is one phase of the evaluative process in which the teacher is left almost entirely to his own resources. Knowledge tests in physical education are rare in the literature, so must be developed locally. Since the acquisition of knowledges and understandings is one of the objectives of physical education, its measurement should be as accurate as possible. The physical education teacher is charged with the responsibility of developing knowledge tests which are valid, reliable, and patterned to fit certain units of instruction. Once such professional skills are acquired, the teacher will build a collection of good knowledge tests. Soon he will have a nucleus of tests in which he has confidence. Revisions will need to be made from time to time, but the basic test structure will be available.

Two pitfalls in test construction seem to have plagued the teacher in the past. One is the quickly constructed test which is either essay in type or composed of a collection of ambiguous true-false statements. The other weakness has been the great emphasis placed on the inclusion of rules questions to the exclusion of questions on technique and strategy. Good tests should reflect the content of the unit of instruction, should be prepared carefully, and should be restudied continually.

Content Balance. The constructor of the test should itemize the types of information which he wishes the test to cover and assign to them certain proportional weightings in the over-all content. These weightings should parallel the weighting each received in the instructional work.

The suggested content balance will change from unit to unit and from sport to sport. Essentially, however, rules probably should never cover over one-quarter of the value of the total test and preferably less. Emphasis should be on the execution of the skills and how to apply them in a game situation. Some basic facts concerning the equipment, the historical background of the sport, and some of the special terms seem appropriate. In some sports, safety is an important aspect of the game and is worthy of some emphasis in a test.

Questions of fact and definition such as might cover rules and terminology are rather simple to construct and measure a certain level of knowledge. Questions of understanding and application of facts are much more difficult to construct and measure the concepts

Table 11–1. Suggested Content Balance of a Test

Content Area	Percentage
Rules	25
Etiquette and Procedures	10
Techniques and Skills	25
Strategy and Tactics	25
Terminology	5
History and Equipment	5
Safety	5
	100

the student has learned. How well a student is able to "know" a game is better measured by how well he can apply his understanding of the game than by how well he can relate facts about the game. Thus the precision of the test instrument and the skill required to construct it are a reflection of how well the teacher is able to test student understanding of a particular activity.

Sources of Items. Good test questions can be gleaned from several sources. The teacher should be alert for such questions and collect them as they appear. The ideas for the questions must come first and then be developed. The teacher's own creativeness and intellectual endeavors will provide many questions. Textbooks, rule books, and sports books are good sources. The questions which the students ask during classes often bring out excellent ideas and their wordage is also worthy of note for future application to test questions. Sample tests from books and research reports supply good ideas for questions and formats. Professional colleagues can be helpful when the instructor is developing written tests. For some reason, there seems to be an unfortunate professional selfishness about test questions. Teachers are usually generous about sharing teaching ideas, rating scales, skills tests, norms, and the like, but much less generous about sharing knowledge tests. Whenever a teacher has the use of a test, he usually has to adapt it to his needs in content, difficulty, format, and the like. It is seldom possible to use a test as it appears, but it does serve to give the teacher a beginning on which to build.

Types of Items. Questions for objective tests are of several types. They each have certain applications and some rules for construction.

1. *Alternate-Response*

   a. Examples of alternate-response questions are True-False, Yes-No, Right-Wrong, and Same-Opposite.

   b. True-False is the most prevalent of this style of question.

   c. They permit a wide range of content coverage in limited space and time.

   d. They are constructed quickly usually, although good true-false questions may require a good deal of time.

   e. They encourage guessing. Guessing can be minimized if the students are told that the questions will be scored by deducting the number wrong from the number answered correctly. An alternative adjustment for guessing would be to subtract the per cent wrong from the number right.

   f. They frequently test for trivial information.

   Example of a poor question: The lines on a tennis court may be no more than 2 inches in width.

   g. They are applicable when only two responses are possible.

   h. They should involve only one concept to be judged.

Example of a poor question: The maximum number of sets in a match shall be five, or where women take part, three.

i. They should be stated in positive terms.

Example of a poor question: A free-style swimmer should not do more than 3 strokes without taking a breath.

j. They should be stated in quantitative instead of qualitative terms.

Example of a poor question: There are several (instead of four) recognized systems of court coverage related to badminton.

k. There should be approximately the same number of questions which are true as there are which are false.

l. They should not be constructed as trick questions.

Example of a poor question: The object rallied in badminton is called a "birdie."

m. No cue words should reveal the correct answer.

Example of a poor question: The side stroke is *always* used as a speed style of swimming.

n. Questions of opinion should be avoided unless the authority is stated.

o. The answers should follow no pattern or sequence.

The True-False format has several variations which can be used to advantage to help the teacher achieve his testing objectives:

a. True or False and tell why.

b. True or False and correct if wrong.

c. True or False or Doubtful choices.

Examples of True-False Questions:

a. Golfers who have holed out may repeat their putts for practice.

b. Trimming a canoe is a matter of balancing the weight of occupants and duffle.

c. One of the chief causes of accidents in rowboats and canoes involves occupants exchanging positions.

*d. Left-handed players may hit the ball on the rounded part of the stick.

*e. A goal may *not* be scored off the stick of a defense player unless it was first touched by the stick of an attacker within the striking circle.

*f. A girl walking with the ball is committing the foul of travelling.

Examples of Alternate Response Questions:

Knowledge Test—First Grade†

Movement Exploration

The teacher will give the directions, read each question and wait for each child to make the appropriate mark or response on his paper.

---

* Used by permission of Miss Paula Drake, Cape Elizabeth High School, Cape Elizabeth, Maine.

† Used by permission of Miss Virginia Hart, Mars Hill College, Mars Hill, North Carolina.

1. Draw a circle around the children who are in a scattered formation.

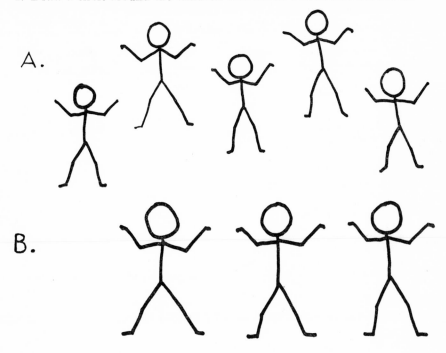

2. Draw a cross mark on the child who is landing softly from a jump.

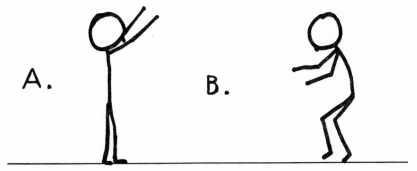

2. *Multiple-Choice*

The multiple-choice style of question has the greatest regard among test constructors. They consider it capable of measuring the applications of facts and thus some of the deeper understandings which the teacher hopes to measure. The question or preliminary statement is known as the stem or the problem. The alternatives listed are known as choices and the incorrect ones are known as distractors or foils.

a. Multiple-choice questions are the most difficult to construct.

b. The multiple-choice format is inappropriate if only two choices are possible.

c. Skill is required to develop plausible yet incorrect choices.

d. Multiple-choice questions require some discriminatory thinking.

e. They may be very easy or very difficult, depending on the closeness or homogeneity of the choices.

f. They require no adjustment in scoring for guessing.

g. The stem should be a complete statement or question.

h. Each possible choice should be plausible.

i. All choices should follow a parallel structure which is grammatically consistent.

j. The choices should all be of about the same length.

k. The answers should follow no pattern.

l. Four plausible choices seem adequate.

m. Each question should have the same number of choices if possible. However, few choices which function is better than having more just for the sake of consistency in format.

n. Each choice should be listed separately.

o. Questions should be stated in the third person.

p. The problem should be simply and concisely presented in the stem.

q. Multiple-choice questions sometimes have as the 4th choice either "Any of these," "All of these," or "None of them." Great care should be taken when using such a choice.

r. The terminology used in the stem should not be repeated in the choices.

s. Negatively stated questions should be minimal, and care should be taken to emphasize the negative words by underlining them.

t. Care should be taken that a question does not give a clue to the answer of some other question in the test. Each item should be independent.

The Multiple-Choice format has several variations:

a. Correct Answer

One answer is correct and the others, while plausible, are definitely incorrect.

Example: Which is the cause of drowning?
1. unconsciousness.
2. shock.
3. panic.
4. suffocation.

b. Best Answer

One answer is preferable. Other choices may be correct but not the best possible response. Questions on strategy lend themselves to this format.

Example: What is the most important factor in determining the height and distance of the flight of the ball?
1. the length of the shaft of the club.
2. the angle of the clubface.
3. the weight of the clubhead.
4. the strength of the player.

c. Multiple Response or Multiple Answer

There is at least one correct answer and there may be more. Two keys are necessary—one to see if all correct answers were selected and another to see that no incorrect answers were selected. Each statement is scored. It is a mistake to choose an incorrect answer just as it is to omit a correct one.

Example: Which square dance calls are examples of the "couple visitor" type figure?
1. Birdie in the Cage.
2. Texas Star.
3. Rip and Snort.
4. Form a Star with a Right-hand Cross.
5. Inside Arch and Outside Under.

Poor Examples and suggestions for revisions:

a. Upon receiving the ball, the player must
1. rotate counterclockwise.
2. let the best server serve.
3. let the man already in the right-hand position serve.
4. rotate clockwise, then let the man in the right-hand position serve.
    What procedure should the team follow when receiving the ball for offensive play?
    The "4" choice is too long in comparison with the other three. The length triggers it as the correct answer.

b. If a ball touches a boundary line
1. it is out-of-bounds.
2. is played over.
3. is good.
4. neither team scores.
Complete the stem and make the choices parallel in structure.
What is the decision when the ball touches a boundary line?
1. it is out-of-bounds.
2. it is replayed.
3. it is good.
4. it is dead.

c. Safety factors for bathing places do not include
1. good bottom.
2. clear runways and decks.
3. swimming areas should be large.
Note that the negative word is underlined for emphasis. Make the choices parallel in structure and grammar and make the stem a complete statement.
Which factor is not essential to a safe bathing place?
1. good bottoms.
2. clear runways and decks.
3. spaciousness.
4. marked areas.

General Examples of Multiple Choice Questions:

*a. Field Hockey   —Advancing the ball means:
1. kicking the ball.
2. hitting the ball forward with the stick.
3. going ahead of the ball down the field.
4. using the wrong side of the stick.

* Used by permission of Miss Paula Drake, Cape Elizabeth High School, Cape Elizabeth, Maine.

b. Tennis

—Why is it important to toss the ball high enough to serve with the arm fully extended?
1. enables the server to hit the ball either to the right or the left of the receiver.
2. enables the server to use the entire body as a lever, thus getting more power behind the ball.
3. eliminates the possibility of hitting the ball into the net.
4. assures the server greater accuracy.

c. Table Tennis

—The receiver returns the serve during a doubles match. Which player is supposed to make the next play on the ball?
1. the server.
2. the server's partner.
3. the receiver's partner.
4. the receiver.

d. Body Mechanics—Which condition is probably the most common postural deviation among high school girls?
1. high shoulder.
2. protruding abdomen.
3. forward head.
4. locked knees

*e. Lacrosse

—What causes the rocking motion of the crosse that is necessary in cradling?
1. twisting the shoulders.
2. keeping both elbows bent.
3. flexing and extending the wrists.
4. keeping the left elbow bent.

f. Badminton

—What is the advantage of the rotation system over the parallel system of doubles play?
1. eliminates many backhand shots.
2. confuses the opponents.
3. provides opportunity for players to see a greater variety of strokes.
4. encourages more cooperation between partners.

†g. Volley Ball

—In which skills will a player increase the efficiency of her play by jumping?
A. Spike
B. Offensive Volley
C. Bump
D. Overhand Serve
E. Block

1. A,B,D,E
2. B,C,D
3. A,B,E
4. A,B

—What provides the majority of force for the bump?
1. The quick armlift and follow through.
2. The redirected force from the incoming ball.
3. The contracting arm and shoulder muscles.
4. The finger and wrist flexion.

—Which statement describes team strategy for coed teams?
1. Women receive serves and set to men for spikes.
2. Men receive serves and set to women for offensive volleys.
3. Men receive serves and pass to women to set to men for spikes.
4. Court position rather than sex determines spiking, passing, and setting assignments.

* *h.* Gymnastics   —Diagrams A, B, C, and D combined illustrate a *continuous* tumbling routine in which there is a fault. Which diagram contains the fault?

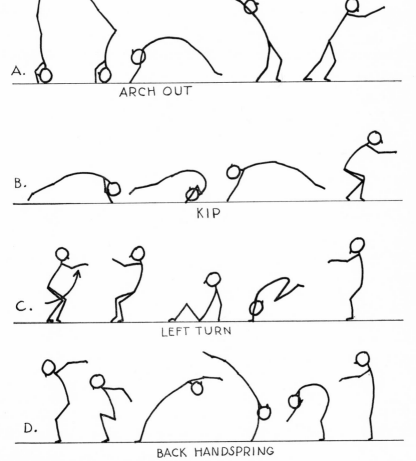

A. ARCH OUT

B. KIP

C. LEFT TURN

D. BACK HANDSPRING

---

* Used by permission of Miss Pat Davis, University of Waterloo, Waterloo, Ontario, Canada.

* *i*. Bowling   —Which principle best relates to the starting position?

  1. first ball delivery, distance from foul line is constant, position from side to side varies.

  2. first ball delivery, distance from foul line varies, position from side to side is constant.

  3. first or second ball delivery, distance from foul line is constant, position from side to side varies.

  4. first or second ball delivery, distance from foul line varies, position from side to side is constant.

3. Matching

Matching statements are applicable to definitions, to personality identifications, and to rules.

a. Matching questions should be homogeneous in content. Terms should not be mixed with personalities in the same question. It would be better to have two short matching questions than one longer one containing a mixture of content.

b. They are likely to measure only memory in contrast to understanding.

c. They are likely to include clues to the correct response.

d. The response column should be arranged in some systematic order such as alphabetically or chronologically.[14]

e. All of the parts of the question should be on one page.[14]

f. Matching questions should probably include at least five and probably not more than 15 items.[14]

g. More responses should be listed than items to be matched.

h. Responses should be in the right-hand column. The answers should be recorded to the left of the left-hand column of the items to be matched.

i. At least two plausible answers for each question should be included in the response column.[14]

Several variations are possible on Matching Questions.

a. Perfect.

The same number of responses are listed as there are items to be matched. This practice is not recommended.

b. Imperfect

There are more choices than are needed. At least two extra choices should be included.

c. *Multiple*

There are two columns of responses and each item to be matched must be answered by one response from each column.

Example of a Matching Question:

Matching—Match the term with the definition. Indicate the letter of the correct response in the first set of brackets on the answer sheet.

---

* Used by permission of Roberta Howells, Western Connecticut State College, Danbury, Connecticut.

34. Down	a. a stroke that makes a return impossible
35. In	b. lost service for the first server in doubles
36. Kill	c. the side which is receiving
37. One Down	d. a fault
38. Out	e. a stroke which initiates each rally
39. Wood	f. a toss
40. Serve	g. shuttlecock
	h. the side which is serving
	i. the long service area
	j. loss of service through failure of the serving side to score.

4. *Classification*

Classification is a type of matching question. There are fewer choices from which to select but there are several items which fit each choice. Classification questions lend themselves to measuring the organization of information and to the relationship of small items to larger concepts.

a. The content should cover material of similar nature.

b. The format is opposite from the matching categories. The short list of classifications is usually given on the right-hand side. The situations are listed in the left-hand column.

For example:

	List of play situations:	Rulings:
	1.	1. Foul
	2. Each play situation	2. Violation
	3. must be judged either a	3. Fair Play
	4. foul, a violation, or a	
	. fair play	
	10.	

c. Care should be taken to be sure each situation fits into one of the categories.

5. *Rearrangement*

Rearrangement questions place emphasis on the order of things. Sequence of a skill execution and chronological order of sporting events would be examples. Questions on history and progression of skill are possible with this format.

a. The order provided should be well scrambled.
b. The unraveled order of each question should follow no pattern.
c. Care should be taken in scoring decisions because an incorrect choice of the first answer may make all the succeeding answers incorrect even though in logical order.

Probably each question should have only a single value. Any error in the sequence would mean a missed question. If a sequence question with 5 parts is allotted 5 points, the weightings in the content balance would become distorted most likely.

Examples of Rearrangement Questions:

Arrange in logical order the following steps in learning to dive.

1. one-leg dive
2. crouched dive
3. standing dive
4. sitting dive
5. kneeling dive

Arrange in proper order the sequence of the tennis serve.

1. reach
2. toss ball
3. back swing
4. follow through
5. contact

6. *Completion*

The completion question provides for a response of one word or perhaps two or three words. Responses longer than this result in less objective and more time-consuming grading practices.

a. Grading is expedited if all the blanks appear in the right-hand column of the page.

b. All acceptable words should be noted on the key by the teacher before the test is given. Acceptance of only one certain word promotes rote learning which may be accompanied by very little understanding.

Example of a Completion Question:

* Two important concepts in the definition of first aid are_____

and_____.

7. *Special Formats*

Sometimes a depth of understanding can be measured better if diagrams, charts, stick figures, symbols, and the like are used in the format of the questions. A diagram could be referred to for the answers for several questions. Strategy questions on court placements are appropriate to this format. Musical symbols and baseball scoring symbols have been used effectively in tests. Stick figures are effective for stunts and tumbling and sports techniques questions. Scoring lines in bowling and in golf are examples of the use of graphics in the construction of test questions. They permit a type of question which might otherwise be difficult to structure, they add variety to the test, and they are challenging to construct.

Final Format. 1. The test should be typed carefully, proofread, and duplicated. A double column of questions will save space.

2. Directions for answering the questions should be stated carefully and thoroughly on the test paper.

* Used by permission of Dr. June P. Galloway, University of North Carolina at Greensboro.

a. True-False

Read each question carefully. If the statement is entirely true, put an X in the first set of brackets; if the statement is wholly or partially false, put an X in the second set of brackets on the answer sheet.

b. True-False

Read each question carefully. If the statement is entirely true, place an X in the blank to the left of the question; if the statement is wholly or partially false, put an 0 in the blank to the left of the question.

c. Multiple-Choice

Read each statement carefully. The questions are worded for right-handed players. Decide which is the one *best* answer and place an X in the brackets on the answer sheet corresponding to the number of the response.

d. Matching

Indicate the letter of the correct response in the first set of brackets on the answer sheet.

3. There should be a double space between questions.

4. No question should be completed by having to turn to the next page of the test.

5. The test should be titled.

The number of questions in a test should be sufficient to assure some degree of reliability, but not so many that few students are able to complete it. Fifty questions is a good "rule of thumb," especially if they are mostly multiple-choice questions.

Test writers seem to be enamored by a test value of 100 points. They arrive at this number either by writing 100 questions or by assigning each question a certain numerical value. For example, multiple-choice questions might be worth 2 points each and true-false questions worth only 1 point. This practice is questionable because it distorts the content emphasis intended for the test. If the rules area is to cover only $\frac{1}{4}$ of the test but each rules question is given a double value, then it is possible, depending on the weightings given the other questions, to put undue stress on this area of the subject content. Tests of 43 questions or of 61 questions, for example, are quite acceptable. Scale the final scores in relation to the total number of questions. There is no magic in the 100-point test except that it may be a little easier to handle mathematically. A test composed of 54 good questions is a far better measuring tool than one containing 100 questions which is prepared less thoughtfully.

Answer Sheets and Keys. The use of answer sheets is recommended for several reasons:

1. They permit the re-use of the test papers.
2. They facilitate scoring the papers.
3. They permit a mark showing the correct answer for later study of the test by the students.
4. They are economical in time and in money.
5. They are convenient to use when doing an item analysis of the test.

Students should be taught how to use an answer sheet. For example, a form answer sheet may provide space for 5 possible responses while a test question may have only 4 choices. Deciding the correct answer is the last one, the student marks the 5th spot on the answer sheet and misses the question. The student should be

EXAMPLE OF ANSWER SHEET FOR 90 QUESTIONS

Name_____ Course_____ Date_____

```
      1  2  3  4  5              1  2  3  4  5              1  2  3  4  5
 1. ( )( )( )(X)( )       31. ( )( )( )( )( )       61. ( )( )( )( )( )
 2. ( )( )( )( )( )       32. ( )( )( )( )( )       62. ( )( )( )( )( )
 3. ( )( )( )( )( )       33. ( )( )( )( )( )       63. ( )( )( )( )( )
 4. ( )( )( )( )( )       34. ( )( )( )( )( )       64. ( )( )( )( )( )
 5. ( )( )( )( )( )       35. ( )( )( )( )( )       65. ( )( )( )( )( )
 .                          .                          .
 .                          .                          .
 .                          .                          .
30. ( )( )( )( )( )       60. ( )( )( )( )( )       90. ( )( )( )( )( )
```

EXAMPLE OF ANSWER SHEET FOR 60 QUESTIONS

Name_____ Activity_____ Date_____

```
 1. 1 2 3 4       16. 1 2 3 4       31. 1 2 3 4       46. 1 2 3 4
    " " " |          " " " "           " " " "           " " " "
    " " " |          " " " "           " " " "           " " " "
    " " " |          " " " "           " " " "           " " " "
 2. 1 2 3 4       17. 1 2 3 4       32. 1 2 3 4       47. 1 2 3 4
    " " " "           " " " "           " " " "           " " " "
    " " " "           " " " "           " " " "           " " " "
    " " " "           " " " "           " " " "           " " " "
    .                 .                 .                 .
    .                 .                 .                 .
    .                 .                 .                 .
15. 1 2 3 4       30. 1 2 3 4       45. 1 2 3 4       60. 1 2 3 4
    " " " "           " " " "           " " " "           " " " "
    " " " "           " " " "           " " " "           " " " "
    " " " "           " " " "           " " " "           " " " "
```

Fig. 11–1. Sample answer sheets.

cautioned about such practices. The use of the answer sheet may take a little more time because the student's attention must be shifted back and forth from the test paper to the answer sheet. It is possible that the use of answer sheets may reduce cheating since the answer is not recorded beside the question.

Most types of questions can be answered on an answer sheet. A stencil cut for the form can be used to replenish the stock whenever more copies are needed. The form should provide for about 60 to 90 questions so it will accommodate a test of almost any length.

Scoring keys for efficient grading can be made. Stencil keys are the type which are superimposed on the answer sheet and which have the correct answer cut out. The grader is able to mark the correct answer, if not already indicated, so the student will know what it should have been when he goes over the test paper later. Strip keys are placed adjacent to the answers. Comparisons are necessary by the grader as he works down the column. The grader should designate the correct answers for any questions missed.

The Evaluation of Objective Knowledge Tests

The evaluation of objective knowledge tests is a procedure which the public school teacher can learn and apply. As a teacher builds a collection of written tests, he will often want to make revisions on them. The teacher would be wise to try to revise one or two tests per year. The work involved in test revision would prevent such a practice for every test administered. Other phases of teaching and of testing would suffer from such over-emphasis on written tests. The teacher will learn to save and label sets of answer sheets so they will be available whenever a test revision is anticipated.

The revision process covers three areas: (1) editing revisions, (2) validity by item analysis, and (3) reliability. Each will be discussed and described so the teacher can perform each step for himself.

Editing. Editing revisions come from close scrutiny of a test. Reading and rereading each question will suggest changes in the structure of the item, in the choices, in the word order, and in the statements which changes in rules and changes in strategy have altered.

A study of the unit outline will suggest ideas for new questions and the deletion of others. The comments of the students will suggest word changes for better clarity of questions. The study of other tests will suggest changes in question format that will improve the question. A growing knowledge of test construction and awareness of the fine points of item construction will make the teacher more and more confident to edit his tests.

Validity. The validity of a written test is the same in concept as the validity of a performance test. A measure of the truthfulness and honesty of the test is indicated. There are at least two types of validity which should be considered. Various authors discuss various kinds using different terms. Here the concern is for empirical validity and statistical validity.

1. *Empirical validity* is achieved if the content of the test is in agreement with the unit of instruction. The test may be studied by several "authorities" who consider its contents in relation to what they consider such a unit should include. The test constructor alone may do this. The test can be compared in content balance with similar tests. If approximately parallel emphasis is evident, validity is assumed. This is face validity, curricular validity, or empirical validity and is often all a teacher will want to insure.

2. *Statistical validity* is a more involved process and answers the more technical question of the internal ability of the test to discriminate between those who "know" and those who "do not know." The process is known as *item analysis*. There are several methods advocated in the literature:

a. *The Flanagan Method* seems to be used most widely in measurement books in physical education and is the one generally taught to college professional students. An item analysis will reveal three qualities about each item in a test: (1) the difficulty of each item, (2) the power of each item to discriminate between the students who know and those who do not, and (3) the amount that each possible response functions by noting the frequency with which each response is chosen.

For purposes of clarity, an example item analysis will be used. The Flanagan method of item analysis operates on the theory that analysis of the answer sheets representing the extreme scores is substantially as efficient as using all of the papers. This decreases the computational work and makes the analysis less tedious.

Flanagan prepared a table in 1939 which provided the correlation coefficients, indicative of an Index of Discrimination, using the upper and lower 27 per cent of the cases. He stated that one of the disadvantages of the procedure was that the extreme cases at the two ends of the distribution did not receive the greater weight they deserved.[6] He recommended that the values near the extremes be counted twice to give them double weight in determining the appropriate proportions of successes and failures. He then suggested that the papers be divided in groups using 9, 20, 42, 20, and 9 per cent of the cases and that the middle 42 per cent be disregarded.[6] The cases in the extreme groups of 9 per cent are each counted as two when adding them to the papers in the next group of 20 per cent. This method requires the selection of 29 per cent of the papers at each end of the distribution. The extreme 9 per cent is given double weight.

After being scored, the papers are arranged in numerical order so the proper number of papers can be counted off. Usually an item analysis should be considered only when there are at least 100 answer sheets available from which to draw the ones to be used in the analysis. Assume that 100 papers are available. Multiply by 29 per cent and get 29. Count off the 29 best papers and the 29 poorest. Consider the top 9 per cent of the papers in the Upper-Upper Group, the next 20 per cent in the Upper Group, the middle 42 per cent set

KNOWLEDGE TEST TABULATION SHEET

Name of Test: 8th Grade Soccer Test   100 papers
29 in Upper Groups, 29 in Lower Groups   38 Possible Maximum

Q	1	2	3	4	5	Omit	D.R.	I.D.	Revise
UU		卌 IIII					29+19		
U		卌 卌 卌 卌 18+20=38÷38 100%					48/58		F
1								.66	
		58% 6+16=22÷38 卌 卌 卌 I					83%		
L	IIII								
LL	卌 I	III							
UU	I	卌 III					25+14		
U	II	卌 卌 卌 II 16+17=33÷38 87%				I	39/58		
2		47% 8+10=18÷38					64%	.42	
L	IIII	卌 卌	II	IIII					
LL	II	IIII	I	II					
UU	卌 III	I					26+26		
U	卌 卌 卌 III 16+18=34÷38 89%	II					52/58		DR ID F
3	89% 16+18=34÷38						90%	.00	
L	卌 卌 卌 III		II						
LL	卌 III		I						
UU	II		III	IIII			13+4		
U	III	III	卌	卌 IIII 8+9=17÷38 45%			17/58		
4				13% 2+3=5÷38			29%	.36	
L	III		卌 卌 IIII	III					
LL	II		卌 I	I					
UU	III		I	卌			10+23		
U	卌 II 6+7=13÷38 34%			卌 卌 III			33/58		ID F
5	79% 14+16=30÷38						57%	-.43	
L	卌 卌 卌 I		III	I					
LL	卌 II		II						

Fig. 11-2. Sample item analysis.

aside, the next 20 per cent in the Lower Group, and the lowest 9 per cent in the Lower-Lower Group. If ties occur, select only the number of papers needed to get 29, selecting at random from the tied group.

Figure 11–2 is a form which can be duplicated to use with item analysis procedures. It will accommodate five questions.

Step 1. Number the question down the Q column.

Step 2. Indicate the correct answer by double framing the appropriate square. Response No. 2 is the correct answer in Question No. 1.

Step 3. Block out the responses which are not used in the question. Most of these questions had 4 choices. Question No. 1 had only 3 choices.

Step 4. Arrange the answer sheets so that only the first 5 questions show and tally them first.

Step 5. Tally first the answers given on the papers for the Upper-Upper 9 per cent and the Lower-Lower 9 per cent. They must be given double weighting so should be tallied separately from the remaining 20 per cent in the Upper Group and the remaining 20 per cent in the Lower Group.

Step 6. Indicate the answers given by the Upper-Upper Group in the very top row of each box. Use the bottom row in the lower half of the box to tally the responses made by the Lower-Lower Group.

Step 7. Tally all of one group first and then tally the other group so tally errors will not be made in switching from group to group.

Step 8. Continue tallying until all questions have been covered. If a test has 39 questions, for example, eight tabluation sheets will be needed.

Index of Discrimination

Step 9. Compute the per cent in the Upper Groups who answered the question correctly. In Question No. 1 of Figure 11–2, the maximum value on which the per cent must be computed is 38. There are only 29 papers in the upper groups, but the uppermost 9 must be given double weighting.

$$\#R = \text{Number Right}$$
$$UU = \text{Upper-Upper Group}$$
$$U = \text{Upper Group}$$
$$L = \text{Lower Group}$$
$$LL = \text{Lower-Lower Group}$$

$$\text{Upper Groups} = \frac{2\,(\#R_{UU}) + \#R_U}{2(\#\text{in }9\%_{UU}) + \#\text{in }20\%_U} = \frac{2\,(9) + 20}{2\,(9) + 20} = \frac{38}{38} = 100\%$$

$$\text{Lower Groups} = \frac{2\,(\#R_{LL}) + \#R_L}{2(\#\text{in }9\%_{LL}) + \#\text{in }20\%_L} = \frac{2\,(3) + 16}{2\,(9) + 20} = \frac{22}{38} = 58\%$$

The maximum value will remain constant for the entire analysis. It will be 38 for all the questions analyzed in this test because 100 papers were used. The weighted sum of the number who answered correctly is divided by the possible maximum to obtain the per cent for the Upper Groups and for the Lower Groups. The possible maximum will be 2(♯ of cases in 9%) + 1(♯ of cases in next highest 20%). The same possible maximum will be used as the constant in the Lower Groups. The double weighting is used for the extreme 9 per cent of the cases only when computing the Index of Discrimination.

Step. 10. Consult the Flanagan Table 11–2 to read out a correlation coefficient. Find 100 per cent, or the closest number to it, on the horizontal axis, and find 58 per cent on the vertical axis. The numbers converge at .66 which is the Index of Discrimination for this item. This particular question has good validity and would be retained if judged on this basis alone. It will be necessary to interpolate to approximate the coefficients for the per cents not given in the table.

Each wrong answer should correlate negatively with the criterion of the total test just as each correct answer should correlate positively. In other words, a greater number of students in the lower groups should select each incorrect answer.

Step 11. Figure all the percentages for the entire test and refer to the Flanagan Table when ready to obtain the coefficient for each of the items. The Index of Discrimination is considered acceptable if over .20. If between .15 and .19 it is questionable and if below .15, the question should be deleted or revised. The average Index of Discrimination for all the items in the test will probably fall between .30 and .40.

Variation of the Flanagan Method

Scott and French[13] report a variation of the Flanagan Method which gives a close approximation of the same results without requiring the same number of computational steps. The number answering correctly in each group is *not* converted into a percentage value.

$$\text{I.D.} = \frac{\text{Number right in upper groups} - \text{Number right in lower groups}}{\text{Number in one group}}$$

Example: Item #2 in Figure 11–2:

$$\text{I.D.} = \frac{25-14}{29} = \frac{11}{29} = .38$$

I.D. computed by the Flanagan Method = .42

Table 11–2. Product Moment Correlation Coefficients Corresponding to Various Proportions of Successes in the 29% Scoring Highest and Lowest*

Percentage of successes in the 29% scoring highest (top 9% weighted 2, next 20% weighted 1)

Percentage of successes in the 29% scoring lowest (bottom 9% counted twice)

	1	2	3	4	5	10	15	20	25	30	35	40	45	50	55	60	65	70	75	80	85	90	95	96	97	98	99
1	00	10	16	21	24	37	45	50	55	59	62	65	67	70	72	74	77	78	81	83	85	87	90	91	92	93	94
2	-10	00	06	11	15	28	36	43	47	52	55	59	62	64	67	70	72	75	77	79	82	85	88	89	90	91	93
3	-16	-06	00	05	09	22	30	37	42	47	51	55	58	61	64	66	69	72	75	77	80	83	87	88	89	90	92
4	-21	-11	-05	00	04	17	26	33	38	43	47	51	54	57	61	63	66	69	72	75	78	81	86	87	88	89	91
5	-24	-15	-09	-04	00	14	23	29	34	40	44	48	51	55	58	61	64	67	70	73	77	80	84	86	87	89	90
10	-37	-28	-22	-17	-14	00	10	17	23	28	32	37	41	45	49	52	56	59	63	66	70	75	80	81	83	85	87
15	-45	-36	-30	-26	-23	-10	00	08	14	19	24	29	33	37	41	45	49	53	57	61	65	70	77	78	80	82	85
20	-50	-43	-37	-33	-29	-17	-08	00	06	12	17	22	26	31	35	39	43	47	52	56	61	66	73	75	77	79	83
25	-55	-47	-42	-38	-34	-23	-14	-06	00	06	11	16	20	25	29	34	38	42	47	52	57	63	70	72	75	77	81
30	-59	-52	-47	-43	-40	-28	-19	-12	-06	00	05	10	15	20	24	28	33	38	42	47	53	59	67	69	72	75	78
35	-62	-55	-51	-47	-44	-32	-24	-17	-11	-05	00	05	10	14	19	24	28	33	38	43	49	56	64	66	69	72	77
40	-65	-59	-55	-51	-48	-37	-29	-22	-16	-10	-05	00	05	10	14	19	24	28	34	39	45	52	61	63	66	70	74
45	-67	-62	-58	-54	-51	-41	-33	-26	-20	-15	-10	-05	00	05	10	14	19	24	29	35	41	49	58	61	64	67	72
50	-70	-64	-61	-57	-55	-45	-37	-31	-25	-20	-14	-10	-05	00	05	10	14	20	25	31	37	45	55	57	61	64	70
55	-72	-67	-64	-61	-58	-49	-41	-35	-29	-24	-19	-14	-10	-05	00	05	10	15	20	26	33	41	51	54	58	62	67
60	-74	-70	-66	-63	-61	-52	-45	-39	-34	-28	-24	-19	-14	-10	-05	00	05	10	16	22	29	37	48	51	55	59	65
65	-77	-72	-69	-66	-64	-56	-49	-43	-38	-33	-28	-24	-19	-14	-10	-05	00	05	11	17	24	32	44	47	51	55	62
70	-78	-75	-72	-69	-67	-59	-53	-47	-42	-38	-33	-28	-24	-20	-15	-10	-05	00	06	12	19	28	40	43	47	52	59
75	-81	-77	-75	-72	-70	-63	-57	-52	-47	-42	-38	-34	-29	-25	-20	-16	-11	-06	00	06	14	23	34	38	42	47	55
80	-83	-79	-77	-75	-73	-66	-61	-56	-52	-47	-43	-39	-35	-31	-26	-22	-17	-12	-06	00	08	17	29	33	37	43	50
85	-85	-82	-80	-78	-77	-70	-65	-61	-57	-53	-49	-45	-41	-37	-33	-29	-24	-19	-14	-08	00	10	23	26	30	36	45
90	-87	-85	-83	-81	-80	-75	-70	-66	-63	-59	-56	-52	-49	-45	-41	-37	-32	-28	-23	-17	-10	00	14	17	22	28	37
95	-90	-89	-87	-86	-84	-80	-77	-73	-70	-67	-64	-61	-58	-55	-51	-48	-44	-40	-34	-29	-23	-14	00	04	09	15	24
96	-91	-89	-88	-87	-86	-81	-78	-75	-72	-69	-66	-63	-61	-57	-54	-51	-47	-43	-38	-33	-26	-17	-04	00	05	11	21
97	-92	-90	-89	-88	-87	-83	-80	-77	-75	-72	-69	-66	-64	-61	-58	-55	-51	-47	-42	-37	-30	-22	-09	-05	00	06	16
98	-93	-91	-90	-89	-89	-85	-82	-79	-77	-75	-72	-70	-67	-64	-62	-59	-55	-52	-47	-43	-36	-28	-15	-11	-06	00	10
99	-94	-93	-92	-91	-90	-87	-85	-83	-81	-78	-77	-74	-72	-70	-67	-65	-62	-59	-55	-50	-45	-37	-24	-21	-16	-10	00

* Flanagan, John C.: *Calculating Correlation Coefficients.* Pittsburgh, American Institute of Research, 1962. Adapted to 5-step interval and used by permission of John C. Flanagan. Copies of the complete table are available from the Institute at 410 Amberson

Difficulty Rating

Step 12. Count all in both groups who answered the question correctly and divide by the total number of papers being used in the analysis. The double weighting for the extreme 9 per cent is not used. See question No. 1 in Figure 11–2.

$$\text{D.R.} = \frac{\#R_U + \#R_L}{N_T} = \frac{\#R_T}{N_T} = \frac{29 + 19}{58} = \frac{48}{58} = 83\%$$

The higher the per cent the easier the question. If the question is answered correctly by over 90 per cent of the students, it is considered too easy. If answered correctly by fewer than 10 per cent of the students, it is considered too difficult. Revisions are indicated for such questions.

Items with Difficulty Ratings of 50 per cent are most desirable because they also discriminate maximally. The average Difficulty Rating for the entire test should be around 50 per cent.

Functioning of Responses

Step 13. Each choice should be appealing enough to be chosen by some of the students. Some authors indicate that at least 3 per cent of the students should use each response. Others list 2 per cent. Question No. 3 in Figure 11–2 shows that no one in either the upper or lower groups selected response No. 4. A revision of this choice is indicated.

Revisions

Step 14. When all the tallying and computational work have been completed, study the results to determine where revisions need to be made.

Step 15. Prepare a summary table of the item analysis to get an over-all picture of the quality of the test. See the one suggested in Figure 11–5.

Step 16. Indicate the revisions necessary in the "Revise" column. Refer to the test to study each question needing attention. Make revisions as they seem indicated.

Step 17. Re-type the test incorporating the revisions and have it ready for another administration. A subsequent item analysis will indicate how effective the revisions have been and will indicate further ones.

Test revision is a continuous, long-term process. Faithfully followed, the steps of revisions will result in a collection of written tests which are valid and reliable measuring instruments.

A closer look at Figure 11–2 reveals certain facts about the five questions treated on the tabulation sheet:

Question No. 1: Choice No. 3 did not function. Three choices were provided and only two of them were active. A true-false format might be better for this question idea. The question was very easy. The "Revise" column shows an F meaning that not all items functioned. The item must be changed for this reason.

Question No. 2: This question stood up pretty well. It discriminated fairly well, it was rather difficult, and all choices functioned. One person, in the upper group, omitted it.

Question No. 3: This question did poorly. As many in the lower groups answered it correctly as did in the upper groups, so the question completely failed to distinguish or discriminate between the better students and the poorer ones. Choices No. 2 and No. 3 were not very tempting and Choice No. 4 did not function at all. It was an easy question. Much revision is needed. Revision is needed because of *D*iffiulty *R*ating, *I*ndex of *D*iscrimination, and *F*unctioning of Items as shown in the last column.

Question No. 4: A difficult question, but it discriminated.

Question No. 5: More of the poorer students answered Question No. 5 correctly than the better or upper group of students. This question measured exactly what the teacher was *not* trying for the test to tell about the students. It definitely needs revision. Choice No. 4 was so attractive to the Upper Groups that the wording may have been misleading or perhaps the key was marked incorrectly. Choice No. 2 was not active so needs some attention. This particular item correlated negatively to what the total test was trying to measure. Response No. 4 reacted inversely. The lower group should choose all the incorrect answers more frequently than the upper group. The correct answers should produce positive correlation coefficients and the incorrect ones should produce negative ones.

b. The *Fan Method*[5] of Item Analysis is similar to the Flanagan Method suggested here but has at least two distinguishing features.

Table 11–3. Item Analysis Table: A table of item-difficulty and item-discrimination indices for given proportions of success in the highest 27 per cent and the lowest 27 per cent of a normal bivariate population*

UPPER PROPORTIONS

LOWER PROPORTIONS

(Table entries give item difficulty index p and discrimination index r for each combination of UPPER PROPORTIONS (rows) and LOWER PROPORTIONS (columns). The table is triangular; each cell shows "p r", and r = 0 along the diagonal where the upper and lower proportions are equal.)

	1		5		10		15		20		25		30		35		40		45		50		55		60		65		70		75		80		85		90		95	
	p	r	p	r	p	r	p	r	p	r	p	r	p	r	p	r	p	r	p	r	p	r	p	r	p	r	p	r	p	r	p	r	p	r	p	r	p	r	p	r
5	5	39	5	0																																					
10	6	47	7	15	10	0																																		
15	8	53	10	24	15	17	15	0																																
20	10	57	12	31	18	20	20	8	20	0																														
25	12	61	14	37	20	25	22	15	25	7	25	0																												
30	14	65	16	42	22	30	25	21	27	13	30	6	30	0																										
35	15	67	18	47	24	35	26	26	30	18	32	12	35	6	35	0																								
40	17	70	20	51	26	39	30	31	32	24	35	17	37	11	40	5	40	0																						
45	19	72	22	55	29	44	31	35	35	28	37	22	40	16	42	11	45	5	45	0																				
50	21	74	24	58	31	48	34	40	37	33	40	27	42	21	45	16	47	10	50	5	50	0																		
55	23	76	26	61	33	51	36	44	39	37	42	31	45	26	47	20	50	15	53	10	55	5	55	0																
60	25	78	29	64	35	55	39	48	42	42	45	36	47	31	50	25	53	20	55	15	58	10	60	5	60	0														
65	28	80	31	67	38	59	41	52	45	46	47	41	50	35	53	30	55	25	58	21	60	16	63	11	65	5	65	0												
70	30	82	33	70	40	62	44	56	47	50	50	45	53	40	55	35	58	31	60	26	63	21	65	17	68	12	70	6	70	0										
75	33	84	36	73	43	66	47	60	50	55	53	50	55	45	58	41	61	36	63	31	66	27	68	22	70	17	73	13	75	6	75	0									
80	36	86	39	75	46	69	50	64	53	59	56	55	58	51	61	46	64	42	66	37	68	32	71	28	73	24	76	18	78	15	80	8	80	0							
85	39	88	45	82	50	73	54	68	56	64	59	61	61	56	64	52	66	48	69	44	71	40	73	35	76	31	78	26	80	21	83	15	85	8	85	0				
90	43	90	50	85	55	77	57	73	61	69	62	65	65	62	67	59	70	55	72	51	74	48	76	44	79	39	81	35	84	30	86	24	88	18	90	10	90	0		
95	50	93	55	88	58	82	61	78	64	75	66	72	69	69	71	67	73	64	76	61	78	58	80	55	82	51	84	47	86	42	88	37	90	31	93	24	95	15	95	0
99	50	93	57	90	61	88	64	86	67	84	70	82	72	80	75	78	77	77	79	76	81	74	83	72	85	70	86	67	88	65	90	61	92	57	94	53	95	47	95	39

UPPER PROPORTIONS

* From *Item Analysis Table* by Chung-Teh Fan. Copyright © 1952 by Educational Testing Service. All rights reserved. Adapted by permission. The original tables, available from the Educational Testing Service, Princeton, New Jersey, are presented in one-interval format and should be consulted for actual item analysis work.

14

401

Fan works with the upper and lower 27 per cent of the papers and makes no provision for double weightings of the very good and very poor papers. In addition, he computes the Difficulty Rating differently. In other methods, all who answered correctly are counted regardless of the group they represent, *i.e.* upper or lower. Fan retains the group identity of the students answering correctly and establishes the difficulty index on the proportions of correct answers in each group. His conversion tables permit the use of the Upper and Lower proportions of those with the correct answers to ascertain both the Difficulty Index and the Index of Discrimination. This is computational efficiency and, according to Fan, a truer indication of the difficulty index. Table 11–3 gives the p (Difficulty Index) values and the r (Index of Discrimination) values for proportions ranging from 5 to 95. As in the Flanagan Table 11–2, either interpolations will have to be made to derive values between the 5 step intervals or the proportions will need to be rounded to the nearest 5th point before entering the table. If the proportion for the Lower 27 per cent is greater than the proportion for the Upper 27 per cent, the same table can be used by switching the axes but the r values will be negative.

c. Wood[15] suggests two other methods which are efficient for the classroom teacher because they require less computational work. They, nevertheless, provide adequate answers to the questions of test and item validity.

Procedure for a Large Number of Answer Sheets

Step 1. One hundred or more answer sheets should be available. Divide the papers into the upper and lower 50 per cent on the basis of the score on the total test.

Step 2. Tally the number of responses to each question for both groups and place in a summary chart as shown in Figure 11–3. A form could be designed to analyze 16 questions in two columns on one page.

Index of Discrimination

Step 3. Compute the per cent in each group who pass each item.

$$P_U = \frac{42}{50} = 84\%$$

$$P_L = \frac{22}{50} = 44\%$$

Step 4. Refer to the chart in Figure 11–4 to determine the correlation of the item to the total test.

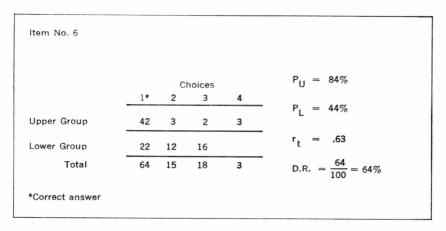

Fig. 11–3.   Tabulation form for the Wood method of item analysis.

Enter 84 on the vertical axis and 44 on the horizontal axis.   The correlation is interpolated at the point where the two numbers intersect on the chart.   The r_t or the *Index of Discrimination* is .63. The correlation is positive if P_U is larger than P_L.   If P_L is larger than P_U, the correlation will be negative and the chart will have to be used by reversing the P_U and P_L scales.   The tallies for the incorrect choices will permit a check on the negative correlations which are as essential to the incorrect choices as the positive ones are to the correct choices.   Use of the chart will show that the correlations for proportions above 99 per cent in either group are very difficult to determine.   The same is true when the proportions are nearing 0 per cent.

The correlation achieved by this method is called a tetrachoric r. It relates one dichotomy to another.   The usual correlation deals with a range of scores, while the tetrachoric accounts for only two categories on each axis.   In this instance, the student is in either the upper or lower group and the question was answered either correctly or incorrectly.   The use of the tetrachoric correlation for item analysis is not acceptable for commercially standardized tests. It has found some use, however, among classroom teachers seeking a method of establishing item validity which requires relatively few computational steps.

Difficulty Rating

Step 5.   Total the number of correct answers by both groups and divide by the total number to get the difficulty percentage of the question.   This is identical to the Flanagan Method.   Referring to the sample in Figure 11–3.

$$\text{D.R.} = \frac{\#R_U + \#R_L}{N} = \frac{42 + 22}{100} = \frac{64}{100} = 64\%$$

The question was fairly easy.

Functioning of Responses

Step 6. The tally for the incorrect choices, or the distractors, will show something of the frequency with which each choice was selected.

Procedure for Small Number of Answer Sheets

Step 1. Count the number of correct answers to each question in the upper group and divide by the number in the group.

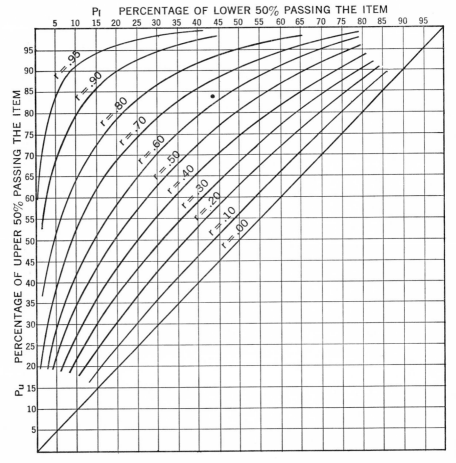

Fig. 11–4. Chart for computing tetrachoric r with the criterion dichotomized at the median. (Wood, Dorothy Adkins, *Test Construction.* Columbus, Ohio, Charles E. Merrill Books, Inc., 1960, p. 85. Used by permission of the publishers.)

Step 2. Count the number of correct answers to each question in the lower group and divide by the number in the group.

Step 3. Sometimes a quick glance of the results will reveal the estimated validity of the item. If a greater proportion of the upper group pass the item, the item correlates positively with the criterion, *i.e.* the total test. When the two percentages are about equal, the item fails to discriminate and serves no useful purpose in the test. If more of the lower group than the upper group pass the item, it correlates negatively with the total test and causes the validity of the total test to decrease.

The results of the tetrachoric correlation, particularly when used on small groups, may be accepted with less confidence because of small sampling errors. Observations of the item tally, such as presented in Figure 11–3, will usually provide sufficient information to help the classroom teacher plan for the revision of items.

Reliability. The *reliability* indicates the *consistency* with which a test can rank the students from good to poor. It is influenced in written tests by several factors. The length of the test, or the number of items, determines the reliability to a great extent. The more items, the greater the reliability will be, excluding such factors as fatigue, boredom, and the like. The reliability is also affected by the ability of the items to discriminate. The testing situation plays an influencing role. The more closely the items measure knowledge in one area of information, the more likely that the reliability will be high.

If the test is too easy, the reliability will be lowered. For example, if a 50-item test has a mean score of 43, the reliability will be low because all the students cluster toward the top of the scale, preventing a normal distribution and a greater range of the scores. The average difficulty level of an entire test should be about 50 per cent of the number of items. When this is the case, the reliability coefficient will give a truer picture of the test consistency.

(*1*) *Assumed Reliability Method.* Many authors believe that a valid test will automatically produce a reliable one. They see no need in computing a statistical reliability coefficient. The classroom teacher is not likely to spend a lot of time determining the reliability of a test unless he is making a concerted effort to get his collection of tests into good shape. If the test has sufficient items, if its content is homogeneous, if its difficulty level is stabilized around 50 per cent, if its scores have a good range, then it is probably safe to assume adequate test reliability.

(*2*) *The Test-Retest Method.* This method requires two administrations of the complete test to the same group. The two scores for each student are correlated and a reliability coefficient is the outcome. A coefficient indicative of the *stability* of the test results.

Sometimes substantial memory and learning factors have undue influence on the coefficient. At times the students are bored with the second administration. They fail to be motivated to perform at their best because they consider the second testing senseless. The test-retest method of establishing reliability is probably more appropriate to various motor tests than it is to written tests. In any case, very careful administrative considerations would have to be made concerning the time element and the motivation of the students.

(3) *The Parallel Forms Method.* The test constructor prepares two tests covering the same topic which are similar in content balance, length, difficulty, and discriminating power. Both forms are administered to the same group, and the two scores are correlated to obtain the reliability. The coefficient indicates the *equivalency* of the two forms. This method rests on the assumption that the two forms are actually parallel. Such a quality is difficult to achieve.

Parallel forms of a test are more prevalent in written tests than in motor tests. Officials' ratings exams are often prepared in two forms so a person may have a second chance if he fails on the first attempt. Parallel forms could be used to measure progress from the beginning to the end of a unit. If the tests are measuring the same thing to the same degree, comparison of the two test scores is reasonable.

The use of parallel forms of written tests by the average classroom teacher is very rare. As more commercially standardized tests become available, this application of tests will be possible.

(4) *The Split-Halves Method.* This method of establishing reliability is one of determining the *internal* consistency of a test.

A single test is administered to a group. Two scores are noted for each paper: one for all the correct even-numbered questions, and one for all the correct odd-numbered questions. A correlation is computed. The r which results is actually the reliability of a test only half the length of the one administered. The Spearman-Brown Prophecy Formula[9] is utilized to predict the reliability for the full length of the test. The use of this formula[9] has been discussed in Chapter 5 on Statistical Techniques and will be applied here.

$$r_{tt} = \frac{2\,r_{hh}}{1+r_{hh}} \qquad\qquad r_{tt} = \text{correlation for the total test}$$

$$r_{tt} = \frac{(2)\,(.65)}{1+.65} = \frac{1.30}{1.65} = .79 \qquad\qquad r_{hh} = \text{correlation obtained on the two halves (}e.g. = .65\text{)}$$

Table 5–7 could be used to make the conversion instead of solving the formula. Items will need to be added to the test if a higher reliability coefficient than .79 is desired.

The results of this procedure are partially influenced by the arrangement of the test items. If all the difficult questions happen to be odd-numbered questions, for example, the reliability coefficient would be adversely affected. The formula operates on the assumption that the difficult items are evenly distributed between the two halves of the test.

(5) *Kuder-Richardson Formula Method.*[12] There are many variations of this formula which have been designed especially for use with written tests. Only one administration of the test is required. The test does not need to be split into odd-even or first and second halves, for example. Therefore, the different results caused by different methods of dividing the test are eliminated. This method does not require the correlation and so reduces the amount of the computational work. It does, however, operate on the same assumptions as the Spearman-Brown Prophecy Formula with regard to item difficulty and discrimination. The Kuder-Richardson formula is considered to provide the lower limit of what the real reliability of a test may be.

$$r_{tt} = \frac{n\sigma_t^2 - M(n-M)}{(n-1)\sigma_t^2}$$

r_{tt} = reliability of total test
n = number of items in test
M = Mean of the scores
σ_t^2 = Standard Deviation of the test scores squared

Example: n = 55 items
M = 30
SD = 8

$$r_{tt} = \frac{(55)(64) - 30(55-30)}{(55-1)(64)}$$

$$= \frac{3520 - 30(25)}{3456}$$

$$= \frac{3520 - 750}{3456}$$

$$= \frac{2770}{3456}$$

$$= .802 \text{ or } .80$$

The teacher will want to know the mean and standard deviation of the test scores anyway. With this information available, the teacher can apply the Kuder-Richardson formula to ascertain the reliability of the test.

None of the methods discussed for arriving at test reliability should be used for speed tests. The introduction of the speed factor is not compatible with the assumptions of the various formulas.

Summary Table

Name of Test_____ Groups Tested_____ Dates_____

No. of answer sheets used in Analysis_____.

Content   *Scores*

    Total number of items_____   Mean _____
        Multiple Choice_____.   Standard
        True-False   _____   Deviation_____
        Matching   _____
        Classification   _____
        Rearrangement _____
        Completion   _____

Validity

	Number	*Per Cent*	*Judgment*
Difficulty Rating (Between 10% and 90%)			
Above 90%	_____	_____	_____
Between 11% and 90%	_____	_____	_____
Below 10%	_____	_____	_____
Index of Discrimination (Above .19)			
Above .19	_____	_____	_____
Between .16 and .19	_____	_____	_____
Below .16	_____	_____	_____
Functioning of Responses (3%)			
All responses function	_____	_____	_____
1 response fails to function	_____	_____	_____
2 responses fail to function	_____	_____	_____
More than 2 fail to function	_____	_____	_____

Reliability

    Method Used   _____
    Coefficient   _____   _____

Comments

Date of Report_____

Test Analyzer _____

Fig. 11–5.   Suggested form-summary table for analysis of written tests.

A teacher should have a file folder for each test which should include a copy of the test, the key, the content analysis, the item analysis, the norms, and a summary table. All of this information will be helpful when he decides to revise the test. It is not wise to file the copies of the test with the key.

Sources of Knowledge Tests

Andrews, Emily R., Helen W. Smith, Mary Lou Paul Squance, and Marion Russell: *Physical Education for Girls and Women*, 2nd ed., Englewood Cliffs, N.J., Prentice-Hall, Inc., 1963. Includes quizzes on 20 different activities.

Blaess, Nancy N.: The Development of an Archery Knowledge Test, MSPE, Springfield College, Springfield, Mass., 1965.

Brown Physical Education Activities Series, Dubuque, Iowa: Wm. C. Brown Co. A test manual is available for each of the 35 activities in the series.

Broer, Marion R., and Donna Mae Miller: Achievement Test for Beginning and Intermediate Tennis, Research Quarterly, *21*, 303–321, October, 1950.

Crickenberger, Margaret E.: Golf Knowledge Test, *Bowling-Fencing-Golf Guide, 1956–58*. Washington, D.C. AAHPER, 1956, pp. 118–122.

Dintiman, George B., and Loyd M. Barrow: *Instruction and Evaluation Manual for Teachers to Accompany a Comprehensive Manual of Physical Education Activities for Men*, New York: Appleton-Century-Crofts Educational Division, Meredith Corporation, 1970. Contains 24 knowledge tests.

Droste, Mildred A.: Written Tennis Tests, *Tennis-Badminton Guide, 1952–1954*. Washington, D.C., AAHPER, 1952, pp. 88–90.

Durocher, Lillian M.: Written Speedball Examinations for Senior High Schools, *Soccer-Speedball Guide, 1956–1958*. Washington, D.C., AAHPER, 1956, pp. 87–89.

Educational Testing Service, AAHPER Cooperative Physical Education Tests for Elementary, Junior High School, and Senior High School, Princeton, New Jersey: Educational Testing Service, 1970.

Ewers, J. B.: Proficiency Examinations in Physical Education for Men at the Ohio State University, Ph.D., Ohio State University, 1963. Contains knowledge tests for 5 activities and for general Physical Education.

Fait, Hollis F., John H. Shaw, Grace I. Fox, and Cecil B. Hollingsworth: *A Manual of Physical Education Activities*, 2nd ed., Philadelphia, W. B. Saunders Co., 1961. Includes tests on 38 different activities.

Goll, Lillian M.: Construction of Badminton and Swimming Knowledge Tests for High School Girls, Unpublished Master's Thesis, Illinois State University, Normal, 1956.

Hambright, Joanne: A Written Knowledge Test for the Fifth Grade Students at Archery Elementary School, MSPE, University of North Carolina at Greensboro, Greensboro, N. C., 1965.

Hennis, Gail M.: Construction of Knowledge Test in Selected Physical Education Activities for College Women, Research Quarterly, *27*, 301–309, October, 1956.

Hewitt, Jack E.: Hewitt's Comprehensive Tennis Knowledge Test—Form A and B Revised, Research Quarterly, *35*, 147–155, May, 1964.

Hodges, Carolyn V.: Construction of an Objective Knowledge Test and Skill Tests in Lacrosse for College Women, MSPE, University of North Carolina at Greensboro, Greensboro, N. C., 1967.

Hooks, E. W.: Hooks' Comprehensive Knowledge Test in Selected Physical Education Activities for College Men, Research Quarterly, *37*, 506–514, December, 1966.

Houndeshell, James D.: An Undergraduate Major's Comprehensive Examination in Selected Physical Education Courses, P. E. D., Indiana University, Bloomington, Indiana, 1968.

Karst, Ralph R.: The Development of Standards of Potential Achievement in Physical Education, Ph.D., U. of Wisconsin, Madison, Wisconsin, 1967.

Ley, Katherine: Construction of Objective Test Items to Measure High Levels of Achievement in Selected Physical Education Activities, Ph.D. in Physical Education, State University of Iowa, Iowa City, Iowa, 1960.

McCutcheon, Sallie: The Construction of an Objective Basketball Knowledge Examination for College Women, MSPE, University of North Carolina at Greensboro, Greensboro, N. C., 1965.

McGee, Rosemary: A Golf Knowledge Test for High School Girls, *Individual Sports Guide, 1952-54.* Washington, D.C., AAHPER, 1952, pp. 109-112.

Moore, Alan C., and I. F. Waglow: Lacrosse Knowledge Test, The Mentor, *6*, 26-27, 36-37, April, 1956.

Palmer, Wendell L.: An Evaluation of a Speed-a-way Knowledge Test, MSPE, Fort Hays State College, Fort Hays, Kansas, 1961.

Power, William Brainerd: A Knowledge Test in Touch Football for Junior High Boys, MSPE, University of California, Los Angeles, 1959.

Seaton, Don Cash, I. A. Clayton, Howard C. Leibee, and L. Messersmith: *Physical Education Handbook.* 5th ed., Englewood Cliffs, N.J., Prentice-Hall, Inc., 1969. Includes written tests on 22 activities.

Wade, Michael G.: A Proficiency Examination for the Foundations of Physical Education (PEM 100) Lecture Materials, MSPE, University of Illinois, Urbana, 1968.

Waglow, Irving Frederick: A Measurement and Evaluation Manual for the Department of Required Physical Education at the University of Florida, Ed.D., New York University, New York, 1964. Contains knowledge tests for 14 activities.

Walker, William P.: The Development of a General Knowledge Inventory Test and a Resource Syllabus for a Foundation Course in Physical Education for College Freshmen, Ph.D., Florida State University, Tallahassee, Florida, 1965.

References

1. AAHPER, *Knowledge and Understanding in Physical Education.* Washington, D.C.: AAHPER, 1969.

2. AAHPER: *Research Methods in Health, Physical Education, Recreation.* 2nd ed., Washingtou, D.C., AAHPER, 1959.

3. Angoff, William H.: Test Reliability and Effective Test Length, Psychometrika, *18*, 1-14, 1953.

4. Ebel, Robert L.: How to Judge the Quality of a Classroom Test. Technical Bulletin No. 7, The Examination Service of the State University of Iowa, Iowa City, Iowa, September, 1955.

5. Fan, Chung-Teh: Notes on Construction of an Item Analysis Table for High-Low 27 Per Cent Group Method, Psychometrika, *19*, 231-237, September, 1954.

6. Flanagan, John C.: *Calculating Correlation Coefficients.* Pittsburgh, American Institute of Research and University of Pittsburgh, 1962.

7. ———: Statistical Method Related to Test Construction, Review of Educational Research, *11*, 109, February, 1941.

8. Green, John A.: *Teacher-made Tests.* New York, Harper & Row, 1963.

9. Guilford, J. P.: *Fundamental Statistics in Psychology and Education.* 4th Ed., New York, McGraw-Hill Book Co., 1965.

10. Lindquist, E. F. (Ed.): *Educational Measurement.* Washington, D.C.: American Council on Education, 1951.

11. Meyers, Carlton R., and T. Erwin Blesh: *Measurement in Physical Education,* New York, The Ronald Press, 1962.

12. Richardson, M. M., and G. F. Kuder: The Calculation of Test Reliability Coefficients Based on the Method of Rational Equivalence, Journal of Educational Psychology, *30*, 681, December, 1939.

13. Scott, M. Gladys, and Esther French: *Measurement and Evaluation in Physical Education.* Dubuque, Iowa, Wm. C. Brown Co., Publishers, 1959.

14. Stanley, Julian C., *Measurement in To-day's Schools.* 4th Ed., Englewood Cliffs, N.J. Prentice-Hall, Inc., 1964.

15. Wood, Dorothy Adkins: *Test Construction.* Columbus, Ohio, Charles E. Merrill Books, Inc., 1960.

Chapter 12
SOCIOPSYCHOLOGICAL MEASURES

Physical Educators have tried to use the holistic approach to the teaching of children. They have concentrated on physical development realizing that mental and social development must accompany it. Categories such as fitness and skill have been used as a convenience to insure identification. The teacher knows they are not developed in a vacuum. The same is true of the often used physical, mental, and social categories or with the psychomotor, cognitive, and affective areas respectively. They all interrelate, react, and influence one another. The learning process develops in all three areas as the education of the student is planned to change behavior. The measures included in this chapter are related to the sociopsychological area or to affective behavior. They are listed in the three categories of Social Measures, Attitude Measures, and Self-Concept Measures as an organizational necessity and not because the student develops these concepts in isolation.

SOCIAL MEASURES

The measures of social factors include such concepts as sportsmanship, leadership, acceptance, behavior, ethics, values, character, and adjustment. The instruments are presented in two categories: first, those which call for the student to make a response about himself; and second, those which call for a response about the students to be made by a teacher or a classmate. When the student makes a response about his own behavior, habits, and beliefs, he becomes aware of some social values worthy of attaining and is more cognizant of them as they occur in physical education situations. Scales used by teachers and classmates also delve into the concepts of behavior, habits, and acceptance but they are assessments of someone else. They differ from the scales filled out by the student because they use an observer who makes the judgment *about* the student.

Johnson Sportsmanship Attitude Scales*

Purpose. To evaluate the sportsmanship attitudes of junior high school boys and girls.

Evaluation. Alternate form sportsmanship attitude scales were developed using the scale-discrimination technique. The reliability coefficient be-

---

* Johnson, Marion Lee: Construction of Sportsmanship Attitude Scales, Research Quarterly, *40*, 312–316, May, 1969. Used by permission of the AAHPER and the author.

tween forms A and B was .856.   The coefficients of reproducibility were .812
and .863 for Forms A and B respectively.   The content is based on football,
basketball, and baseball situations.   The data represent 167 boys and girls
in the 7th, 8th, and 9th grades.[8]

Level and Sex.   Junior high school boys and girls.

Uses.   To ascertain sportsmanship attitude status.
To study changes in attitude.
To use as discussion points in class.

Directions.   This booklet contains several statements describing events
that happen in sports and games.   Read each statement carefully and
decide whether you approve or disapprove of the action taken by the person.   Circle the ONE response category that tells the way you feel.
PLEASE COMPLETE *EVERY* ITEM.

Example: A pitcher in a baseball game threw a fast ball at the batter
to scare him.

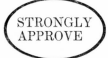

    STRONGLY   STRONGLY
     APPROVE   APPROVE   DISAPPROVE   DISAPPROVE

(If you strongly approve of this action by the pitcher, you would circle
the first response category as shown.)

The four responses can appear either after each item or an answer sheet
can be used.

The Scales: Form A

1. After a basketball player was called by the official for traveling, he
    slammed the basketball onto the floor.
2. A baseball player was called out as he slid into home plate.   He
    jumped up and down on the plate and screamed at the official.
3. After a personal foul was called against a basketball player, he shook
    his fist in the official's face.
4. A basketball coach talked very loudly in order to annoy an opponent
    who was attempting to make a very important free throw shot.
5. After a baseball game the coach of the losing team went up to the
    umpire and demanded to know how much money had been paid to
    "throw" the game.
6. A basketball coach led the spectators in jeering at the official who made
    calls against his team.
7. After two men were put out on a double play attempt, a baseball coach
    told the players in his dugout to boo the umpire's decision.
8. As the basketball coach left the gymnasium after the game, he shouted
    at the officials, "You lost me the game; I never saw such lousy officiat-
    ing in my life."
9. A basketball coach put sand on the gym floor to force the opponents
    into traveling penalties.
10. A football coach left the bench to change the position of a marker
    dropped by an official to indicate where the ball went out of bounds.
11. During the first half of a football game a touchdown was called back.
    At halftime, the football coach went into the official's dressing room
    and cursed the officials.
12. A football player was taken out of the game for unsportsmanlike con-

duct. The player changed jerseys and the coach sent him back into the game.

13. Following a closely played basketball game, the coach of the losing team cursed his boys for not winning.
14. After a baseball game the losing team's coach yelled at spectators to "Go get the Ump!"
15. A baseball coach permitted players to use profanity loud enough for the entire park to hear when the players did not like a decision.
16. The basketball coach drank alcoholic beverages while supervising his basketball team on a trip.
17. A college football player was disqualified for misconduct. While on the way to the sideline, the player attacked the official.
18. During a time-out in a basketball game, the clock was accidentally left running. The coach whose team was behind ran over to the scoring table and struck the timekeeper.
19. After a basketball player was knocked into a wall, his coach rushed onto the court and hit the player who had fouled.
20. After a baseball player had been removed from the game, the coach met him at the sidelines and hit him.
21. After a runner was called out at first base, the baseball coach went onto the field and wrestled the umpire down to the ground.

Form B

1. During a basketball game the B team coach sat on the bench and called loudly to the officials telling them who to watch for fouls.
2. Repeated complaints and griping came from the football players on the bench toward the officials when fouls were called on their team, and the coach did nothing to stop this action.
3. After a basketball game the hometown coach made fun of the visiting team's playing ability.
4. A football coach took time out and came onto the playing field and accused referees of cheating his team.
5. During a football game a player made an error that resulted in a touchdown for the opponents. The coach ran onto the field and bawled out the player in front of the fans.
6. After a questionable foul was called against a football player, his coach went onto the field and refused to leave when the referee told him to do so.
7. During a basketball game the coach of the losing team yelled that the officials had been "paid off" by the opposing team.
8. A baseball coach acted as referee for an important game and called in favor of his team.
9. A basketball coach installed a light to blind the opponents when they were shooting at a goal.
10. After a third baseman caught a ball which put a player out, the opposing coach cursed the third baseman.
11. A football coach used profane language during workouts and in conversation with the boys.
12. A baseball coach cursed loudly after a runner was called out on first base.
13. After a football game a player attacked the official who had taken him out of the game. The coach covered up for the player and said the player had not done such a thing.

14. At a basketball game students in a balcony spat on the opposing team and coach.
15. A basketball coach went onto the court and shook an official who had called fouls against his team.
16. After a football game, the captain of the winning team was hit by the captain of the losing team when the winner tried to shake hands.
17. A baseball coach instructed his players to file their cleats to sharpen them in order to injure opponents.
18. A football coach stepped to the sideline in front of the player's bench and kicked an opposing player who had just made a tackle.
19. Between innings the coach of the losing baseball team grabbed the umpire and threw him to the ground.
20. Before a baseball game a coach went into the umpire's dressing room and offered him money to help his team win.
21. In a football game the visiting team was penalized for roughing the kicker. The coach of the visiting team rushed onto the field and hit an official.

Scoring: Each of the items is stated negatively, *i.e.* to illustrate a poor act of sportsmanship. Scoring values would be 0 for Strongly Approve, 1 for Approve, 2 for Disapprove, and 3 for Strongly Disapprove. There is a maximum of 63 points on each form. The higher the total value, the more the student disapproves of unsportsmanlike events and consequently, the better his sportsmanship attitude.

Behavior-Attitude Check List*

Purpose. To provide a self-appraisal of everyday behavior in a physical education class.

Level and Sex. Developed for high school girls but adaptable for use with boys.

Uses. To give periodically during the year.
To motivate development of good habits.
To stimulate awareness of what constitutes good behavior.

The Check List

Name_____ Date_____

Directions: Read each statement and think how it will describe your behavior. Put a check in the column that tells most nearly what statement is correct for you.

Always	Often	Seldom	Never	SELF-DIRECTION
				1. I work diligently even though I am not supervised.
				2. I practice to improve the skills I use with least success.
				3. I follow carefully directions that have been given me.

* Teachers Guide to Physical Education for Girls in High School. Compiled by Genevie Dexter, State Department of Education, State of California, Sacramento, 1957, p. 318. Used by permission of the Department.

Always Often Seldom Never

4. I willingly accept constructive criticism and try to correct faults.
5. I play games as cheerfully as I can.
6. I appraise my progress in each of my endeavors to learn.

Social Adjustment

1. I am considerate of the rights of others.
2. I am courteous.
3. I am cooperative in group activities.
4. I accept gladly responsibility assigned me by a squad leader.
5. I accept disappointment without being unnecessarily disturbed.
6. I expect from the members of my group only the consideration to which I am entitled.

Participation

1. I am prompt in reporting for each class.
2. I dislike being absent from class.
3. I ask to be excused from an activity only when it is necessary.
4. I do the best I can regardless of the activity in which I am participating.
5. I give full attention to all instructions that are given in class.
6. I encourage others with whom I am participating in an activity.

Care of Equipment and Facilities

1. I use equipment as I am supposed to use it.
2. I return each piece of equipment to its proper place after using it.
3. I avoid making my dressing area untidy.
4. I arrange my clothes neatly in my locker.

Personal Attractiveness

1. I am particular about my personal appearance.
2. I take a shower after I have participated in any vigorous activity.
3. I wear clean clothes in physical education.
4. I dress appropriately for each activity.
5. I bathe regularly even during my menstrual period.

Outcomes of Sports: An Evaluation Check-Sheet*

Purpose. To measure the outcomes of sports so players, coaches, administrators, and parents may know.

Level and Sex. Designed for use with secondary school boys in varsity sports activities.

Scoring. There are a possible 100 points on the check sheet.

Uses. To use as a departure for discussion at the beginning of the season. To use at the end of the season.
To use with constituents in public relations efforts.

OUTCOME OF SPORTS: AN EVALUATION CHEEK-SHEET

	(5) A Very Great Deal	(4) A Great Deal	(3) Somewhat	(2) Very Little	(1) Not at All
1. To sacrifice my own personal "whims" or desires for the good of the group or team?					
2. To test myself—to see if I could "take it," endure hardship and "keep trying" to do my best even under adversity?					
3. To overcome awkwardness and self-consciousness?					
4. To recognize that the group can achieve where the individual alone cannot?					
5. That each team member has a unique or special contribution to make in the position he plays?					
6. To share difficult undertakings with my "buddies" (teammates) because of struggling together for a goal?					
7. To respect the skill and ability of my opponents and be tolerant of their success?					
8. To make friendships with boys from other schools and to maintain good guest-host relationships in inter-school games?					
9. To feel that the school team helped break up "cliques" and factions in the school by developing common loyalty and community of interests?					

* Cowell, Charles C.: Our Function is Still Education!, The Physical Educator, *14*, 6–7, March, 1957. Used by permission of the Phi Epsilon Kappa Fraternity.

	(5) A Very Great Deal	(4) A Great Deal	(3) Somewhat	(2) Very Little	(1) Not at All
10. To consider and practice correct health and training routine such as proper eating, sleeping, avoidance of tobacco, etc.?					
11. To "take turns" and to "share"?					
12. To develop physical strength, endurance and a better looking body?					
13. To be loyal and not "let my buddy, the coach, team, or school down"?					
14. To give more than I get—not for myself but for an ideal or for one's school, town, or country?					
15. To develop a sense of humor and even to be able to laugh at myself occasionally?					
16. To think and act "on the spot" in the heat of a game?					
17. To understand the strategy—the "why" of the best methods of attack and defense in games?					
18. To understand and appreciate the possibility and limitations of the human body with respect to skill, speed, endurance, and quickness of reactions?					
19. That in sports there is no discrimination against talent? It is performance and conduct and not the color of one's skin or social standing that matters.					
20. That nothing worthwhile is accomplished without hard work, application, and the "will to succeed"?					

Peterson Social Efficiency Scale*

Purpose. To evaluate social efficiency in 9 sub-areas and as a total concept.

Evaluation. This scale was devised by using 2 character and personality trait actions from the McCloy[9,10] rating scale, 11 trait actions from O'Neel's[12] scale and 25 from Blanchard's[2] rating scale. The use of sub-

* Peterson, Beverly A.: A Comparison of the Social Efficiency of Selected Groups of Tenth- and Twelfth-Grade Girls, M.A., San Diego State College, 1965. Used by permission of the author.

categories was designed to aid in the validity of the instrument.   The scale was developed using 200 10th and 12th grade girls.

Level and Sex.   Secondary school girls.

Uses.   To identify areas in which social efficiency needs enhancing.   To use as an instrument for evaluation by the instructor, by classmates, and to compare results with a self-evaluation.

Directions.   Ratings are based on behavior frequencies.   The rater circles the appropriate numbers on the form.

The Instrument.

BEHAVIOR RATING SCALE

Name of Person Rated_____ Grade——— Age__

Name of Rater _____ School _____

Personal Information	No Opportunity To Observe	Frequency of Observation					Score
		Never	Seldom	Fairly Often	Frequently	Extremely Often	
Leadership 1. She is popular with classmates .		1	2	3	4	5	
2. She shows intellectual leadership in the class		1	2	3	4	5	
3. She schemes, works underhandedly to get her way		5	4	3	2	1	
4. She advances ideas to which group pays attention		1	2	3	4	5	
Positive Active Qualities 5. She quits on tasks requiring perseverance.		5	4	3	2	1	
6. She exhibits aggressiveness in her relationship with others . . .		1	2	3	4	5	
7. She shows initiative in assuming responsibility in unfamiliar situations		1	2	3	4	5	
8. She is alert to new opportunities .		1	2	3	4	5	
9. She gives of her best efforts even when the team is losing . . .		1	2	3	4	5	

Personal Information	No Opportunity To Observe	Frequency of Observation					Score
		Never	Seldom	Fairly Often	Frequently	Extremely Often	
10. She avoids disagreeable duties through excuses, fake injuries, etc.		5	4	3	2	1	
Positive Mental Qualities 11. She shows keeness of mind . .		1	2	3	4	5	
12. She volunteers ideas		1	2	3	4	5	
Self-Control 13. She grumbles over decisions of classmates		5	4	3	2	1	
14. She takes a justified criticism by teacher or classmate without showing anger or pouting . . .		1	2	3	4	5	
15. She controls herself when provoked.		1	2	3	4	5	
16. She swears freely		5	4	3	2	1	
Cooperation 17. She is loyal to her group . . .		1	2	3	4	5	
18. She discharges her group responsibilities well		1	2	3	4	5	
19. She is cooperative in her attitude toward the teacher		1	2	3	4	5	
20. She hogs the ball (or other equipment)		5	4	3	2	1	
21. She plays to the gallery . . .		5	4	3	2	1	
Social Action Standards 22. She makes loud-mouthed criticisms and comments . . .		5	4	3	2	1	
23. She respects the rights of others		1	2	3	4	5	

Personal Information	No Opportunity To Observe	Frequency of Observation					Score
		Never	Seldom	Fairly Often	Frequently	Extremely Often	
24. She makes fun of others who like games she does not like . . .		5	4	3	2	1	
25. She razzes, teases, or bullies opponents		5	4	3	2	1	
26. She acts like a good sport toward opponents		1	2	3	4	5	
Ethical Social Qualities 27. She cheats		5	4	3	2	1	
28. She is truthful		1	2	3	4	5	
29. She takes decisions, wins, and losses in good spirit		1	2	3	4	5	
30. She "crabs" about officiating . .		5	4	3	2	1	
Qualities of Efficiency 31. She seems satisfied to "get by" with tasks assigned		5	4	3	2	1	
32. She is dependable and trustworthy		1	2	3	4	5	
33. She works conscientiously to perfect her form in sports . . .		1	2	3	4	5	
34. She thinks ahead of the play . .		1	2	3	4	5	
Sociability 35. She is liked by others		1	2	3	4	5	
36. She makes a friendly approach to others in the group		1	2	3	4	5	
37. She is chosen by others of group as preferred companion in some activity		1	2	3	4	5	
38. She shows timidity, hurt feelings, oversensitiveness		5	4	3	2	1	

Scoring: The circled values are summed and divided by the number of items (38) to get an index of social efficiency. This can be done for each part of the scale as well as for the total scale. The best possible score would be a five and the poorest would be a one for each item.

Cowell Social Adjustment Index*

Purpose. To measure the positive and negative behavioral trends of each student.

Evaluation. The validity was based on the ability of the scale to distinguish between junior high school boys who made good or poor social adjustment in physical education. The reliability was reported to be .82.

Level and Sex. The Index was developed for junior high school boys but is appropriate for use with all secondary school boys and girls.

Scoring. The total differential score for the Form A items minus the corresponding scores for the Form B items are added to give the raw score. A high plus score is indicative of good social adjustment; a minus score is indicative of poor social adjustment.

* Cowell, Charles C.: Validating an Index of Social Adjustment for High School Use. Research Quarterly, *29*, 7–18, March, 1958. Used by permission of the AAHPER.

The Index

FORM A

Date:_____ Grade:____

School: _____ Age:____

_____ Describer: _____
Last name   First name

Instruction: Think carefully of the student's behavior in group situations; check each behavior trend according to its degree of descriptiveness.

	Descriptive of the Student			
Behavior trends	*Markedly* (*3*)	*Some— what* (*2*)	*Only slightly* (*1*)	*Not at all* (*0*)
1. Enters heartily and with enjoyment into the spirit of social intercourse.				
2. Frank, talkative and sociable, does not stand on ceremony.				
3. Self-confident and self-reliant, tends to take success for granted, strong initiative, prefers to lead.				
4. Quick and decisive in movement, pronounced or excessive energy output.				
5. Prefers group activities, work or play, not easily satisfied with individual projects.				
6. Adaptable to new situations, makes adjustments readily, welcomes change.				
7. Is self-composed, seldom shows signs of embarrassment.				
8. Tends to elation of spirits, seldom gloomy or moody.				
9. Seeks a broad range of friendships, not selective or exclusive in games and the like.				
10. Hearty and cordial, even to strangers, forms acquaintanceships very easily.				

FORM B

Date:_____ Grade:_____

School: _____ Age:_____

_____ Describer: _____
Last name   First name

Instruction: Think carefully of the student's behavior in group situations; check each behavior trend according to its degree of descriptiveness.

Behavior trends	*Descriptive of the Student*			
	Markedly (−3)	*Some-what* (−2)	*Only slightly* (−1)	*Not at all* (−0)
1. Somewhat prudish, awkward, easily embarrassed in his social contacts.				
2. Secretive, seclusive, not inclined to talk unless spoken to.				
3. Lacking in self-confidence and initiative, a follower.				
4. Slow in movement, deliberative or perhaps indecisive. Energy output moderate or deficient.				
5. Prefers to work and play alone, tends to avoid group activities.				
6. Shrinks from making new adjustments, prefers the habitual to the stress of reorganization required by the new.				
7. Is self-conscious, easily embarrassed, timid, or "bashful."				
8. Tends to depression, frequently gloomy or moody.				
9. Shows preference for a narrow range of intimate friends and tends to exclude others from his association.				
10. Reserved and distant except to intimate friends, does not form acquaintanceships readily.				

A Subjective Rating Scale for Social, Personal, and Emotional Development*

Purpose. To rate the social, personal, and emotional development of children in the first six grades.

Uses. To use every marking period.
To follow the progress of development of very young children.

* Physical Education—Guide for North Dakota Elementary Schools, Grades 1–6. Department of Public Instruction, Bismarck, North Dakota, 1960, p. 17. Used by permission of the Department.

THE RATING SCALE

A subjective Rating Scale for Social, Personal, and Emotional Development

Name of Student _____ Year _____

Check each basic factor each marking period and record final mark on left (See example on Interest).

Basic Factors	Definition of Basic Factors	Final Mark Abv. Ave.	Final Mark Ave.	Final Mark Bel. Ave.	Above Average Marking Period 1	2	3	4	5	6	Average Marking Period 1	2	3	4	5	6	Below Average Marking Period 1	2	3	4	5	6
Interest	Concern for the activity	X					X	X	X	X	X	X					X					
Effort	Conscientious exertion to achieve																						
Self-Control	Ability to control inner feelings																						
Dependability	Reliability and trustworthiness																						
Cooperation	Works together for the common good																						
Attention	Concentrates on activities at hand																						
Fair Play	Plays according to rules																						
Sportsmanship	Good loser and gracious winner																						
Appearance	Proper speech and dress																						
Leadership	Followed because of respect for achievement and essential worth																						
Followership	Follows leaders well because of respect for leaders' ability																						
Self-Adjustment	Integrated total being for a balanced happy personality																						
Group Adjustment	Adjustment of the Individual to others in the group																						

Nelson Leadership Questionnaire*

Purpose. To identify the leaders as perceived by coaches and by teammates.

Evaluation. A "guess who" kind of questionnaire, as suggested by Cattell and Eber[3], was developed by Nelson to be used by coaches and team members.

Level and Sex. High school varsity basketball players.

Uses. To identify leaders and non-leaders on basketball teams according to coaches' opinions and teammates' opinions. To study the agreement of the two groups in identifying leaders. To discuss factors of leadership. To foster individual counseling.

Directions and Coach's Questionnaire:

INSTRUCTIONS—Coach's Questionnaire

The same names can be used any number of times and in all cases give your first and second choice for each question.

1. Who are the most popular men on your squad?
   1. _____ 2. _____

2. Which players on the team know the most basketball, in terms of strategy, team play, etc.?
   1. _____ 2. _____

3. Of all the players on your team, who exhibits the most poise on the floor during the crucial parts of the game?
   1. _____ 2. _____

4. Who are the "take charge" men on your squad?
   1. _____ 2. _____

5. Who are the most consistent ball handlers on your squad?
   1. _____ 2. _____

6. Who are the most consistent shooters on your squad?
   1. _____ 2. _____

7. Who are the most valuable players on your squad?
   1. _____ 2. _____

8. Who are the two players who play "most for the team"?
   1. _____ 2. _____

9. Which players have the most overall ability on the squad?
   1. _____ 2. _____

10. Who are the most likable players on the squad?
   1. _____ 2. _____

* Nelson, Dale O.: Leadership in Sports, Research Quarterly, *37*, 268–275, May, 1966. Used by permission of the AAHPER and the author.

11. Which players do you think would make the best coaches?

1. _____ 2. _____

12. If you were not present for practice which players would you place in charge of the practice?

1. _____ 2. _____

13. Who are the players endowed with leadership qualities?

1. _____ 2. _____

14. Who are the players least endowed with leadership ability?

1. _____ 2. _____

Directions and Player's Questionnaire:

INSTRUCTIONS—Player's Questionnaire

Do not sign your name to the questionnaire. Fill in the name or names of the squad members that, in your opinion, best fit the question. Give your first and second choice in all cases. *Do not use your own name* on any of the answers. The names of the same players can be used any number of times and your answers will be kept confidential.

1. If you were on a trip and had a choice of the players you would share the hotel room with, who would they be?

1. _____ 2. _____

2. Who are the most popular men on the squad?

1. _____ 2. _____

3. Who are the best scholars on the squad?

1. _____ 2. _____

4. Which players on the team know the most basketball, in terms of strategy, team play, etc.?

1. _____ 2. _____

5. If the coach were not present for a workout which players would be the most likely to take charge of the practice?

1. _____ 2. _____

6. Which players would you listen to first if the team appeared to be disorganized during a crucial game?

1. _____ 2. _____

7. Your team is behind one point with 10 seconds remaining in the game and you could pass to anyone on the squad. Who would it be?

1. _____ 2. _____

8. Of all the players on your team, who exhibits the most poise on the floor during the crucial parts of the game?

1. _____ 2. _____

9. Who are the "take charge" men on your team?

1. _____ 2. _____

10. Who are the most consistent ball handlers on your squad?

1. _____ 2. _____

11. Who are the most consistent shooters on your squad?

1. _____ 2. _____

12. Who are the most valuable players on your squad?

1. _____ 2. _____

13. Who are the most unselfish players who are interested most in the team as a whole and who play most "for the team"?

1. _____ 2. _____

14. Which players have the most overall ability on the squad?

1. _____ 2. _____

15. Who are the most likable players on the squad?

1. _____ 2. _____

16. Which players on your team have influenced you the most?

1. _____ 2. _____

17. Which players have actually helped you the most?

1. _____ 2. _____

18. Which players do you think would make the best coaches?

1. _____ 2. _____

19. Which players do you most often look to for leadership?

1. _____ 2. _____

20. Who are the hardest workers on the squad?

1. _____ 2. _____

Scoring: No particular scoring method is recommended. Probably the frequency with which various players are listed would be one way to summarize the information.

Cowell Personal Distance Scale*

Purpose. To measure a student's degree of harmony with his social group and his social growth from year to year. To ascertain an index of acceptance.

Evaluation. The validity, judged by using a "Who's Who in My Group" test as the criterion, was .84. The reliability was reported to be around .90.

*Cowell, Charles C.: Validating an Index of Social Adjustment for High School Use, Research Quarterly, *29*, 7–18, March, 1958. Used by permission of the AAHPER.

The Scale

Cowell Personal Distance Scale

What to do	I would be willing to accept him:						
If you had full power to treat each student in this group as you feel, just how would you consider him? Just how near would you like to have him to your family? Every student should be checked in some one column. Circle your own name and be sure you check every student in one column only.	Into my family as a brother	As a very close pal	As a member of my gang or club	On my street as a next-door neighbor	Into my class at school	Into my school	Into my city
	1	2	3	4	5	6	7
1. Stanley Whitaker							
2. James Southerlin							
3. Parvin Schriber							
.							
.							
15.							

Level and Sex. Developed for use with a class of boys and girls.

Scoring. The maximum distance is valued 7 and the minimum 1. The index of acceptance is determined by adding all of the weighted scores and dividing this sum by the number of ratings, *e.g.*, if all 50 students checked a given student in the first column (into my family as a brother or sister) his index would be $50 \times 1 = 50 \div 50$ or 1.00. Dropping the decimal, his index would be 100. The lower the index the greater the degree of acceptance by the group. When used for girls, the "him" would be changed to "her," and "brother" to "sister."

Cook Sociometric Status Index*

Purpose. To measure the extent to which a student is chosen by fellow classmates for a specific functional situation, *i.e.*, selecting a softball team, selecting a group to go camping, etc.

Level and Sex. Junior and Senior High School boys and girls.

Uses. To measure the status of individuals within a group. To relate status to other measures such as skill, fitness, or attitude.
To use as a basis for individual counseling.

Directions. A choice situation must be present. Selecting a softball team, as in the Allerdice study[1], will be used as the example. Ask the students to list, in order of preference, the five girls within their own physical education class whom they would like to have on their softball team. The first girl listed would be the first choice, and so on through five choices. The students then list, below the five choices, anyone whom they do not want on their team. The students are furnished 3 x 5 cards to write their choices and rejections. The students are asked to list a minimum of 3 choices and a maximum of 5 choices.

Scoring. A first choice receives 5 points, 2nd choice receives 4 points, 3 points for 3rd choice, 2 points for fourth choice, and 1 point for 5th choice. The points are totaled for each student and the following formula is used to compute the Status Index:

$$\text{S. I.} = \frac{\text{Total Choice Points} - \text{Total \# of Rejections}}{\text{Number in class} - 1}$$

Example: $\text{S. I.} = \dfrac{5-1}{18} = .22$ This particular student received a third

choice, a fourth choice, and one rejection in a class of 19 students.[1]
The higher the index score, the more desired the student is for the defined situation.

Social Measures—Additional Sources

Barrow, Harold M.: Social Evaluation Score Card, Unpublished Study, Wake Forest University, Winston-Salem, North Carolina, 1956.

* Allerdice, Mary Ellen: The Relationship Between Attitude Toward Physical Education and Physical Fitness Scores and Sociometric Status, MA, State University of Iowa, 1963.

Biddulph, Howell G.: Athletic Achievement and the Personal and Social Adjustment of High School Boys, Research Quarterly, *25*, 1–8, March, 1954.

Bogardus, E. S.: A Social Distance Scale, Sociological and Social Research, *17*, 225–271, 1933.

Bovyer, George: Children's Concepts of Sportsmanship in the Fourth, Fifth, and Sixth Grades, Research Quarterly, *34*, 282–287, October, 1963.

Burdg, Barbara: My Democratic Skills: Self Evaluation, located in Latchaw, Marjorie, and Camille Brown, *The Evaluation Process in Health Education, Physical Education, and Recreation.* Englewood Cliffs, N.J., Prentice-Hall, Inc., 1962, pp. 113–115.

Cowell, Charles C.: An Abstract of a Study of Differentials in Junior High School Boys Based on the Observations of Physical Education Activities, Research Quarterly, *6*, 129–136, December, 1935.

————: Contributions of Physical Activity to Social Development, Research Quarterly, *31*, 286–306, May, 1960.

Dawley, Dorothy J., Maurice E. Troyer, and John H. Shaw: Relationship Between Observed Behavior in Elementary School Physical Education and Test Responses, Research Quarterly, *22*, 70–76, March, 1951.

Fulton, Ruth, and Elizabeth Prange: Motor Learning of Highly Chosen and Unchosen Teammates and Friends, Research Quarterly, *21*, 116–131, May, 1950.

Hale, Patricia Whitaker: Proposed Method for Analyzing Sociometric Data, Research Quarterly, *27*, 152–161, May, 1956.

Haskings, Mary Jane: Problem-Solving Test of Sportsmanship, Research Quarterly, *31*, 601–606, December, 1960.

How is Your Physical Education Coming Along? NEA Journal, *44*, 353, September, 1955.

Jones, Harold E.: Physical Ability as a Factor in Social Adjustment in Adolescence, Journal of Educational Research, *40*, 287–301, December, 1946.

Kehr, Geneva B.: An Analysis of Sportsmanship Responses of Groups of Boys Classified as Participants and Non-Participants in Organized Baseball, Doctoral Dissertation, New York University, 1959.

McAfee, Robert A.: Sportsmanship Attitudes of Sixth, Seventh, and Eighth Grade Boys, Research Quarterly, *26*, 120, March, 1955.

McGraw, L. W., and J. W. Tolbert: Sociometric Status and Athletic Ability of Junior High School Boys, Research Quarterly, *24*, 72–76, March, 1953.

Nelson, Jack D., and Barry L. Johnson: Effects of Varied Techniques in Organizing Class Competition Upon Changes in Sociometric Status, Research Quarterly, *39*, 634–639, October, 1968.

New York State Social Efficiency Scale, Secondary Physical Syllabus, Bulletin No. 1062, State Department of Education, Albany, New York.

Skubic, Elvira: A Study in Acquaintanceship and Social Status in Physical Education Classes, Research Quarterly, *20*, 80–87, March, 1949.

Smith, Hope, and Marguerite A. Clifton: *Physical Education—Exploring Your Future*, Englewood Cliffs, N.J., Prentice-Hall, Inc., 1962, Social-Emotional Maturity Profile, pp. 77–78.

Todd, Frances: Sociometry in Physical Education, Journal of Health, Physical Education, and Recreation, *24*, 23–24, May, 1953.

Williams, Roger L.: A Forced Choice Rating Scale for Coaches, Unpublished Master's Thesis, University of Illinois, Urbana, 1961.

Yarnall, C. D.: Relationship of Physical Fitness to Selected Measures of Popularity, Research Quarterly, *37*, 286, May, 1966.

Social Measures—References

1. Allerdice, Mary Ellen: The Relationship Between Attitude Toward Physical Education and Physical Fitness Scores and Sociometric Status, MA, State University of Iowa, Iowa City, 1963.
2. Blanchard, B. E., Jr.: A Behavior Frequency Rating Scale for the Measurement of Character and Personality in Physical Education Classroom Situations, Research Quarterly, *7*, 56–66, May, 1936.

3. Cattell, Raymond B., and Herbert W. Eber: *Handbook for the Sixteen Personality Factor Questionnaire*, Champaign, Illinois: The Institute for Personality and Ability Testing, 1957 edition with 1964 supplementation.
4. Cook, Lloyd A.: An Experimental Sociographic Study of a Stratified Tenth Grade Class, American Sociological Review, *10*, 252–264, April, 1945.
5. Cowell, Charles C.: Our Function is Still Education! The Physical Educator, *14*, 6–7, March, 1957.
6. ————: Validating an Index of Social Adjustment for High School Use, Research Quarterly, *29*, 7–18, March, 1958.
7. Dexter, Genevie, Compiler: *Teachers Guide to Physical Education for Girls in High School.* Sacramento, California State Department of Education, 1957.
8. Johnson, Marion Lee: Construction of Sportsmanship Attitude Scales, Research Quarterly, *40*, 312–316, May, 1969.
9. McCloy, Charles H.: Character Building Through Physical Education, Research Quarterly, *1*, 41–61, October, 1930.
10. McCloy, Charles H., and Ferene Hepp: General Factors or Components of Character as Related to Physical Education, Research Quarterly, *28*, 269–278, October, 1957.
11. Nelson, Dale O.: Leadership in Sports, Research Quarterly, *37*, 268–275, May, 1966.
12. O'Neel, F. W.: A Frequency Rating Scale for the Measurement of Character and Personality in High School Physical Education Classes for Boys, Research Quarterly, *7*, 67–76, May, 1936.
13. Peterson, Beverly A.: A Comparison of the Social Efficiency of Selected Groups of Tenth- and Twelfth-Grade Girls, MA, San Diego State College, 1965.
14. *Physical Education—Guide for North Dakota Elementary Schools, Grades 1–6*, Department of Public Instruction, Bismarck, 1960.

ATTITUDE MEASURES

Attitudes are predispositions to actions and so their proper development is important to the total development of the individual. They are acquired concurrently with activity and often have tremendous influence on performance. Not every student can be a championship performer but each can develop a favorable attitude toward activity.

Mercer Attitude Inventory*

Purpose. To evaluate the attitude of high school girls toward psychological, sociological, and moral and spiritual values of physical education experiences.

Evaluation. This inventory is an adaptation of the one developed by Galloway[4] for use with college women. The revision has a reliability of .92 and a validity coefficient of .74 computed against a criterion of a self-rating scale.

Level and Sex. Developed for use with high school girls. Adaptable for use with all secondary school students.

* Mercer, Emily-Louise: An Adaptation and Revision of the Galloway Attitude Inventory for Evaluating the Attitudes of High School Girls Toward Psychological, Moral-Spiritual, and Sociological Values in Physical Education Experiences, Unpublished Master's thesis, The Woman's College of the University of North Carolina, 1961. Used by permission of the author.

Scoring. The bracket positions on the answer sheet represent the various degrees of agreement with the statement.

(1) Strongly disagree
(2) Disagree
(3) Neutral or undecided
(4) Agree
(5) Strongly agree

Both positive (+) and negative (—) statements are included in the inventory. For the positively stated statements (see the coded answer key), the best answer on the answer sheet would be a 5, indicating a very strong agreement with the statement.

For the *positive* statements, the answer is scored as it is recorded. For example, if the person taking the inventory marked a 5, his score would be a 5, if he marked a 4, his score would be a 4.

Example from scoring key:

$$1 \quad 2 \quad 3 \quad 4 \quad 5$$
$$(\ ) \ (\ ) \ (\ ) \ (\ ) \ (x)$$

The *negatively* stated statements are scored in the reverse manner. The best answer for a negatively stated statement would be placed in the first set of brackets, indicating strong disagreement with the statement; and therefore, a positive attitude.

Example from scoring key:

$$5 \quad 4 \quad 3 \quad 2 \quad 1$$
$$(x) \ (\ ) \ (\ ) \ (\ ) \ (\ )$$

For the *negative* statements, the answer is scored in reverse. For example, if the person taking the inventory marked in the first set of brackets, his score would be 5, if he marked in the second set, his score would be 4, and the like. For ease in scoring the statements, it is good to mark the values of the statements on the scoring key. The answer sheet cannot be printed in this manner because the person taking the inventory would be able to detect the key immediately.

The final score is the total of all the values for the 40 items. There is a possible 200 points.

The Inventory

MERCER ATTITUDE INVENTORY

1. Physical education activities are likely to be emotionally upsetting to many girls.
2. The saying, "Rules are made to be broken," is true in highly competitive sports.
3. It would be better to study than to spend time in physical education classes.
4. Physical education contributes nothing toward character development.
5. Girls who are skilled in active games and sports are not popular with boys.
6. Social dancing helps one to improve in grace and poise.
7. Competitive activities break down emotional self-controls.
8. Physical education classes are not looked forward to with enthusiasm.
9. Learning to accept situations as they are rather than as they should be is learned through participation in competitive sports.

10. An appreciation for art and beauty can be learned from physical education.
11. Archery is an activity in which one learns to score honestly.
12. Opportunities for making friends are provided more in other classes than in physical education.
13. Feelings of joy and happiness may be expressed through physical activities.
14. Girls who excel in sports are not as intellectual as other girls.
15. A team is composed of individuals each working for her own particular good.
16. The spending of money for "exercise" and "play" is unnecessary and wasteful.
17. There is no apparent spiritual basis for physical education.
18. Working together as a team does not reduce the value of human relationships.
19. Being dishonest in calling balls good or bad in tennis is not related to personal integrity and honesty.
20. Physical education is not related to any other subject in the school program.
21. Learning to play by the rules of the game is not related to learning good moral and spiritual conduct.
22. Participation in competitive games and sports gives an opportunity for self-control.
23. Girls who enjoy physical activities are "unfeminine."
24. Individual student interests are not considered in physical education classes.
25. Accepting defeat graciously is not learned from participation in games and sports.
26. Physical education activities offer many opportunities for emotional expression.
27. Accepting your own capabilities is learned from participation in physical education.
28. Physical education activities do not provide opportunities for learning moral and spiritual values of living.
29. Physical education should be required in grades 1–12, and in college.
30. Just playing is not as important as having instruction in physical education.
31. A team should play according to the rules regardless of how unfairly the opposing team plays.
32. Associating with others in physical education activities is fun.
33. Physical education should be concerned with the learning of physical skills.
34. Physical activities are embarrassing for girls who are not skilled.
35. Each player on a team should play in every game regardless of her skill.
36. Physical education makes important contributions to the mental health of an individual.
37. Physical education offers little of importance to the general education of high school girls.

15

38. No opportunities are offered for students to become leaders in the physical education classes.
39. Physical education activities provide no opportunity for learning emotional control.
40. Physical education activities develop socially desirable standards of conduct.

Scoring Key

Code	Strongly Disagree	Disagree	Neutral	Agree	Strongly Agree	Code	Strongly Disagree	Disagree	Neutral	Agree	Strongly Agree	Code	Strongly Disagree	Disagree	Neutral	Agree	Strongly Agree
— 1.	5 ( )	4 ( )	3 ( )	2 ( )	1 ( )	—14.	5 ( )	4 ( )	3 ( )	2 ( )	1 ( )	+27.	1 ( )	2 ( )	3 ( )	4 ( )	5 ( )
— 2.	5 ( )	4 ( )	3 ( )	2 ( )	1 ( )	—15.	5 ( )	4 ( )	3 ( )	2 ( )	1 ( )	—28.	5 ( )	4 ( )	3 ( )	2 ( )	1 ( )
— 3.	5 ( )	4 ( )	3 ( )	2 ( )	1 ( )	—16.	5 ( )	4 ( )	3 ( )	2 ( )	1 ( )	+29.	1 ( )	2 ( )	3 ( )	4 ( )	5 ( )
— 4.	5 ( )	4 ( )	3 ( )	2 ( )	1 ( )	—17.	5 ( )	4 ( )	3 ( )	2 ( )	1 ( )	+30.	1 ( )	2 ( )	3 ( )	4 ( )	5 ( )
— 5.	5 ( )	4 ( )	3 ( )	2 ( )	1 ( )	+18.	1 ( )	2 ( )	3 ( )	4 ( )	5 ( )	+31.	1 ( )	2 ( )	3 ( )	4 ( )	5 ( )
+ 6.	1 ( )	2 ( )	3 ( )	4 ( )	5 ( )	—19.	5 ( )	4 ( )	3 ( )	2 ( )	1 ( )	+32.	1 ( )	2 ( )	3 ( )	4 ( )	5 ( )
— 7.	5 ( )	4 ( )	3 ( )	2 ( )	1 ( )	—20.	5 ( )	4 ( )	3 ( )	2 ( )	1 ( )	—33.	5 ( )	4 ( )	3 ( )	2 ( )	1 ( )
— 8.	5 ( )	4 ( )	3 ( )	2 ( )	1 ( )	—21.	5 ( )	4 ( )	3 ( )	2 ( )	1 ( )	—34.	5 ( )	4 ( )	3 ( )	2 ( )	1 ( )
+ 9.	1 ( )	2 ( )	3 ( )	4 ( )	5 ( )	+22.	1 ( )	2 ( )	3 ( )	4 ( )	5 ( )	+35.	1 ( )	2 ( )	3 ( )	4 ( )	5 ( )
+10.	1 ( )	2 ( )	3 ( )	4 ( )	5 ( )	—23.	5 ( )	4 ( )	3 ( )	2 ( )	1 ( )	+36.	1 ( )	2 ( )	3 ( )	4 ( )	5 ( )
+11.	1 ( )	2 ( )	3 ( )	4 ( )	5 ( )	—24.	5 ( )	4 ( )	3 ( )	2 ( )	1 ( )	—37.	5 ( )	4 ( )	3 ( )	2 ( )	1 ( )
—12.	5 ( )	4 ( )	3 ( )	2 ( )	1 ( )	—25.	5 ( )	4 ( )	3 ( )	2 ( )	1 ( )	—38.	5 ( )	4 ( )	3 ( )	2 ( )	1 ( )
+13.	1 ( )	2 ( )	3 ( )	4 ( )	5 ( )	+26.	1 ( )	2 ( )	3 ( )	4 ( )	5 ( )	—39.	5 ( )	4 ( )	3 ( )	2 ( )	1 ( )
												+40.	1 ( )	2 ( )	3 ( )	4 ( )	5 ( )

Kneer Attitude Inventory and Diagnostic Statements*

Purpose. To measure attitudes toward physical education.
To explore the specific aspects of the facilities, program, and leadership which students either like or dislike.

Evaluation. The Kneer Inventory was adapted from the one developed by Wear[3] for college men. The reading ability level was geared to the 8th grade and above. The scale correlated .84 with the Wear Attitude Inventory serving as the validity criterion and .87 and .89 with graphic self-ratings of attitude. The reliability coefficient was .95.

Level and Sex. The inventory was revised to make its reading level at 8th-grade comprehension and to clarify certain statements found to be ambiguous to high school girls. It may prove equally satisfactory for boys.

Scoring and Answer Key. The first 40 items comprise the attitude inventory and are scored as follows:

The positive statements are valued as
strongly agree	5
agree	4
neutral or undecided	3
disagree	2
strongly disagree	1

The negative statements are valued as
strongly agree	1
agree	2
neutral or undecided	3
disagree	4
strongly disagree	5

A copy of the answer sheet should be keyed with the values marked above each row of brackets since the negative and positive statements are interspersed in the listing. The answer sheet indicates the statements which are positive and negative. The value each answer should have is given above the set of brackets which would be punched out in the key. The key superimposed on an answer sheet would help the instructor count the number of 5's, 4's and the like and put them in the upper right-hand box of the student's paper to get the total score. Thus a 100 per cent strongly positive attitude will receive a score of 200, a mean positive score is 160, a mean neutral score is 120, a mean negative score is 80 and a mean strongly negative score is 40.

The last 30 statements are the diagnostic statements which are all scored like the positive statements; that is, the 5 sets of brackets are valued at 1, 2, 3, 4, 5 across the answer sheet.

Two scores result: one for the attitude inventory which covers the first 40 items, and one for the diagnostic statements which covers statements numbered 1 to 30. The two scores are *not* added together.

* Kneer, Marian E.: The Adaptation of Wear's Physical Education Attitude Inventory for Use with High School Girls, Unpublished Master's thesis, Illinois State Normal University, Normal, 1956. Used by permission of the author.

The Inventory

KNEER ATTITUDE INVENTORY AND DIAGNOSTIC STATEMENTS

A. Attitude Inventory

DIRECTIONS—*Please read carefully!* Below you will find some statements about physical education. We would like to know how you feel about each statement. You are asked to consider physical education only from the standpoint of its place as an activity course taught during a regular class period. No reference is intended in any statement to interscholastic or intramural athletics. People differ widely in the way they feel about each statement. There are no right or wrong answers.

You have been provided with a separate answer sheet for recording your reaction to each statement. (a) Read each statement carefully, (b) go to the answer sheet, and (c) opposite the number of the statement place an "x" in the square *which is under* the word (or words) which best expresses your feeling about the statement. After reading a statement you will know at once, in most cases, whether you *agree* or *disagree* with the statement. If you *agree*, then decide whether to place an "x" under "agree" or "strongly agree." If you *disagree*, then decide whether to place the "x" under "disagree" or "strongly disagree." In case you are undecided (or neutral) concerning your feelings about the statement, then place an "x" under "undecided." Try to avoid placing an "x" under "undecided" in very many instances.

Wherever possible, let your own personal experience determine your answer. Work rapidly. Do not spend much time on any statement. This is not a test, but is simply a survey to determine how people feel about physical education. Your answers will in no way affect your grade in any course. In fact, we are not interested in connecting any person with any paper—so please answer each statement as you actually feel about it. BE SURE TO ANSWER EVERY STATEMENT.

1. If for any reason a few subjects have to be dropped from the school program, physical education should be one of the subjects dropped.
2. Students can better understand each other after meeting and playing together in physical education activities.
3. Physical education activities provide no chance for learning to control strong feelings, such as anger.
4. Taking part in lively physical activities gets one interested in using good health habits.
5. Physical education is one of the more important subjects in helping to teach and practice acceptable rules of behavior with other people.
6. Time spent in dressing, showering, and playing in physical education class could be more valuable if spent in other ways.
7. Very active play works off harmful strong feelings, such as anger.
8. A person's body usually has all the strength it needs without taking part in physical education activities.
9. I would take physical education only if it were required.
10. Taking part in physical education activities tends to make one more likable and better able to get along with other people.
11. Taking part in physical education gives no help in developing the ability to feel calm in strange situations.

12. Physical education in most schools does not receive the stress that it should.

13. Because physical skills seem very important in youth, it is necessary that a person be helped to learn and to improve such skills.

14. Physical education classes are poor in chances to learn how to get along with other people.

15. Exercises taken regularly are good for one's general health.

16. A person would be better able to control his feelings if he did not take part in physical education.

17. An average amount of skill in active games or sports is not necessary for leading the fullest kind of life.

18. It is possible to make physical education a valuable subject if a wide variety of useful activities is offered.

19. Physical education does more harm than it does good.

20. Developing a physical skill will relax your mind.

21. Meeting and playing with others in some physical education activity is fun.

22. Physical education classes provide nothing which will be of value outside of class.

23. Physical education classes provide no chances for learning to respect the rights of others which will help one to become a better citizen.

24. There should not be over two one-hour periods per week given to physical education in schools.

25. Physical education situations are among the poorest for making friends.

26. Belonging to a group, for which opportunity is provided in team activities is a desirable experience for a person.

27. Physical education is not valuable enough to make it worth the time spent.

28. Physical education is an important subject in helping a person gain and keep all around good health.

29. Physical education skills will add to the joy and pleasure of living.

30. No definite good results come from taking part in physical education activities.

31. People get all the physical exercise they need in just taking care of their daily work.

32. Taking part in team sports during physical education is helpful in learning how to get along with people and how to make friends.

33. All who are physically able will profit from an hour of physical education each day.

34. Physical education activities tend to upset a person's feelings—for example, make him angry.

35. Physical education is helpful in building up enough extra strength and in improving the ability to keep going for daily living.

36. Physical education should be included in the program of every school because it helps a person to think better and to control strong feelings, such as anger.

37. Physical education makes one less friendly by encouraging people to be better than others in many of the activities.

38. I would advise anyone who is able to take physical education.
39. Taking part in sports, games, and dance makes for a better understanding of life, and increases the enjoyment of it.
40. Physical education class is a waste of time in improving health.

B. Diagnostic Statements

DIRECTIONS TO STUDENTS—Same as for Attitude Inventory (A)

1. Our physical education activities are fun.
2. Many of the games we play during physical education class are a waste of time.
3. I enjoy physical education class when team games are taught.
4. I enjoy physical education class when dance activities are taught.
5. I enjoy physical education class when individual games are taught.
6. Various physical education activities that we take part in have helped me develop leadership.
7. Many of our physical education activities may be played when not in school.
8. Our physical education activities will improve physical fitness.
9. I would like a greater variety of physical education activities to be offered.
10. I would like more health instruction.
11. We have enough indoor play space.
12. We have enough outdoor play space.
13. We have enough dressing room space.
14. We have enough shower room space.
15. We have enough clothes storage space.
16. Our gym is clean and pleasant.
17. Our shower room is clean and pleasant.
18. Our dressing room is clean and pleasant.
19. Our outdoor play space is clean and pleasant.
20. We have enough playing equipment.
21. Our physical education teacher is friendly.
22. Our physical education teacher teaches us a lot.
23. Our physical education teacher allows us to share in planning class.
24. Our physical education teacher treats everyone in class very fairly.
25. Our physical education teacher gives special help to those needing it.
26. We are given enough time for dressing and showering.
27. Our grading system in physical education is fair.
28. Our physical education class time is too short.
29. Our physical education classes are not too large.
30. Our physical education uniform is pleasant to wear and comfortable.

Answer Sheet and Key

	Attitude		Diagnostic Statements	
	N	Value	N	Value
Name_____	5_____ _____		5_____ _____	
Class _____	4_____ _____		4_____ _____	
Date _____	3_____ _____		3_____ _____	
Instructor_____	2_____ _____		2_____ _____	
	1._____ _____		1_____ _____	
	Total _____		Total _____	

Strongly Disagree Disagree Neutral Agree Strongly Agree

```
          5 4 3 2 1                5 4 3 2 1                1 2 3 4 5
 1  ( )( )( )( )( )      24  ( )( )( )( )( )       7  ( )( )( )( )( )
          1 2 3 4 5                5 4 3 2 1
 2  ( )( )( )( )( )      25  ( )( )( )( )( )       8  ( )( )( )( )( )
          5 4 3 2 1                1 2 3 4 5
 3  ( )( )( )( )( )      26  ( )( )( )( )( )       9  ( )( )( )( )( )
          1 2 3 4 5                5 4 3 2 1
 4  ( )( )( )( )( )      27  ( )( )( )( )( )      10  ( )( )( )( )( )
          1 2 3 4 5                1 2 3 4 5
 5  ( )( )( )( )( )      28  ( )( )( )( )( )      11  ( )( )( )( )( )
          5 4 3 2 1                1 2 3 4 5
 6  ( )( )( )( )( )      29  ( )( )( )( )( )      12  ( )( )( )( )( )
          1 2 3 4 5                5 4 3 2 1
 7  ( )( )( )( )( )      30  ( )( )( )( )( )      13  ( )( )( )( )( )
          5 4 3 2 1                5 4 3 2 1
 8  ( )( )( )( )( )      31  ( )( )( )( )( )      14  ( )( )( )( )( )
          5 4 3 2 1                1 2 3 4 5
 9  ( )( )( )( )( )      32  ( )( )( )( )( )      15  ( )( )( )( )( )
          1 2 3 4 5                1 2 3 4 5
10  ( )( )( )( )( )      33  ( )( )( )( )( )      16  ( )( )( )( )( )
          5 4 3 2 1                5 4 3 2 1
11  ( )( )( )( )( )      34  ( )( )( )( )( )      17  ( )( )( )( )( )
          1 2 3 4 5                1 2 3 4 5
12  ( )( )( )( )( )      35  ( )( )( )( )( )      18  ( )( )( )( )( )
          1 2 3 4 5                1 2 3 4 5
13  ( )( )( )( )( )      36  ( )( )( )( )( )      19  ( )( )( )( )( )
          5 4 3 2 1                5 4 3 2 1
14  ( )( )( )( )( )      37  ( )( )( )( )( )      20  ( )( )( )( )( )
          1 2 3 4 5                1 2 3 4 5
15  ( )( )( )( )( )      38  ( )( )( )( )( )      21  ( )( )( )( )( )
          5 4 3 2 1                1 2 3 4 5
16  ( )( )( )( )( )      39  ( )( )( )( )( )      22  ( )( )( )( )( )
          5 4 3 2 1                5 4 3 2 1
17  ( )( )( )( )( )      40  ( )( )( )( )( )      23  ( )( )( )( )( )
          1 2 3 4 5
18  ( )( )( )( )( )                                24  ( )( )( )( )( )
          5 4 3 2 1                1 2 3 4 5
19  ( )( )( )( )( )       1  ( )( )( )( )( )      25  ( )( )( )( )( )
          1 2 3 4 5
20  ( )( )( )( )( )       2  ( )( )( )( )( )      26  ( )( )( )( )( )
          1 2 3 4 5
21  ( )( )( )( )( )       3  ( )( )( )( )( )      27  ( )( )( )( )( )
          5 4 3 2 1
22  ( )( )( )( )( )       4  ( )( )( )( )( )      28  ( )( )( )( )( )
          5 4 3 2 1
23  ( )( )( )( )( )       5  ( )( )( )( )( )      29  ( )( )( )( )( )

                         6  ( )( )( )( )( )      30  ( )( )( )( )( )
```

439

Edgington Attitude Scale for High School Freshman Boys*

Purpose. To measure the attitudes of high school freshman boys toward physical education. Four objectives were identified:

> Physical Development
> Motor Development
> Mental Development
> Human Relations

"The concepts for the statements used in this attitude scale were selected from the areas of the four general objectives and were intended to measure the extent to which the student attitudes indicated these objectives were being achieved."[3]

Evaluation. The scale was revised three times, once after a jury had ruled on the favorableness or unfavorableness of each item. The remaining items were administered to 107 9th grade boys. Likert's method of internal consistency was used to study the items. The second administration involved 109 different 9th grade boys. Again items were dropped which did not meet the standard of internal consistency. The final form included 66 items of the 125 original ones. Construct validity was established by comparing the scores of the 15 boys selected by their instructors as having the most favorable attitude and the scores of the 15 boys with the most unfavorable attitude. The Chi Square results were significant at the 1 per cent level of confidence.

The reliability coefficient for the final form was .92 computed on the split-halves and the Spearman-Brown Prophecy Formula.

Level and Sex. Designed for 9th grade boys. Probably suitable for secondary school boys and girls.

Uses. To ascertain favorable and unfavorable attitudes.

To strengthen favorable attitudes and remove or change unfavorable ones.

To reduce unfavorable attitudes because they are "obstacles to learning."

To alter instruction because of attitudes and to alter attitudes through instruction.

Directions

Attached you will find a list of statements about physical education. Feelings about these statements vary among people. There are no right or wrong answers. Please answer each statement according to your own feelings about physical education.

Please put your answers on the provided answer sheet. You are to cross out the box on the answer sheet to indicate how strongly you agree or

---

* Edgington, Charles W.: Development of an Attitude Scale to Measure Attitudes of High School Freshman Boys Toward Physical Education, Ed.D., Colorado State College, Greeley, 1965. Used by permission of the University of Northern Colorado and the author.

disagree with each statement. The numbers in the boxes on the answer sheet are there to guide you. They stand for the following:

+3 = Very strongly agree   −3 = Very strongly disagree
+2 = Strongly agree   −2 = Strongly disagree
+1 = Agree   −1 = Disagree

PLEASE BE SURE TO ANSWER EVERY STATEMENT.

The Scale:

ATTITUDE SCALE FOR HIGH SCHOOL FRESHMAN BOYS

1. Physical education is mainly concerned with muscle building.

2. Physical education should be eliminated from the curriculum.

3. Physical education is too strenuous for the average student.

4. Knowledge of various sports learned in physical education helps students to become more understanding spectators.

5. Physical education should develop in students an understanding of the importance of exercise to health.

6. Respect for human personality should be one of the qualities sought in a physical education class.

7. Credit should not be given for physical education.

8. Physical education has little value and should be eliminated.

9. Skills learned in physical education are of value in social life.

10. Cooperation is not necessary in physical education activities.

11. Physical education is not as important as other academic classes.

12. Emotional expressions can be brought under control through participation in games.

13. Physical education helps students to develop poise.

14. The main purpose of physical education is to cause fatigue in students.

15. Physical education should not be considered a part of general education.

16. The intellectual processes are related to the physical processes of the body.

17. Physical education should be a required subject.

18. Physical education should introduce only activities that are useful during the teen-age years.

19. Grades should not be given in physical education.

20. A student should learn to respect his opponent in physical education.

21. Physical education helps students adapt to group situations.

22. Physical education does little in developing desirable standards of conduct.

23. Tolerance, obedience, and respect for the rights of others are learned in physical education.

24. Physical education should be an elective subject after the ninth grade.

25. Exercise is of little importance in maintaining good health.

26. There is a scientific basis for physical education.

27. To participate in games is undignified.

28. Physical education once or twice a week is inadequate.

29. Written tests should be given in physical education.

30. Physical education is mainly concerned with team games.

31. Physical education should be required in every grade.

32. Students have little opportunity in physical education to receive recognition and status.

33. Physical education classes provide opportunities to make friends.

34. Physical conditioning is an important part of the physical education class.

35. No real learning takes place in a physical education class.

36. Physical education is harmful if an individual is physically weak.

37. Credit should be given for physical education.

38. Physical education has little to offer for the unskilled individual.

39. Varsity athletes should be excused from physical education classes.

40. The program in physical education should be organized so there is progression in the learning of skills.

41. Calisthenics should be eliminated from physical education.

42. Participants in physical education learn to cooperate as members of the group.

43. Physical education is important in the growth and development of students.

44. The physical education program should include activities leading to sports appreciation.

45. Activities in physical education offer students opportunities to make quick decisions and responses.

46. Physical education contributes to physical development.

47. Physical education should be a relaxation period between academic classes.

48. The activities in the physical education program do little to develop physical fitness.

49. The program in physical education is the same year after year.

50. Students get all the physical activity they need outside of school.

51. Taking a long walk would be a good substitute for physical education.

52. Learning the rules of activities is an important part of physical education.

53. The rules of sportsmanship should be practiced in physical education.

54. Physical education is not an important phase of education.

55. There is little carry-over value from physical education.

56. Physical education classes should not be free play periods.

57. Flexibility is important in physical education.

58. Some calisthenics should be included in physical education.

59. Physical education is needed for a complete education.

60. Little intelligence is required for physical education.

61. Physical education classes should provide challenging activities.

62. Physical education is a waste of time in school.

63. Individual sports learned in physical education can be useful in later life.

64. Physical education is mainly for the physically gifted.

65. Coordination can be developed in physical education.

66. Strength cannot be developed in physical education.

Scoring: A six-point scale is used. The statements are scored as follows:

Response	Values for Favorable or Positive Statements	Values for Unfavorable or Negative Statements
(a) Very Strongly Agree	6	1
(b) Strongly Agree	5	2
(c) Agree	4	3
(d) Disagree	3	4
(e) Strongly Disagree	2	5
(f) Very Strongly Disagree	1	6

The statements are keyed so the instructor can prepare a scoring key similar to the one suggested for the Mercer scale. The plus and minus signs should not appear on the copy which the student uses.

The top possible score, showing a very favorable attitude, would be 396 and the lowest possible score would be a 66. Anything above 264 would indicate an attitude on the favorable side.

Scoring Key:

	VSA	SA	A	D	SD	VSD
− 1.	1 ( )	2 ( )	3 ( )	4 ( )	5 ( )	6 ( )
− 2.	1 ( )	2 ( )	3 ( )	4 ( )	5 ( )	6 ( )
− 3.	1 ( )	2 ( )	3 ( )	4 ( )	5 ( )	6 ( )
+ 4.	6 ( )	5 ( )	4 ( )	3 ( )	2 ( )	1 ( )
+ 5.	6 ( )	5 ( )	4 ( )	3 ( )	2 ( )	1 ( )
+ 6.	6 ( )	5 ( )	4 ( )	3 ( )	2 ( )	1 ( )
− 7.	1 ( )	2 ( )	3 ( )	4 ( )	5 ( )	6 ( )
− 8.	1 ( )	2 ( )	3 ( )	4 ( )	5 ( )	6 ( )
+ 9.	6 ( )	5 ( )	4 ( )	3 ( )	2 ( )	1 ( )
−10.	1 ( )	2 ( )	3 ( )	4 ( )	5 ( )	6 ( )
−11.	1 ( )	2 ( )	3 ( )	4 ( )	5 ( )	6 ( )
+12.	6 ( )	5 ( )	4 ( )	3 ( )	2 ( )	1 ( )
+13.	6 ( )	5 ( )	4 ( )	3 ( )	2 ( )	1 ( )
−14.	1 ( )	2 ( )	3 ( )	4 ( )	5 ( )	6 ( )
−15.	1 ( )	2 ( )	3 ( )	4 ( )	5 ( )	6 ( )
+16.	6 ( )	5 ( )	4 ( )	3 ( )	2 ( )	1 ( )
+17.	6 ( )	5 ( )	4 ( )	3 ( )	2 ( )	1 ( )
−18.	1 ( )	2 ( )	3 ( )	4 ( )	5 ( )	6 ( )
−19.	1 ( )	2 ( )	3 ( )	4 ( )	5 ( )	6 ( )
+20.	6 ( )	5 ( )	4 ( )	3 ( )	2 ( )	1 ( )
+21.	6 ( )	5 ( )	4 ( )	3 ( )	2 ( )	1 ( )
−22.	1 ( )	2 ( )	3 ( )	4 ( )	5 ( )	6 ( )
+23.	6 ( )	5 ( )	4 ( )	3 ( )	2 ( )	1 ( )
−24.	1 ( )	2 ( )	3 ( )	4 ( )	5 ( )	6 ( )
−25.	1 ( )	2 ( )	3 ( )	4 ( )	5 ( )	6 ( )
+26.	6 ( )	5 ( )	4 ( )	3 ( )	2 ( )	1 ( )
−27.	1 ( )	2 ( )	3 ( )	4 ( )	5 ( )	6 ( )
+28.	6 ( )	5 ( )	4 ( )	3 ( )	2 ( )	1 ( )
+29.	6 ( )	5 ( )	4 ( )	3 ( )	2 ( )	1 ( )
−30.	1 ( )	2 ( )	3 ( )	4 ( )	5 ( )	6 ( )
+31.	6 ( )	5 ( )	4 ( )	3 ( )	2 ( )	1 ( )
−32.	1 ( )	2 ( )	3 ( )	4 ( )	5 ( )	6 ( )
+33.	6 ( )	5 ( )	4 ( )	3 ( )	2 ( )	1 ( )

	VSA	SA	A	D	SD	VSD
+34.	6 ( )	5 ( )	4 ( )	3 ( )	2 ( )	1 ( )
−35.	1 ( )	2 ( )	3 ( )	4 ( )	5 ( )	6 ( )
−36.	1 ( )	2 ( )	3 ( )	4 ( )	5 ( )	6 ( )
+37.	6 ( )	5 ( )	4 ( )	3 ( )	2 ( )	1 ( )
−38.	1 ( )	2 ( )	3 ( )	4 ( )	5 ( )	6 ( )
−39.	1 ( )	2 ( )	3 ( )	4 ( )	5 ( )	6 ( )
+40.	6 ( )	5 ( )	4 ( )	3 ( )	2 ( )	1 ( )
−41.	1 ( )	2 ( )	3 ( )	4 ( )	5 ( )	6 ( )
+42.	6 ( )	5 ( )	4 ( )	3 ( )	2 ( )	1 ( )
+43.	6 ( )	5 ( )	4 ( )	3 ( )	2 ( )	1 ( )
+44.	6 ( )	5 ( )	4 ( )	3 ( )	2 ( )	1 ( )
+45.	6 ( )	5 ( )	4 ( )	3 ( )	2 ( )	1 ( )
+46.	6 ( )	5 ( )	4 ( )	3 ( )	2 ( )	1 ( )
−47.	1 ( )	2 ( )	3 ( )	4 ( )	5 ( )	6 ( )
−48.	1 ( )	2 ( )	3 ( )	4 ( )	5 ( )	6 ( )
−49.	1 ( )	2 ( )	3 ( )	4 ( )	5 ( )	6 ( )
−50.	1 ( )	2 ( )	3 ( )	4 ( )	5 ( )	6 ( )
−51.	1 ( )	2 ( )	3 ( )	4 ( )	5 ( )	6 ( )
+52.	6 ( )	5 ( )	4 ( )	3 ( )	2 ( )	1 ( )
+53.	6 ( )	5 ( )	4 ( )	3 ( )	2 ( )	1 ( )
−54.	1 ( )	2 ( )	3 ( )	4 ( )	5 ( )	6 ( )
−55.	1 ( )	2 ( )	3 ( )	4 ( )	5 ( )	6 ( )
+56.	6 ( )	5 ( )	4 ( )	3 ( )	2 ( )	1 ( )
+57.	6 ( )	5 ( )	4 ( )	3 ( )	2 ( )	1 ( )
+58.	6 ( )	5 ( )	4 ( )	3 ( )	2 ( )	1 ( )
+59.	6 ( )	5 ( )	4 ( )	3 ( )	2 ( )	1 ( )
−60.	1 ( )	2 ( )	3 ( )	4 ( )	5 ( )	6 ( )
+61.	6 ( )	5 ( )	4 ( )	3 ( )	2 ( )	1 ( )
−62.	1 ( )	2 ( )	3 ( )	4 ( )	5 ( )	6 ( )
+63.	6 ( )	5 ( )	4 ( )	3 ( )	2 ( )	1 ( )
−64.	1 ( )	2 ( )	3 ( )	4 ( )	5 ( )	6 ( )
+65.	6 ( )	5 ( )	4 ( )	3 ( )	2 ( )	1 ( )
−66.	1 ( )	2 ( )	3 ( )	4 ( )	5 ( )	6 ( )

Penman Physical Education Attitude Inventory for Inner-City Junior High School Girls*

Purpose. To adapt the Wear attitude inventory to make it appropriate for use with students in an inner-city environment.

Evaluation. Judges were used to study the appropriateness, clarity, and vocabulary of the statements. Reliability coefficient was .92 using the Spearman-Brown Prophecy Formula. Validity coefficient was .64 using a graphic self-rating scale as the criterion. Data were based on responses from 204 girls in the 7th, 8th, and 9th grades in 2 inner-city junior high schools in Detroit.

Level and Sex. Junior high school girls.

Uses. To measure the attitudes of disadvantaged students toward physical education.

Directions:

Please Read Carefully—On the next two pages you will find some statements about gym. There are no right or wrong answers. People are very different in the way they feel about each statement.

You have been given a separate answer sheet for putting down how you feel about each statement. (*a*) Read each statement carefully, (*b*) go to the answer sheet, and (*c*) next to the number of the statement place an "X" in the square *which is under* the word (or words) which tells best how you feel about the statement. After reading a statement you will know at once, in most cases, whether you *agree* or *disagree* with the statement. If you *agree* then decide whether to place an "X" under "agree" or "strongly agree." If you *disagree*, then decide whether to place the "X" under "disagree" or "strongly disagree." If you don't know how you feel about the statement, then place an "X" under "undecided." Try not to place an "X" under "undecided" too many times.

Wherever possible, let your experience help you decide how to answer. Work as fast as you can. Don't spend too much time on any one statement. This is *not* a test, it's just a way of finding out how you feel about gym. Your answers *will not* affect your grade. Please answer each statement as you really feel about it. BE SURE TO ANSWER EACH STATEMENT.

The Instrument:

ATTITUDE STATEMENTS

1. If some classes have to be dropped from your class program, gym should be one of them.

2. Playing together in gym helps us to understand one another better.

3. In gym we learn how to control feelings.

4. Playing hard in gym gets girls interested in using good health habits.

5. Gym is one of the more important subjects in helping to set up and keep good rules for getting along.

---

*Penman, Mary M.: An Adaptation of Wear's Physical Education Attitude Inventory for Inner-City Junior High School Girls, M. Ed., Wayne State University, Detroit, Michigan, 1967. Used by permission of Wayne State University and the author.

6. Time spent in getting ready for, and taking part in gym, could be used better in other ways.

7. Playing hard helps to work off bad feelings.

8. A girl's body is usually strong enough without taking part in gym.

9. I would take gym only if I had to.

10. Taking part in gym activities helps make you a nicer person.

11. Gym should be given more time in schools.

12. Because play skills are important when you are young, you should be helped to get and improve your skills.

13. Regular exercise is good for your health.

14. Skill in games and sports is not necessary to have the best kind of life.

15. Developing a skill in gym helps rest the mind.

16. Taking part with others in a gym class is fun.

17. Gym doesn't give me anything that can be used outside of class.

18. Two hours a week is enough time to spend in gym.

19. A gym class is one of the worst places for making friends.

20. Being part of a group that gets the chance to play as a team is a good experience.

21. Not enough good comes from gym to make it worth the time.

22. Gym is important in helping a person become healthy and stay that way.

23. Skills learned in gym class help make life worthwhile.

24. Nothing really good comes from taking part in gym.

25. We get all the exercise we need just going to school and doing our work.

26. Because it helps your mind and body, gym should be a part of every school's program.

27. Gym makes it harder to get along with others because some people try to be better than others.

28. I would tell anyone who had the chance, to take gym.

29. Taking part in gym gives one a better outlook on life.

30. Gym is a waste of time as far as improving health is concerned.

Scoring: The attitude scale has a five point scoring system with 5 indicating a strongly favorable attitude, 1 indicating a strongly unfavorable attitude, and 3, the mid-point, indicating an undecided attitude. The 30 statements are coded with a plus or minus sign. If the code is +, a Strongly Agree response is worth 5 points, etc. If the statement is coded with a —, a Strongly Disagree response would be worth 5 points etc. The individual items are scored and then summed to get a total score. On the thirty item inventory, the highest possible score is 150 and the lowest is 30. A score of 30 indicates a totally unfavorable attitude, between 31–60 an unfavorable attitude, between 61–90 that the respondent is undecided, 91–120 a favorable attitude, and from 121–150 a very favorable attitude.

Scoring Key:

	SA	A	U	D	SD			SA	A	U	D	SD
− 1.	1	2	3	4	5		+16.	5	4	3	2	1
+ 2.	5	4	3	2	1		−17.	1	2	3	4	5
+ 3.	5	4	3	2	1		−18.	1	2	3	4	5
+ 4.	5	4	3	2	1		−19.	1	2	3	4	5
+ 5.	5	4	3	2	1		+20.	5	4	3	2	1
− 6.	1	2	3	4	5		−21.	1	2	3	4	5
+ 7.	5	4	3	2	1		+22.	5	4	3	2	1
− 8.	1	2	3	4	5		+23.	5	4	3	2	1
− 9.	1	2	3	4	5		−24.	1	2	3	4	5
+10.	5	4	3	2	1		−25.	1	2	3	4	5
+11.	5	4	3	2	1		+26.	5	4	3	2	1
+12.	5	4	3	2	1		−27.	1	2	3	4	5
+13.	5	4	3	2	1		+28.	5	4	3	2	1
−14.	1	2	3	4	5		+29.	5	4	3	2	1
+15.	5	4	3	2	1		−30.	1	2	3	4	5

(Each item provides five response blanks: ( ) ( ) ( ) ( ) ( ))

Dell Attitude Scale for High School Freshman Athletes*

Purpose. To measure primarily the attitudes of self-control, sense of responsibility, and respect for others.

Evaluation. The Flanagan Discriminatory Index was used to establish validity. The reliability coefficient was .91 for 100 8th grade boys who wanted to become high school athletes.

Level and Sex. Designed for 9th grade athletes. Might be usable with all secondary age boys.

Uses. To aid coaches in guiding high school freshmen who have indicated an interest in athletics.

Directions. "This is not a test which measures knowledge or how much you know. This is a scale which measures your attitude toward certain areas of athletics which are very essential toward becoming a successful athlete.
There are five choices: Strongly Agree, Agree, Undecided, Disagree, or

* Dell, Donald L.: An Attitude Scale for High School Freshman Athletes, MSPE, Illinois State University, Normal, 1965. Used by permission of the author.

Strongly Disagree.   Indicate on the answer sheet your opinion concerning the statement.

Are there any questions?—If there are no further questions, you may begin."

The Instrument:

1. I often find myself daydreaming when I should be studying.
2. You should be able to call your coach by his first name.
3. A good time for horseplay is when the coach is instructing a teammate.
4. A coach doesn't like you if he is constantly criticizing you.
5. The responsibility for leaving the host's dressing room neat and clean lies solely with the manager.
6. If your team is far in the lead, it is permissible to clown around.
7. You have a right to be angry if the coach takes you out of a game just before you have broken the school scoring record.
8. An athlete must follow a healthy nutritional diet only on game nights.
9. If I don't like a teammate, I'll just ignore him on and off the playing floor.
10. An athlete must show respect for all his teachers.
11. Minor cheating is permissible if it results in victory.
12. Players could perform much better if fans were not present.
13. Officials sometimes cause teams to lose games.
14. An athlete must realize his body has limitations.
15. An opponent can never be a friend.
16. To be a success in high school, you must belong to a special group or clique.
17. Slamming the basketball on the floor and pounding the mat are healthy outlets for one's emotions.
18. The coach should not offer criticism to the captain of the team.
19. School equipment that is damaged is easily replaced.
20. If I saw a chance to go into a theater without paying, I would take advantage of the situation.
21. A boy who is unreliable but well coordinated should expect to play often in varsity competition.
22. A boy who can outslug his opponent is courageous.
23. A good athlete should stay as far away from weak athletes as possible.
24. Athletic success is not always measured in the score book.
25. Teachers often make unreasonable requests.
26. Practice isn't fun unless you can occasionally horse around.
27. The superintendent has no right taking disciplinary action against an athlete.
28. I am very disturbed when someone watches me work.
29. An excellent athlete can win a game single-handed.
30. A gentleman is soft and could never become an athlete.
31. Patience is a virtue of a good athlete.
32. You should be allowed to let your uniform shirt tail hang down over your trousers.

33. If you are ruled ineligible because of grades, the coach should talk to the teacher and convince him to change the grade.

34. Officials frequently call violations against me which I do not deserve.

35. You should try to play even though you are sick.

36. I rarely pay compliments to people.

37. When your teammate loses his temper, help him get back at his opponent.

38. A coach should leave the first five in until the school scoring record has been broken, regardless of the competition.

39. Acquaintances made through athletics are a great benefit of athletics.

40. When faced with failure, a true athlete will lose his temper.

41. Teachers should give athletes special privileges because they represent the school and put in many extra hours of practice.

42. If an opponent has a violent temper, do everything possible to cause him to lose his temper.

43. An easily irritated boy makes a good competitor.

44. If you are elbowed by an opponent, wait for your chance and elbow back.

45. My parents are always finding fault with my actions.

46. The conduct of the athlete outside of competition is none of the coach's business.

47. If you are taken out of a game, you should throw your towel to the floor in disgust at yourself.

48. You should pay no attention to criticism regardless of its merit.

49. I enjoy being at home with my parents.

50. A true athlete always keeps track of the points he has scored during the game.

51. Fans should never tell me what I'm doing wrong.

52. If a spectator is riding an athlete, the athlete should give the spectator a dirty look to keep him quiet.

53. My father and I understand each other.

54. I should work at the best of my ability at all times to make my parents proud of me.

Scoring. The range of scores is from 1 to 5. The most favorable attitude for each statement is scored either strongly agree or strongly disagree. If the answer is strongly agree, then a strongly agree response will be worth 5 points, agree (4), undecided (3), disagree (2) and strongly disagree (1). If the correct answer is strongly disagree, then a strongly disagree response will be worth 5 points, disagree (4), undecided (3), agree (2), and strongly agree (1). The Scoring Key is coded with a + or − to indicate if the answer should be strongly agree or strongly disagree. These code marks should not appear either on the scale or the answer sheet which the student sees.

The final score is determined by the addition of the point values for the 54 statements. After a raw score is obtained for each student, the scores are placed in a frequency distribution. The scores in the upper 27 per cent are scored *Good*, the middle 46 per cent *Average*, and the lower 27 per cent *Poor*.

Scoring Key:

	SA	A	U	D	SD			SA	A	U	D	SD
	1	2	3	4	5			1	2	3	4	5
− 1.	( )	( )	( )	( )	( )		−28.	( )	( )	( )	( )	( )
	1	2	3	4	5			1	2	3	4	5
− 2.	( )	( )	( )	( )	( )		−29.	( )	( )	( )	( )	( )
	1	2	3	4	5			1	2	3	4	5
− 3.	( )	( )	( )	( )	( )		−30.	( )	( )	( )	( )	( )
	1	2	3	4	5			5	4	3	2	1
− 4.	( )	( )	( )	( )	( )		+31.	( )	( )	( )	( )	( )
	1	2	3	4	5			1	2	3	4	5
− 5.	( )	( )	( )	( )	( )		−32.	( )	( )	( )	( )	( )
	1	2	3	4	5			1	2	3	4	5
− 6.	( )	( )	( )	( )	( )		−33.	( )	( )	( )	( )	( )
	1	2	3	4	5			1	2	3	4	5
− 7.	( )	( )	( )	( )	( )		−34.	( )	( )	( )	( )	( )
	1	2	3	4	5			1	2	3	4	5
− 8.	( )	( )	( )	( )	( )		−35.	( )	( )	( )	( )	( )
	1	2	3	4	5			1	2	3	4	5
− 9.	( )	( )	( )	( )	( )		−36.	( )	( )	( )	( )	( )
	5	4	3	2	1			1	2	3	4	5
+10.	( )	( )	( )	( )	( )		−37.	( )	( )	( )	( )	( )
	1	2	3	4	5			1	2	3	4	5
−11.	( )	( )	( )	( )	( )		−38.	( )	( )	( )	( )	( )
	1	2	3	4	5			5	4	3	2	1
−12.	( )	( )	( )	( )	( )		+39.	( )	( )	( )	( )	( )
	1	2	3	4	5			1	2	3	4	5
−13.	( )	( )	( )	( )	( )		−40.	( )	( )	( )	( )	( )
	5	4	3	2	1			1	2	3	4	5
+14.	( )	( )	( )	( )	( )		−41.	( )	( )	( )	( )	( )
	1	2	3	4	5			1	2	3	4	5
−15.	( )	( )	( )	( )	( )		−42.	( )	( )	( )	( )	( )
	1	2	3	4	5			1	2	3	4	5
−16.	( )	( )	( )	( )	( )		−43.	( )	( )	( )	( )	( )
	1	2	3	4	5			1	2	3	4	5
−17.	( )	( )	( )	( )	( )		−44.	( )	( )	( )	( )	( )
	1	2	3	4	5			1	2	3	4	5
−18.	( )	( )	( )	( )	( )		−45.	( )	( )	( )	( )	( )
	1	2	3	4	5			1	2	3	4	5
−19.	( )	( )	( )	( )	( )		−46.	( )	( )	( )	( )	( )
	1	2	3	4	5			1	2	3	4	5
−20.	( )	( )	( )	( )	( )		−47.	( )	( )	( )	( )	( )
	1	2	3	4	5			1	2	3	4	5
−21.	( )	( )	( )	( )	( )		−48.	( )	( )	( )	( )	( )
	1	2	3	4	5			5	4	3	2	1
−22.	( )	( )	( )	( )	( )		+49.	( )	( )	( )	( )	( )
	1	2	3	4	5			1	2	3	4	5
−23.	( )	( )	( )	( )	( )		−50.	( )	( )	( )	( )	( )
	5	4	3	2	1			1	2	3	4	5
+24.	( )	( )	( )	( )	( )		−51.	( )	( )	( )	( )	( )
	1	2	3	4	5			1	2	3	4	5
−25.	( )	( )	( )	( )	( )		−52.	( )	( )	( )	( )	( )
	1	2	3	4	5			5	4	3	2	1
−26.	( )	( )	( )	( )	( )		+53.	( )	( )	( )	( )	( )
	1	2	3	4	5			5	4	3	2	1
−27.	( )	( )	( )	( )	( )		+54.	( )	( )	( )	( )	( )

Football Playing Ability and Attitude Rating Scale*

Purpose. To indicate football playing ability and an attitude toward the activity.

Uses. This is an example of a scale that can be combined with skill performance tests to arrive at a more comprehensive picture of the ability of the player.

The Scale

Name of rater	Date	Name of ratee

Condition

6	5 4	3 2	1
Excellent shape; plays hard every minute, good wind.	Fair shape; must take a breather now and then.	Can't keep up; obviously in poor condition.	

Aggressiveness

6	5 4	3 2	1
Very agressive; the first to start work; always tries hard; never quits.	Quits when he could have made a block or tackle; never eager to go to work.	Half-heartedly tries to block or tackle; last man to go to work.	

Perseverance

6	5 4	3 2	1
Constantly works to improve fundamentals and condition.	Works only when coaches are near.	Seldom tries to improve self.	

Team play

6	5 4	3 2	1
Always plays for the team to win; never thinks of his own glory.	Plays to suit himself; not for team as a whole.	Plays for the fans or for personal publicity or gain.	

* Adapted by David H. Hardy from Kenneth L. Meyer, Located in Cowell, Charles C., and Hilda M. Schwehn: *Modern Principles and Methods in High School Physical Education.* Boston, Allyn & Bacon, Inc., 1958, pp. 296–297. Used by permission of the publishers.

Name of rater	Date	Name of ratee

Attitude toward coaches

6	5	4	3	2	1

Listens to coaches at all times; carries out their instructions.	Listens to coaches, but does as he pleases.	Does not listen to the coaches.

Plays position

6	5	4	3	2	1

Knows every duty well; should be first string easily.	Average; does a steady job.	Can't carry out requirements of position.

Blocking

6	5	4	3	2	1

Skilled; accurate; good body control.	Average; does a steady job.	Unreliable; can't handle body; misses key blocks.

Tackling

6	5	4	3	2	1

Vicious and deadly; they stay tackled.	Will usually get his share.	Tackles half-heartedly.

Football "know-how"

6	5	4	3	2	1

Analyzes in a hurry; knows what to do when defensive and offensive situations change.	Slow to realize situation has changed; misses blocks or defensive shifts.	Never makes adjustments to new situations.

Attitude Measures—Additional Sources

Adams, R. S.: Two Scales for Measuring Attitude Toward Physical Education, Research Quarterly, *34*, 91–94, 1963.

Bowman, Mary: Relationship Between Student and Parent Attitudes and Skills of Fifth-Grade Children, Doctoral Dissertation, State University of Iowa, Iowa City, Iowa, 1958.

Brown, Ruth Eileen: A Use of the Semantic Differential to Study the Feminine Image of Girls Who Participate in Competitive Sports and Certain Other School-Related Activities, Ph.D., Florida State University, Tallahassee, 1965.

Callahan, Barbara Louise: Self-Determination Measurement in Physical Education, MSPE, University of California, Los Angeles, 1962.

Campbell, Donald E.: Student Attitudes Toward Physical Education, Research Quarterly, *39*, 456–462, October, 1968.

———: Wear Attitude Inventory Applied to Junior High School Boys, Research Quarterly, *39*, 888–893, December, 1968.

Carr, Martha G.: The Relationship Between Success in Physical Education and Selected Attitudes Expressed in High School Freshmen Girls, Research Quarterly, *16*, 176–191, October, 1945.

Cowell, Charles C., and A. H. Ismail: Validity of a Football Rating Scale and Its Relationship to Social Integration and Academic Ability, Research Quarterly, *32*, 461–467, December, 1961.

Drinkwater, Barbara: Development of an Attitude Inventory to Measure the Attitude of High School Girls Toward Physical Education as a Career for Women, Research Quarterly, *31*, 575–580, December, 1960.

Gibson, William Garnet: Evaluation of Outdoor Education Using Guttman Scales and Sociometric Analysis, MA, University of Alberta, Edmonton, Alberta, Canada, 1966.

Harres, Bea: Attitudes of Students Toward Women's Athletic Competition, Research Quarterly, *39*, 278–284, May, 1968.

Johnson, Warren R.: An Approach to Attitude Studies in Health and Physical Education, The Physical Educator, *18*, 20–22, March, 1961.

Kenyon, Gerald S.: Assessing Attitudes Toward Sport and Physical Activity, Proceedings, First International Congress of Psychology of Sport, Rome, Italy, April 24, 1965.

————: Six Scales for Assessing Attitude Toward Physical Activity, Research Quarterly, *39*, 566–574, October, 1968.

Karst, Ralph Roland: The Development of Standards of Potential Achievement in Physical Education, Ph.D., University of Wisconsin, Madison, Wisconsin, 1967.

Lakie, William L.: Expressed Attitudes of Various Groups of Athletes Toward Athletic Competition, Research Quarterly, *35*, 497–503, December, 1964.

McGee, Rosemary: Comparison of Attitudes Toward Intensive Competition for High School Girls, Research Quarterly, *27*, 60–73, March, 1956.

McPherson, B. D., and M. S. Yuhansz: An Inventory for Assessing Men's Attitudes Toward Exercise and Physical Activity, Research Quarterly, *39*, 218–219, March, 1968.

Meyne, Robert H.: A Situation Response Attitude Scale for College Men Physical Education Majors, PED, Indiana University, Bloomington, Indiana, 1964.

Moawad, Hassan Sayed: A Situation-Response Physical Education Attitude Scale for the Sophomore High School Boys, Doctoral dissertation, Indiana University, Bloomington, Indiana, 1960.

Moyer, L. J., J. C. Mitchem, and M. M. Bell: Women's Attitudes Toward Physical Education in the General Education Program of Northern Illinois University, Research Quarterly, *37*, 515–519, December, 1966.

O'Brian, Carol K.: The Relationship Between Personality and Attitude Toward Physical Activity, MSPE, University of Wisconsin, Madison, Wisconsin, 1966.

Ray, Barbara J.: Attitudes of High School Girls and Their Parents Toward Physical Education, DPE, Springfield College, Springfield, Mass., 1968.

Rice, S.: Attitudes and Physical Education, Journal of Health & Physical Education, *17*, 224, April, 1946.

Richardson, Charles E.: Thurstone Scale of Measuring Attitudes of College Students Toward Physical Fitness and Exercise, Research Quarterly, *31*, 638–643, December, 1960.

Scott, Phebe M.: Attitudes Toward Athletic Competition in Elementary Schools, Research Quarterly, *24*, 353–361, October, 1953.

Sheehan, Thomas J.: The Construction and Testing of a Teaching Model for Attitude Formation and Change Through Physical Education, Ph.D., Ohio State University, Columbus, 1965.

Wear, C. L.: The Evaluation of Attitudes Toward Physical Education as an Activity Course, Research Quarterly, *22*, 114–126, March, 1951.

Attitudes Measures—References

1. Cowell, Charles C., and Hilda M. Schwehn: *Modern Principles and Methods in High School Physical Education.* Boston: Allyn & Bacon, Inc., 1958.

2. Dell, Donald L.: An Attitude Scale for High School Freshman Athletes, MSPE, Illinois State University, Normal, Illinois, 1965.
3. Edgington, Charles W.: Development of an Attitude Scale to Measure Attitudes of High School Freshman Boys Toward Physical Education, Ed.D., Colorado State College, Greeley, Colorado, 1965.
4. Galloway, June P.: An Exploration of the Effectiveness of Physical Education Experiences in the Development of Attitudes of College Women Toward Sociological, Psychological, and Spiritual Values as Related to These Experiences, M.Ed., University of North Carolina at Greensboro, 1959.
5. Kneer, Marian E.: The Adaptation of Wear's Physical Education Attitude Inventory for Use with High School Girls, Illinois State University, Normal, 1956. Microcard PSY 64.
6. Mercer, Emily-Louise: An Adaptation and Revision of the Galloway Attitude Inventory for Evaluating the Attitudes of High School Girls Toward Psychological, Moral-Spiritual, and Sociological Values in Physical Education Experiences, M.Ed., University of North Carolina at Greensboro, 1961.
7. Penman, Mary M.: An Adaptation of Wear's Physical Education Attitude Inventory for Inner-City Junior High School Girls, M.Ed., Wayne State University, Detroit, Michigan, 1967.
8. Wear, Carlos L.: Construction of Equivalent Forms of an Attitude Scale, Research Quarterly, *25*, 113–119, March, 1955.

SELF-CONCEPT MEASURES

Self-concept measures relate to the student's perception of himself. They are ascertained indirectly sometimes by comparing the way a student thinks about himself with the way he would like to be. These scales represent some of the more recent measurement tools developed for use in physical education. Their implementation reflects the trend of using movement experiences as one avenue of self-understanding. The student should be able to know himself as he moves just as he should know himself as he thinks and as he relates to others; in fact, they are all interwoven.

Adjective Check List for Physical Education*

Purpose. To measure the student's feeling about himself. To measure the student's feeling about how he thinks the teacher feels about him.

Evaluation. The Adjective Check List presented here is an adaptation suggested by Reynolds[6] of the 50-item one constructed by Davidson and Lang.[1] Reynolds' study shows these 34 adjectives probably more related to the field of physical education because they were significant in his study of maturity, physique, body size, muscular strength, endurance, motor ability, and intelligence. The original work by Davidson and Lang shows the appropriateness of the words for vocabulary level, shows the words are either definitely favorable or unfavorable, and shows words commonly used to describe how people feel and think of others.

Level and Sex. The scale was developed on a sample of junior high school students. Davidson and Lang consider it appropriate for upper elementary groups. Reynolds used it with 13-year-old boys.

* Reynolds, Robert M.: Responses of the Davidson Adjective Check List as Related to Maturity, Physical, and Mental Characteristics of Thirteen-Year-Old Boys, Ed. D., University of Oregon, Eugene, Oregon, 1965. Used by permission of the author.

Uses. To measure the student's feelings and thoughts about himself.
To measure how a student thinks his teammates think and feel about him.
To measure how a student thinks a teacher thinks and feels about him.
To measure how a teacher feels and thinks about a child or a group of children.
To compare the student's feelings with the way he thinks others feel about him.

Directions:

Method 1: These are words that are often used to describe young people. Pick the ones that apply to you.

Method 2: These are words that are often used to describe young people. Check the first column if the trait applies to you most of the time, the middle column if the word is like you about half of the time, and the column on the right if the trait is seldom or almost never like you.

Method 3: These are words that are often used to describe young people. Check the first column if you think the teacher feels this way about you most of the time, the middle column if you think she thinks you are like this trait about half of the time, and mark the column on the right if you think she would almost never think the trait described you.

The Check List:

____BAD	____FRIENDLY	____A PEST
____BOSSY	____GENEROUS	____QUIET
____BRAT	____A HARD WORKER	____SELFISH
____BULLY	____KIND	____A SHOW OFF
____CARELESS	____A LEADER	____SILLY
____CHEERFUL	____NOT EAGER TO	____A SISSY
____CLEAN	LEARN	____A SLOPPY
____CLEVER	____LOVING	WORKER
____CLUMSY	____MEAN	____A SMART
____A CRY-BABY	____NERVOUS	ALECK
____DEPENDABLE	____NOT ALERT	____A SORE LOSER
	____OUTSTANDING	____SMART
		____STUPID
		____UNHAPPY

Scoring:

Method 1: Several alternative ways can be used to study the responses.
    a. Each trait could be analyzed for the entire class. For example, how many of the students thought "Selfish" characterized them? Did more boys than girls consider themselves selfish?
    b. Analyze how many of the 34 traits were checked. What is the ratio of favorable to unfavorable traits?
    c. Analyze if there is any change in the traits checked either after a school year or a particular unit.

Methods 2 and 3: A favorable word is assigned a score of 3 when it is checked in the "most of the time" column, a score of 2 for "half of the time," and 1 for "seldom or almost never." For unfavorable words, the scoring is reversed.

The total score, the Index of Favorability, is obtained by adding the scores of all the words and dividing the total by 34, the number of traits. The higher the index, the more favorable the child's perception either of himself or of the way he thinks others feel toward him. Theoretically, the index can range from 1.00 to 3.00.[1]

Scoring Key: To be used with Methods 2 or 3.

SCORING KEY

Feeling Tone		Most of the Time	Half of the Time	Seldom or Almost Never
Favorable *Unfavorable*				
U	Bad	1	2	3
U	Bossy	1	2	3
U	Brat	1	2	3
U	Bully	1	2	3
U	Careless	1	2	3
F	Cheerful	3	2	1
F	Clean	3	2	1
F	Clever	3	2	1
U	Clumsy	1	2	3
U	A Cry Baby	1	2	3
F	Dependable	3	2	1
F	Friendly	3	2	1
F	Generous	3	2	1
F	A Hard Worker	3	2	1
F	Kind	3	2	1
F	A Leader	3	2	1
U	Not Eager to Learn	1	2	3
F	Loving	3	2	1
U	Mean	1	2	3
U	Nervous	1	2	3
U	Not Alert	1	2	3
F	Outstanding	3	2	1
U	A Pest	1	2	3
F	Quiet	3	2	1
U	Selfish	1	2	3
U	A Show Off	1	2	3
U	Silly	1	2	3
U	A Sissy	1	2	3
U	A Sloppy Worker	1	2	3
U	A Smart Aleck	1	2	3
U	A Sore Loser	1	2	3
F	Smart	3	2	1
U	Stupid	1	2	3
U	Unhappy	1	2	3

How I See Myself Scale*

Purpose. To obtain an estimate of the child's view of himself

Evaluation. Gordon defines self-concept "as the way a child reports on himself."[3:3] The scale was developed from material in Jersild's *In Search of Self*[4] and later examined by factor analysis using nearly 9,000 school children in north central Florida public schools in grades three through twelve. The factor structure identified several sub-scales such as Teacher-School, Physical Appearance, Interpersonal Adequacy, Autonomy, Academic Adequacy, Emotions, Physical Adequacy, and Body-Build.

Reliability ranged from .162 to .89 for various age and school groups. The instrument is recommended for comparisons between groups of children and not for individual diagnosis. Content validity, based on the material by Jersild, and construct validity are presented by Gordon. He recommends the scale for use, at this time, for either descriptive or research study of groups, rather than for individual diagnosis. Normative data were presented for children from grades 3–12 by sex, race, and social class.

"A basic assumption underlying this scale is that the self-concept is not a unitary trait. That is, it doesn't really pay to talk about the child's self-concept as though it were a single thing. Rather, the position here is that the child has several concepts of himself which are to some degree interrelated in a unifying organization but which are discreet enough to be measured separately. On the face of it the scale measures the child's view of his body, of his peers, of his teachers, of his school, and of his own emotional control."[3:4]

Level and Sex. For boys and girls grades 3–12.

Uses. To measure the self-concept of a class.

To compare the self-concept of a class before and after instructional units or at the beginning and end of a school year.

To compare the self-concept of boys and girls.

Directions. I would like to explain this scale to you.

Let me emphasize that this is not a test to see how much you know or do not know about something. These questions are all about you. They are to learn how you see yourself most of the time. There are no right or wrong answers. We are only interested in what you think about yourself.

I am going to ask you to think about yourself for a little while before you write anything. I want you to think of how you are most of the time . . . not how you think you ought to be—not how the teacher thinks you ought to be . . . not how you want to be or your parents or friends want you to be. No—this is to be how *you* yourself feel you are *most* of the time.

Now—let's look at the papers.

Look at No. 1. On one side it has "Nothing gets me mad" and on the other side "I get mad easily and explode." If you feel that nothing gets you too mad most of the time, you would circle the 1. If you feel that most of the time, you get mad easily and explode, you would circle the 5. If you feel you are somewhere in between, you would circle the 2, 3, or 4.

* Gordon, Ira J.: *A Test Manual for the How I See Myself Scale.* Gainesville, Florida: Florida Educational Research and Development Council, 1968. The scale originally appeared in *Studying the Child in School* by Ira J. Gordon, John Wiley and Sons, Inc., Publishers, 1966. The scale is available for purchase directly from the author and is used here with the permission of the author and John Wiley & Sons, Inc.

Look at No. 2. It is different. On one side it has "I don't stay with something till I finish." If you feel that most of the time you don't stay with things and finish them, you would circle a 1. If you feel that most of the time you do stay with things and finish, you would circle a 5. If you feel you fit somewhere in between, you would circle the 2, 3, or 4. It is important to see that some of these mean one thing on the left side, some of them mean another. So it is very important to think about each statement as I read it. I will answer any questions you need answered, so feel free to ask them.

Remember, we want how you yourself feel. We want you to be honest with us in your answer. Remember, it is how you feel most of the time.

The Scale—Elementary Form:

How I See Myself

1. Nothing gets me too mad	1 2 3 4 5	I get mad easily and explode
2. I don't stay with things and finish them	1 2 3 4 5	I stay with something till I finish
3. I'm very good at drawing	1 2 3 4 5	I'm not much good in drawing
4. I don't like to work on committees, projects	1 2 3 4 5	I like to work with others
5. I wish I were smaller (taller)	1 2 3 4 5	I'm just the right height
6. I worry a lot	1 2 3 4 5	I don't worry much
7. I wish I could do something with my hair	1 2 3 4 5	My hair is nice-looking
8. Teachers like me	1 2 3 4 5	Teachers don't like me
9. I've lots of energy	1 2 3 4 5	I haven't much energy
10. I don't play games very well	1 2 3 4 5	I play games very well
11. I'm just the right weight	1 2 3 4 5	I wish I were heavier (lighter)
12. The girls don't like me, leave me out	1 2 3 4 5	The girls like me a lot, choose me
13. I'm very good at speaking before a group	1 2 3 4 5 1 2 3 4 5	I'm not much good at speaking before a group
14. My face is pretty (good looking)	1 2 3 4 5	I wish I were prettier (good looking)
15. I'm very good in music	1 2 3 4 5	I'm not much good in music
16. I get along well with teachers	1 2 3 4 5	I don't get along with teachers
17. I don't like teachers	1 2 3 4 5	I like teachers very much
18. I don't feel at ease, comfortable inside	1 2 3 4 5	I feel very at ease, comfortable inside
19. I don't like to try new things	1 2 3 4 5	I like to try new things

20. I have trouble controlling my feelings   1 2 3 4 5   I can handle my feelings

21. I do well in school work   1 2 3 4 5   I don't do well in school

22. I want the boys to like me   1 2 3 4 5   I don't want the boys to like me

23. I don't like the way I look   1 2 3 4 5   I like the way I look

24. I don't want the girls to like me   1 2 3 4 5   I want the girls to like me

25. I'm very healthy   1 2 3 4 5   I get sick a lot

26. I don't dance well   1 2 3 4 5   I'm a very good dancer

27. I write well   1 2 3 4 5   I don't write well

28. I like to work alone   1 2 3 4 5   I don't like to work alone

29. I use my time well   1 2 3 4 5   I don't know how to plan my time

30. I'm not much good at making things with my hands   1 2 3 4 5   I'm very good at making things with my hands

31. I wish I could do something about my skin   1 2 3 4 5   My skin is nice-looking

32. School isn't interesting to me   1 2 3 4 5   School is very interesting

33. I don't do arithmetic well   1 2 3 4 5   I'm real good in arithmetic

34. I'm not as smart as the others   1 2 3 4 5   I'm smarter than most of the others

35. The boys like me a lot, choose me   1 2 3 4 5   The boys don't like me, leave me out

36. My clothes are not as I'd like   1 2 3 4 5   My clothes are nice

37. I like school   1 2 3 4 5   I don't like school

38. I wish I were built like the others   1 2 3 4 5   I'm happy with the way I am

39. I don't read well   1 2 3 4 5   I read very well

40. I don't learn new things easily   1 2 3 4 5   I learn new things easily

The Scale—Secondary Form:

How I See Myself

1. I rarely get mad   1 2 3 4 5   I get mad easily

2. I have trouble staying with one job until I finish   1 2 3 4 5   I stick with a job until I finish

3. I am a good artist   1 2 3 4 5   I am a poor artist

4. I don't like to work on committees   1 2 3 4 5   I enjoy working on committees

5. I wish I were taller or shorter   1 2 3 4 5   I am just the right height

6. I worry a lot   1 2 3 4 5   I seldom worry

How I See Myself (continued)

7. I wish I could do something with my hair　　1 2 3 4 5　　My hair is nice-looking

8. Teachers like me　　1 2 3 4 5　　Teachers dislike me

9. I have a lot of energy　　1 2 3 4 5　　I have little energy

10. I am not good at athletics　　1 2 3 4 5　　I am good at athletics

11. I am just the right weight　　1 2 3 4 5　　I wish I were lighter or heavier

12. The girls don't admire me　　1 2 3 4 5　　The girls admire me

13. I am good at speaking before a group　　1 2 3 4 5　　I am poor at speaking before a group

14. My face is very pretty (good looking)　　1 2 3 4 5　　I wish my face were prettier (better looking)

15. I am good at musical things　　1 2 3 4 5　　I am poor at musical things

16. I get along very well with teachers　　1 2 3 4 5　　I don't get along well with teachers

17. I dislike teachers　　1 2 3 4 5　　I like teachers

18. I am seldom at ease and relaxed　　1 2 3 4 5　　I am usually at ease and relaxed

19. I do not like to try new things　　1 2 3 4 5　　I like to try new things

20. I have trouble controlling my feelings　　1 2 3 4 5　　I control my feelings very well

21. I do very well in school　　1 2 3 4 5　　I do not do well in school

22. I want the boys to admire me　　1 2 3 4 5　　I don't want the boys to admire me

23. I don't like the way I look　　1 2 3 4 5　　I like the way I look

24. I don't want the girls to admire me　　1 2 3 4 5　　I want the girls to admire me

25. I am quite healthy　　1 2 3 4 5　　I am sick a lot

26. I am a poor dancer　　1 2 3 4 5　　I am a good dancer

27. Science is easy for me　　1 2 3 4 5　　Science is difficult for me

28. I enjoy doing individual projects　　1 2 3 4 5　　I don't like to do individual projects

29. It is easy for me to organize my time　　1 2 3 4 5　　I have trouble organizing my time

30. I am poor at making things with my hands　　1 2 3 4 5　　I am good at making things with my hands

31. I wish I could do something about my skin　　1 2 3 4 5　　My skin is nice-looking

32. Core is easy for me　　1 2 3 4 5　　Core is difficult for me

33. Math is difficult for me　　1 2 3 4 5　　Math is easy for me

34. I am not as smart as my   1 2 3 4 5   I am smarter than most of
     classmates   my classmates

35. The boys admire me   1 2 3 4 5   The boys don't admire me

36. My clothes are not as nice   1 2 3 4 5   My clothes are very nice
     as I'd like

37. I like school   1 2 3 4 5   I dislike school

38. I wish I were built like the   1 2 3 4 5   I like my build
     others

39. I am a poor reader   1 2 3 4 5   I am a very good reader

40. I do not learn new things   1 2 3 4 5   I learn new things easily
     easily

41. I present a good appearance   1 2 3 4 5   I present a poor appearance

42. I do not have much confi-   1 2 3 4 5   I am full of confidence in
     dence in myself   myself

Scoring. Items on this scale were randomly reversed so that there would be a decrease in the tendency of a student to simply go down the 5 column in making his responses. The first step in scoring, therefore, is the conversion of items so that five always represents the positive end of the scale. This means that on the elementary form items 1, 3, 8, 9, 11, 13, 14, 15, 16, 21, 22, 25, 27, 28, 29, 35, and 37 are reversed; and on the secondary scale, in addition, item 41 is reversed. The score (on a factor) represents the sum of the items. The higher the score, the more positive the child's report on himself.

Nelson Self-Concept Statements*

Purpose. To measure the relationship between the self-concept as it actually is and the ideal or desired self-concept.

Evaluation. Most early work with self-concept was used in psychotherapy. More recently it has been used with school groups. Nelson's self-concept statements are taken from Doudlah's[2] work on college women and adapted for use with 8th grade girls. Doudlah credits Rogers[7,8] for the original self-concept Q-sort statements. The Q-sort technique is a forced choice method with the following characteristics as described by Sakers:[9]

"(1) The Q-sort test is easy to administer, score, and correlate.
(2) The interpretation of each test statement is left to the individual, therefore no predetermined value judgment is forced upon the subject.
(3) The Q-sort technique allows the investigator to clearly measure, in the form of correlation, the relationship between the self and the ideal self." [9:36]

* Nelson, Sara Marie, "An Investigation of the Relationship Between the Real Self-Concept-Ideal Self-Concept and the Motor Ability of Eighth Grade Girls in Physical Education," M. Ed., University of North Carolina at Greensboro, Greensboro, North Carolina, 1966. Used by permission of the author.

MYSELF AS I AM*

1.
Describes
Me Best

a. ——
b. ——

2.
Describes
Me Very
Well

a. ——
b. ——
c. ——
d. ——
e. ——

3.
Describes
Me Well

a. ——
b. ——
c. ——
d. ——
e. ——
f. ——
g. ——
h. ——
i. ——

4.
Describes
Me Rather
Well

a. ——
b. ——
c. ——
d. ——
e. ——
f. ——
g. ——
h. ——
i. ——
j. ——
k. ——
l. ——
m. ——

5.
Somewhat
Like Me

a. ——
b. ——
c. ——
d. ——
e. ——
f. ——
g. ——
h. ——
i. ——
j. ——
k. ——
l. ——
m. ——
n. ——
o. ——
p. ——
q. ——

6.
Describes
Me Rather
Poorly

a. ——
b. ——
c. ——
d. ——
e. ——
f. ——
g. ——
h. ——
i. ——
j. ——
k. ——
l. ——
m. ——

7.
Describes
Me Poorly

a. ——
b. ——
c. ——
d. ——
e. ——
f. ——
g. ——
h. ——
i. ——

8.
Describes
Me Very
Poorly

a. ——
b. ——
c. ——
d. ——
e. ——

9.
Describes
Me Worst

a. ——
b. ——

Name ————
Section ————

* Note: The second answer sheet would be entitled "My Ideal Self."

Level and Sex. Developed for 8th grade girls. Probably appropriate for all secondary school girls and could be adapted for use with secondary school boys.

Uses. To ascertain the discrepancy between the real self-concept and the desired self-concept.

To study this discrepancy in light of change from time to time and in relation to other factors such as a unit of instruction, movement-concept, or body-image concept.

Directions and Answer Sheet. You have received two answer sheets and a group of 75 statements. You will notice to the left of each statement two columns, Column A and Column B. You will be using each of these statements twice. The first time you use the statement you will be concerned with Column A and the white answer sheet titled "Myself as I am." After you study the 75 statements you have to choose two that describe you best and place the number of those statements under the appropriate heading on the white answer sheet. If you think #4 (I feel secure within myself) is one of these, write #4 in a blank in column 1 and place a check mark under Column A beside statement #4 so you will know you have used it. You are to place the number for each of the 75 statements under one of the nine columns. All 75 statements must be used. You may not use a statement more than once on the white answer sheet, and you may not place more numbers in a column than there are lettered spaces.

When you have completed the white answer sheet, you will then do the same thing on the blue answer sheet. This time, however, you will check each statement off as you use it under Column B and use the 75 statements to describe your "Ideal Self."

Q-Sort Statements—Self-Concept

1. It is easy for me to talk about my feelings.
2. Most of my troubles are not my own fault.
3. I feel happy much of the time.
4. I am sure of myself.
5. It's quite important for me to know how I seem with others.
6. I cover up my real feelings.
7. I often feel as if trying to live in this world is just too much for me.
8. I have confidence in myself.
9. I look forward to a better life and this keeps me going now.
10. I have courage and the willingness to keep trying.
11. I usually like people.
12. I know I can do any job I set for myself.
13. I am full of life and good spirits.
14. I feel free. Nothing stands in my way.
15. I can stand up for my rights if I need to.
16. My decisions are not my own. I feel controlled by others.
17. I am liked by most people who know me.
18. I am ashamed of myself.
19. I often have new ideas and think of new ways of doing things.
20. I don't change the way I am to suit everyone I really like.
21. I can get started on my own. I don't need a push.
22. Everything I want has to be perfect. I don't like a halfway job in anything.
23. It takes everything I've got just to keep going.

24. I am shy.
25. Basically I like myself.
26. I depend on others. I am no one by myself.
27. I'm often afraid of the things that might happen to me.
28. I'm very sure of myself. I can always count on my own strength, ideas, and brains.
29. I am intelligent.
30. I have a feeling I slide away from some things I don't want to face.
31. I am different from others.
32. I forgive easily because I don't hold grudges and try to "get even."
33. Sometimes I'm jealous of the good things some people seem to have.
34. I am satisfied with myself.
35. I often need to make excuses for myself, or else I'd think I was no good.
36. I am worth loving.
37. I back away whenever I get in a real tough spot.
38. I understand myself.
39. I have a feeling of hopelessness.
40. I often feel as if I dislike everything and everybody.
41. I feel helpless.
42. I feel as if everything is in a mess and I can't straighten it out.
43. I don't think I can change myself because I've been this way too long.
44. I feel as if almost everyone I know is a better person than I am.
45. I'm just no good at any time.
46. I feel I can handle almost any problem that comes up in my life.
47. I can't see any way out, and I don't know what to do next.
48. I look forward with pleasure to living the rest of my life.
49. I am pretty sociable, and really enjoy being with people.
50. I get pleasure out of life.
51. Most people I know just don't live up to what I think they should be.
52. I think I'm better than most of the people I know.
53. I get upset when old and familiar things are changed.
54. I'm a pretty calm and relaxed person. Few things really bother me.
55. I think I'm lucky most of the time.
56. I think first of myself because other people don't mean much to me.
57. I can't always be myself. Sometimes I have to pretend to be someone I'm not.
58. Most of the time I keep to myself. It is not easy to get to know me.
59. I do care for others and want them to be happy.
60. I really have a chip on my shoulder. I don't get along well with anyone.
61. I'm very careful of what I do or say, not because this means much to me, but because other people's good opinions of me are important.
62. I really am disturbed—close to the breaking point.
63. It seems to me I'm always in the wrong. I just can't be good enough for some people.
64. I am sure that the way I feel about most things and most people is the right way to feel.
65. I am kind and gentle.
66. Most people like me because I'm warm and friendly to them.
67. I can't do things easily. I have to keep pushing myself.
68. I've learned to do what I'm told and not ask questions or talk back.
69. I feel able to make up my own mind and stick to it if I want to.
70. I'm not afraid if something new comes up. I can get along almost anywhere.
71. I just wish I could be someone else and forget all about me.

72. I can't really tell anyone what I'm like inside.
73. I feel that there is nothing I can't do if I set my mind to it.
74. People can count on my being about the same all the time. I don't change very much.
75. I am conscientious and honorable. I can be depended upon.

Score Sheet:

Columns

statements

	1	2	3	4	5	6	7	8	9	D	D²
1				A	B					1	1
2					A		B			2	4
3		B	A							2	4
4											
5											
6											
7											
8											
9											
10											
11											
12											
13											
14											
15											
16											
17											
18											
19											
20											
21											
22											
23											
24											
25											
26											
27											
28											
29											
30											
31											
32											
33											
34											
35											
36											
37											
38											
39											
40											

	1	2	3	4	5	6	7	8	9	D	D²
41											
42											
43											
44											
45											
46											
47											
48											
49											
50											
51											
52											
53											
54											
55											
56											
57											
58											
59											
60											
61											
62											
63											
64											
65											
66											
67											
68											
69											
70											
71											
72											
73											
74											
75											

16

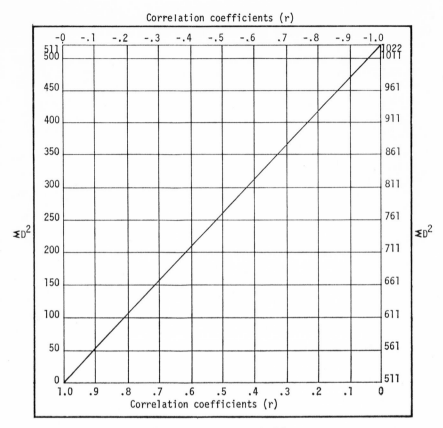

Fig. 12-1. Nomograph ($^{2:62}$)

Scoring. To read r, the correlation coefficient, for any sum of D^2 up to 511, the nomograph is entered from the left at the level of D^2 sum. By proceeding to the diagonal line and then down the value of r is read off the positive scale. If the sum of D^2 is within the 511–1022 range, the nomograph is entered from the right and the value of r is read off the top (negative) scale.$^{2:25}$ The nomograph is appropriate for any Q-Sort containing 75 items.

The smaller the discrepancies, the larger the correlation coefficient and the better the agreement or relationship between "Myself As I Am" and "My Ideal Self."

Doudlah Movement-Concept Statements*

Purpose. To determine the relationship between a student's movement-concept and what she would ideally like her movement-concept to be.

* Doudlah, Anna May: The Relationship Between the Self-Concept, the Body-Image, and the Movement-Concept of College Women with Low and Average Motor Ability, MSPE, University of North Carolina at Greensboro, Greensboro, N. C.. 1962. Used by permission of the author.

Evaluation. "Movement-concept is used to denote that view an individual has of himself as a physically mobile entity."[2:16] The group of statements was constructed by Doudlah and submitted to a 7-man jury to judge on the basis of their relevancy in helping a college freshman evaluate her OWN body-image and movement-concept.

Seventy-five statements were selected at random from the ones judged relevant.

Level and Sex. Developed for college women. May be appropriate for secondary school girls.

Uses. To enable the student to become more aware of her movement-concept.

To study changes in movement-concept.

To relate movement-concept to other factors such as Body-Image and Self-Concept.

Directions and Score Card.

1. You will be given a packet of 75 statements and 2 answer sheets.
2. Sort the statements into three piles:
   a. On the left the statements which are "least like" you.
   b. An in-between pile of statements.
   c. On the right the statements which are "most like" you.
3. Sort the statements further into 9 categories. Place the statement number for only 2 items in the 1st column, the statement numbers of 5 statements in column 2, continuing until you have used all the statements and filled in all the blocks on the answer sheet. Statements which are "least like" you will be noted toward the number one side of the answer sheet. Statements which are "most like" you will be indicated toward the number nine side of the answer sheet.
4. Statements in each column have the same value regardless of their order.
5. You will complete two sorts:
   Sort One: Sort the statements from the point of view of how you see yourself at this exact moment in time. This is called the self-sort.
   Sort Two: Sort the statements from the point of view of how you would ideally like to be. This is called the ideal-sort.

Q-Sort Statements—Movement-Concept

1. I am able to push a heavy object (like a piano) without difficulty.
2. My movements are described as slow.
3. Hanging by my arms is difficult for me.
4. I cannot keep up with the class when we do sit-ups.
5. Fine movements (like typing) are difficult for me.
6. Modern dance scares me.
7. I have difficulty getting my arms and legs to work together when I swim.
8. I like to move to music.
9. I take average size steps when I walk.
10. I have difficulty with balance when standing on one leg.
11. I doubt my ability to make baskets when playing basketball.
12. I feel discouraged about my physical ability.

13. I like to do stretching type exercises.
14. I try to get out of physical activity.
15. I have stiff joints.
16. Physical activity has always been important to me.
17. I feel hopeless when playing a game.
18. I am afraid to swim in deep water.
19. I fatigue easily.
20. I judge my physical performance by the best players in the class.
21. I can move as well as anyone.
22. I feel adequate when playing volleyball.
23. I really don't move well.
24. Sports scare me.
25. I feel confident about being able to learn new physical activities.
26. I feel embarrassed when doing exercises.
27. I am able to do heavy physical work.
28. I prefer doing things with my hands.
29. I like difficult physical tasks.
30. Jumping is no problem for me.
31. Physical fitness is unimportant to me.
32. I learn physical skills easily.
33. I throw a ball with accuracy.
34. I am able to meet the physical demands of everyday living.
35. I can be described as an energetic person.
36. I like to do big sweeping movements.
37. I usually use the handrail when going down the stairs.
38. I have difficulty climbing up a rope.
39. I stumble a lot when walking.
40. I have no difficulty carrying a wooden chair.
41. I like to do flowing kinds of movements.
42. I have difficulty with exercises which require me to move my arms and legs at the same time.
43. I like to swim.
44. I have fun playing on a team.
45. I like people who are active.
46. I make strong physical demands on myself.
47. I feel good when I move.
48. I am usually not able to do as well as others on the team.
49. I am physically fit.
50. I am easily discouraged when learning new movements.
51. I have difficulty catching large objects.
52. I can bounce a ball with ease.
53. I am interested in knowing how I perform physically.
54. I am really a good player.
55. I drop things.
56. I have trouble remembering dance steps.
57. I feel awkward when carrying large objects.
58. I perform best when doing small coordinated movements.
59. I like sports where I play against one other person.
60. I usually lose at sports.
61. I bowl with ease.
62. Controlling the ball in bowling is no problem for me.
63. I am a good swimmer.
64. I am afraid of falling.
65. My movements are inhibited.

66. I am average in physical skill.
67. I like to do hard physical work.
68. I like to be active.
69. I frequently bump into things.
70. My movements are brisk and sharp.
71. I have no difficulty keeping time with the music when I dance.
72. I feel helpless when faced with a physical task.
73. I have always been proud of my physical ability.
74. Physical activity bothers me. I would rather do something else.
75. I am well coordinated.

Scoring and Score Sheet. See the description for scoring the Nelson Self-Concept Q-Sort Statement on page 466.

Answer Sheet:

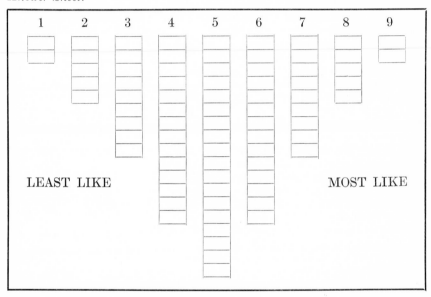

Doudlah Body-Image Statements*

Purpose. To measure the discrepancy between the body-image as perceived by the student and the body-image she would like to have.

Evaluation. The statements were developed by Doudlah[2] using the jury method to determine relevancy of statements. The Q-Sort technique was used to measure differences in body-image as perceived and as desired.

Level and Sex. Developed for college women. Probably suitable for secondary school girls. Could be adapted for use with boys.

Uses. To make the student aware of a body-image concept.

* Doudlah, Anna May: The Relationship Between the Self-Concept, the Body-Image, and the Movement-Concept of College Women with Low and Average Motor Ability, MSPE, University of North Carolina at Greensboro, Greensboro, N. C., 1962. Used by permission of the author.

To study differences between body-image at a certain time and a desired or ideal body-image.

To relate body-image to self-concept and to movement-concept.

To study changes in body-image concept after units of instruction or a year of physical education.

Directions and Answer Sheet. See Directions for Nelson Self-Concept Statements on page 463 or Doudlah Movement-Concept Statement on page 467.

Q-Sort Statements—Body-Image

1. I am good looking.
2. I enjoy having my picture taken.
3. I feel uneasy when I sit facing a group.
4. Heels make my legs look better.
5. I usually wear flat heeled shoes.
6. I am particular about the length of my skirts and dresses.
7. I am sophisticated.
8. People notice me when I enter a room.
9. I often notice people staring at me.
10. I enjoy looking at myself in the mirror.
11. Being well dressed is important to me.
12. I can appear sophisticated when I want to.
13. I dislike fat people.
14. I inherited my body build and therefore cannot do much about the way I look.
15. I enjoy being a girl.
16. I am concerned about the shape of my legs.
17. I get upset when my face breaks out.
18. I feel sorry for people who are homely.
19. My complexion has never been a problem.
20. Having a clear complexion is important to me.
21. I feel sorry for the girl who has a skin problem.
22. Physical activity is important to me.
23. My shoulders are broad.
24. I have good posture.
25. I feel most comfortable doing small restricted movements.
26. I am poised.
27. I am muscular.
28. I feel good in the clothes I wear.
29. I often wished I looked like someone else.
30. My physical appearance bothers me.
31. I often think about how I appear to others.
32. I look like an average person.
33. I wish I could wear the kind of clothes other girls wear.
34. I like to wear tight fitting clothes.
35. I wish I could do something about my size.
36. I am ashamed of my appearance.
37. I have big feet.
38. It is important for me to know I am physically attractive.
39. Weight control is difficult for me.
40. I think a lot about my physical appearance.
41. I am underweight.
42. I have nice teeth.
43. I have skinny arms.

44. I usually weigh more than I think I do.
45. I like to dress up because it gives me a good feeling.
46. My hair has always been a problem to me.
47. My hands are strong.
48. I have thick ankles.
49. I have expressive eyes.
50. My smile is warm and friendly.
51. I am sensitive about my size.
52. I am awkward.
53. I am well proportioned physically.
54. I spend a great deal of time on personal grooming.
55. Comments made in a group about physical appearance usually bother me.
56. I like to be told how I look.
57. I really don't care how I look.
58. I usually wear tight fitting sweaters.
59. I rarely think about my body.
60. I look good in shorts.
61. I feel fat.
62. I am too tall.
63. I have heavy thighs.
64. I look good in a bathing suit.
65. I like to talk about my appearance.
66. People are judged by their physical appearance.
67. I have ugly legs.
68. I have skinny legs.
69. My physical size makes me stand out.
70. I have big hips.
71. I like to learn about my body.
72. I am satisfied with the way I look.
73. I have small muscles.
74. I have big bones.
75. I am physically attractive.

Scoring and Scale Sheet. See scoring procedures described for Nelson Self-Concept Statements on page 466.

Self-Concept Measures—Additional Sources

Beatty, Walcott H., Ed.: *Improving Educational Assessment—An Inventory of Measures of Affective Behavior.* Washington, D.C.: Association for Supervision and Curriculum, N. E. A., 1969.

Belzer, Edwin G.: Effect of Physical Activity Upon Body Image as Measured by an Aniseikonic Technique, M. A., University of Maryland, 1962.

Clifton, Marguerite A., and Hope M. Smith: Comparison of Expressed Self-Concepts of Highly Skilled Males and Females Concerning Motor Performance, Perceptual and Motor Skills, *16*, 199–201, February, 1963.

Duke, James E. : Changes in Self-Concept Following a One-Week Resident Outdoor Education Experience, M.S. in Recreation and Parks, Pennsylvania State University, 1968.

Elbaum, Isabel: Body Image and Motor Development, MSPE, University of California, Los Angeles, 1964.

Engel, M., and W. J. Raine: A Method for the Measurement of the Self-Concept of Children in the Third Grade, Journal of Genetic Psychology, *102*, 125–138, March, 1963.

Felker, Donald W.: Relationship Between Self-Concept, Body Build, and Perception of Father's Interest in Sports in Boys, Research Quarterly, *39*, 513–517, October, 1968.

Flynn, Kenneth W.: Responses on the Davidson Adjective Check List as Related to Maturity, Physical, and Motor Ability Characteristics of Sixteen Year Old Boys, Ed. D., University of Oregon, Eugene, Oregon, 1967.

Gottesman, Eleanor, and W. E. Caldwell: The Body Image Identification Test, Journal of Genetic Psychology, *108*, 19–34, March, 1966.

Hunt, Valerie V., and Mary Ellen Weber: The Body Image Projective Test, Journal of Projective Techniques, *24*, 3–10, 1960.

McBee, Dorothy Carolyn: Self Conceptualization in Movement, MSPE, University of California, Los Angeles, 1962.

Piers, Ellen V., and Dale B. Harris: Age and Other Correlates of Self-Concept in Children, Journal of Educational Psychology, LV, No. 2, 91–95, 1964.

Shadduck, Ione G.: Self Concept of Appearance and Movement in Space: An Index for Fifth Grade Children, MA, Michigan State University, Lansing, Mich., 1964.

Smith, Hope M., and Marguerite A. Clifton: Sex Differences in Expressed Self-Concepts Concerning the Performance of Selected Motor Skills, Perceptual and Motor Skills, *14*, 71–73, February, 1962.

Sugarman, A. Arthur, and Frank Haronian: Body Type and Sophistication of Body Concept, Journal of Personality, *32*, 380–394, September, 1964.

Sullivan, Linda: Relationship Between Self—and Measured Perception of Physical and Personality Characteristics, MSPE, Springfield College, Springfield, Mass., 1965.

Tessier, Florence Annette: Self-Inventory for Movement Education, MSPE, University of California, Los Angeles, 1962.

Vincent, William J., and Don S. Dorsey: Body Image Phenomena and Measures of Physiological Performance, Research Quarterly, *39*, 1101–1106, December, 1968.

Woods, Marcella D.: An Exploration of Developmental Relationships Between Children's Body Image Boundaries, Estimates of Dimensions of Body Space, and Performance of Selected Gross Motor Tasks, Ph.D., Ohio State University, Columbus, Ohio, 1966.

Worchel, P., and B. L. McCormick: Self-Concept and Dissonance Reduction, Journal of Personality, *31*, 588–599, December, 1963.

Yeatts, Perline P., and Ira J. Gordon: Effects of Physical Education Taught by a Specialist on Physical Fitness and Self-Image. Research Quarterly, *39*, 766–770, October, 1968.

Self-Concept Measures—References

1. Davidson, Helen H., and Gerhard Lang: Children's Perceptions of Their Teacher's Feelings Toward Them Related to Self-Perception, School Achievement, and Behavior, Journal of Experimental Education, *29*, 107–118, December, 1960.

2. Doudlah, Anna May: The Relationships Between the Self-Concept, the Body-Image, and the Movement-Concept of College Women with Low and Average Motor Ability, MSPE, University of North Carolina at Greensboro, Greensboro, N. C., 1962.

3. Gordon, Ira J.: *A Test Manual for the How I See Myself Scale*, Gainesville, Florida: Florida Educational Research and Development Council, 1968.

4. Jersild, A. T.: *In Search of Self*. New York: Teachers College Bureau of Publications, 1952.

5. Nelson, Sara Marie: An Investigation of the Relationship Between the Real Self-Concept—Ideal Self-Concept and the Motor Ability of Eighth Grade Girls in Physical Education, M. Ed., University of North Carolina at Greensboro, Greensboro, N. C., 1966.

6. Reynolds, Robert M.: Responses of the Davidson Adjective Check List as Related to Maturity, Physical, and Mental Characteristics of Thirteen-Year-Old Boys, Ed. D., University of Oregon, 1965.

7. Rogers, C. R.: *Client-Centered Therapy*. Boston: Houghton-Mifflin, 1952.

8. Rogers, C. R., and Rosalind F. Dymond: *Psychotherapy and Personality Change*. Chicago, The University of Chicago Press, 1954.

9. Sakers, Amy E.: The Relationships Between a Selected Measure of Motor Ability and the Actual-Ideal Self-Concept, Body-Image and Movement-Concept of the Adolescent Girl, MAPE, University of Maryland, College Park, Md., 1968.

Part III. EVALUATION OF THE PROCESS

Chapter 13
INTRODUCTION TO PROCESS
EVALUATION

The two aspects of education—the product and the process—have been discussed in Chapter 1. There it was explained that society examines values and selects those which it considers desirable. A physically educated person is one of the desirable values of society and, like so many other lofty goals, when attained, is the result of educational endeavor. In order to be sure that the qualities of a physically educated person are achieved, the physical educator establishes objectives to serve as points of reference. The achievement of the product through these points of reference necessitates further the establishment of the educational processes. These are the prescribed ways and means by which the desired results are obtained. There must be acceptable standards in each aspect of the process. These processes and their acceptable standards are significantly important because the objectives for the product are difficult or impossible to achieve when the processes are inadequate.

After the processes have been prescribed, the standards set and the procedures implemented, it is good educational practice to evaluate these procedures to determine how well they measure up to the prescribed standards and to find out how effective they have been in satisfying the listed objectives which have been established for the product. Measurement determines the worth of the program in terms of the objectives and selected values. After measurement there is a follow-up to re-appraise the aims and objectives and to revise or strengthen those areas of process which were discovered to be weak as a result of the analysis of the test data. This replanning of the process requires re-evaluation and a repetition of the entire cycle. Thus, process evaluation, as has been pointed out in Chapter 1, is part of an on-going cycle with measurement, analysis, and prescription following each other in a continuous sequential pattern.

Process in Relation to Product

The *process* may be measured in one of two ways. First, it may be measured first hand when measurement techniques are applied directly to process components; or second, it may be measured indirectly by measuring the status and achievement of the product. Total evaluation would consist of data collected from both sources. This measurement of product has been discussed in Part II of this text and the factors of the product and the means of measuring them were discussed specifically in Chapter 6, page 115. When the student is measured directly, his learnings and accomplishments should in a sense reflect the quality of the process because there is an assumed cause-effect relationship between them whereby the product is inextricably related to the process. A good process should be reflected through a superior product.

It is not enough, however, to assume that product and process are inexorably related. This question is frequently asked by general educators and critics of physical education, "Does physical education educate?" In other words, does the product of physical education when manifested by student status in, and progress toward desirable outcomes relate to the process when it is revealed by the attainment of the school program in recognized standards? Some people question that physical education can show that its product and process are related, and physical educators have been challenged to submit evidence to support the claim that good programs are producing desirable, tangible, and measurable results in the product. A number of investigators, including Bookwalter, have provided this evidence.[2]

Bookwalter and associates have shown that achievement in the objectives of physical education at the secondary school level is directly related to the standards of physical education according to the LaPorte Health and Physical Education Score Card.[3] This study shows that in all the areas tested except attitudes the process of physical education is causal to product.[4,6] Achievement of students in the objectives of physical education is highly related to the school's attainment in acceptable standards. If students score high on tests of fitness, skill, knowledge, and attitude, it may reasonably be expected that there is a good program behind such achievement. Also, if the school physical education process is rated high on score cards pertaining to the standards of physical education, it might logically be expected that its students in general will score well on achievement tests. However, as Bookwalter points out, while physical education does educate, it does not educate automatically. The amount of progress and achievement in physical education is dependent upon the degree to which a school has attained recognized standards in administration and instruction. In summary, it would seem necessary for the physical educator to know his purposes and the standards set up for his process and then to measure the status and progress of this process in order to see how nearly it is meeting the accepted standards. Then, and only then, is he prepared to submit to those who request it and to those who need it, tangible evidence that good programs produce good results.

Values of Process Evaluation

The purpose of measuring the physical education process has several points of departure and there are a number of values accruing from such procedures.

Adequacy. One of the first values to accrue is that of revealing the *adequacy* of the program. The procedures of evaluation lead to the identification of status, and since the objectives for process are designed to move from a given status to an improved one, measurement of progress toward desirable outcomes is a corollary to identification of status. In fact, the procedures of evaluation themselves may be excellent means of helping to achieve progress. This revealing of adequacy or lack of it is valuable knowledge. Generally, it can be given in terms of percentages or some other quantitative measure. For example, Bookwalter's study shows that programs throughout the country are only 28 per cent effective.[3] However, a final index of this type is not the most important value to accrue from measurement.

Inservice Training. A second value is *inserive training*. The use of evaluation tools both educates and motivates physical education personnel. When measuring techniques are applied to the process, they tend to focus the attention of the personnel who use them on the elements of a sound program. For example, when an evaluation tool is applied to the process, it demands a thorough study of the standards which are involved as criteria and a basic understanding of those essential components which constitute a good program. This knowledge of program construction and standard evaluation is of great value to those using the measurement techniques, and is one of the most important outcomes to accrue from the actions of evaluation. Staff members and administrators are inevitably forced to analyze not only their own programs but also themselves, their methods, and the environment in which they work. They engage in discussions of the facts revealed by the evaluation and in cooperative action they make observations and reveal their impressions. This self-analysis or self-study by school personnel of themselves and their program and its surroundings is certain to provide them with a better perspective of their particular situation and an appreciation of good programs in general. In reality, their program is displayed to them for the first time and in some instances in a graphic and objective manner. For example, the LaPorte Score Card employs a profile.[8] Here attention is directed toward the significant deviations of the process from the standards which have been set forth for comparisons. Since in-service training is inherent in the use of most measuring techniques, this work with program evaluation is excellent on-the-job training for staff members. In fact, this value alone is worth the cost in time for such evaluation.

Follow Up. A third value is apparent. There is a follow up to evaluation. This experience and training on the part of leadership should result in *positive action*. It should result in a better planned, a better administered, and a better taught process. Ultimately, of course, these things will be reflected in a better product. When personnel have become aware of weaknesses which have been revealed or uncovered by measurement, they can prescribe such alterations as seem necessary to improve the situation. Those areas of process subject to change in view of the existing conditions can be studied further and adjustments made. Such adjustments generally concern the manner in which the program is organized and conducted. The administrator should be alert to this need for evaluating his total program and searching for means to improve it. These evaluation results can be used as administrative support for making improvements in those phases of the process over which he has control, including such factors as facilities, equipment, program, and staff. These same results can also serve as guides to the teachers and supervisors who work with the administrator as together they set about improving the various aspects of the process for which they have responsibilities.

Factors in Process Evaluation

This measurement of status and progress in physical education outcomes has become a many-faceted procedure not only with regard to the product but also the process. Generally, when the product is evaluated, the student is measured directly as described in Part II of this textbook through one of the many techniques which are available and also described in Part II. When this product is measured, the part method is employed and various factors are, in effect, isolated and evaluated. In many cases these factors may be measured more or less objectively by the numerous objective techniques. There are many such tools to identify the level of achievement in the factors of fitness, motor ability, sport skills, and knowledge. The use of these tools lends results which are rather precise and definite. This is not to deny the fact that many facets of the product are qualitative and qualitative techniques involving observation and judgment must be used to measure them.

The process of physical education, like the product, is made up of basic factors or components. The type of product which is desired determines in a large measure the nature and the extent of these factors. When the factors of the process of physical education are measured, precise and exact measurement instruments are frequently not available just as is the case with some factors of the product. Subjective techniques must be used to measure these procedures. The procedures of the process are complex and many-faceted and total evaluation of them is difficult. It is frequently not possible to dichotomize. Since many factors of the process are qualitative in nature, measurement results to a certain extent must be based on subjectivity, although most of the techniques are objectified as much as possible. In general, factors of process may be identified under such headings as philosophy, organization and administration, staff, program of activities, instruction, facilities and equipment, and participation. Each of these particular factors has its specific elements or items. These factors are associated with standards and criteria which have been established for each component. Measurement will determine the degree of compliance of each factor and its specific elements with the standards. Classification of the aspects of process is a relative matter, but for purposes of this textbook only the main factors will be discussed.

While there are many facets of the process which can be evaluated, in general it is fragmented into four categories for study: evaluation of the staff (teacher), the curriculum, methodology, and the total process.

Staff Evaluation. The National Education Association states that more time and research money have gone into studies related to teacher evaluation than any other facet of education.[15] It is a controversial topic and has not been popular with teachers. However, with the explosion of knowledge and the greater demands on the student for learning, there is a correspondingly greater responsibility for the teacher to teach more effectively. In the future there will be a greater premium on effective teaching. The current emphasis on knowledge and academics and their extension into the realm of the affective domain will force administrators to learn where this good teaching is taking place and equally where poor teaching exists. This discovery process involves evaluation in one form or another.

Teacher evaluation can be dichotomized into two categories with respect to uses: (1) *for the improvement of instruction,* and (2) for *sound administrative decisions affecting the teacher* such as salary, promotion, tenure, re-employment, placement, and transfer.[14] This latter use, especially salary and promotion, has generally been referred to as "merit rating." This does not mean, however, that the two uses are dichotomous and refer to two different things. Even when evaluation is used for merit, it is presumably an incentive toward improvement in teaching. Therefore, the one overriding goal of teacher evaluation is *improvement of teaching*.

Since many of the studies reported in the literature concern merit ratings, some attention might be directed toward this topic for a brief discussion. On the surface, merit ratings seem logical since the purpose behind them appears to be consistent with the democratic premise that all men should be paid what they are worth. No professional or administrator could oppose this tenet in principle. In practice, however, this principle has not always been operable. Some form of teacher evaluation is needed in order to move away from the "sacred white cow"—training and number of years of experience—which has dominated education as an easy way out for administrators when salary, promotion and other administrative decision are involved. The merit system, while it must not be confused as being synonymous with teacher evaluation, appears to have failed in the past because there seemed to be no adequate basis for estimating a teacher's worth which could be agreed upon. Also, there seemed to be no acceptable way of adequately and fairly measuring this worth after it had been established.

Advocates of teacher evaluation believe the idea is sound and can be implemented under right conditions. The NEA supports a belief that the teaching profession has a commitment to evaluate the quality of its services.[12] Recognizing the difficulties that must be overcome and aware of failures in the past, it recommends that teacher evaluation programs be developed through identification of the following three things: (1) What are the factors that determine professional competency? (2) What are the methods or techniques of evaluating these identified competencies? (3) What are the ways of recognizing professional competence after it has been identified?[13]

When teacher evaluation programs are instituted, there are some questions which must be answered such as "why" evaluate in the first place, "who" does the evaluation, "how" is the process implemented, and "what" is the basis for evaluation? The first question has already been answered.

Who Evaluates? In the past most teacher evaluation has been done by administrators and supervisors. In some instances the teacher's own peers have shared in a limited sense. While parents have rarely been involved in formal evaluation, they do make evaluations and often the evaluators are very much conscious of the parents' opinion. Students have always evaluated the teacher either in a formal or an informal way. Informally, they do it by either registering for the good class so as to avoid the bad, or finding the sinecure which would allow them the best chance of a passing grade with the least amount of effort. However, today's students are the most intellectual, most perceptive and the best prepared academically of any students in history. They are capable of making sound judgments and it is no longer possible to ignore them when the purpose of evaluation is improvement of teaching.

However, the most important person to share in evaluation is the teacher who is being evaluated. Whether the teacher is being evaluated for merit or for improvement in teaching, the most important educational value to accrue is improvement of his teaching where he becomes a better teacher because of the evaluation. If improvement in teaching is to occur, it can come about only through the teacher's own effort and initiative. Ultimately self-evaluation must take place. The teacher must evaluate himself and in the light of information he gets from others plus his own analysis of himself, he tries to improve his teaching performance and skills.

How is Evaluation Done? There seem to be certain well defined steps in the implementation of a teacher evaluation program. *First,* the initial planning must be a cooperative effort between the teachers and administrators at which time the criteria for the basis of evaluation are developed—the characteristics of a good teacher. It may well be that different sets of criteria will be needed for the evaluation of teachers in the different disciplines since they will vary according to job analysis for the different subject matter areas. *Second,* the evaluation instrument itself must be designed and constructed. These instruments vary all the way from homemade techniques to the devices shown in Chapter 17. In some cases the more objective techniques are used, while in others the more subjective types are preferred. The most common device is the rating scale but check lists and open ended narrative types are frequently used.[11] *Third,* the next step is the evaluation itself. The general principles to follow here is a more positive approach whereby the teacher's strengths are spotlighted rather than the weaknesses. This approach seems to be necessary in order to offset the problems of low morale created by the traditional merit system. This does not mean that weakness cannot be revealed and discussed at the proper time.

In the evaluation itself there are certain crucial steps which are necessary. *First,* there should be a self-evaluation by the teacher usually on a check list or rating scale form designed for that purpose. *Second,* the teacher is evaluated by one or more evaluators. This could be the administrator, supervisor, departmental chairman, a peer associate, or even an outside evaluator. *Third,* there should be a time for review and discussion between the teacher and the evaluators. Certainly this meeting should be carried on in an atmosphere of mutual concern and trust if possible. *Fourth,* there should be a follow-up where the emphasis is on self-correction by the teacher in the light of the evaluation results.

At this stage there are perhaps three more steps which could be added for a total program of evaluation. *First,* after teacher evaluation there should always be a procedure for adjudication of disputed evaluations especially if some form of the merit system is involved.[14] This right of appeal in the event of disagreement would seem to be in keeping with the democratic idea of evaluation for worth. *Second,* a system of evaluation is never perfect. It must be constantly reviewed and re-structured. Therefore, a continuous evaluation of the evaluating system should be encouraged with both teachers and administrators involved. *Third,* evaluation is a two-way process. There should be an evaluation of the administrators by the teachers. This plan would undoubtedly be a factor in better morale.

Some of the methods which have been used include observations, conferences, comments, from parents' evaluation of students, record of student achievement, and rating scales (see Chapter 17).

What is the Basis for Evaluation? One of the most difficult facets of evaluation of the teacher concerns establishing the factors of professional competency. There have been long lists of these used in the past and they do not easily fall into well defined categories. However, for the sake of expediency, they have been assigned to the following four categories:[10] *PERSONAL QUALITIES* such as character, personality, poise, social amenities, grooming, sense of humor, health, vitality, patience, self control, friendliness, fairness and the like. *TEACHING PERFORMANCE* such as knowledge of subject matter, instructional skills, guidance and counseling concern and skill, classroom atmosphere, emotional climate, evaluation and the like. *PROFESSIONAL QUALITIES* such as ethics, pride in the profession, support of authorized policies, desire for improvement, willingness to take advantage of in-service training opportunities, further study and the like. *RELATIONSHIPS* with the students, parents, staff, administration, community and professional personnel and associations.

Curriculum Evaluation. Curriculum building is a continuous dynamic ongoing process. It is a part of the education cycle which starts with the formulation of objectives, continues with the establishment of the program and methodology, and ends with the evaluation of results. This entire cycle is repeated again and again. The curriculum building process has been referred to by Cassidy as a merry-go-round with many riders.[5] These riders include administrators, supervisors, teachers, specialists, students, and parents, and they all share in the various facets of the process. The curriculum itself is in a constant state of being re-studied, revised, and rebuilt. The basis for any orderly but ongoing improvement is evaluation.

Every school must provide for some ongoing permanent study for the purposes of this evaluation. Since the process is a cycle there must be some force or machinery to keep the cycle moving.

This is usually performed by a curriculum committee which could even be the original committee which first developed the curriculum with new riders from time to time. However, the committee should represent the entire staff and should keep the lines of communication open so that all staff members may relate and share in the re-study and revision. In small schools the entire staff can serve as a committee.

Evaluation can be carried out on a formal or an informal basis. In the formal approach there are techniques designed to measure the various aspects of the curriculum such as rating scales, score cards or inventories. On the more informal approach, the staff reviews, discusses and appraises these same aspects in terms of how they think their objectives have been met. Also, evaluation can be done directly or indirectly. In the indirect type of approach, it is the student who is measured by the many type tests which have been discussed in Part II of this book. In this approach it is assumed that the product reflects the quality of the curriculum. A good program should produce a quality student who is moving toward the ideal of a physically educated person. In the direct approach both the formal and the informal techniques may apply. The less formal plan lends itself to curriculum re-study and evaluation because it is closely related to curriculum study and construction. The informal approach reviews the curriculum by seeking answers to certain relevant questions such as: Are the objectives being met? Is the program of activities varied enough? Does the program show enough progression and sequential arrangement of learning experiences? Is there articulation between levels? Is the curriculum adapted to the age and sex needs of boys and girls? Does it provide a balanced program of activities? Is it flexible enough to meet the changing circumstances? These and many other questions must be answered.

In the more formal approach the rating scale and score card shown in the next chapter can be used to measure the curriculum phase of the process. Perhaps there is need for both the formal and informal approach to evaluation of curriculum.

Evaluation of Methodology. Another important facet of process evaluation is methodology or the instructional process. It is difficult to separate the teacher from the teaching act, just as it is difficult to separate them both from the curriculum. Thus, this section on evaluation of methodology is highly related to the two preceding sections. However, this factor is more concerned with the methods and materials which are employed by staff members as they make use of equipment and facilities to make the curriculum function. It is also concerned with the actual techniques of teaching the class, class management, class administrative details, demonstrations, explanations, and drill techniques. Also involved are the materials which are used such as audio-visual aids, charts, models, chalk board, bulletin boards, rules books, textbooks and reference books. Also involved are the uses made of courses of study, student leadership, and evaluation since evaluation is an integral part of the teaching and instructional procedures.

In a well-organized and conducted program of physical education these established ways of approach to teaching, the instructional procedures, and the methods of doing things need to be evaluated. They need to be reviewed, discussed and revised much in the same manner as the curriculum. The informal discussion attack is best suited to this problem although in many cases an alert staff with initiative want to research the best methods of teaching.

Evaluation of the Total Process. Instead of evaluating the various aspects separately, there is an approach to the total process for measurement. Some purposes make it necessary to learn about the total situation which would include not only the leadership, curriculum and methodology, but also such facets as philosophy, the organization and administration aspects, equipment, outdoor and indoor facilities, intramurals, interschool athletics, and participation which involves time requirements and the uses made of it.[9]

There are numerous tools which can be used for evaluating this total process. In general, the devices which have been employed are in the form of check lists or rating scales. In a rating scale, for example, the standards which have been included conform to the accepted standards established by experts in physical education. The scale is constructed with categories so they can be checked to indicate the extent of compliance with the accepted standard. This may be just a plain "yes" or "no" or in some cases a third category of "U" added for undecided. In others, the categories may be a simple three-point scale or a five-point scale. The points on the scale are usually defined to indicate the degree of compliance with the standard.

The purpose of most of these tools is to reveal weaknesses. When these weak areas have been revealed, attention can be given to ways and means of *improvement*. Therefore, the primary purpose of such evaluation is process improvement. In some cases the evaluation is done as a step toward *accreditation*. These criteria tools are available at the elementary, the secondary, and college levels. They are designed so that an individual, a staff, or an evaluation team may apply them. Generally when a school seeks accreditation on the basis of an evaluation by a team of evaluators, the physical education staff is required to do a self-study and an evaluation. This self-evaluation is then used by the evaluators as a part of their total evaluation.

However, since evaluation is a constant ongoing process and as many people should share in it as possible, the rating scale or check list is not the final answer. Another facet of evaluation is through the students. What the students think and how they view the total program can be found through rating scales and through interest questionnaires. The data, when obtained from these sources, should be used to supplement information from other facets of the evaluation processes. Student evaluation, although not always highly reliable and valid, does provide a more complete picture and has the added advantage of involving the student in an active way in the evaluation and curriculum construction processes.

Uses of Process Evaluation

There are many uses for results of process evaluation. Primarily, of course, the end result of all measurement in physical education is to serve the needs of the students because ultimately the final criterion of program worth is the way it affects student growth and development. However, a more immediate end of process measurement is the improvement of the process itself. In addition to these more general reasons for process measurement, there are a number of more specific uses.

Measurement of Status and Progress. The basic use of measurement is to secure the data which are necessary to *reveal the status of the program*—its relative quality and effectiveness. If re-evaluation is done and comparisons are made with previous measurements, *there is an identification of progress.* The measurement of this rate of progress or improvement is an important outcome of evaluation. If measurement is made annually and a profile, graph, or chart is constructed of the findings, a graphic picture is available to show how some aspects of the process have moved closer to the standards which have been established.

Comparisons. Evaluation always involves comparisons and these comparisons are made in relation to certain criteria with well-established standards. Probably the most basic use in this area is to make comparisons with established standards in order to show how present programs stand with respect to the ideal program or with a previous measurement of the same program to show progress and achievement. Other frequent uses are to compare the effectiveness of an existing program with another program and the program in one locale with programs in another. In any event, it is essential that comparisons be made with acceptable educational standards if the program outcomes are to be effectively evaluated.

Identification of Strengths and Weaknesses. When measurement results are compared with norms or standards, certain aspects of the process are revealed. Such comparisons will basically reveal two conditions: First, they might show in what aspect or aspects the standards are met or surpassed. Second, they may show need and weaknesses. Both approaches have great value. In some cases, a profile is used to set up measurement data and to indicate needs in a graphic and quantitative manner. Probably the most practical result of comparisons is the uncovering of weaknesses, which, when pinpointed, can furnish the focal point of the follow-up. This follow-up is most important because what happens to the program after measurement is far more important than the measurement itself or its results. On the basis of significant weaknesses which are revealed by measurement, the process can be changed and strengthened. Some results can be used to show a need in the factors of personnel and facilities. On the basis of these revealed needs, requests can be made for additional staff members or equipment and facilities to carry on the program in an effective manner. Measurement results may also be used to gather material and supporting evidence to justify an existing program which has already been in operation, a pilot project, or a particular technique in use at the present time. Also, they may be used to indicate the needs for new procedures or the use of new materials.

Indication of Teacher Effectiveness and Methods of Teaching. In addition to the appraisal of the program and tools, it is frequently important to find the answer to the question of how good the teacher is. How effective are his methods and his teaching skills? How effective are the materials which he uses, such as graphic arts, instructional media, etc.? Does he have a good teaching personality? Are his students motivated to scale greater heights? Does he lead his students into assuming greater responsibility and into making a self-analysis? Is he developing leadership and citizenship? Can he teach skills and does he inculcate a desire on the part of his students to be fit?

Motivation. One of the uses of program appraisal is motivation. Such self-evaluation and self-analysis, which are necessary in program and personnel evaluation, are bound to have stimulating effects. It should encourage staff members individually and as a group to strive for greater efficiency and to put out more effort. Process evaluation results will furnish them with materials and knowledge which can lead them to self-improvement. This in turn will lead to the up-grading of other factors of the process, and eventually have its effect in producing a better product.

Contribution to Research. Many times process evaluation is carried out in schools as a part of a research project. These studies naturally make contributions to the field in numerous ways. Probably the best known such project in recent years is a national survey of health and physical education in high schools supervised by

Karl W. Bookwalter and mentioned previously in this chapter.[1] From 1950–1954, 2600 schools selected through random sampling techniques in 26 states were surveyed. LaPorte's Health and Physical Education Score Card No. II was used as a basis of evaluation.[7] While each survey was a separate study in itself, all used similar techniques and their results could be compared and combined. When these data from the various studies were combined, a most dramatic and revealing picture is presented of the status of physical education at the secondary school level on a national basis. The median national score was only about 28 per cent of possible.[3] Results of such studies have many uses in themselves, including interpretation of the program, justification for more emphasis, serving as a basis for curriculum construction, and serving as a basis for making general and specific recommendations to teachers and administrators.

Administrative Understanding and Support. It is no secret that in the field of physical education one of the weak areas has been in public relations. The very nature of its activities and the climate in which it operates have led to misunderstandings and false beliefs. Also, the leadership in the past has not always been of the best quality and the conduct of many programs has not been conducive to a universal appreciation and acceptance of the field. This lack of appreciation for the needs and outcomes of physical education and the misunderstanding of its program frequently are shared by school administrators. Along with other media the results of process evaluation can be used to interpret the program to the school administrator and gain his understanding and support. If program objectives are to be achieved, not only must this understanding and support of the school administrator be available, but also that of the community.

Techniques

The importance of process evaluation has become more evident in recent years. There are numerous tools which have been employed. In general, the techniques which have been most used are the check list and rating scale. The majority of the instruments in these two areas of measurement are constructed along the same pattern. Standards are included in the instruments which conform to the accepted standards in physical education. These standards are grouped in numerous ways, but in general they are grouped under the factors which have been discussed in this chapter. The extent of compliance with the listed standards is generally determined by the use of category scales. These categories may be either "yes" or "no" or a three- or a five-point progressive scale. The point scales are usually defined in order to portray the degree or extent of compliance. The answers are generally helpful in focusing attention to weaknesses in the process and the primary purpose is the improvement of those areas found to be weak. Most tools are designed so that either an individual, a staff, or an evaluation team may evaluate the various factors of the program. Such criteria are available at the elementary, the secondary, and the college levels. These evaluation techniques are highly related to curriculum. Since all curricula should be dynamic and subject to frequent change and revision in the light of changing conditions, process evaluative criteria also need to be constantly reviewed and brought up to date according to the most recent standards.

One of the accepted ways of evaluating the physical education process is through the students. This is a different point of view and should provide interesting and valuable information. Just as students provide one of the best media of publicity for schools, they should also provide an excellent means of evaluating certain aspects of the program. However, just as students do not always report events and school happenings as they occur and certain allowances must be made in interpreting their school news, allowances must also be made in interpreting the results of student evaluation of school processes. Therefore, when this technique is used alone, it does not provide enough information for total appraisal. When it is used in conjunction with other tools, it does provide a more complete picture and it further enables the students to share in not only the process of evaluation but also in curriculum construction. There are a number of interest and attitude inventories which can be used. The Kneer Adaptation of Wear's Physical Education Attitude Inventory and Diagnostic Statements is perhaps one of the best examples of this type.[7]

References

1. Bookwalter, Karl W.: A National Survey of Health and Physical Education for Boys in High Schools, 1950–54. *Professional Contributions*, American Academy of Physical Education, No. 4, 1955, pp. 1–11.
2. ————: Physical Education Educates, The Physical Educator, *14*, 43–44, May, 1957.
3. Bookwalter, Karl W., and Carolyn W.: Purposes, Standards, and Results in Physical Education, Bulletin of the School of Education, Indiana University, *38*, No. 5, September, 1962, Bloomington, p. 26.
4. Calhoun, R. A.: A Comparison of Program Objectives of Selected Rated High School Physical Education Programs in Indiana. Unpublished P.E.D. Thesis, School of Health, Physical Education, and Recreation, Indiana University, Bloomington, 1956.
5. Cassidy, Rosalind: *Curriculum Development in Physical Education*. New York, Harper and Brothers, Publishers, 1954.
6. DeVoll, C. H.: An Analysis of the Boys' Health and Physical Education Program in Selected Secondary Schools in Wisconsin. Unpublished P.E.D. Thesis, School of Health, Physical Education, and Recreation, Indiana University, Bloomington, 1956.

7. Kneer, M. E.: The Adaptation of Wear's Physical Education Attitude Inventory for Use with High School Girls, Unpublished M.S. in Education Thesis. Illinois State Normal University, 1956.
8. LaPorte, Wm. Ralph, (Edited by Cooper, John M.): *The Physical Education Curriculum.* Los Angeles, College Book Store, 1955, pp. 72–87.
9. Larson, L. A., and R. D. Yocom: *Measurement and Evaluation in Physcial, Health, and Recreation Education.* St. Louis, The C. V. Mosby Co., 1951.
10. McGee, Rosemary: The How and What of Teacher Evaluation. Unpublished Report, Southern District Convention AAHPER, Memphis, Tennessee, 1959.
11. National Education Association: Classroom Observation Record. Research Memo 1962–31, NEA Research Division, Washington, D.C.
12. National Education Association: Policy Statements on Salaries for School Personnel: Research Memo 1968–12, NEA Research Division, Washington, D.C.
13. National Education Association: Merit Provisions in Teachers' Salary Schedules, 1967–68: NEA Research Division, Washington, D.C.
14. National Education Association: Guidelines for the Evaluation of the Classroom Teacher: NEA Research Division WP 62–30, Washington, D.C.
15. National Education Association: Merit Provisions in Teachers' Salary Schedules, 1967–68. NEA Research Memo, NEA Research Division, Washington, D.C.

Additional References

1. AAHPER, CPEA, and NAPECW: Physical Education for College Men and Women (Report of joint conference 1954 and revised 1959). Washington, D.C., AAHPER, 1959, pp. 30–33.
2. AAHPER: Your Community—School-Community Fitness Inventory, National Education Association, Washington, D.C., 1959, pp. 14–28.
3. Bookwalter, Karl W. (Edited by Carolyn W. Bookwalter and Robert J. Dollgener): *A Score Card for Evaluating Undergraduate Professional Programs in Physical Education.* Bloomington, Indiana University, 1962.
4. Blesh, T. E.: Evaluative Criteria in Physical Education. Unpublished Doctor's dissertation, New Haven, Yale University, 1945.
5. ———: Evaluative Criteria in Physical Education, Research Quarterly, *17*, 114–126, May, 1946.
6. Carr, Martha G., and Karl W. Bookwalter: Standards for High School Health and Physical Education Programs, Research Council National Survey Project. (Presented at Miami Convention of the AAHPER, 1960.)
7. Educational Policies Commission: Checklist on School Athletics, School Athletics, Washington, D.C., National Education Association, 1954, pp. 88–97.
8. Jackson, Chester O.: How Does Your Physical Education Program Rate? Journal of Health, Physical Education, and Recreation, *25*, 21–22, June, 1954.
9. LaPorte, W. D.: *Health and Physical Education Score Card No. I for Elementary Schools.* Los Angeles, College Book Store, University of Southern California, 1955.
10. ———: *Health and Physical Education Score Card No. II for Junior and Senior High Schools and for Four Year High Schools.* Los Angeles, College Book Store, University of Southern California, 1955. (May be purchased through College Book Store, University of Southern California, both Score Card No. I and No. II).
11. ———: Health and Physical Education Score Card No. I for Elementary Schools, *The Physical Education Curriculum,* Sixth Edition (Edited by John M. Cooper). Los Angeles, College Book Store, University of Southern California, 1955, pp. 66–71.
12. ———: Health and Physical Education Score Card No. II for Junior and Senior High Schools, *The Physical Education Curriculum* 6th Ed. (Edited by John M. Cooper). Los Angeles, College Book Store, University of Southern California, 1955, pp. 72–86.
13. Minnegan, Donald: Criteria of a Good Physical Education Program for Boys in the Senior High School. Unpublished Doctor's dissertation, Washington, D.C., George Washington University, 1947.
14. National Study of Secondary School Evaluation: Evaluative Criteria—Physical Education for Girls, 1960 Edition, Washington, D. C.

15. ———: Evaluative Criteria—Physical Education for Boys, 1960 Edition, Washington, D.C.
16. Neilson, N. P., and Glen W. Arnett: *A Score Card for Use in Evaluating Physical Education Programs in Elementary Schools*, Salt Lake City, Utah, University of Utah Press, 1955.
17. Ohio Association for Health, Physical Education, and Recreation: *Evaluative Criteria for Physical Education.* (Approved by State Department of Education.) Columbus, 1957.
18. Schooler, V. E.: Standards for Facilities for Athletics, Health, Physical Education, and Recreation for Secondary Boys. Doctor's dissertation, Bloomington, Indiana University, 1950.
19. State of Arkansas: A Physical Education Check List for Secondary Schools. *A Guide for Secondary Schools* (Revised). Little Rock, Division of Instructional Services, State Education Department, 1957, pp. 28–34.
20. State of Florida: A Check List—An Evaluation in Physical Education. Bulletin 5A, Tallahassee, State Department of Education, 1961.
21. State of New York: *Check List for Physical Education.* Albany, Division of Health and Physical Education, State Education Department.
22. State of North Carolina: *Athletics in the Public Schools.* Raleigh, State Department of Public Instruction, North Carolina, 1954, pp. 18–27.
23. State of Utah: *A Score Card for Evaluation of Physical Education Programs for High School Boys.* Salt Lake City, Department of Public Instruction, Utah, 1949.

Chapter 14

TECHNIQUES OF PROCESS EVALUATION

Laporte Health and Physical Education Score Cards*

Purpose. To measure status and progress in the process of physical eduction.

Evaluation. Score cards have been validated through the jury technique.

Level. Score Card No. I is for the elementary school and Score Card No. II is for Junior and Senior High Schools and for Four Year High Schools.

General Procedure. 1. Score cards can be ordered from College Book Store, University of California, Los Angeles.
2. Ratings can be made by the members of the school administrative staff assisted by the staff of physical education.
3. Each item is to be checked 1, 2, or 3 according to whether it is fair, good, or excellent. A score of zero may be given.
4. All ratings must be made in as objective manner as possible without prejudice.
5. In cases where exact standards are listed and the situation is an approximate condition, equivalent scores should be estimated.

Uses. The first fact revealed is the status of the program according to the standards set up in the score card. When the profile is used, this status is revealed in a graphic manner. Status data can be used to compare one's school with the ideal program, with the national norms shown in Figure 14–1, p. 507, or with a previous survey of one's own school. When the data are thus set up, they can be interpreted to school administrators and the community in order to gain support for those phases of the process which need strengthening.

Health and Physical Education Score Cards

No. II—Secondary Schools

Instructions for Use of Score Cards

Nature of Cards. These cards are intended as measuring devices for purposes of evaluating the physical education program and the general health, recreation, and safety provisions of an entire school. The rating should be made by the school principal himself or by his official representative assisted by the physical education instructor. The purpose is to

* LaPorte, W. R., John M. Cooper, ed.: Health and Physical Education Score Card No. II for Junior and Senior High Schools, *The Physical Education Curriculum*. Los Angeles: College Book Store, University of Southern California, 1955, pp. 72–86. (Copies may be purchased from the College Book Store, University of Southern California, Los Angeles.) Adapted by permission of John M. Cooper and the College Book Store.

center attention upon the characteristics of a good program and to provide opportunity for a school to compare its offering somewhat objectively with these characteristics. The evaluation should serve to disclose significant weaknesses that are subject to improvement, rather than to present merely a critical rating of the school.

The Rating Standards. The standards presented in these score cards are based on the 23-year intensive study by the Committee on Curriculum Research of the College Physical Education Association. Preliminary score cards were formulated by the chairman from the committee findings, and submitted for critical evaluation to a selected jury of 150 leading state, city, and rural supervisors and administrators of physical education throughout the United States. Their varied criticisms served as the basis for reconstructing the cards in preliminary form in 1938.

After 12 years of experience with the cards in rating state, county, and city school systems, the chairman conducted a re-evaluation survey in the fall of 1950. A jury of specialists was again asked to re-examine the Score Card standards for needed changes. A number of modifications were proposed which appear in the revised Score Cards presented herewith.

In order to keep the standards as flexible as possible for adaptation to schools of all sizes, it was necessary to resort to subjective scoring for some items. It was also necessary in some cases, for the sake of brevity, to include a number of important characteristics under a single standard.

No. II—For Secondary Schools

I. *Program of Activities*

Possible Score = 30.   Actual Score =

1. Content of core and elective programs is distributed over gymnastics, rhythms, aquatics, individual sports (including defense activities), and team sports.
   (Not less than 6% of time to each of the five types = 1; not less than 9% = 2; not less than 12% = 3)
                                                                      Score_____

2. Program calls for systematic class instruction in activity fundamentals on the "block" or "unit of work" basis (continuous daily instruction in an activity for from 3 to 6 weeks).
   (Definite, but unsystematic instruction = 1; systematic instruction in other than block program = 2; systematic block instruction = 3)
                                                                      Score_____

3. Daily participation in physical and/or health education class instruction periods of from 45 to 60 minutes is required of *all* students.
   (Two days a week = 1; four days = 2; five days = 3)
                                                                      Score_____

4. Participation in intramural sports in addition to class instruction is available for all students.
   (Fair program = 1; good = 2; excellent = 3)
                                                                      Score_____

5. Detailed yearly program (course of study, including special objectives) for each grade level is on file in Principal's Office and activity schedules are posted on gymnasium office bulletin boards.
(Fair program = 1; good = 2; excellent = 3)

Score_____

6. A course of study committee (men and women) gives consideration, at least annually, to needed revisions in the program.
(Fairly active = 1; active = 2; very active = 3)

Score_____

7. Provision is made for adequate maintenance and sanitation of school grounds, plant, and classrooms.
(Fair = 1; good = 2; excellent = 3)

Score_____

8. A modern health instruction program is maintained under expert leadership in *physical education*, in *home economics*, or in *general science*, or is *correlated* through several departments. (Separate course in one department = 1; fairly well correlated = 2; completely correlated, with co-ordinating director = 3)

Score_____

9. A comprehensive safety education program is maintained, emphasizing safety habits and practices, safety codes, and safety standards, in all departments.
(Fair program = 1; good = 2; excellent = 3)

Score_____

10. Definite efforts are made to encourage faculty recreational activity and to improve the health status of teachers.
(Fair results = 1; good = 2; excellent = 3)

Score_____

II. *Outdoor Areas*

Possible Score = 30.   Actual Score =

1. Total available unobstructed field and court playing space for school and community use varies from four to fifteen or more acres, according to size of school.

(Minimum of four acres—an area equal to one small soccer field, seven tennis courts, and one hard baseball field—and one additional acre for each added unit of five hundred students* [boys and girls] = 1; minimum of six acres, and one additional acre for each additional unit of four hundred students = 2; minimum of eight acres, and one additional acre for each additional unit of three hundred students = 3)

Score_____

* Explanation: Four acres for first 500 students; five acres for 1,000, etc.

2. Sufficient playing fields are marked off and equipped (for multiple use in field hockey, field ball, soccer, softball, speed-ball, touch football, et cetera) to accommodate all outside peak load classes (both boys and girls).
(Fair facilities = 1; good facilities = 2; excellent facilities = 3)

Score_____

3. Court areas (for separate or multiple use in archery, bad-minton, handball, horseshoes, paddle tennis, tennis, et cetera) are marked off and equipped to accommodate both boys' and girls' classes in all court activities offered.
(Fair facilities = 1; good facilities = 2; excellent facilities = 3)

Score_____

4. Field and court areas are surfaced with materials that are resilient, non-slippery, firm and as nearly dustless as possible, and have suitable slope for good drainage in rainy weather. At least 20% of area should be paved for multiple court game use, with blacktop (bitumals or asphalt concrete).
(Hard packed clay or decomposed granite, plus 20% black-top = 1; calcium chloride, plus 20% blacktop = 2; good turf, plus some dirt area, plus 20% blacktop = 3)

Score_____

5. Jumping pits and field apparatus are protected by sawdust, sand, or dirt kept soft.
(Dirt kept soft = 1; sand = 2; sawdust = 3)

Score_____

6. Field, court, and diamond areas are kept clean and well marked; are without hazardous obstructions; and are laid out to provide maximum relief from sun glare.
(Fair condition = 1; good = 2; excellent = 3)

Score_____

7. Maintenance work on fields and courts is done by workmen other than instructors or students.
(Partly by others = 1; mostly = 2; entirely = 3)

Score_____

8. All play areas are fenced off from streets, with subdivision fences where necessary for safety and control.
(Partly fenced = 1; all fenced from street = 2; all fenced, with subdivisions = 3)

Score_____

9. Play areas are bordered by attractive trees, shrubbery, and vines; and in warm climates are equipped with shaded tables and seats.
(Fair condition = 1; good = 2; excellent = 3)

Score_____

10. Play areas are lighted for night use for community recreation programs.
(Fair lighting = 1; good = 2; excellent = 3)

Score_____

III. *Indoor Areas*

Possible Score = 30.   Actual Score =

1. One or more gymnasium areas sufficient for boys' and girls' inside class activities (according to size of school) (for common use, for apparatus, boxing, corrective, fencing, gymnastics, rhythms, tumbling, and wrestling) are available and are appropriately equipped, and properly heated, lighted, and ventilated.
(Standards approximately met = 1–2; fully met = 3)

Score_____

2. Gymnasium floors are of hardwood; lines are properly painted; walls are smooth and clear; painting is a light neutral color; radiators and drinking fountains are recessed; ceiling height is between 18 and 22 feet.
(Standards approximately met = 2; entirely met = 3)

Score_____

3. Additional classrooms, appropriately equipped for theory instruction and health education classes, are provided in the building or conveniently adjacent.
(One room = 2; two or more rooms = 3)

Score_____

4. Special rooms for coeducational social activities are appropriately furnished.
(Classroom or gymnasiums partly furnished = 1; well-furnished separate rooms = 3)

Score_____

5. A rest room for boys (equipped with cots, pads, blankets, and sheets), adequate to handle peak load use of building, is provided for use in injury or illness, or for rest periods.
(One cot for 100 boys in peak load = 1; 1 cot for 75 boys = 2; one cot for 50 boys = 3)

Score_____

6. A rest room for girls, with equipped cots adequate to handle peak load use of building, is provided for use in injury or illness, or for rest periods.
(One cot in peak load for 50 girls = 1; one cot for 30 girls = 2; one cot for 20 girls = 3)

Score_____

7. Rest rooms each for men and women faculty members are provided with appropriate dressing rooms and showers.
(Satisfactory facilities for women only = 2; for both men and women = 3)

Score_____

8. An equipment office is provided in both boys' and girls' locker rooms properly arranged for issuing towels, suits, and supplies for both indoor and outdoor use.
(Satisfactory office for one only [boys or girls] = 1–2; satisfactory for both = 3)

Score_____

9. Properly equipped instructors' offices (separate for men and women), with suitable facilities for medical examinations, are available, in good locations for adequate supervision of student activities.

(Well-equipped offices but poorly located for supervision = 1; well-equipped, with good supervision of one major activity area = 2; well-equipped, with supervision of two or more major activity areas = 3)

Score_____

10. The combined inside facilities (including classrooms, gymnasiums, and special rooms) are adequate to handle all classes (boys and girls), inside, during bad weather.

(Approximately = 1-2; entirely = 3)

Score_____

IV. *Locker and Shower Areas*

Possible Score = 30.   Actual Score =

1. Locker rooms (sunny and well ventilated) provide free floor space, exclusive of lockers, adequate to care for peak load of use. (Peak load equals largest number of students dressing in any one class period.)

(8 sq. ft. per pupil = 1; 10 sq. ft. = 2; 12 sq. ft. = 3)

Score_____

2. Individual locker facilities are provided for all students.

(Box lockers or narrow vertical lockers = 1; combination box and dressing lockers = 2; half length standard size lockers or self-service basket system, combined with full-length dressing lockers for peak load = 3)

Score_____

3. Adequate lock protection is provided for lockers or baskets.

(Key locks = 1; permanent combination locks = 2; high-grade combination padlocks = 3)

Score_____

4. Continuous supervision by either equipment clerks or instructors is provided for locker areas while in use by students.

(Fair supervision = 1; good = 2; excellent = 3)

Score_____

5. Boys' dressing areas are of the open aisle type, with fixed benches in the aisles; girls' areas offer choice of closed booth or open aisle.

(Standards approximately met = 2; fully met = 3)

Score_____

6. Boys' shower rooms are of the "gang" type, with adequate drying room capacity; girls' areas offer choice of "gang" type or closed booth type.

(Standards approximately met = 2; fully met = 3)

Score_____

7. Shower rooms provide 8 to 12 square feet of floor area per shower head, and sufficient showers to take care of peak load adequately.
(Five students per shower at peak load = 1; four per shower = 2; three per shower = 3)
Score_____

8. Hot water is thermostatically controlled to prevent scalding; shower heads are at neck height; liquid soap dispensers are provided in all shower areas.
(Standards approximately met = 2; fully met = 3)
Score_____

9. Adequate toilet facilities are available in separate areas immediately adjoining locker and shower rooms (accessible directly to playground); and contain adequate bowls, urinals, washbasins (conforming to established standards for the peak load); hot and cold water, liquid soap dispensers, drinking fountains, mirrors, wastebaskets, and paper towels or drying machines.
(Fair facilities = 1; good = 2; excellent = 3)
Score_____

10. Floors are washed daily with antiseptic solution; and antiseptic footbaths are provided for optional use, to aid in control of foot ringworm.
(Standards approximately met = 2; fully met = 3)
Score_____

V. *Swimming Pool*

Possible Score = 30. Actual Score =

1. Adequate swimming facilities are available for all students (both boys and girls).
(Off-campus facilities, closely adjoining = 1; small pool [less than 1250 sq. ft.] on school grounds = 2; large pool [over 1250 sq. ft.] on school grounds = 3)
Score_____

2. Pool construction provides proper acoustics; suitable scum gutters; nonslip decks; white tile or other light finish on sides and bottom; underwater lighting if pool is used at night; bottom of pool clearly visible at all times of operation.
(Standards approximately met = 1–2; fully met = 3)
Score_____

3. Pool is equipped with adequate machinery for heating, filtering, and sterilizing water, and for maintaining it in conformity with established health standards.
(Fair equipment = 1; good = 2; excellent = 3)
Score_____

4. Standard tests are made daily for air temperature, water temperature, water acidity, and residual chlorine content and, at least weekly, for bacterial content of water.
(Score = 3)
Score_____

5. Pool is equipped with standard safety devices and is protected by control doors which are kept locked at all times except when life guard or instructor is on duty.
(Score = 3)

Score_____

6. Swimmers are required to enter pool through a water foot bath, opening from the shower rooms; to visit toilet and take supervised soap shower baths before entering; and are not permitted in pool with colds or skin infections.
(Standards approximately met = 2; fully met = 3)

Score_____

7. Spectators in street shoes are not permitted on pool decks but are provided with appropriate gallery space.
(Score = 3)

Score_____

8. Use of pool facilities is distributed equally between men and women students.
(Approximately met = 3)

Score_____

9. All life guards and swimming instructors are required to hold the Senior Red Cross Life Saving Certificate or the Examiner's Certificate.
(Score = 3)

Score_____

10. Pool is available for community recreational use when not required for school purposes, particularly during summer months.
(Score = 3)

Score_____

Note: Schools without campus pools or adjacent facilities, if they conduct and stress swimming campaigns, may score up to maximum of 15 points for swimming pool, as follows: (annual "learn to swim" campaign, in cooperation with Red Cross or other agency, reaching successfully 25% of student body = 5; campaign reaching 50% of student body = 10; campaign reaching 75% of student body = 15)

Score_____

VI. *Supplies and Equipment*

Possible Score = 30.   Actual Score =

1. Adequate supply of balls (in good condition) and similar equipment is available for class instruction in all team activities offered.
(One ball, or other item, for every ten members of average size class = 1; one for every eight members = 2; one for every six members = 3)

Score_____

2. Class sets of supplies for individual or dual sports are provided for class instruction in all activities offered (archery, badminton, handball, golf, horseshoes, table tennis, squash, tennis, et cetera).
(Individual supplies for each member of average size class = 2; for each member of peak load class = 3)

Score_____

3. All class supplies are kept repaired and in good condition (balls clean and well inflated, bats taped) both for efficiency and safety.
(Fair condition = 1; good = 2; excellent = 3)

Score_____

4. All students wear appropriate uniforms in activity classes.
(Uniform furnished by themselves = 1; provided by school, and fee charged = 2; provided by school, without charge = 3)

Score_____

5. Towels and swimming suits or trunks (where needed) are made available.
(Furnished by student = 1; by school with fee = 2; by school without charge = 3)

Score_____

6. Swimming suits and towels are laundered daily, and uniforms weekly.
(By student at home = 1; by school, with fee = 2; by school, without charge = 3)

Score_____

7. Adequate first aid supplies are available at all times in a first aid room, or in instructors' offices and equipment offices.
(Fair supplies = 1; good = 2; excellent = 3)

Score_____

8. Adequate equipment clerks (other than instructors) are provided at all activity hours to handle equipment and supplies (including towel dispensing).
(Volunteer student help [not for phys. ed. credit] = 1; paid student help = 2; full-time equipment clerk = 3)

Score_____

9. Piano and pianist, or phonograph, and other necessary musical accompaniment equipment are furnished for dancing classes.
(Fair equipment and service = 1; good = 2; excellent = 3)

Score_____

10. Activity supplies are available for community recreation use outside of school hours.
(Score = 3)

Score_____

VII. *Medical Examinations and Health Service*

Possible Score = 30.   Actual Score =

1. Medical examining, advisory, and emergency service is provided by school physicians with co-operative arrangements for handling handicapped and problem cases in school or public clinics or by private medical practitioners.
   (Adequate volunteer service by community physicians = 2; part-time paid school physician, or [in schools of 2,000 or more] one or more full-time physicians = 3)
                                                          Score_____

2. Trained school nurse service is provided for both school and home visitation purposes, by either part-time or full-time nurses according to size of school.
   (Fair service = 1; good service = 2; excellent service = 3)
                                                          Score_____

3. A comprehensive examination by the school physician (assisted by physical education instructors) is required of every student at least once in each school level (example, junior high); and includes at least a careful check for orthopedic and postural defects, vision, hearing, nose, mouth, throat, teeth, heart, lungs, nutrition, skin, nervous condition, and possible hernia.
   (Once in school level = 2; two or more times in school level = 3)
                                                          Score_____

4. No student is permitted to participate in strenuous class or athletic activity without a satisfactory medical examination.
   (Score = 3)
                                                          Score_____

5. A permanent, continuous, progressive health record is maintained and passed on for each child and is used as a basis for advice and follow-up health service.
   (Fair = 1; good = 2; excellent = 3)
                                                          Score_____

6. On basis of medical examination children are classified into three divisions, or equivalent: A, average normal for unlimited participation; B, subnormal, with temporary or permanent limitation to restricted activity; C, offered individual or corrective treatment, supplementing normal program.
   (Fair = 1; good = 2; excellent = 3)
                                                          Score_____

7. Assignment to rest, restricted, or individual activity, or excuse from required normal physical education activity (for other than temporary illness) is approved by the school physician in consultation with the physical education department head.
   (Score = 3)
                                                          Score____

8. Students returning after influenza or other serious illness are inspected by the school physician or nurse and assigned to a modified program until their condition justifies resumption of normal activity; students sent home in case of illness or accident are accompanied by an adult.
(Standards approximately met = 1–2; fully met = 3)

Score_____

9. A health examination is made by the school physician of all teacher applicants; followed by a periodic examination every 3 years thereafter; and a careful inspection of all teachers returning to duty after illness of 2 weeks or more.
(Standards approximately met = 1–2; fully met = 3)

Score_____

10. Nonmedical teachers or school officers are never permitted to diagnose or treat health disorders; but a close co-operation is maintained between physical education teachers and the school physician.
(Score = 3)

Score_____

VIII. *Modified-Individual (Corrective) Activities*

Possible Score = 30.   Actual Score =

1. Adequate modified and individual activity classes, with limited enrollment, are provided for students incapacitated for normal participation or needing special postural or orthopedic correction (classes B and C).
(Maximum of 30 students per instructor = 1; 25 students per instructor = 2; 20 students per instructor = 3)

Score_____

2. All modified and individual activity cases are properly classified and grouped within classes for effective instruction and guidance, according to their condition.
(Fair = 1; good = 2; excellent = 3)

Score_____

3. Extreme types of restricted cases are assigned to periodic rest periods, in addition to the modified activity, with appropriate reductions in academic program, where needed.
(Fair = 1; good = 2; excellent = 3)

Score_____

4. Adequate facilities are provided for suitable games for modified cases (table tennis, deck tennis, horseshoes, croquet, archery, shuffle board, et cetera).
(Fair facilities = 1; good = 2; excellent = 3)

Score_____

5. Adequate facilities for handling individual activity cases are available either within the school or in a central corrective center, accessible to several schools (or the equivalent).
(Fair facilities = 1; good = 2; excellent = 3)

Score_____

6. All teachers assigned to handle individual activity (corrective) classes have had technical training in corrective and therapeutic work.
(Fair training = 1; good = 2; excellent = 3)

Score_____

7. In individual activity instruction, emphasis is placed upon practicing the directed exercises at home, frequently, with the co-operation of parents; and upon maintaining good postural alignments at all times.
(Fair = 1; good = 2; excellent = 3)

Score_____

8. All individual activity cases are encouraged to participate also in modified class activities for which they are fitted, and are returned to normal activity as soon as their condition permits.
(Fair = 1; good = 2; excellent = 3)

Score_____

9. Wherever possible, interesting activities of the sports, gymnastic, aquatic, or rhythmical types are used in place of corrective drills, to secure postural and corrective results.
(Fair results = 1; good = 2; excellent = 3)

Score_____

10. Normal students, who are temporarily incapacitated for strenuous activity because of accident, operation, or serious illness, are assigned to modified activity, under supervision (either in their regular period or in a special class), until school physician or nurse approves their return to regular class work.
(Score = 3)

Score_____

IX. *Organization and Administration of Class Programs*

Possible Score = 30.   Actual Score =

1. All persons coaching teams, or handling physical education classes, or community recreation activities under school supervision are properly certified to teach in the state and have had extensive training and/or experience in physical education.
(All certified and experienced = 2; all with a major or minor = 3)

Score_____

2. Teachers are active in professional organizations such as the American Association for Health, Physical Education, and Recreation, attend professional meetings, subscribe to professional magazines, and maintain a good supply of late professional books in library.
(Fairly active = 1; active = 2; very active = 3)

Score_____

3. Instructors stress co-ordinated teaching; combining with performance fundamentals, the necessary rules, team strategy, social and ethical standards, health and safety factors; and attempt to adapt program to outside recreational needs and interests.
   (Fair = 1; good = 2; excellent = 3)

   Score_____

4. Frequent opportunity is provided for coeducational activity, either in class instruction or in recreational participation.
   (Mild encouragement = 1; coeducational intramural sports = 2; coeducational elective class instruction = 3)

   Score_____

5. Instructional classes for normal students are limited in size for effective instruction purposes.
   (Maximum of 45 students per instructor = 1; 40 students per instructor = 2; 35 students per instructor = 3)

   Score_____

6. Teacher class assignments (including after school responsibilities such as team coaching and playground direction, unless these involve additional salary) are sufficiently limited for adequate instruction.
   (Maximum load six hours per day = 2; five hours per day = 3)

   Score_____

7. Testing for final grade in activity classes is distributed over (1) performance skills, (2) knowledge of rules and strategy, (3) social attitudes (citizenship), (4) posture and body mechanics (or equivalent).
   (Fair tests = 1; good = 2; excellent = 3)

   Score_____

8. Students are not permitted to substitute clerical work, janitor work, towel dispensing, or piano playing, et cetera, in place of physical education class activity.
   (Score = 3)

   Score_____

9. Healthful living (health education instruction) is offered in concentrated instruction periods, in appropriate departments, in addition to coordinated health counseling in other departments. Classes meet in quiet, comfortable classrooms, not in locker rooms or on bleachers.
   (Equivalent of at least 2 hours per week for one semester in each level = 1; equivalent of 5 hours per week for one semester in each level = 2; equivalent of 5 hours per week for two semesters in each level = 3). (If substituted for an activity class = 0)

   Score_____

10. Assignment to activity classes is based on age, physical condition, skill development, need, and interest.
(Assigned at random according to free period = 0; by grades = 1; by medical diagnosis and grade = 2; by medical diagnosis, degree of development and skill, need and interest = 3)

Score_____

X. *Administration of Intramural and Interschool Athletics**

Possible Score = 30.   Actual Score =

1. Both intramural and interschool sports programs (for boys and girls) are budgeted and financed from school funds; and ticket selling for contests is discouraged or prohibited.
(Partly financed, and sale discouraged = 1; fully financed, and sale to students prohibited = 2; fully financed, and public admitted free to contests = 3)

Score_____

2. Students are classified for competitive purposes on basis of three-point classification plan (or equivalent) in addition to medical examination, in order to reduce hazards and to minimize inequalities between opponents.
(Fair classification = 1; good = 2; excellent = 3)

Score_____

3. Instruction, coaching, and officiating of athletics is handled by women instructors for girls, and by men instructors for boys, with close cooperation between the two in coeducational activities and joint sports days; use of athletic facilities is equitably divided between boys and girls.
(Standards approximately met = 2; fully met = 3)

Score_____

4. Well-organized sports (play) days are staged periodically under trained and experienced leadership with major emphasis on carry-over types of sports.
(Sports days for girls and boys separately = 2; both separate and joint sports days for boys and girls = 3)

Score_____

5. Noon-hour activities (where time is available beyond adequate period for unhurried eating) are carefully supervised and limited to modified sports of physiologically defensible types.
(Fair organization and supervision = 1; good = 2; excellent = 3)
(If no time available, score = 1)

Score_____

* NOTE: Schools that do not sponsor interschool athletics should double the score on items 1–5, and leave out items 6–10.

6. Interschool competition for girls (when conducted) is under strict supervision and control of well-trained women instructors; is conducted according to girls' rules; and is limited chiefly to interschool sports (play) days.
(Standards approximately met = 2; fully met = 3)

Score_____

7. Interschool competition for boys is restricted largely to local leagues; without overnight travel; no state (or larger) championships; no postseason games; not over seven games in football season; not over sixteen games in basketball season; other sports with appropriate limits; and with from 2 to 3 weeks of preliminary practice preceding first contest.
(Standards approximately met = 2; fully met = 3)

Score_____

8. Students are eligible for interschool competition only between fourteenth and nineteenth birthdays; for not more than four years in any one sport; and for not more than one major sport in a given semester or term.
(Standards approximately met = 2; fully met = 3)

Score_____

9. Interscholastic athletic policies are determined by school administrators and physical education instructors or by regularly constituted school athletic leagues; and game officials are selected from experienced school people as far as possible.
(Mostly = 2; entirely = 3)

Score_____

10. School officials provide necessary traffic and safety protection to and from and during interschool contests; and maintain school physician in attendance at all major athletic contests.
(Standards approximately met = 2; fully met = 3)

Score_____

Scoring Procedure. The rating standards are intended to represent a range from a very poor program to a superior-excellent program. (For example, in the No. II Scorecard, 100 = poor program; 200 = fair-good; 300 = excellent.) If desired, the scores can be reduced to percentages, as indicated in the summary sections. In most cases, a given item should range from one to three points if the program is at all acceptable. If it does not approximate even one point, however, the score should be listed as zero. Scores should represent the unprejudiced judgment of the rater in order to give a reasonably fair picture of the program.

Items have not been weighted relatively (except a few in the elementary card), because it is almost impossible to determine comparative values, where all factors are of great importance. Only the most significant characteristics of program content, facilities, or administrative procedures have been included in these standards, hence each one is of great importance.

Profile Chart. It is suggested that after all ratings have been completed the total score under each of the major divisions be inserted on the Score Card summary chart on the next page. These scores may then be spotted at the appropriate points under the several headings in the following profile chart. These points may then be connected by lines and the resulting profile will indicate graphically the strong and weak points in the institution's rating. Those items which appear below the 15-point line will be considered "poor"; those between 15 and 20, "fair"; those between 20 and 25, "good"; and those between 25 and 30, "excellent."

	I	II	III	IV	V	VI	VII	VIII	IX	X
	PROGRAM	OUTDOOR AREAS	INDOOR AREAS	LOCKER	SWIM. POOL	SUPPLIES	MEDICAL EXAMS.	MODIFIED ACTIVITY	ORIG. AND ADMIN.	ATHLETICS
30 Excellent→										
25 Good→										
20 Fair→										
15 Poor→										
10 Very Poor→										
5										
0										

Score Card

HEALTH AND PHYSICAL EDUCATION SCORE CARD
No. II
FOR JUNIOR AND SENIOR HIGH SCHOOLS AND
FOUR-YEAR HIGH SCHOOLS

Name of School_____Address_____

Jr., Sr., or 4-Yr. School_____Principal_____

Rating for school year_____Rated by_____Date_____

Number of students enrolled: boys_____girls_____

	Possible Score	Actual Score
Score Card Summary		
I. Program of Activities..................	30	
II. Outdoor Areas.......................	30	
III. Indoor Areas.........................	30	
IV. Locker and Shower Areas..............	30	
V. Swimming Pool......................	30	
VI. Supplies and Equipment...............	30	
VII. Medical Examinations and Health Service	30	
VIII. Modified-Individual (Corrective) Activities	30	
IX. Organization and Administration of Class Programs.............................	30	
X. Administration of Intramural and Inter-school Athletics......................	30	
TOTAL POSSIBLE SCORE	300	Total Actual____

Percentage Score (Actual ÷ 3) = _____

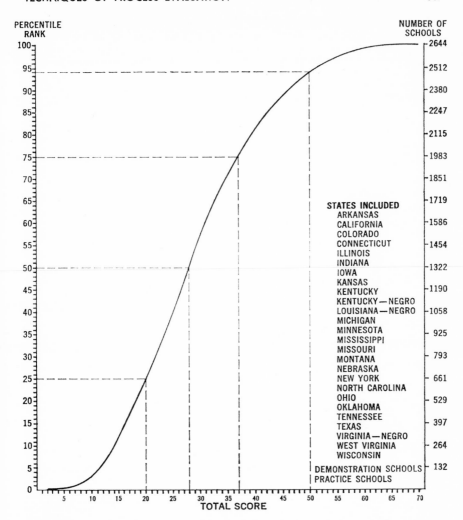

Fig. 14–1. Bookwalter's National Norms for LaPorte Score Card No. II. Cumulative frequency for determining percentile rank on health and physical education score card No. II. Based upon 2644 schools, 1950–1954.

Norms*

Under the direction of Karl W. Bookwalter, national norms have been provided for the LaPorte Health and Physical Education Score Card No. II. These norms may be obtained from the cumulative frequency curve and data shown in Figure 14–1 by observing the following steps:

1. All possible scores on the LaPorte self-survey score card are summed. There is a possible total score of 300 points on the 100 items.

* Adapted by permission. Bookwalter, K. W., and Carolyn W. Bookwalter: *Purposes, Standards, and Results in Physical Education.* Bulletin of School of Education, Indiana University, Bloomington, *38*, No. 5, 11–13, September 1962.

2. This total score is divided by three to secure the percentage of the possible score.
3. At the bottom of the norm table presented in Figure 14–1, is shown the percentage scale of all possible scores. The percentage for any self-study score made by a school survey may be found by following along this scale.
4. From the point on the scale where the percentage is located, a line is drawn perpendicular to the base line until it reaches the cumulative frequency curve.
5. From this point on the frequency curve a line is then drawn parallel to the base line until it joins the percentile rank scale on the left.
6. At the point where this horizontal line connects with the percentile rank scale, the percentile rank of the self-study school is located.
7. This percentile rank shows the per cent of the schools nationally that are exceeded by the self-study school.
8. Bookwalters' national survey of high school programs for boys shows that nationally the schools were but 28% effective for the total program. When this 28% is located on the base line and the perpendicular and horizontal lines are put in place, the percentile rank of 50 is found.
9. In the event a school staff is interested in setting a higher standard for its total program and selects, for example, a percentile rank of 75, this standard may be located on the scale to the left. From this point the horizontal and perpendicular lines may be drawn in the reverse order to 3 and 4 above and the percentage of 37 is obtained. This percentage may be multiplied by three to obtain the needed raw score on the score card.

New York State Check List for Physical Education*

Education assumes a responsibility to pass on our cultural and social inheritance and to equip children and youth physically, mentally and emotionally for living in a changing world. This process involves (1) recognition of the needs of the individual in terms of the principles of pupil growth and development, (2) organization and administration of the curriculum for most effective use in the realization of its purposes as established by these needs, and (3) continuous evaluation of the program to insure systematic progress toward the realization of the objectives of physical education and the purposes of education.

Physical education recognizes this concept of education and has a unique contribution to make in meeting these needs for the self-realization of the individual through the activities in its program. The beneficial effects of exercise and activity, however, are produced only when activities of the right type and amount are provided under qualified personnel. The methods and techniques used in the conduct of these activities need to be such that not only are these physical and organic needs met but opportunity is provided for growth in the development of social behaviors, habits, attitudes, emotional stability.

In order for individuals to function as contributing members of a democracy it is essential that they learn self-discipline in relation to the group through the development of those qualities which are essential to

* State of New York. Check List for Physical Education. Albany, New York, Division of Health, Physical Education, New York State Education Department. Used by permission of the State Education Department.

democratic living such as cooperation, leadership, fellowship, good sportsmanship etc. It is also essential that they develop (1) strength to be ready for tasks encountered in everyday routine and in emergencies, (2) stamina to continue necessary tasks without undue fatigue, and energy to participate in recreation activities after a day's work, (3) cardio-respiratory endurance for sustained effort in activities involving motion of the entire body, (4) agility to be able to make wide ranges of movement easily, (5) speed to be able to move rapidly when personal safety demands it, (6) control to coordinate body movement skillfully, (7) knowledge and skill in a wide variety of recreational activities to insure continued participation.

The check list has been prepared to help school officials and interested citizens' groups to judge their physical education programs in terms of the basic elements needed to reach the objectives stated above and to stimulate planning in terms of pupil needs and local conditions. It should enable communities to identify the strength and weaknesses of their physical education programs and to direct attention to areas needing further study and action for improvement.

These elements are grouped under eight main headings:

Program activities	Personnel
Program planning	Facilities
Evaluating	Safety and sanitation
Scheduling	Budget

I. The program provides a broad variety of activities to serve all pupils.

1. Informal activities such as singing games, simple circle games, creative activities (games of invitation and imagination) and games of hunting, fleeing and chasing type. Yes____ No____
2. Games of simple organization such as kickball, dodgeball, relays etc. Yes____ No____
3. Team games, such as basketball, volleyball, softball, soccer etc. Yes____ No____
4. Individual and dual games, such as badminton, tennis, horseshoes etc. Yes____ No____
5. Gymnastics, such as stunts, tumbling, apparatus. Yes____ No____
6. Rhythms and dancing, such as folk, square, social. Yes____ No____
7. Winter sports, such as skating, skiing, snowshoeing. Yes____ No____
8. Body mechanics and correctives. Yes____ No____
9. Swimming and water safety. Yes____ No____
10. Extraclass, interschool and intramural activities (boys and girls)
    a. An organized extraclass program is provided for pupils in upper elementary grades. Yes____ No____
    b. All athletic activities are an integral part of the physical education program. Yes____ No____
    c. The intramural program is well organized and attractive to the extent that most of the pupils willingly participate. Yes____ No____
    d. Girls' interschool activities are limited to sports days, invitation games and other invitation activities. Yes____ No____. Girls' rules are used in the conduct of these activities. Yes____ No____
    e. Interschool activities for boys below the seventh grade are limited to sports days and invitation games. Yes____ No____

II. The program is planned in terms of community needs and of the growth and development needs of pupils.

1. The purposes of education and objectives of physical education are used to guide planning. Yes____ No____
2. The activities are introduced at the appropriate grade and growth level. Yes____ No____
3. There is a written master plan which provides for progression and continuity in the instruction. Yes____ No____
4. Planning for the program is shared by administrator and staff. Yes____ No____ By staff and pupils. Yes____ No____. With citizens' groups. Yes____ No____

III. Provision is made for evaluating the program by determining the growth and progress of pupils.

1. Records of pupil status and progress are maintained with reference to the following:
   a. Physical fitness. Yes____ No____
   b. Knowledge and skill in activities. Yes____ No____
   c. Social growth and group relationships. Yes____ No____
2. Appropriate evaluative methods are used to determine pupil progress in the above-mentioned items.
   a. Recognized standards. Yes____ No____
   b. Teacher-made tests or measures. Yes____ No____
   c. Anecdotal report. Yes____ No____ Teacher observation. Yes____ No____

IV. The school schedule provides for the following:

1. A daily period of physical education instruction for each pupil. Yes____ No____
2. Pupils grouped for such instruction according to their grade or growth level. Yes____ No____
3. Classes of uniform size. Yes____ No____ Small enough to provide good working groups (a maximum of 40 pupils is recommended). Yes____ No____
4. Additional classes for those who need remedial (corrective) work. Yes____ No____
5. Restricted program for pupils physically unable to participate in regular program of activities. Yes____ No____
6. Equitable scheduling of facilities between boys and girls for both class and extraclass activities. Yes____ No____

V. Qualified personnel is provided to conduct a well-rounded program.

1. Sufficient personnel is provided to meet the class instruction and laboratory requirements in accordance with the needs of pupils as outlined in the Regulations of the Commissioner. (A physical education teacher for each 240 elementary or 190 secondary pupils is recommended.) Elementary: Yes____ No____ Secondary: Yes____ No____
2. A qualified director (where there are five or more on the staff) or a department head (four or less on staff) is available to provide necessary administrative and supervisory services. Yes____ No____

3. Continuous professional growth of staff is provided for through:
   a. Regular staff conferences. Yes____ No____
   b. Attending general faculty meetings. Yes____ No____
   c. Attending local, zone and state meetings and workshops. Yes____ No____
   d. Recent graduate study in physical education and related fields. Yes____ No____
   e. A well-equipped professional library. Yes____ No____
   f. Professional visits to observe programs in other schools. Yes____ No____
4. Girls' program is conducted by a woman teacher. Yes____ No____
5. Additional faculty assistance is provided for intramural program.
   Girls: Yes____ No____ Boys: Yes____ No____
   For interschool program.
   Girls: Yes____ No____ Boys: Yes____ No____

VI. The physical education and recreation facilities permit a well-rounded program for all pupils.

1. Teaching station indoors for every 240 pupils enrolled. Yes____ No____
2. Sufficient dressing space for largest class. Yes____ No____
3. Dressing locker for each pupil in largest class. Yes____ No____
4. A gymnasium storage locker for every pupil enrolled above the 4th grade. Yes____ No____
5. At least one shower head for every five pupils in the largest class. Yes____ No____
6. A well-drained, suitably located body-drying area. Yes____ No____
7. Storage space for apparatus. Yes____ No____ Equipment and supplies. Yes____ No____
8. Suitable office space for each physical education teacher. Yes____ No____
9. A swimming pool. Yes____ No____
10. Remedial (corrective) room. Yes____ No____
11. All-weather paved area adjoining building for primary grades' use. Yes____ No____
12. Separate apparatus and play area for smaller children. Yes____ No____
13. Separate playing fields for Intermediate grades. Yes____ No____ Secondary girls. Yes____ No____ Secondary boys (class and intramurals). Yes____ No____ Interschool sports. Yes____ No____
14. Court area for tennis. Yes____ No____ Badminton. Yes____ No____ Volleyball. Yes____ No____
15. Area for archery. Yes____ No____ Horseshoe pitching. Yes____ No____ Golf instruction. Yes____ No____
16. Shed or other building for the storage of outdoor equipment. Yes____ No____
17. The elementary school is planned to function as a neighborhood center and the high school as a community center. Yes____ No____ This planning is shared with citizens' groups. Yes____ No____ Park officials. Yes____ No____ Planning officials. Yes____ No____

VII. Provisions are made for healthful and safe conduct of physical education activities.

    1. A thorough annual medical examination is provided for all pupils. Yes____ No____

    2. All candidates for interschool teams are given a special examination at the beginning of each sport season. Yes____ No____

    3. Subsequent examinations within each sport season are given when needed. Yes____ No____

    4. All participants in the more vigorous sports are provided with adequate protective equipment. Yes____ No____

    5. There is a regular safety check on all equipment and apparatus. Yes____ No____

    6. Gymnasium floor is kept clear of apparatus and equipment when not in use. Yes____ No____

    7. Good care, proper use and orderly storage of equipment are provided. Yes____ No____

    8. Fields are properly maintained for maximum and safe use. Yes____ No____

    9. Clean and sanitary conditions prevail in all areas. Yes____ No____

    10. An appropriate towel service is provided. Yes____ No____

    11. Protection Plan or other accident insurance coverage is provided for the physical education classes. Yes____ No____ Interschool teams. Yes____ No____ Intramural groups. Yes____ No____

VIII. The physical education budget is adequate and there is an equitable distribution of funds between the different activities of the program.

    1. The annual budget request for physical education is prepared on the basis of a careful inventory and the complete needs of the program to be provided for the school year. Yes____ No____

    2. Essential equipment is available for physical education. Yes____ No____ If not, the purchase of needed items is planned for. Yes____ No____ Available instructional supplies are satisfactory in quantity to permit maximum and simultaneous pupil participation in any one activity. Yes____ No____ The supplies provided permit instruction in a broad variety of activities. Yes____ No____

    3. Sufficient funds have been allocated for travel, protective equipment and other necessary expense in connection with: Boys' interschool activities. Yes____ No____ Boys' intramural activities. Yes____ No____ Girls' invitation games. Yes____ No____ Girls' intramural activities. Yes____ No____

    4. Funds are provided for attendance at professional meetings and conferences by staff members. Yes____ No____

Means' Physical Education Instruction Evaluation*

In an effort to improve the quality of physical education instruction, you are asked to complete the following questionnaire. Listed below are certain qualities considered important to good teaching. Read each item carefully. Circle the appropriate number on the scale at the right of each

---

* Means, Richard K.: A Teacher Appraisal Scale, Journal of Health, Physical Education and Recreation, *31*, 36–37, May–June, 1960. Adapted by permission.

item. The extreme right end of the scale (5) represents outstanding characteristics, the extreme left side (1) inadequate instruction. Judge the instructor and his instruction by other physical education courses you have completed. Comments on low or high ratings will be appreciated.

1—poor; 2—fair; 3—average; 4—good; 5—superior

Personal Characteristics

1. APPEARANCE: clean, well-groomed, fashionable, well-dressed, no noticeable peculiarities or annoying mannerisms.   1 2 3 4 5
2. PHYSICAL CONDITION: generally fit and healthy; good carriage, build, and posture.   1 2 3 4 5
3. SPEAKING ABILITY: clear, well-modulated voice, poise, good pronunciation and command of words.   1 2 3 4 5
4. TEMPERAMENT: even disposition and nature, attentive, self-controlled, good sense of humor.   1 2 3 4 5
5. SELF-ASSURANCE: secure, self-respected, confident without conceit, assured in expression and action.   1 2 3 4 5
6. CHARACTER: honest, fair, high values and ideals, ethical behavior, sound philosophy, and integrity.   1 2 3 4 5
7. JUDGMENT: common sense, thinking ability, ability to make sound decisions and deductions, solves problems intelligently.   1 2 3 4 5

Comments:

Teacher-Student Relations

1. ATTITUDE TOWARD STUDENTS: understanding, enthusiastic, considerate, interested in problems.   1 2 3 4 5
2. RESPECT FOR STUDENTS: sympathetic regard for student views, complimentary when feasible.   1 2 3 4 5
3. CONCERN FOR STUDENTS: for health and safety, for student progress, regard for individual differences.   1 2 3 4 5
4. DEPENDABILITY: trustful, reliable, prompt, accurate, respectful of confidences.   1 2 3 4 5
5. MATURITY: emotionally stable, accepts commendation and suggestions gracefully, handles emergencies well.   1 2 3 4 5
6. DEMOCRATIC: sociable, encouraging, accepts group decisions, sympathetic but firm, fair.   1 2 3 4 5
7. PLANNING AND EXPERIENCES: systematic, long-range planning, cooperative opportunities, leadership experiences, experimentation.   1 2 3 4 5
   1 2 3 4 5

Comments:

Class Considerations

1. COURSE ORGANIZATION: well constructed, logical progression of learning experiences, correlation with total program, carry-over value.   1 2 3 4 5

2. METHODS OF TEACHING: variety of techniques,   1   2   3   4   5
up-to-date, balance, informality, flexibility.
3. KNOWLEDGE OF SUBJECT: competent, thor-   1   2   3   4   5
ough, aware of new developments in field, scientifically
accurate.
4. EVALUATION AND GRADING: clear and continu-   1   2   3   4   5
ous evaluation method of skill and knowledge, variety
of appraisal techniques, understanding by group.
5. OBJECTIVES OF COURSE: cooperatively formu-   1   2   3   4   5
lated, clear and understood, realistic, achievement
possibilities.
6. EXPLANATIONS AND DEMONSTRATIONS: 1   2   3   4   5
clear and meaningful, timely, well adapted to subject,
easily interpreted, illustrative, adequate usage of
equipment and facilities.
7. COURSE IMPROVEMENT: willing to experiment   1   2   3   4   5
with new ideas, alert to suggestions, continuously
seeking revision, improvement, progress.

Comments:

References

1. LaPorte, W. R., and John M. Cooper, ed.: Health and Physical Education
Score Card No. II for Junior and Senior High Schools, The Physical Education
Curriculum. Los Angeles: College Book Store, University of Southern California,
1955, pp. 72–86.
2. Means, Richard K.: A Teacher Appraisal Scale, Journal of Health, Physical
Education and Recreation, *31*, 36–37, May–June, 1960.
3. State of New York. Check List for Physical Education. Albany, New York,
Division of Health, Physical Educaton, New York State Education Department.

Part IV. Classification, Grading and Rating Scales

Chapter 15
CLASSIFICATION IN PHYSICAL EDUCATION

Philosophy

One of the important uses of measurement in physical education is classification. Classification may be defined as the placement of individuals into groups for a particular purpose. The chief purpose of classification or grouping in the schools is to equate or group students on the basis of similarities with respect to certain characteristics, abilities, needs, or previous experience in order to increase learning and facilitate instruction. In physical education there are a variety of purposes and the instructor must know what these purposes are, how they may be achieved, and recognize when they have been met. Each of these purposes is more readily achieved by a grouping of students in relation to that specific purpose. For example, one of the purposes of education and physical education is to provide for the principle of individual differences. This purpose can be achieved in whole or in part only if students are grouped according to their needs and abilities. The instructor, however, must be aware of the limitation of all classification systems. These techniques are merely for convenience, and while in theory they divide groups into well-defined categories, in practice there always will be the twilight zone where there will be borderline cases and overlapping of characteristics and needs. At the onset the instructor must recognize the need to make exceptions for those who do not fit into the categories.

Generally, the purposes of classification will require homogeneous grouping, although there are times when the situation is best met with heterogeneous grouping. In any event such groupings are made according to scientific, educational principles and imply a knowledge of the status and primary abilities of students. Fortified with such knowledge the instructor may group students for many purposes. Mention has been made already that it is possible to classify students in such manner that the principle of individual differences will become more operable in the educational process. One of the keys in the implementation of this principle is an effective system of grouping students into similar or dissimilar groups. There are a number of approaches to classification and ways of grouping to accomplish the purposes.

In the area of the physical, very little of this grouping of students has been done other than by sex and sometimes by grade. In general, classes have been sectioned on the basis of administrative convenience. Quite the reverse is true in the academic area where tests of intelligence and achievement have become the rule rather than the exception in the placement of students in classes. The usual procedure in physical education is to assign the student to a class period which most conveniently fits his class schedule, or what is more condemning, the schedule of the administration. It is only chance that would place him in a class where he would have the advantage of fair or even competition, and where there would be a challenge to his ability. When this indiscriminate placement prevails in the scheduling of classes, the student abilities vary from the lowest to the highest, and a similar situation exists with respect to student size and experience. This presents an almost impossible teaching climate and it must necessarily follow that achievement levels for most students will be lower. This situation exists partly because of administrative misunderstanding and partly from professional apathy. While the ideal situation may not be found too often, some form of classification can be provided if the teacher is alert to the needs of the students and is motivated by high standards of instruction. Classification is one of the keys in helping students gain maximum benefits from the limited time that is available.

Purposes of Classification

There are several purposes of classification. Among the most important are: equalize competition, facilitate instruction, provide for program continuity, and serve the health and safety needs of the students.

Equalizes Competition. Perhaps the first use of classification is for equalizing competition in games, contests, and sports. The classification of students into like groups for competition in many sports and games has many advantages. Probably the most important advantages center around such factors as safety, health, interest, and class morale. This purpose applies equally as well to intramurals and to the instructional program.

Facilitates Instruction. Second, classification facilitates instruction by determining student needs through measurement and then gearing the program to fit these needs. Heterogeneity presents obstacles to instruction which are overcome to a great extent by homogeneous grouping. A more desirable teaching situation is created when students in a class have similar abilities so the instructor may direct his teaching toward the total group. If, through status measurement, the instructor can know what level students are currently occupying, he can plan a better program for them and set more definite goals. The loss of prestige sometimes felt by the low skilled when they are placed in classes for the so-called "fundamentals" is more than offset by the increased efficiency in instruction. Equally important is the opportunity which is presented to extend the upper limits of achievement for the gifted. When students in a class have a range of ability from high to low, the instructor must develop three or more lesson plans and then he must make them all operable in one teaching period; or, he takes the easy way out and directs his teaching at one of the levels in particular. What this level is will depend on the philosophy of the instructor but in any event the other two levels will suffer. If these three levels could be grouped into separate classes, instruction would be much more effective.

Provides for Program Continuity. Third, classification is essential for the continuity of the program. Continuity implies that program content for any one student from grade one through grade twelve be a comprehensive, progressive series of experiences from the simple to the complex for all groups. The instructor uses one experience as a basis for a subsequent one, but he does this at each level of ability. Without classification by grade there can be little continuity or progression from year to year for the individual student or the total group. Classification by grade provides for a sequence of program activities and a certain amount of continuous homogeneity. Permanent or complete homogeneity is impossible to achieve because the student is an entity and responds as a whole whereas classification is always done on the basis of one or a few tests which only measure parts of the whole. It is obvious that students who are similar in the characteristics or traits measured may be dissimilar in the many others which may either directly or indirectly affect the measured characteristics.

While it is never possible to attain permanent or lasting homogeneity, students will tend to have a great deal in common as their background and experience in the instructional process achieve a measure of uniformity. Classification by grade could in a sense be classification by experience. The first time an activity is presented, it can be taught at an elementary level. The second time it is presented, it can be approached at a more advanced level. If it is going to be presented three times, the second such presentation could be at an intermediate level. Indiscriminate placement of students with all grade levels in one class would require that an activity be taught on the elementary level each time it is presented, and thus eliminate any progression in the program from one year to the next.

Serves Health Needs and Promotes Safety. Fourth, a form of classification is essential to serve the health needs of students and to insure their safety. Proper grouping always starts with the medical examination and continues by serving the students of lesser abilities. Such grouping would tend to equalize such factors as age, size, and maturity, and protect the students, especially in contact-type activities.

Values of Classification

Interest. As a result of classification, several values accrue. First, student interest is generally greater, since competition is usually keener when teams and individuals are evenly matched. When the skillful compete against the skillful, and the duffer against the duffer, a good situation prevails. Both groups extend themselves and learning takes place more rapidly because students gain more satisfaction from their efforts. Both groups attain a measure of success and are challenged in their own way. Challenge and success are needed by all students if they are to be highly motivated and interested. Classification into homogeneous groups facilitates a differentiation between groups, but at the same time provides sufficient variety within the group to challenge and stimulate. The teacher should recognize that some heterogeneity is valuable in class. Frequently, progress for one student may be greater when he competes with someone more skillful than he. However, a more basic principle of learning is that the student must feel adequate and secure. If there is too wide a range in abilities, this situation will not prevail.

Socialization. Second, socialization is more likely to occur when students are equated and are learning and playing in homogeneous groups. Grouping by grade or age tends to put students together who are nearer the same physiological age than does indiscriminate grouping. Since students of the same physiological age tend to play together and seek companionship together, a more favorable social atmosphere prevails. Students who are not socially well adjusted to their group are generally unhappy. When students are not equated in such factors as strength, skill, and fitness, one individual or group generally has an unfair advantage and the development of social efficiency is difficult. Social values are taught as well as caught, and just as skills are more easily taught in a group with similar abilities, so are social learnings. The low-skilled students especially need a different type of emotional adjustment than do the average and the highly skilled, and similar grouping provides a more conducive atmosphere for it to take place.

Class Morale and Spirit. Third, class morale and spirit are better when there are no extremes. It is difficult to maintain esprit de corps in a class when student abilities run the gamut. Those in the lower ranges grow timid and tend to become withdrawn and discouraged, while those in the upper ranges lose interest because opportunities in relation to their abilities are limited and thus they are not fully challenged. The gifted or those with much previous experience will receive greater motivation and their morale will be higher if their instruction can be started at a more advanced level where they do not have to repeat the basic fundamentals which are necessary for those of lesser experience or ability. When students are unclassified, class instruction is generally geared to the level of the average, and the extremes tend to be neglected. Similar grouping in a class fosters democracy and a democratic atmosphere fosters high morale and spirit.

Realization of Objectives. Fourth, program objectives are more fully realized. Students at all levels achieve more, and thus the outcomes established for the program are more nearly attained. Outcomes for a heterogeneous group would of necessity be somewhat vague and nebulous, easily reached by some and unattainable for others. Classification could provide the basis for more exact goals for the different levels and provide goals which are within the range of accomplishment for all. At the same time, evaluation takes on more meaning since it can be designed and interpreted in terms of these more exact goals.

Teaching Effectiveness. Fifth, the effectiveness of teaching is materially increased. When students are classified into groups of similar abilities and needs, it is possible to accomplish a great deal more in the same amount of time. All students tend to be similar at the start, and in general tend to make progress at similar rates of speed. The group can be taught as a whole in most cases, and the methods and materials do not have to be directed at so many widely different needs. The program of activities and instructional procedures can more easily be adapted to meet the needs of the particular ability level. The progress need not proceed too rapidly for the low-skilled student nor hold back the gifted. The gifted group will attain higher levels of achievement because they will not only be starting at a more advanced point but will move ahead more rapidly because they are gifted.

Student Needs. Sixth, the needs of the student will more adequately be met. This can be done because a program is adapted to the needs of the individual. When suitable classification devices are administered, they generally place students into three distinct groups. If classification is done on the basis of motor ability, a program can be planned to fit the needs of the gifted, the average, and the low skilled. If classification is done on the basis of experience, a different program can be planned for the advanced, the intermediate, and the beginner. The student in the lower ranges will be motivated to do better and will learn faster because he receives more individual attention from the instructor and more satisfaction from his physical education experience. The student in the upper ranges will be challenged to greater effort, since he, too, will have the advantage of both advanced instruction, program content, and good competition. His competition is stiffer, he is not retarded by the average or the low skilled, and he can receive his share of the instructional time. The needs of the average will, also, be met more adequately for the same reasons. These students are neither retarded by the non-stimulating atmosphere which surrounds the mediocre, nor are they discouraged by the standards of excellence displayed by the gifted.

Approaches to Classification

There are several steps in the implementation of an effective classification program. There is some choice of implementation procedures on the part of the instructor, but his choice should always be made with certain factors in mind. Some of these factors are: (1) the purpose of the physical education experience; (2) the purpose for which classification is needed; (3) the nature and size of the group to be classified; (4) the equipment and facilities available; and (5) the time necessary for test administration. The instructor must be aware that no single device or method will suffice for a permanent classification scheme. Best results are obtained when several factors are considered and several approaches used. Even then, there will be exceptions to the rule when a student obviously does not belong in the category where the classification instrument has placed him. These exceptions will stem from many factors including student motivation, educability, past experience, age level, determination, interest, native ability, and hard work. In the final analysis, the instructor uses his judgment and makes the necessary adjustments by moving the exception to the rule up or down in the grouping as the situation may dictate. It is an important principle that no classification device will function perfectly. Any grouping is subject to change and there will always be need for teacher judgment in making adjustments and changes when they are necessary.

Medical Examination. The first step in screening for purposes of classification is the medical examination, and it is a prerequisite to all succeeding steps. The medical examination will screen out a small percentage of students who have handicaps and disabilities and who should not be required to participate in the required program of instruction. This group should not be excused entirely from activity, but should have a program planned to care for the individual needs of each person. All of the students not screened out by the medical examination should take the regular program.

Grade or Level. After the medical examination has screened out the corrective or adapted group, the next step, and perhaps the simplest classification device, is to group students by grade in school. This grouping has a fair relationship with age and with experience, although the nature of the physical education program in most situations has been such that nothing can be taken for granted in the way of past experience. This method does work satisfactorily for the elementary school, and is a commonly accepted procedure at that level. It can be made to work at the secondary level if progression is adhered to from grade seven through twelve. Since classification by grade is done in other subject matter areas, it is realistic to continue the practice in physical education.

Sex. An extension of the class or grade classification is to group by sex. It is a commonly accepted principle in physical education to divide the sexes for most physical education activities after the fourth grade. No grouping is needed by sex for certain activities which are recognized as co-educational in nature. When co-educational activities are not indicated, classification by sex is necessary.

Ability. Students may be grouped first by the medical examination, next by grade in school, and then by sex, if necessary. A fourth ingredient can be introduced at this point which will insure that more of the purposes and values of classification will be realized. This ingredient is ability. The medical exam and the grade in school are necessary as a basis for this grouping. If the activity in question is not of a co-educational nature, then classification by sex is probably necessary, too. The next step involves ability grouping. For the junior and senior high school levels, grouping is more functional when it is based on all four of the steps. Implementation of the first three steps is easy to accomplish. This fourth step is more complex and needs careful study of the purpose behind grouping and the various techniques to be employed. There are two approaches to classifications by ability.

Subjective Judgment

The first approach is through the use of subjective judgment. This method can be a rank-order affair, or perhaps a more general grouping based on ratings. This approach has one definite disadvantage. It is essential that the instructor should know the abilities of his group when this method is used. Such knowledge is hardly feasible early in the school year, since the instructor will not have had enough time to acquaint himself sufficiently with the abilities of students. Most coaches use this approach at one time or another as they "cut" squads or select starting line-ups.

Objective Tests

The second approach is through the use of some objective measurement. Practically any type of test in physical education can be used to classify students. The test to be used for classification will depend chiefly on the purposes of the instructor. However, the size and nature of the group and the local situation may have some influence. Certainly, some tests are far superior to others in efficiency and many of the tests are not interchangeable. No test will do the job completely. After the test, the instructor must use his judgment. Students should be moved up or back in classification groups at the beginning if it is obvious they are exceptions to the results, or during the period of instruction if their progress is faster or slower than that of their group. In general, this objective approach is accomplished in two ways: (1) grouping for specific ability, and (2) grouping for general activity.

1. *Specific Ability Grouping.* The equating may be done on the basis of specific ability or sport skill. If swimming is the activity to be taught, students should be grouped on the basis of swimming skill; or, if basketball is the sport, a basketball skill test may be used. Such grouping is the most effective method of classification and more accurately differentiates between the various ability levels. However, there are some definite handicaps in the use of such techniques. First, grouping by special ability in one activity generally will not carry over to another activity. Skill learning is specific and will not transfer except when there are identical components. After a season of baseball the player is no better swimmer than he was when he started his training in baseball. Second, if this method of equating is to be used, re-classification must take place each time an activity changes. This is ineffectual as a part of the instructional process because it is time-consuming and difficult to administer if the activity changes frequently. However, if the activity is to be continued over a long period of time such as a semester or a year, this method is quite satisfactory. It also may be feasible to use in a class where the activities change, if the activity does not change too often and if inter-class grouping is employed. Grouping by specific ability rates high in administrative economy, and is more efficient in screening than are methods of general classification such as fitness, strength, or motor ability. The results of such tests will clearly indicate where the students are, at the elementary, the intermediate, or the advanced level of a specific sport or activity.

2. *General Grouping.* The equating may be done for general activity. This is a survey-type program where several activities are presented and these activities change frequently. Perhaps they may change as often as every two or three weeks. In this method

of grouping, classification is done on the basis of some general ability or quality such as fitness, strength, motor ability, or age, weight, and height. This approach does not measure achievement in a particular sport, but indicates a level of achievement in general motor skills, or a probable capacity for performance after a period of practice and instruction in a particular sport. It is present status or capacity but is based on both innate ability and achieved ability through experience. One who scores high on such a test will generally do well in a specific sport. This method works best in the physical education program where the activity changes periodically. Students are tested prior to being scheduled in a class and are classified into groups and kept together for a semester or the entire year. Only one classification is required per year. While this method is neither as effective nor as accurate as the specific grouping by particular sport skills, it is far less time-consuming and does rate acceptably high from the standpoint of efficiency. This method can be used for classification in the instructional program, and in the intramural program, or for classification within the class. There are two forms of equating for general ability.

(1) *Age, Height, Weight, and Physique.* First, the students may be grouped according to age, height, and weight, some combination of these, or by body build or type of physique. These methods are rough techniques which are useful only because they can be applied quickly and could serve as a basis for initial classification. At best, such classification indicates only probable ability of students. Such methods will function effectively only to the extent that the instructor recognizes they equalize only the factors of age, height, weight, body build, or physique. They do not equalize such important factors as native ability, interest, or experience. However, there is a relationship between age, height and weight, and performance in physical education activities. As the child grows older, he gains in weight and height. These gains generally are accompanied by an increase in strength, power, agility, and coordination. It is agreed that any method of classification based on age, height, and weight is a rough measure and should be used only when a quick and tentative grouping is needed. Sometimes this method may present the only practical way to grouping. If the instructor understands the inadequacy of his instrument and if he makes allowances for its weaknesses, it can be useful. Probably the most important use of age, height, weight classification indices is concerned with the construction of norms. Many motor ability and fitness tests have scale scores or other norms set up for the various age, height, weight classes. When the three factors of age, height, and weight are taken into consideration, a much fairer and more meaningful test score is obtained.

The two best known methods of classification in this category are: (1) McCloy's Classification Index[8] and (2) Neilson and Cozens Classification Index.[13]

(a) *McCloy's Classification Index.* McCloy has proposed the following three classifications for the indicated levels:

HIGH SCHOOL
Classification Index I = 20 (age in years) + 6 (height in inches) + weight in pounds.
COLLEGE MEN
Classification Index II = 6 (height in inches) + weight in pounds.
ELEMENTARY SCHOOL
Classification Index III = 10 (age in years) + weight in pounds.

These indices are related, but one may observe that age has been omitted at the college level, and height at the elementary level. Height was found to be a negligible factor in Classification Index III, and age was of no significance in Classification Index II. The Wetzel Grid[18] is helpful in computing Classification Index I and also II when weight is added. After each student's index has been computed, he is grouped in categories according to A, B, C, D, etc. according to Table 15–1.

For example our student, Jerry, is 12 years old, is 60 inches tall, and weighs 92 pounds. His physical education class is to be grouped for participation in touch football. His Classification Index is 20(12) +6(60) +92 or a score of 692. Referring to Table 15–1 at the top of the chart, it is found that Jerry would be classified into group "E" for his participation.

(b) *Neilson and Cozens Classification Index.* The classification scheme developed by Neilson and Cozens is quite similar to McCloy's and is highly related to it as shown by a very high correlation. In this method the exponent system is used with age, height, and weight being related to numbers in an exponent column. These exponents are shown in Table 15–2 for boys and girls grades 5 through 8, and in Table 15–3 for boys in high school.

To illustrate in the case of Jerry who is 12 years old, 60 inches tall, and weighs 92 pounds. His exponents are: height—10, age—5, and weight —7. His total exponent value is 22. This exponent value of 22 places Jerry in the D classification.

(c) *Wetzel Grid.*[18] One of the weaknesses of the two classification schemes described in (a) and (b) is that they fail to take into consideration body type. One's body type or physique is sometimes more important in his performance in motor skills than is his age, height, and weight. The Wetzel Grid (see page 353, Chapter 10) has been used successfully to classify men at the college level and offers possibilities at the elementary and secondary school levels.

Table 15–1.   McCloy Classification Index Divisions*

CLASSIFICATION INDEX-ELEMENTARY SCHOOL
Range 515–875

Class	For a Small Group	Class	For a Larger Group
A	800 and over	A	800 and over
B	770	B	775
C	740	C	750
D	710	D	725
E	680	E	700
F	650	F	675
G	620	G	650
H	619 and under	H	625
		I	600
		J	599 and under

CLASSIFICATION INDEX—JUNIOR HIGH SCHOOL
Range 540–900

Class	
A	875 and over
B	845
C	815
D	785
E	755
F	725
G	695
H	665
I	664 and under

CLASSIFICATION INDEX—HIGH SCHOOL
Range 685–955

Class	For a Small Group	Class	For a Larger Group
A	890 and over	A	900 and over
B	860	B	875
C	830	C	850
D	800	D	825
E	770	E	800
F	740	F	775
G	739 and under	G	750
		H	725
		I	724 and under

* From: *Tests and Measurements in Health and Physical Education*, 3rd. Ed., by Charles Harold McCloy and Norma Dorothy Young.   Copyright, 1954, Appleton-Century-Crofts, Inc.   Reproduced by permission of Appleton-Century-Crofts.

Table 15–2.   Neilson and Cozens Classification Chart for Boys and Girls Grade Five Through Grade Eight*

Exponent	Height in Inches	Age in Years and Months	Weight in Pounds	Sum of Exponents	Class
1	50 to 51	10 to 10–5	60 to 65	9 & below	A
2	52 to 53	10–6 to 10–11	66 to 70	10 to 14	B
3		11 to 11–5	71 to 75	15 to 19	C
4	54 to 55	11–6 to 11–11	76 to 80	20 to 24	D
5		12 to 12–5	81 to 85	25 to 29	E
6	56 to 57	12–6 to 12–11	86 to 90	30 to 34	F
7		13 to 13–5	91 to 95	35 to 38	G
8	58 to 59	13–6 to 13–11	96 to 100	39 & above	H
9		14 to 14–5	101 to 105		
10	60 to 61	14–6 to 14–11	106 to 110		
11		15 to 15–5	111 to 115		
12	62 to 63	15–6 to 15–11	116 to 120		
13		16 to 16–5	121 to 125		
14	64 to 65	16–6 to 16–11	126 to 130		
15	66 to 67	17 to 17–5	131 to 133		
16	68	17–6 to 17–11	134 to 136		
17	69 & over	18 & over	137 & over		

* Neilson, N. P.: *An Elementary Course in Statistics, Tests and Measurements in Physical Education.* Palo Alto, National Press Publications, 1960, pp. 65. Courtesy of the author.

(2) *Ability Tests.* Second, students may be grouped on the basis of general test scores. These generally fall into three types: motor ability, strength, or fitness. Ability tests take more time to administer than the age, weight, height combination methods, but they are more effective classifiers. The type of test used will depend to a large extent on the philosophy of the instructor, and what his aims and objectives of physical education are, and his purpose for grouping. Generally this type of classification is best implemented through the use of a motor ability test. Motor ability testing has several uses, but probably the most important use is

Table 15–3. Neilson and Cozens Classification for Secondary School Boys*

Exponent	Age	Height	Weight	Exponent	Age	Height	Weight
9			53–59	24	11:9–12:2	$49\frac{1}{2}$–$51\frac{1}{2}$	147–153
10			60–65	25	12:3–12:8	52 –$53\frac{1}{2}$	154–159
11			66–71	26	12:9–13:2	54 –$55\frac{1}{2}$	160–165
12	Class	Sum of Exp.	72–78	27	13:3–13:8	56 –$57\frac{1}{2}$	166–171
13			79–84	28	13:9–14:2	58 –$59\frac{1}{2}$	172–178
14	F	69 & below	85–90	29	14:3–14:8	60 –62	179–184
15	E	70–74	91–96	30	14:9–15:2	$62\frac{1}{2}$–64	185–190
16	D	75–78	97–103	31	15:3–15:8	$64\frac{1}{2}$–66	191–up
17	C	79–82	104–109	32	15:9–16:2	$66\frac{1}{2}$–68	
18	B	83–87	110–115	33	16:3–16:8	$68\frac{1}{2}$–$70\frac{1}{2}$	
19	A	88 & over	116–121	34	16:9–17:2	71 –$72\frac{1}{2}$	
20			122–128	35	17:3–17:8	73 –$74\frac{1}{2}$	
21			129–134	36	17:9–18:2	75 –up	
22	10:9–11:2	47 down	135–140	37	18:3–18:8		
23	11:3–11:8	$47\frac{1}{2}$–49	141–146	38	18:9–19:2		

* Neilson, N. P.: *An Elementary Course in Statistics, Tests and Measurements in Physical Education.* Palo Alto, National Press Publications, 1960, pp. 68. Courtesy of the author.

selecting the students at either end of the continuum. The test is given and those in the upper ranges, such as the upper quartile or the upper 20 per cent, are placed in classes for the physically "gifted" student. Those students in the lower ranges, such as the lower quartile, or the lower 20 per cent, can be placed in classes which are frequently referred to as "fundamentals." In any event both groups profit by such placement.

Motor ability, while not a permanent quality and improves with training, experience, and maturity, is a relative quality. Individual differences in students will tend to remain the same throughout the school level. Therefore, a motor ability test need not necessarily be administered each year for results to be valid and useful. Probably the best arrangement is the administration of such a battery at the beginning of the 4th, 7th, and 10th grades. (See Chapter 7, p. 157, for an appropriate motor ability test.)

Other Methods. It is possible to classify students on the basis of other factors as well as the ones already discussed. The instructor has a free rein in the selection of techniques, but should have a good reason for whatever technique he selects. The following factors have been used successfully:

Interest. In a recreational type program interest alone is a good method. Where teaching is not an important aspect, and where differences in ability are not important, or where such differences

18

may be eliminated by handicapping, as in golf, this method works quite adequately. The elective program at the college level is to some extent based on this idea. However, it must be recognized that interest may provide only temporary homogeneity. Lasting interest is generally related to how well one plays an activity. As some students fail to achieve the measure of success to which they aspire, they tend to become discouraged, lose interest, and drop out of activity.

Experience. Previous experience has been used as a basis for grouping in sports instruction. Of course, it is recognized that previous experience in physical education varies a great deal more than it does in the academic field. Where it can be assumed that all students have had similar experiences, this method is a means of grouping for certain activities. For example, this method might be suitable for such activities as rhythms and tumbling and stunts. If this approach is to function most effectively, however, there must be a certain amount of uniformity in the previous instructional process. The time factor alone is not an adequate basis for judging the adequacy of past experience.

Grades (Marks). Grades indicate how a student stands in his group not only with respect to the other students, but also in relation to the standards which have been set in the established objectives. The teacher may use these grades to classify his students into both homogeneous or heterogeneous groups. When a grading system rates high in the criteria established for grading (See Chapter 16, p. 536), grades might conceivably provide an excellent basis for classification for the second semester especially.

Combinations. Sometimes two or more tests may be used for purposes of classification. A combination of age, weight, and height, and a test of either motor ability or fitness might be employed. The chart to follow shows the various categories into which students might be divided on the basis of McCloy's Classification Index[8] (see page 526), and the Indiana Physical Fitness Test.[17]

All boys with a Classification Index above 715, and a fitness score of 61 are in the group "C" category. All boys with a Classification

CLASSIFICATION INDEX

		644 Down	*645 to 714*	*715 Up*
INDIANA PHYSICAL	61 Up	A	B	C
FITNESS	40 to 60	D	E	F
SCORE	39 Down	G	H	I

Index below 644 and a physical fitness score of below 39, are in category "G." Categories A, B, D, E, F, H, and I can be found in the same way by checking the limits vertically and horizontally. The way the limits are set up at the present time in the chart, categories D, E, F, B, and H, will tend to run larger in number of students than categories A, C, G, and I. However, if the limits of Classification Index and Fitness were to be arranged so that each of the three levels would include one third of the group, each of the categories would be approximately even in number. For example, Jerry's score on the Indiana Physical Fitness Test is 51 and his Classification Index is 692. Reading across horizontally according to the fitness scores and down vertically according to the Classification Index it is found that Jerry is in the "E" category.

Interclass Grouping. As has been pointed out, two of the main uses of classification are for increasing the effectiveness of teaching, and for equalizing competition. This presents a problem on the basis of one ability grouping within the same class period for an average size class. Ideally, of course, classification tests should be administered before registration so that when classes are scheduled, the student could be placed in homogeneous groups at the beginning. This practice of classifying the entire group of students into homogeneous groups is a desirable one. However, in today's schools where adequate scheduling presents an almost insurmountable problem in most situations, such grouping is rarely feasible. The resourceful teacher, when faced with this eventuality, can meet the challenge by classifying within the group. Satisfactory results may be achieved by the instructor when he is faced with a heterogeneous situation by administering some classification test such as a motor ability test. On the basis of the test scores he can group his students two ways, horizontally and vertically.

The vertical grouping is done by placing students into homogeneous groups, or squads, while the horizontal grouping is done by placing the students into heterogeneous groups. This can be implemented in the following way. The class scores are placed into a frequency distribution or ranked from high to low. If the scores are ranked from high to low, the ranks can be placed in a table as follows:

	A	B	C	D	E	F	(For Teaching)
Red	1	12	13	24	25	36	
White	2	11	14	23	26	35	
Blue	3	10	15	22	27	34	
Green	4	9	16	21	28	33	
Yellow	5	8	17	20	29	32	
Black	6	7	18	19	30	31	

(For Competition)

In the first instance the class is divided into squads designated, for instance, as A,B,C,D,E,F. These squads are for the purpose of teaching. Each group is made up of students who have similar abilities, thus making instruction easier and more effective. This grouping is generally used at the beginning of the physical education period when the instructor wishes to emphasize instruction and teach the fundamentals of sports through drills. An instructor who is a good organizer and who is willing to train and make use of student leaders can enhance his instruction and bring about more learning on the part of all groups.

In the second instance, the class is divided into squads designated as Red, White, Blue, Green, Yellow, and Black. These squads are made up of students of varying abilities, some good, some average, and some below average. This grouping is used for the purpose of competition. Since each squad has a fair share of each ability level, the competition is equalized. It is necessary for the student to know that he is a member of one squad for learning, and one squad for playing. This system works best when there is a good student leadership program. At times, in the example above during the instructional phase of the class, the floor would resemble a six-ring circus with trained squad leaders in charge of each ring.

Grouping within the class is somewhat less complicated in the medium and large schools where there are a number of instructors and enough teaching stations to accommodate three or four classes at one period. In this instance, 75 to 125 students (this number could be even more if the average class size is more than 35) and 3 or 4 instructors are assigned to each class period. Classification tests are administered to the large group, and on the basis of test results, the students are classified into ability levels and an instructor assigned to each different group. A program can then be planned to serve the needs of each ability level. If this method is combined with the classification by grade, a very good situation prevails. Students who progress faster or slower than their group may easily be shifted to another class in the same period without upsetting the class schedules. The success of this method depends primarily on the number of instructors and teaching areas available.

Proficiency Tests. Proficiency testing is another facet of measurement which is related to classification. It is, in fact, a method of classification since it actually divides students into categories on the basis of test data. In general proficiency tests are used for two purposes: (1) placement, and (2) exemption. These tests have several uses and numerous approaches. They can be applied in (1) the professional physical education program for competency of the major student; (2) they can be used in the institution's basic instruction program in physical education to measure the general student's proficiency in the basic requirement; and (3) they can be used in the *nongraded* school for the elementary and secondary student. In the first two instances, proficiency tests may serve as either exemption programs or for advanced placements. In the third instance they are used to measure progression from one proficiency level to a higher one.

These techniques will no doubt be used more often in the future. The explosion of the college population has placed a burden on the basic instruction program. Not only staff but also facilities and equipment are taxed in many instances beyond normal limits. One answer to large numbers in the basic requirement is to exempt the more gifted physically so that more time, space and leadership can be devoted to those who need instruction most.

In the professional training programs more is expected of the major student as time passes. Since the demands on his time are greater, he should not be expected to spend valuable time in repeating skills which he can already perform adequately. In both of the above uses the procedure compares with current educational trends in other subject matter areas.

Below the college level, proficiency tests will probably find more use in the nongraded school which is an innovation that eliminates the traditional placement of the student in school by grades. Pupil progress and promotion in the traditional sense have been replaced by a program of continuous progress whereby each student moves through the educational spectrum at his own pace. In this nongraded school there are levels which generally correspond to the primary, elementary, junior high school, and senior high school levels but there are no grades within these levels. Proficiency tests are needed to evaluate a student's status so that he may move on to a higher level if he can demonstrate proficiency. Little has been done in this area for the field of physical education, however. Physical educators will need to learn much more about student needs and characteristics in the future. For example, when is the best time to begin tennis and how proficient should the student be before he can progress on to the more advanced level?

In the basic instruction program at the college level proficiency tests are used in a number of ways. In general, most of these tests involve both skills and knowledges. The most common approach is to administer the knowledge test first. Only those students who meet the standards on the written tests are permitted to continue with the skill portion of the exempt program. Standards are usually set locally in these tests and those students who meet the standards are handled in one of two ways. First, it may be presumed that they have met the requirement and they are exempted from further participation. Second, there are many values from participation in well planned and conducted programs of physical education other than skills and knowledges. Therefore, the student is not excused from the requirement entirely but is permitted to elect the activity in which he may wish to specialize. In some cases, proficiency in a stipulated number of activities is required and he may demonstrate proficiency and pass out of some but must meet certain requirements in others. Institutions which administer classification tests sometimes permit only those students who score above the 75th or 80th percentiles on the classification test to have the privilege of exemption tests.

After a student has met the standards established for knowledge and understanding, he may continue with the skill proficiency. His skill performance can be determined in one of two ways. First, skill tests (see Chapter 13) may be administered and standards set for exemption. Second, and perhaps the most commonly used, exemption is to be granted by an instructor, usually a specialist in the particular activity. This may be done by the instructor observing the student's performance and giving him a rating; or in the case of some activities, the instructor may actually participate with the student in the activity. Regardless of which method is used, empirical standards have to be set. Ultimately standards of proficiency are really left to subjective judgment as to when a competency is demonstrated.

Under the impact of burgeoning enrollments, proficiency tests seem to be expedient as well as educational. However, it seems that few students are being exempt. Those who may want to be exempt, cannot meet the standards, while those who can, rarely want to.

Proficiency testing for the professional student presents a slightly different problem. In the first place any institution initiating a testing program for exemption is confronted with several issues. First, it must determine what are the activities which the professional should know and perform. After these activities have been determined, the next step involves the establishment of standards. What are the levels of performance in the selected activities needed for exemption? In general each institution must not only decide on the activities for exemption but also on the level of competency necessary for exemption. Levels of performance may be categorized in several ways. Perhaps the best known is a three category scale involving (1) *beginners*, (2) *intermediate*, and (3) *advanced*. In some cases two other categories may be added at the opposite ends of the scale involving (0) *fundamentals* and (4) *enriched*.

Arrasmith has suggested that the "intermediate level" of skill performance be selected as the standard for exemption along with a "high level" in the area of knowledge.[2] However, these levels continue to be vague and until definite norms can be established for each activity, such standards will depend somewhat on the interpretation placed on them by each individual instructor in each institution. For those activities which do not lend themselves to objective skill tests, rating scales may be developed with the above five categories.

The proficiency test for the major student should come as early in the student's career as possible. In the event that the student cannot meet the level of competency required, he has options about meeting his deficiency. He may register for an activity course in each of his weak areas, or he may work on his skills outside of class during the school year or during vacation and ask for a re-examination.

References

1. Adams, E. E.: The Study of Age, Height, Weight, and Power as Classification for Junior High School Girls, Research Quarterly, *5*, 95–99, May, 1934.
2. Arrasmith, J.: An Exemption Testing Program, Journal of Health, Physical Education and Recreation, *41*, 83–85, April, 1970.
3. Barrow, H. M.: Classification in Physical Education, The Physical Educator, *17*, 101, 1960.
4. Bovard, J. F., F. W. Cozens, and E. P. Hagman: *Tests and Measurements in Physical Education*, 3rd Ed., Philadelphia, W. B. Saunders Co., 1949, pp. 114–123.
5. Cozens, F. W., and N. P. Neilson: Age, Height, and Weight as Factors in the Classification of Elementary School Children, Journal of Health and Physical Education, *3*, 21, December, 1932.
6. Cozens, F. W., M. H. Trieb, and N. P. Neilson: The Classification of Secondary School Boys for Purposes of Competition, Research Quarterly, *7*, 36, March, 1939.
7. McCloy, C. H.: *The Measurement of Athletic Power*. New York, A. S. Barnes & Co., 1932.
8. McCloy, C. H., and Norma Dorothy Young: *Tests and Measurement in Health and Physical Education*, 3rd. Ed., New York, Appleton-Century-Crofts, Inc., 1954. p. 59.
9. Lockhart, Aileene, and Jane A. Mott: An Experiment in Homogeneous Grouping and Its Effect on Achievement in Sports Fundamentals, Research Quarterly, *22*, 58–62, March, 1951.
10. Miller, K. T.: The Wetzel Grid as a Performance Classifier with College Men, Research Quarterly, *22*, 63–70, March, 1951.
11. ———: A Critique on the Use of Height-Weight Factors in the Performance of College Men, Research Quarterly, *23*, 402–416, December, 1952.
12. Neilson, N. P.: *An Elementary Course in Statistics, Tests and Measurements in Physical Education*. Palo Alto, National Press Publications, 1960, pp. 65–68.
13. Neilson, N. P., and F. W. Cozens: *Achievement Scales in Physical Activities for Boys and Girls in Elementary and Junior High Schools*. New York, A. S. Barnes & Co., 1934.
14. Rousey, Merle A.: The Physical Performance of Secondary School Boys Classified by the Grid Technique. Doctor's Dissertation, Bloomington, Indiana University, 1949.
15. Standbury, Edgar: A Simplified Method of Classifying Junior and Senior Boys into Homogeneous Groups for Physical Education Activities, Research Quarterly, *12*, 765–776, December, 1941.
16. Stein, J. U.: Better Basketball Through Skill Classification, Journal of Health, Physical Education and Recreation, *28*, 10–11, November, 1957.
17. State of Indiana: High School Physical Education Course of Study, Bulletin No. 222, Department of Public Instruction, Indiana, 1958, pp. 170–177.
18. Wetzel, Norman C.: *Instruction Manual in the Use of the Grid for Evaluating Fitness*. Cleveland, NEA Services, 1941.

Chapter 16

GRADING IN PHYSICAL EDUCATION

Philosophy

Grades are symbols used to denote student progress and achievement. While grading is not the same thing as measurement, it is related. It is not so broad in its scope, nor so comprehensive in its approach since it is only one of the purposes of measurement. The process of grading employs many of the same techniques used in evaluation, and there is a close relationship between established objectives, effective measurement, and the reporting of student achievement toward those objectives. Measurement techniques are employed in the school process as a means to an end rather than as ends in themselves. Grading, while it may be an end of measurement, is in itself a means to an end and should be based on some rational approach. Grades should not become goals in and of themselves. Rather, they should be symbols of achievement or progress toward established goals.

The grading of educational endeavors is receiving much attention and criticism currently. There is probably no quarrel with the need to assess achievement and for the students to know about their accomplishments and status. The methods and uses, however, have been questioned. The primary complaint is that the symbol, the grade, is emphasized more than the learning. Or, as McQuire says, "We must abolish the grading system and replace it by another means of evaluation that has less tendency to dominate the educational process."[23] The "symbolic replacement for knowledge"[11] seems unfair in several aspects. Many students and parents consider a "C" grade an unsatisfactory grade; "B" and above denotes success and anything below is tantamount to failure. Grading is distracting to teachers, as well as students, who sometime spend more time on grading procedures than on teaching. Grades add to the drop-out rate in high schools because the success cut-off point is interpreted by students to be between "B" and "C." There is some research to show that grades are a good predictor of success in school but not a good predictor of success after school.[3] Yet grades follow a person throughout life, often creating misleading stumbling blocks difficult to overcome. Grades destroy student self-confidence and create a dislike for subjects in which students receive low grades.[17] Grades encourage cheating. They are a deterrent to independent study and creative pursuits. "When grades become the substitute for learning, and when they become more important than what is learned, they tend to lower academic standards. As long as grades remain as important as they are, few students will study any course material that will not be covered on a test and thus lead directly to a grade."[11]

Educators are agreed that there should be evaluation and assessment but they question the use of fear and pressure as the motivation for learning. The uses of the grade or assessment should be to have the student realize his own performance, not to punish him, but rather to demonstrate to the student the need for a definite relationship between achievement and responsibility.[30]

A change from the traditional schemes would mean the use of better measuring instruments, more emphasis on other forms of appraisal than tests,[10] less emphasis on failure, better counseling programs, more individual conferences, and more reasonable student-teacher ratios.[7] Several alternatives have been suggested:

1. **Descriptive evaluations about strengths and weaknesses.** These statements would cover such areas as skill development, interpersonal relationships, and responsibility. They would require considerable time to prepare; time would need to be alloted to teachers for this purpose. If the philosophy behind the evaluative scheme and the statements is educationally responsible, the time devoted to their formulation would be justified.

2. **Individual conferences.** Such conferences might follow testing sessions in skill and knowledges and would be used for analytical remarks. The testing results would not be used for determining grades translated into A, B, C, D, and F or perhaps even Pass-Fail, but would be used to help each student understand his achievement. Individual conferences could also be used in conjunction with descriptive statements serving the purpose of "report cards."

3. **Grades Without Failures.** The usual appraisal methods would be used as a basis for informing the student of his status. There would be no failing grades unless a student made no effort.

4. **Evaluation by classmates or peer groups.** Subjective ratings of skill performance, contributions to the team, sportsmanship, and such factor could involve students in the evaluation process. Guidelines would need to be established covering such topics as impartiality, analysis of skills to be observed, definitions of personal qualities, and the use of rating scales. Probably several students should be involved in the ratings for each student. Both the raters and the student being rated could learn from these experiences. The ratings identify important concepts and inform the student of his status in each. These ratings could lead to discussions between the

raters and the rated and between the teacher and the raters and the rated. There is some evidence to show that peer ratings can have a high degree of consistency, can show good agreement with instructor ratings, and that they provide a more typical grade distribution than self-ratings.[5]

5. **Self-evaluations.** Self-evaluations could be made on each assignment or test as well as on the unit as a whole. The research findings are mixed. Some have found students prone to evaluate themselves higher than justified, especially when first adopting this system.[17] Others have reported self-ratings worthy of consideration when guidelines are established and when individual conferences are conducted to discuss the self-assigned grades. Filene[9] experimented with this procedure and set forth the following guidelines:

On test or exams: (1) concentration on issues
                   (2) adequate evidence
                   (3) coherence
                   (4) inclusiveness
                   (5) originality

On the course: (1) weightings for the various parts of the course
                       were stated
                   (2) a 2-fold standard was stated:
                       Grade yourself
                       (a) by what you put into the course in terms of
                           effort and interest
                       (b) by what you got out of the course relative to
                           what was to be gotten

Filene considered the system workable and advocated self-evaluations until the final exam. He hoped this would "preserve the idealistic principle of self-grading within the pragmatic framework of the system."[9]

One teacher, reporting on the use of this system in a high school class in Oregon, had not had a single student take advantage. "But even if one did, so what? Would it be better for a teacher to have issued failing grades, perhaps causing the student to become totally disenchanted with school and drop out? If grades, used as a club, is our chief means of motivating students, we had best take a long look at our own competence as teachers. Our primary function as educators should be to make learning a meaningful experience. If evaluation or grading must take a back seat to accomplish this, so be it."[17]

Prevalent grading systems using letter grades, percentages, or numerical levels can be improved if there is wise use of good instruments to assess progress and if the grades are used as guidance information to help students become involved in learnng. Even these standard systems could be improved if some alternative methods were used in conjunction with them, and if teachers could convince administrators that grades are not necessary to achieve a healthy learning situation.

Grading in physical education is unique in many respects. Physical educators maintain that physical education should adhere to the same standards and practices observed by other disciplines which give academic credit toward graduation and promotion. Since physical education also has educational content, it must accept this responsibility of academic credit. It is generally classified as a laboratory subject where the usual classroom work, recitation, and homework are not the primary bases of grades. The traditional techniques of grading used in the classroom, while they may be relatively simple and mechanical, are seldom applicable to physical education classes. If one accepts the principle that physical education is an education through the physical, then learning in physical education becomes a many-faceted process as a multiplicity of objectives is pursued. Some of these learnings are difficult to evaluate; they make grading in physical education the unique process it has become. In spite of the many types of learning in physical education, the final grade has become a single index as in all other subjects.

Purposes

Physical education has an over-all aim of optimum development of the student through movement experiences into a physically, mentally, and socially effective person. This aim is a major objective of education. Physical education is a phase of education. To achieve this over-all aim, objectives have been established to serve as guides and to indicate direction. Traditionally, grades have been used to indicate the student's achievement in terms of the stated objectives.

Grading systems must become reliable symbols of student achievement in the objectives and be based on some objective evidence of achievement such as performance scores or valid rating scales. In many instances, no grades at all would be better than hastily-arrived-at, subjective ones which have little meaning and cannot be defended. Students have little respect for a grade which they do not deserve whether it is low or high. The chances of a meaningless or misleading grade occurring should be reduced to a minimum. Grades serve the following individuals, and have several purposes.

Students. Grades are useful to the student because they indicate to him how he ranks in his group with respect to the standards which have been set concerning the established objectives. Also, grades may serve to motivate him to greater effort. They influence his attitude toward physical education. It is recognized that the way a student feels toward physical education is affected by his grade. There is one danger inherent in grades for the student. Grades are based on achievement toward the established objectives. Since the grades themselves are frequently more tangible than the goals they represent, they sometimes become ends for the student rather than means. Grades are often the primary object which the student seeks, while he should be more interested in his degree of progress toward the objectives and outcomes which they represent.

Parents. Grades are necessary so that parents may follow the progress and achievement of their children. Grading is an important public relations medium. Parents can be informed concerning the objectives of physical education, and then be furnished with facts concerning their children's progress in reaching the objectives. Grades, besides indicating to the parents the status of their children, also serve as a means of informing them concerning the purposes and objectives of physical education. Grades probably offer the most important link between the parent and the school. Jerry's parents will be interested in a report of his progress and achievement in physical education if that report truly represents Jerry's status in relation to other 12-year-old boys.

Teachers. Grades serve a manifold purpose for the teacher. First, they encourage him to make a competent evaluation of each student, thus providing a more comprehensive understanding of the individual. Second, they furnish him with information for use in guidance. Students are interested in their performance. It is the job of the teacher to counsel the student who seeks information about ways of improving. Third, the teacher is furnished with data which can be used to evaluate the efficiency of his program and the quality of his teaching. The teacher may use grades for classification of students into homogeneous groups. Grades reflect a teacher's philosophy of education, his professional attitude, his objectives, and the principles to which he holds.

Administrators. Grades have become absolutely necessary for the school administration. Because of the public's confidence in the validity of grades, frequently grade points furnish the basis for many administrative decisions. They are used as a basis for graduation and promotion, for academic honors, for college entrance, and for guidance. They represent pupil progress and achievement, and they become a part of the permanent records of the school. Physical education grades should be considered along with all academic grades in such matters as college admission, scholastic honors, and academic societies.

MEASURABLE FACTORS

There is no standard method of grading. All good systems have certain characteristics in common, and are based on certain well-established criteria. For a clearer picture of grading, it is necessary to start with some basic beliefs. The system of grading reflects the basic beliefs and philosophy of the grader. The kind of grades, or whether there will be grades at all in physical education, will depend on the instructor's individuality. If his aim is to develop the physical only, the grades will be based on physical skills and ability alone. If his aim is to develop the individual through the physical, then in addition to physical skills and achievement, grades will be based on attitude, knowledge, understanding, appreciation, and perhaps still other factors. If a program is to pursue the recognized, well-rounded objectives of physical education, the grade must become a composite of a number of factors from several areas. For the sake of expediency, most factors are grouped under the psychomotor, cognitive, and affective domains. Procedures for evaluating each factor must be determined. Learning in physical education is both quantitative and qualitative. Some procedures of grading will be objective with a quantitative concept. Others will be subjective with a qualitative concept. Certainly a large proportion of a student's grade should be based on objective tests which measure the skills acquired, the fitness developed, and the knowledges learned. For many characteristics concerning a physically educated person, there are no objective measuring devices. Rating devices, objectified as much as possible, should be employed. In the final analysis, however, both qualitative and quantitative measures must be resolved into a single index grade.

Psychomotor Factors. Probably the most commonly used factors employed for grading purposes in this area are skill in the activity, fitness, motor ability, and game performance. These factors can be weighted as logic would dictate. They are generally weighted according to the time allotted each.

In the skills area, the grade for each sport might be determined on the basis of the following: a skill test, team work if the sport is a team sport, tournament in individual sports, and a subjective analysis of the student's ability to play the sport. When skill tests are not feasible, the student's ability in the various skills of the sport can be measured by rating devices.

Cognitive Factors. In the mental area, the grade should be based on knowledges and understandings pertaining to rules, performance, strategy, techniques, history, place in program, health, and information concerning physiology, fitness, and conditioning. Tests of knowledge and understanding over sports, exercise, and fitness are generally of the objective type. While standardized tests may be employed, the well constructed, homemade type are better for local use.

Affective Factors. In the social area, the student's grade should be based on an evaluation of the student's social behavior in the physical education environment. The grade should consist of a subjective evaluation of such factors as attitude, appreciation, sportsmanship, cooperation, citizenship, leadership, and sociability.

Social qualities are graded best on the basis of observation and rating by both the teacher and students themselves. There are two possibilities where students are involved in making ratings. The students either may rate themselves, or they may rate each other. These self-appraisal records must be used judiciously, however, since some students tend to rate themselves too severely and some too leniently. There are numerous check lists and rating scales which may be used. These devices are invaluable for measuring such subjective factors as responsibility, leadership, and sportsmanship.

When grades are given subjectively by the instructor, care must be taken that they are not based on vague factors and awarded carelessly. Subjective evaluation without the aid of guides such as rating scales or check lists is a technique which starts with an image in the mind of the instructor, and ends with a comparison of each individual student with that image. This sounds simple. It requires a mental picture of correct performance or behavior. This mental picture is the criterion against which the student is evaluated. However, when it is the sole means of grading, it becomes very complex since there are many items in a number of activities at several graded levels. This complexity makes subjective evaluation most difficult, and at the same time most unreliable. As has been pointed out several times, the subjective can be made more reliable only when it is objectified, and this is best done through rating scales and check lists.

Questionable Factors. Other items such as effort, improvement, attendance, showers, uniforms, interest, and punctuality have been used. These seem out of place and are questioned as important factors in grading. They should be considered as matters to be covered by departmental policies and not as a part of grading procedures. Grades which represent hygiene, showers, and uniforms are held by many to be inconsistent with modern philosophy and should be eliminated. These factors are important and should be emphasized, but they should not become major factors in grades. Grades based on these items would be entirely misleading to both parents and administrators.

The practice of grading partly on *attendance* is not an uncommon approach. There are pros and cons regarding any system of grading which includes this factor. Those who would reduce a grade because of excessive absences argue that the student cannot hope to achieve the objectives of the course, especially the more intangible ones, if he is not there. Those who are opposed to grading directly on attendance contend that absences from class will be reflected in the achievement of the student anyway, and thus attendance is an inconsequential factor. It is probably true that the final status of any student in well-organized programs of physical education will be somewhat lower as a result of absences. Attendance could be viewed as an administrative problem having no connection with the objectives of physical education. As such it would have no direct influence on the student's grade.

Grades which are based on *improvement* are questioned by some. A grade is usually given on the basis of status, at a particular time, in the objectives of the course. If physical education is to be accepted in the academic family, then its grades must be reports of measures of status. Improvement is definitely included as part of status, but the grade should be based on status and not on the degree of gain. It is difficult to evaluate improvement. The increment of gain varies in value. It becomes increasingly more difficult to improve as one moves nearer the ultimate. For example, it is easy for the learner to cut his golf score 10 strokes from 120 to 110, but most difficult for the 80 shooter to reduce his score to 70. There is another weakness in grading on improvement by means of objective tests. If the student knows his grade is based in part on improvement, he may not do his best on the first administration of the test so that his range of improvement will be greater. Some argue that this should be reflected in the student's social grade, but it is sometimes difficult to tell when a student is not trying to do his best.

Effort is another factor mentioned frequently in any discussion of the grading process. The idea behind using effort as a factor of grading is that it serves to motivate students toward greater effort. It is similar to improvement and is almost as difficult to evaluate. In the early stages of learning, it is easy to identify the effort being put forth by the learner. Many times in order to accomplish a little, the learner must expend a great amount of effort. However, as he becomes more proficient, he is able to accomplish more with less effort. As he approaches the ultimate, the work load seems to be accomplished with ease. The record breaker in a mile run usually comes in with his knees high and in full stride, while the last-place man invariably is plodding along like a workhorse. We say the highly skilled athlete makes his activity look easy. It is almost impossible to attach a value to such levels of effort. It does make sense, however, to grade on status, which can be evaluated and which is definitely related to effort. This relationship is indirect but apparent. Effort is invariably reflected in the status of the student and in his level of achievement.

Criteria for Grades

Relation to Objectives. Grades must be determined in relation to the objectives which have been formulated. It is necessary to determine what each student should achieve at each grade level. A student's grade should then indicate his degree of proficiency in the established objectives of the program. For example, a student's attainment on a fitness test would indicate, in part at least, his proficiency in the recognized objective of organic efficiency and his grade should reflect this attainment. Not only should this grade be determined in relation to the objectives, but also in relation to the importance of these objectives. In determining a grade in physical education, the instructor generally groups objectives into areas such as physical, mental, and social, or technical, associated, and concomitant or psychomotor, cognitive, and affective. There is no agreement as to how these areas are weighted, but logic should be followed. The final grade would be a combination of these areas into a single index and would be indicative of the total achievement of the student.

Validity. Next, the grade must have validity. This simply means that the grade truthfully measures the qualities or factors intended. Grades should honestly represent the achievement for which they are purportedly a symbol. The validity of most grading systems is lowered somewhat by the fact that the physical educator must measure the immeasurable or the difficult to measure if he is to be consistent with the idea that grades must be related to objectives. Frequently, the intangibles are more valuable in the quest for fine living than the measurable qualities. For example, such qualities as team spirit and a willingness to sacrifice oneself for the good of the group are very important in team games and sports, but it is difficult to assign a degree of attainment to them. Validity can never be as high as desired in grading. When the intangibles are objectified, something is inevitably lost in the process in the same manner that something is lost when a circle is squared or when a poem is translated.

Reliability. Grades must have reliability. The system must report consistently whatever it does report. The reliability of the grading system may be determined by asking the question, "Will the instructor using this system be apt to obtain the same grade for students on the same performance if re-figured?" An affirmative answer means that the system has reliability.

Objectivity. Grades should have some degree of objectivity. Objectivity in grading means the degree to which two or more instructors will arrive at the same grade when they have access to the same information. This implies, of course, that objective tests should be used when they are available in order to eliminate bias and subjective opinion. Present thought, however, recognizes that all important objectives of physical education cannot be measured in quantitative terms. When no objective tests are available to measure a particular factor, subjective methods must be used, but these methods should be objectified as much as possible. Even when objective tests are used, the subjective is not entirely eliminated in grading since levels of achievement are arbitrarily set by the instructor. Most successful athletic coaches operate through use of subjective techniques in the selection of squads and starting line-ups. There are numerous techniques which may be employed in the appraisal of subjective factors (see Chapter 17, p. 555).

Understandability. Grades must be understandable to the student and to his parents and should be easily interpreted by the teacher. Students must know the basis on which the grades will be given and they must understand how the system operates. The student should have an idea of what his grade will be before he gets it. Some time should be devoted to the explanation of grades. Interpretation is best accomplished through the results of objective tests interpreted in relation to levels on a scale. Such tests and accompanying interpretation leave little doubt about what a grade actually indicates.

Weightings. Since all factors in grading are not of equal importance, it is common procedure to weigh the measurable elements according to their relative importance. The final answer in weighing the various factors must be determined logically by the teacher in accordance with the needs of the student and the emphasis in the course. The weight of the factor as a part of the total grade should relate to the emphasis placed on it in the program and its comparative importance in producing a physically educated person. There is no general agreement, but there must be an adequate sampling of all the experiences presented in the course. Properly weighted factors should result in a single index grade for each student. This grade would be most representative of the student's real achievement. For example, when the instructor is grading on fitness, sport skill, knowledge, and attitude, he might assign the following respective weights: 2, 3, 2, 1.

Various Weighting Combinations

Psychomotor	Cognitive	Affective
50%	25%	25%
50%	30%	20%
40%	35%	25%
50%	40%	10%
60%	30%	10%

There is no agreement about how the three areas of psychomotor, cognitive, and affective are weighted. For reasons of logic, the psychomotor grade is generally weighted heaviest, and the affective grade lightest. The weighting would reflect relative emphasis among objectives and the philosophy of the grader.

Discrimination. Grades should discriminate between levels of performance. This criterion would generally eliminate the two category systems of grading such as pass-fail and satisfactory-unsatisfactory. Levels of performance are relative matters and have to be handled in an empirical way. These levels must be established high enough so that the gifted will be challenged and low enough so that the poorly skilled will not be discouraged. There should be no massing of grades at either the higher or lower levels in unselected groups. When physical handicaps place a restriction on the degree of proficiency a student can attain in fitness or sports skills, some adjustment should be made. This procedure applies only to the handicapped, and not to differences due to innate ability. The handicapped student should have the opportunity to receive a fair and encouraging grade within the range of his handicap when he is placed in the remedial phase of the program.

Standards of Attainment. After the factors have been determined and weighted, standards of attainment should be established in each of them. There should be a norm or scale of performance and some point or points along the way to indicate levels of achievement. These levels are then transmitted into grades. The levels are generally established with reference to some criteria or desired characteristics of these factors. Respect is shown for grades when they are based on modern performance tests, knowledge tests, and ratings of unmeasurable factors. The establishment of levels of performance, however, is generally an arbitrary affair and the lines drawn depend on the philosophy of the teacher and the local situation.

Where possible, standards should be set up in all performance tests. The best means is through use of some type of score which can be employed to reduce all variables to a common denominator. This enables the instructor to compare and add all the items. This may best be accomplished through the use of T-scores, standard scores, or six sigma scores (see Chapter 5, p. 80). These scores are based on the standard deviation and indicate the deviation of the score from the mean. These scores enable the teacher to make a composite of the scores of tests on several factors and to weight these factors according to their importance. Other means of setting up standards are through the use of percentiles and percentages. Qualities which cannot be measured quantitatively may be rated and these results can be converted to T-scores also.

If physical education grades are to be accepted on the same level with grades of other subjects in grade points and scholastic honors, a normal spread in grades is essential. If there is a massing of grades at the top levels, the standards are too low and the better students are not being challenged. Also, there will be no discrimination between the excellent and the good, and perhaps the good and the higher-average. If there is a massing of grades at the lower end of the continuum, quite the reverse is true—there will be no discrimination between the poor and the average. In either event, the grades do not differentiate between levels of ability and achievement. It is a sound principle that performance of a sufficiently large group of unselected students at any given level invariably resembles the normal curve.

Administrative Economy. The grading system must operate within the framework of time, cost, and personnel. The most important consideration concerns time. The system should not require too much clerical work. A teacher's first duty is to teach. An undue amount of his time should not be spent in implementing a complicated grading system. A grading system should work as a tool to improve instruction and not to hinder it. The objectives to be used as a basis for grading must be kept to a minimum. Too many factors complicate the picture. Many factors add very little to the evaluation of the student's grade. For example, when the factors of attendance, hygiene, uniforms, and showering are added to the more commonly recognized factors of fitness, sports skill, knowledge, and sportsmanship, very little is added if these first-listed factors are weighted according to their importance. They are irrelevant and inconsequential and could be discarded without lowering the validity of the grade.

Methods of Grading

Any method of grading which is based on sound philosophy and well established criteria will serve. One of the essential requirements of any grading system is that the instructor be able to justify the grade that has been awarded. While it is necessary to adhere to certain criteria and principles in grading, there is no standardized method or technique, and there probably should not be any. There are many difficulties to be overcome in evolving a grading system, but when a system is set up on some rational basis in the light of the local program and philosophy, many of these difficulties resolve themselves. There are numerous methods of grading but in general they all end up similar to one of these three types: (1) the more conventional letter grade such as A, B, C, D, and F; (2) the two-category pass-or-fail method; and (3) the descriptive type.

Letter Grades. Letter grades expressed as A, B, C, D, and F and number grades expressed as 1, 2, 3, 4, and 5 are essentially the same type. Whereas the number grades have not been used as extensively as the letter grades, the letter grades frequently must be converted to numbers when grade points are computed. Letter and number grades when adminstered in an acceptable manner may meet most of the criteria laid down in this chapter. Letter grades may be grouped into the following categories:

Percentage Method. Many test scores are reported in the form of percentages. Teachers are in the habit of working with percentages. They understand these scores and can interpret them to the students. Percentages are converted generally into letter grades. One method of using percentage scores is to divide the attained score by the highest possible score and multiply by 100. For example, if Jerry scores 33 on a test where 40 is the highest possible score, the score of 33 divided by 40 and multiplied by 100 equals 82 per cent. Another approach is to convert raw scores made on the various tests into letter or number grades by means of the percentage system. The instructor can arbitrarily assign percentages for each of the grade or number levels. For example, he might assign the following distribution of grades: A-7 per cent; B-24 per cent; C-38 per cent; D-24 per cent; and F-7 per cent. In a class of approximately 100 students, the top seven students will be awarded a grade of A, the next 24 a grade of B and the like. While this system is considered to be one of the most common approaches to grading, it is not recognized as a good system. Many educators believe there is no justification for grading on the curve. Standards should be set and if students achieve them, they should receive commensurate grades. If this system is to be used, however, the assigned percentages must be used as a guide and not as a standard from which there can be no deviation. Perhaps there are natural divisions in the distribution of scores which, if adhered to, will make the grades awarded seem more logical and much fairer. Table 16–1 indicates some possible choices of techniques in this system.

Numerical Method. The numerical method is similar to the percentage system. In this case, numerical scores are awarded and

Table 16–1. Table of Percentages for Grade Levels

Grade	Grade	Grade	Grade	Possible Per Cent	Possible Per Cent	Possible Per Cent
5	4	A	E	10	7	15
4	3	B	S	20	24	20
3	2	C	M	40	38	30
2	1	D	I	20	24	20
1	0	F	F	10	7	15

these scores in turn are converted to letter grades. For example, the following scale for scores may be established: 95–100, A; 88–94, B; 80–87, C; 70–79, D; below 70, F. The system of converting the numerical grade to a letter grade relieves the instructor of having to differentiate between such levels of performance as a 90 and 91. However, this may work as a handicap since this finer discrimination is sometimes needed to show small amounts of progress by the student. For example, when a student is at the lower range of C and makes even a fair amount of progress but not enough to raise his level to a B, he may feel that a grade of another C does not indicate any progress on his part and he may become discouraged. Another disadvantage of this system is that the degree of difficulty of the measuring instrument must be appropriate to the group. If the test is too difficult, there will be no one in the upper ranges, particularly the A's. If it is too easy, there may be far too many students scoring in the upper ranges.

Standard Deviation Method. In order to overcome some of the disadvantages of the first two methods of grading described, the standard deviation technique is employed. If this technique is to be used, however, there must be a sufficient number of students from an unselected group. The use of the standard deviation always assumes a normal distribution. This technique is implemented by securing the mean and standard deviation of all scores in the group to be graded and applying Table 16–2. A variation of this method is applied on page 293 in connection with a football skills battery.

The percentages of 7, 24, 38, 24 and 7 approximate the curve of normal distribution and, when they are used as a part of the standard deviation technique, make allowances for many of the shortcomings of other systems of grading. There are three definite advantages of this system: (1) it permits grades in one factor to be added to grades in another; (2) it permits scores on one test to be compared with scores on another; and (3) it permits weighting of different items in order to take into consideration their importance. This method has been employed very little in the grading system of

Table 16–2. Table for Assigning Grades by Standard Deviation Technique

Per Cent of Group	Standard Deviation Range	Rating	Grade
7	$1.5\,\sigma$ or more above mean	Excellent	A
24	Between $+.5\,\sigma$ and $+1.5\,\sigma$	Good	B
38	Between $+.5\,\sigma$ and $-.5\,\sigma$	Average	C
24	Between $-.5\,\sigma$ and $-1.5\,\sigma$	Inferior	D
7	$1.5\,\sigma$ or more below the mean	Failure	F

schools, but it should be used a great deal more in the light of its high rating in the criteria of grading systems. Teachers who use the standard deviation technique for arriving at grades may report them in the usual traditional form as shown in Table 16–2.

One problem concerning letter grades is arriving at an average for the single index final mark. One approach is to assign some point value to each letter. When the student's several letter grades are converted into numerical scores and summed, a numerical total is obtained. This total may be averaged by dividing it by the number of grades or it may be used as an index itself and treated further. It is generally true that when several grades are averaged to arrive at a final index, the grades tend to be grouped toward the middle and there are too many C's and, thus, too little discrimination. One way to prevent this from occurring is to place all totals in a frequency distribution. Final indexes may then be arrived at by assigning limits. This generally is done by the percentage method. Some possible percentages are shown in Table 16–1. A system of conversion for letter grades into numerical values is shown in Table 16–3. For example, Jerry made grades of B—, A, C+, and B+. When these grades are referred to the table, they may be converted into scores of 8, 12, 7, and 10. The total is 37. This number is tallied in a frequency distribution along with the totals for all the students in Jerry's class and then the final grades are derived.

Pass or Fail. A second method of grading is the two-category pass-fail type, or satisfactory-unsatisfactory. In some instances, a third category, exceptional, is added. This method is used rather widely in physical education classes. It fails to measure up to many of the listed criteria of grading which have been discussed previously in this chapter. For example, it does not discriminate; it is difficult to interpret; and it does not conform to an established distribution of grades. It falls far short of reporting student status and progress toward the objectives of physical education. There is considerable move to this system because it takes the pressure of grades off students. If it is used, it should be supplemented with student conferences to discuss achievement toward the various objectives of physical education.

Table 16–3. Conversion Table for Averaging Letter Grades

A+ — 13	C+ — 7
A — 12	C — 6
A— — 11	C— — 5
B+ — 10	D+ — 4
B — 9	D — 3
B— — 8	D— — 2
	F — 1

Descriptive Statements. A more recent innovation of reporting achievement in the schools is through use of some descriptive techniques. Teachers write comments about the progress, achievement, and problems of the students. These comments are in the form of descriptive words, phrases, or sentences which give an analysis of what the instructor knows about the progress of each student. They frequently are more meaningful to parents and students than are the more traditional grades. Some descriptive phrases or words frequently used are excellent, good, fair, unsatisfactory, improving, needs, applying, seems unable, showing progress toward, average, etc. These words or phrases may be in the form of a check list or rating scale and evaluation may be made in an objective or a subjective manner. This method can become more elaborate and take the form of a short anecdotal record in which an analysis is written of the student's status and achievement. There is no doubt of the value of this scheme, but for the instructor with a large number of students in his classes, such reports are prohibitive because of the burden of time. Also, it is relatively easy to describe the very good performer and the poor performer, but it becomes increasingly more difficult to describe the many who are in the large middle-average group. In these many instances, the descriptive anecdotal method could become a perfunctory and meaningless device.

Some progressive reports are in the form of a letter to the parents. One kind of report lists the aims and objectives of the course and then follows up with an appraisal of the amount of progress of the student in relation to the objectives. This report is informative and meaningful to both the student and the parent. It is a means of informing the parents concerning the objectives of physical education and at the same time provides a report of the student's status in terms of the objectives. Disadvantages center around the criterion of administrative economy. This method does require careful and frequent observations of the student, and a great deal of time in the preparation of the letters. If the teacher load is too heavy, this method is not workable. In some cases, letters to the parents may be form letters in mimeograph style. These could be used to explain the objectives, the program, specific tests, evaluation and grading, and other techniques. Each letter could be accompanied by some type of grade for the student, or perhaps a rating in a number of the more pertinent factors.

Sample Systems of Grading

Several sample systems of grading are presented in the succeeding paragraphs. Each system observes most of the criteria laid down in this chapter but at the same time is flexible enough to meet the needs of most local situations. It is best for the individual school to develop its own system based on the criteria listed in the preceding pages and in accordance with its own philosophy and program.

Moriarty[26] has suggested a system in which four general factors have been selected as a basis of the final grade. These factors are potential ability, achievement, attitude, and knowledge. The letter grades A, B, C, D, and F are used with respective numerical values of 5, 4, 3, 2, and 1. The four factors are weighted as follows: achievement—3, potential ability—2, knowledge—2, and attitude—1. The following example shows the grade awarded to a student in each of the four areas with their weightings and final grade.

Factor	Weighting	Grade	Points
Sports Skill	3	A (5)	15
Physical Fitness	2	B (4)	8
Knowledge	2	C (3)	6
Attitude (Social)	1	B (4)	4
TOTAL WEIGHTS	8	TOTAL	33

When the total score of 33 is divided by the total weights of 8, a score of approximately 4 is obtained. Referring back to the numerical value of each letter grade, one finds that the final grade is B.

Another system, a bit more elaborate, divides the final grade into three areas with the following weightings: Psychomotor—5, Cognitive—3, and Affective—2. The psychomotor grade is made up of peer ratings of skill, teacher ratings of skill, skill tests, and a fitness test. The cognitive grade is derived from a knowledge test on the unit of instruction. The affective area is assessed by both student and teacher ratings. The following example shows the grades awarded to a student in each area, and his final mark.

Area	Weight of Area	Factor	Weight of Factor	Grade of Factor	Points
Psychomotor	5	Fitness	1	A	12
		Sports Skills	2	C	12
		Peer Rating of skill	1	B	9
		Teacher Rating of skill	1	B	9
Cognitive	3	Knowledge Test	3	A	36
Affective	2	Student Rating	1	A	12
		Teacher Rating	1	B	9
	10		10		99

If the student receives an A in all factors, a total weighted score of 120 would result. The instructor has several ways of converting the 99 weighted total into a grade:

1. determine the percentage: 99 ÷ 120 = 82.5%
2. divide the total by the number of weightings:
   99 ÷ 10 = 9.9. Table 16-3 shows 9.9 equal to a grade of B+.
3. Place all the total weightings for the class in a frequency distribution and determine the appropriate places in the distribution to designate either the various grade levels, or the pass-fail cut-off line, or the qualitative levels expressed in good, fair, excellent, etc.

Another alternative would be to write a descriptive statement: "Jerry keeps himself in good physical condition. His fitness scores are in the top quartile. He is able to apply his exceptional insight into the strategies of volley ball to enhance average skill performance in the game. He sometimes performs less well, however, on skills tests. His classmates consider him a valuable member of the team. Jerry's attitude has improved from the soccer to the volley ball unit. This may be due partially to his above average skill in volley ball."

References

1. Bard, Bernard: The Death of the Report Card, Ladies' Home Journal, pp. 160–161, October, 1970.
2. Boyd, Clifford A.: A Philosophy of Assigning Grades in Physical Education Classes. The Physical Educator, *14*, 64–65, May, 1957.
3. Boyle, P. P.: Functional Dilemmas In the Development of Learning, Sociology of Education, *42*, 71–90, Winter, 1969.
4. Broer, Marion R.: Are Our Physical Education Grades Fair? Journal of Health, Physical Education, and Recreation, *30*, 27, March, 1959.
5. Burke, R. J.: Some Preliminary Data on the Use of Self-Evaluation and Peer Ratings in Assigning University Course Grades, Journal of Educational Research, *62*, 444–448, July, 1969.
6. Callon, Ruth: Marks or Misjudgments? The Physical Educator, *12*, 125–126, December, 1955.
7. Cummins, P.: De-escaluate Grades, Journal of Secondary Education, *45*, 188–191, April, 1970.
8. Fairfield, Paul: Credit for Physical Education, New York State Journal of Health, Physical Education, and Recreation, *10*, 36–38, June, 1958.
9. Filene, P. G.: Self-Grading: An Experiment in Learning, Journal of Higher Education, *40*, 451–458, June, 1969.
10. Garth, Warner D.: Marks—How Much Do They Mean? PTA Magazine, pp. 2–4, April, 1969.
11. Glasser, William: *Schools Without Failure*, New York, Harper & Row, Publishers, 1969.
12. Grigson, W. H.: The Physical Education Report Card, The Physical Educator, *16*, 56–61, May, 1959.
13. Gustafson, Willam F.: A Look at Evaluative Criteria in Physical Education, The Physical Educator, *20*, 172–173, December, 1963.
14. Handy, D. T., and Marjorie Latchaw: Value of Academic Grades in Estimating Student Teaching Success, Research Quarterly, *28*, 347–351, December, 1957.

15. Hatfield, Robert W.: A Study of Grading Procedures and Practices in Physical Education, M.A., Washington State University, 1965.
16. Hooks, Edgar W., Jr.: Now, Cross Your Heart, Is Your Grading System Honest? North Carolina Education, pp. 14–15, 35–36, December, 1969.
17. Jackson, Charles D.: Students Grade Themselves, Today's Education, pp. 24–25, October, 1970.
18. Jackson, E. L.: The Improvement of Marking in College Physical Education, The Physical Educator, *14*, 140–142, December, 1957.
19. Jensen, Clayne: Improve Your Marking System in Physical Education, The Physical Educator, *19*, 97–98, October, 1962.
20. Kindsvatter, Richard: Guidelines for Better Grading, Clearing House, *43*, 331–334, February, 1969.
21. Massey, B. H.: The Use of T-Scores in Physical Education, The Physical Educator, *10*, 20–21, March, 1953.
22. McCraw, Lynn W.: Principles and Practices for Assigning Grades in Physical Education, Journal of Health, Physical Education, and Recreation, *35*, 24–25, February, 1964.
23. McQuire, B. P.: Grading Game, Today's Education, *58*, 32–34, March, 1969.
24. Miller, K. D.: A Plea for the Standard Score in Physical Education, The Physical Educator, *8*, 49–50, May, 1951.
25. Milton, Ohmer: What It Is . . . I Measure I Do Not Know, Educational Record, *49*, 160–165, Spring, 1968.
26. Moriarty, Mary J.: How Shall We Grade Them? Journal of Health, Physical Education, and Recreation, *25*, 27, January, 1954.
27. Waglow, I. F.: A Measurement and Evaluation Manual for the Department of Required Physical Education at the University of Florida, Ed.D., New York University, 1964.
28. ———: Marking in Physical Education, Journal of Health, Physical Education, and Recreation, *25*, 48, May, 1954.
29. ———: The Comparison of Marks and Marking Systems, The Physical Educator, *13*, 22–23, March, 1956.
30. Winkler, J. E.: Grading, Peabody Journal of Education, *46*, 350–351, May, 1969.
31. Wright, Logan, and Patsy K. Wright: An Instrument for Evaluation of Skill in Women's Physical Education Classes, Research Quarterly, *35*, 69–74, March, 1964.

Chapter 17

RATING SCALES IN PHYSICAL EDUCATION

Introduction

A principle of measurement is that anything which exists, exists in amounts, and if it exists in amounts, it can be measured.[6] This does not imply, however, that all measurement is accurate and objective. It is important, also, to remember another salient principle of measurement which presents the idea that not all measurement is perfect.[6] Many important variables concerning physical education cannot be measured objectively. No one has yet accurately measured such qualities as courage, desire to win, confidence, poise, spirit, esprit de corps, loyalty, or beauty of sunset, although one frequently is aware that all of these exist in varying degrees. Yet most of these qualities and many others are outcomes of the recognized objectives of physical education and a concept of measurement suggests that all objectives and important outcomes be evaluated even though some are difficult to measure. While these variables do not lend themselves to accuracy in measurement, they, and many similar qualities, may be far more important in living a good life than are many of the more tangible and objectively measured traits. The entire area of the affective domain involving interests, attitudes, appreciations, ideals, values and social behavior in general falls into this category.

When no objective measurement exists for a quality, or when the existing devices for measurement are not administratively feasible or practical, or when it appears expedient to supplement objective measurement by subjective opinion, observation techniques are used. Rating devices are one of the best methods for recording observations and focusing the attention of the teacher on the more important aspects of the variables being observed. All teachers make use of ratings in some form or another even though they may not be aware of it at the time. Ratings are based on subjective opinions and estimates, and such subjective decisions must be made many times daily in the physical education program as teachers and coaches work with the "whole" student. The rating scale itself is a tool used to help the teacher or coach understand better what he is looking for and to identify the degree or amount of the trait under observation. These rating devices are neither as accurate nor as reliable as most objective tests, but are more so than a pure guess or random judgment made by the teacher without the help of a scale or check list to guide him. No apologies need be made for the use of subjectivity in the measurement program. In the final analysis all tests, including objective tests, are based to a great extent on subjective opinion. This is true because all tests are validated by means of a criterion and most criteria eventually revert to the consensus of experts and thus, in the final analysis, are based on subjectivity.

Rating scales are a valuable tool in a testing program. Many of them are prepared and used locally and never appear in the literature. The majority of these are adapted to a particular situation and group, and fulfill a specific need. In general, rating scales serve a multiplicity of purposes and may be applied both to the product and the process. In addition to providing a means of more accurately evaluating the many intangible factors of physical education, they also may provide a more effective means of measuring student achievement in skill and form in athletics. For example, in addition to measuring attitudes toward physical education and facets of social behavior, including sportsmanship, ratings scales are used to measure performance skills and form in such activities as gymnastics, diving, and the dance. A semi-objective measurement may be made of highly specialized skills found in most team and individual sports, and when form is being judged in activities like golf, swimming, and tumbling, such devices are almost the only means of measurement. In some sports there are no objective tests to measure certain important abilities. For example, there is no test to measure the rebound in basketball. This ability, and many others, if it is to be measured for any of the various purposes of measurement, must be measured by ratings. The many subjective traits and qualities inherent in the area of the affective domain are also objectified to a great extent through ratings.

The rating scale is frequently more economical in time than is a more valid objective measure. Since time is such a valuable adjunct in the daily program, this item becomes an important consideration in the teaching process. In addition to being a timesaver in the measurement of psychomotor and affective learnings, rating scales provide the instructor with a wealth of other knowledge. When they are applied to the product, they provide the teacher with a better understanding of his students. If he is to use the rating scale correctly, he must observe each individual carefully, and thus he becomes well acquainted with his students on a more personal basis. The use of rating scales enables the teacher to focus his attention on the more important facets of an activity or behavior so he tends not to "major in the minors." Good scales can be constructed only after the teacher has made a thorough analysis of the qualities and activities which he wishes to measure. He is forced to make a better analysis of skills and techniques and to understand the nature of social behavior and attitudes. Movement patterns can be identified more readily through study and repeated practice of observing. The golf or tennis professionals can easily spot incorrect techniques because of their long association with their teaching. Attitudes and appreciations can also be revealed to a greater extent. This greater insight into movement and social behavior undoubtedly enables one to become a better teacher.

The process of physical education is an area where measurement is needed badly but where it has been somewhat sporadically applied until recently. Since the process consists of many aspects which are constantly changing, rating devices and check lists form almost the sole means of evaluation. In this area they are used to bridge the gap between total subjectivity and objectivity. There are some excellent tools in this area which are being used to measure the various aspects of the educational process. (See Chapters 13 and 14.)

For best results, the physical educator must use both objective tests and subjective ratings in his measurement of the product. The usual practice is to employ objective measurements when they are available and when they have administrative feasibility and then to supplement them with ratings. When the activity as a whole is being evaluated, the use of ratings should be considered. Sometimes ratings are far more effective in the testing of game situations than are skill tests. Frequently, the highest scorers on skill tests are not always the best players in the game situations. A skill test is but a part of a whole. This "whole" combines many facets into one, including skill, knowledges, fitness, and attitudes. These facets are all used in a game situation to give a performance quality. This game performance or quality can be measured only by some type of subjective measurement. All coaches use ratings either consciously or subconsciously to select their squads, choose their starting line-ups, and evaluate their opponents.

The teacher should approach ratings with a knowledge of their limitations and an understanding of how they can be made more effective if they are to be used. Accuracy of rating is limited by the experience the rater has in its use, by his understanding of the students to be rated, by his knowledge of the particular instrument to be employed, and by his understanding of the factor or item to be rated. This last mentioned requirement is a most important consideration. The teacher or coach cannot judge reliably what he does not know or understand. The teacher or coach must know the materials with which he works and be qualified in the activities in his field. He must "know his stuff." If his ratings are to be accurate, he must observe the basic rules for rating, give his attention to the job before him, and proceed with his ratings in as objective a manner as possible. Experience in doing ratings increases one's insight into making good judgments. Therefore, he should have practice in exercising his habits of observation. The more meaningful his practice, the better he becomes at the job of rating.

Steps in Construction of Rating Devices

In the construction of homemade rating devices, intelligent and careful preparation is necessary if the instruments are to be valid and reliable. The following steps are not pertinent to all scales, but are essential to most types.

Determination of Purpose for Rating. First, the *purpose* of ratings should be known before they are prepared. This might include grading, classification, motivation, guidance, measurement of progress, program evaluation, and research, or perhaps a combination of these. The purpose will determine several things concerning the scale, but especially its range in terms of divisions or points on the scale. Classification might require but two divisions, while grading would require at least five. Program evaluation might require three. If greater discrimination is required, seven and even ten divisions may be used. An example is in the rating of swimming and gymnastics where a scale of ten is used. Also, the purpose of the rating generally will determine the type of category to be used, such as numerical, descriptive, or graphic. The purpose will further dictate whether single rating forms or a group form will be employed, and whether a student's rating is made according to his group or an ideal.

Determination of Traits and Definitions. Second, the *quality*, *trait*, or *activity* to be measured must be *determined* and its basic factors *isolated* and *defined* carefully. Selection of these factors or items may be made by analyzing the whole activity or behavior into its components and using the important ones in the rating scale. For example, if basketball is the activity to be measured, it could be analyzed into such factors as dribbling, shooting, passing, footwork, etc., and each of these items could be rated separately. When this is done, however, each quality must be clearly defined and described in relation to the situation in which it will be used and in as objective terms as possible. If it is feasible, the descriptions should be stated in specific terms of action and behavior rather than as general concepts of action and behavior. The more specific the item, the more objective and reliable the rating result, since it will be more clearly understood by the rater. Frequently, the item can best be understood if it is stated in a negative manner. For example, when "Professional Interest" is being described, the question, "Does not shirk responsibility" is easily understood. Each trait or factor may be given a weighting in terms of its importance, difficulty, frequency, or time allotment. This problem, like grading, is a relative matter and is frequently difficult to implement.

Divisions of Traits into Sub-traits. Third, if a factor to be measured is of a *complex nature*, it is perhaps best to break it into smaller units and *rate each separately*. For instance, in the above example, shooting may be broken down into several types of shots and each rated separately, or each shot might be divided into its fundamental parts, such as grip, stance, take off, ball release, and follow-through. Passing can be handled the same way. Hitting in baseball has frequently been analyzed into fundamental parts for rating. This rating of sub-items adds to validity. Also, the sub-item may be weighted in the same manner as described in the preceding paragraph. Since the ball release in the long jump shot is more important than the stance, it might be weighted twice as heavily, or since the shift of weight in the baseball swing is more important than the position of the hands in the grip, it might receive a heavier weighting. An example of this type of complex skill broken into its component parts is shown in Figure 17–1.

Selection of Categories. Fourth, the rating device should be divided into points on the scale called categories. This sets the range of the instrument. These categories may be simple dichotomous types, such as pass and fail, yes and no, or good and bad. Usually, however, measurement, as life itself, is not quite that simple. The human entity is difficult to dichotomize. In fact, all human traits and abilities are in the form of a continuum, although for convenience, classifications have been arbitrarily set. If more than two categories are required, the usual number is five. Excellent, good, average, poor, and failure; or always, often, sometimes, seldom, or never are commonly used divisions. For most purposes the five-category scale is entirely adequate and provides optimum validity. Frequently, the two-category scale leads to questions relative to the borderline cases. When this occurs, the scale may be converted to three categories by adding a third category, such as "undecided," "uncertain," "not sure," or "questionable." Also, since many raters tend not to use the extremes, it sometimes is well to consider the use of a seven-point scale when five divisions are desired. In this instance, the two extremes at either end of the scale are combined with the adjacent categories for a five-category scale. However, logic will generally help determine the limits for the range in order to afford easy administration without losing validity. In

Name_____ Age_____ Date_____
        Last   First   Middle

	Points
KEY: Varsity Caliber	5
Good	4
Average	3
Fair	2
Poor	1

SUGGESTED CHECKLIST

____1. STANCE AND STRIDE

Stance   Stride
  Body is fairly erect   Striding foot slides
  Body faces the plate   Back foot remains anchored
  Hips and shoulders are level   Stride is short—6 to 10 inches
  Knees are slightly bent   Stride is away from inside
  Weight is equally distributed   pitches
  Bat covers the plate   Stride is toward outside
  Hitter is relaxed   pitches
  Arms are free
  Head of the bat is held above the handle
  Bat is held steady in a cocked position

____2. SHIFT IN WEIGHT AND ROTATION OF HIPS

At Start of Swing
  Weight is shifted to the rear foot
  Hips are rotated toward the catcher
During Swing
  Weight is shifted to the front foot
  Hips rotate sharply to the left

____3. FOLLOWING BALL AND MAKING CONTACT
  Head is held steady
  Ball is hit sharply
  Head tracks the ball until last split second
  Swings at strikes, takes balls

____4. COMPLETE SWING
  Loose arm action
  Swing is parallel to the ground
  Wrists snap at contact
  Wrists roll after contact
  Swing is against the stride
  Body leans in the direction the ball is hit
  Bat head is usually ahead of the wrists when ball is hit
  Swing is smooth and coordinated

_____RAW SCORE TOTAL

_____T-SCORE

Fig. 17–1.   Rating form for hitting.   (Courtesy of G. E. Hooks,
Wake Forest University, Winston-Salem, North Carolina.)

general, the range on the scale is related to the degree of discrimination and the degree of discrimination is inherent in the purpose. The greater the degree of distinction, the greater should be the number of categories.

These categories or points on the scale may be defined or undefined. It is best, however, if they are clearly and concisely defined and limited. The definition should be specific and should describe the standards or levels of achievement at each point on the scale for each of the items being rated in terms of the particular group of students. For example, what does "excellent" mean when applied to dribbling for the junior high school boy? An indefinitely described or defined category would limit the accuracy of the rating and thereby lower the validity of the instrument. However, categories should not be described in too much detail because then it becomes more difficult to place a performer in any one category. A category may be established to conform to the curve of normal distribution if there is need for as many as five divisions. This can be done by indicating the number of performers to be placed in each of the categories. The characteristics of each of these categories should be spelled out. In the example of basketball ability, the categories could be 1, 2, 3, 4, and 5, with 5 indicating varsity ability, 1 the novice, and 2, 3, and 4 the in-between groups. Of course these categories must be in terms of the age, sex, or grade of the group being rated. Category definitions or descriptions should reveal graduated amounts of the traits being observed not only at each level on the scale but also between the scales designated for the different age and sex groups. For example, one cannot expect as much from a group of junior high school players on a basketball or a field hockey rating as from a group of high school students and the descriptions of the categories should reveal these differences.

Use of Number Values for Points on the Scale. Fifth, the need for arriving at a single index grade suggests the use of numerical values for the categories in some scales. This permits the data to be tabulated, classified, and statistically treated. Even when numbers are not used directly in the rating device itself, the teacher may empirically assign the categories with number values for his own purpose. Figure 17–1 shows a rating scale with number categories. If the situation does not call for numerical scores, however, the use of numbers is superfluous, since categories are generally described anyway. Once again the use of number values in the scale depends on the preparation of the rating.

Preparation of the Rating Sheet. Sixth, the rating or check sheet should be prepared before the rating period. There are a number of types from which to select. Some types are standardized but many are teacher-made for local use and for a particular purpose.

The important thing here is accuracy and ease of scoring. Rating forms may be classified another way—according to whether they are designed to rate a single student per form or a number of students on the same form. If the trait is complex and a group is being measured, rating forms can be mimeographed so that each student's status or achievement can be recorded on an individual form. Figure 17-1 shows this type of scale. However, it is possible to have a score or rating sheet for the entire class and it frequently resembles a roll sheet. This type scale is shown below.

SOCIAL EVALUATION SCORE CARD

NAME OF STUDENT	Traits	Sportsmanship	Enthusiasm	Attitude	Effort	Language	Sociability	Responsibility	Appearance	Leadership	Care of Equip.	Total

In either case, the same definition of items and categories can be placed on the rating forms. When raters are provided with these rating forms in advance, they may orient themselves in the nature of the device.

Rules for Use of Ratings

There are some basic rules and precautions to be observed in the use of ratings. Some mistakes may be avoided by attention to the following suggestions.

Combined Ratings. The combined rating of several raters with assurance is more valid than that by a single rater. It is an old saying that there is safety in numbers and this certainly applies to ratings. When more than one rater is being used, an average of their scores may be taken and a composite rating obtained. If five or more raters are used, the scores of the middle three only are sometimes employed for averaging. Sometimes a better spread in scores is obtained if the raters' scores for each student are summed rather than averaged.

Precautions in Ratings. Ratings are just as valid as the observations on which they are based. Raters must be aware of certain influences which tend to lower the validity of their ratings. They must exercise caution against the "halo effect" which includes liking a student because of some factor or factors extrinsic to the quality being measured. These influences might include such characteristics as politeness, helpfulness, popularity, enthusiasm, and just plain "apple polishing." Because of these factors the instructor tends to rate the student higher in the quality under examination than he deserves. Also, the reverse could be true and the student could be given a lower rating than he deserves for quite the opposite reasons. Raters should not be influenced by physical appearance and personality except when these things are being rated. Raters must also be aware that ratings made by persons of the same sex as that of the student being rated are generally more valid than if the ratings were made by raters of the opposite sex. Therefore, when the opposite sex is being rated, added precautions must be taken to be fair and impartial.

Degree of Assurance. Raters should have a high degree of assurance if their ratings are to be used. This degree of assurance is probably in proportion to the number of opportunities the raters have had to observe the students in the situations requiring rating. This is especially true in the area of the affective. Opportunities to make observations must be made available and raters should not judge until they have had the necessary opportunities. Some rating

Degree of Assurance 0 --- pure guess 1 --- some knowledge 2 --- fair knowledge 3 --- positive assurance	Degree of Assurance	Excellent	Good	Average	Below Average	Inferior	No Opportunity to Observe
DEPENDABILITY (Highly reliable & punctual, with integrity)							
RESOURCEFULNESS (Has initiative, originality, & adaptability)							
SELF CONTROL (Poise, dignity, tact, & Control of emotions)							
COOPERATION (Ability to work with others loyally)							
LEADERSHIP (Popular, friendly, aggressive & responsible)							

devices provide a category to specify the rater's degree of assurance (see page 563) while others merely provide a space for the rater to check that he has had no opportunity to observe this area. There is a high relationship between the degree of assurance or basis for judgment and validity of ratings.

Judgments Made During Performance. If the performance is being rated, judgment should be made as the activity is being performed. The teacher cannot trust to memory on such things. Also, the rating should be made on the basis of observation at the time and not on previous knowledge or experience. Each performer must be given a sufficient number of opportunities to show what he can do, and sufficient time must be allotted to the rating period.

Rating of Multiple Items. Ratings are more valid in a rating scale with multiple items if each item is rated for all students instead of all items for one student. For example, if students are being rated in swimming, all would be rated first on the crawl stroke before any would be rated on any other stroke. In a tumbling class each student would be rated on the back roll before any would be rated on the front roll. It is easier for the teacher to keep in mind the definitions of items and categories when one item is rated for all the students before moving on to the next.

Discussions of Ratings by Raters. If more than one rater is being used, several precautions are needed. First, the raters must be sure they have the same anchor points. Ratings are more valid if the several raters will discuss their ratings together. This is especially true at the very beginning of the rating period. If wide differences appear in the results, the entire technique being employed should be thoroughly reviewed and perhaps revised. At least a discussion of results will enable raters to get together on their anchor points.

Equalization of Competition for Ratings. If ratings depend on competition between individuals or teams from a group, care should be taken to equalize the individuals or teams in abilities as much as possible. Otherwise, the ratings may well be unfair. If tennis under game conditions is being rated, a superior player pitted against an average one will make the average player appear even poorer than he actually is and it might be difficult for him to get a fair rating. By the same token the better player might look so good against the duffer that he might be overrated.

Mechanics and Climate for the Rating Period. If observations are to be carried on with accuracy, the mechanics of the setting should receive careful attention. The raters should be placed in the best position for an unobstructed view with as few distractions as possible. For example, in rating swimming, the rater must be above the subject in order to observe the various type kicks. A poor vantage point for raters will lower the objectivity of results, and thus the reliability and validity. Raters should be given sufficient time to make their ratings. Hurried observations will also lower validity. Ratings have little significance unless they are based on valid observation.

Training of Raters. If ratings are to be valid, the raters must have training. This training is aside from the fact that the rater must "know his stuff" as a coach and teacher and be expertly qualified in the activity to be rated. Training takes two forms. First, the rater must know the mechanics of the device which is to be employed. The typical rating device is not very complicated. The rater merely has to apply the simple mechanics. However, he must not be lulled into complacency because of the ease with which rating scales can be checked. While checking the form is easy, making good judgments prior to the checks is more difficult. Thus, the second step in training is how to make good judgments for recording on the rating device. Naturally, all of the suggestions and precautions mentioned in the preceding paragraphs should be understood and carried out in the rating process. The rater must understand that he is to be completely unbiased and impartial. He must keep his attention on the traits being rated at the time. He must not be influenced by previous impressions, and he should know whether he is rating students according to their particular group or according to an ideal. Generally, the purpose of the rating will dictate the approach. Also, he should occasionally refer to his definitions of items and categories to see that he is being consistent in their application to each student. All of this training must be in advance of the rating period and it is helpful if some practice in rating is provided for the raters.

Interpretation of Ratings to Students. After the ratings have been made, if they are to be most useful, the student must be informed of the outcome and his standing interpreted to him. This job is easier if the students are familiarized with the rating tool during a brief orientation period. The purpose of the test and the nature of the rating device could be explained to them at that time. Interpretation of ratings to the students offers an opportunity for teaching and should not be neglected. This is the time to stimulate the student to greater heights and to help him plan his program for improvement. However, the teacher should never lose sight of the fact that ratings are based on subjective opinion and do have their shortcomings which the student should understand. Some rating scales are developed so that the students can rate themselves. (See "Outcomes of Sports: An Evaluation Check-Sheet" by Cowell in Chapter 12, p. 416.) These self-appraisal scales are probably more unreliable, but frequently may be worth more to the student than

a teacher's rating. Also, there are scales where students may rate
each other.

Types of Rating Devices

There are several types of rating scales which are adapted for use
in physical education. Several of these are merely variations or
elaborations of others. These devices designate categories for different levels of ability or varying amounts of a quality. Generally,
five categories are enough, but if greater discrimination is desired
seven categories or even ten may be employed. Five category scales
frequently take the form of excellent, good, average, inferior, and
failure; or always, often, sometimes, seldom, and never; most, many,
some, a few, and none; or just plain A, B, C, D, F. In order to
encourage raters to make use of all the categories in a scale, it is
sometimes necessary to indicate the number of students to be assigned in each category or the percentage of students. This practice
insures greater reliability. Rating scales may be loosely categorized
into the following types:

Student-to-Student Rating Scales. This device selects five
students from the group being rated and assigns them degrees or
per cents of the qualities being evaluated. This enables the raters
to see a picture in the form of a living model of the various levels
of achievement or status in the trait, quality, or activity. The best
student is placed at the top, the poorest at the bottom, and the
typically average at the middle. Then two additional students are
selected. One is placed midway between the poorest and the average
and the other is placed midway between the average and the best.
All students in the group to be measured are then compared with
the five standards. In essence, this is another form of category
rating with students or players representing the described levels.
One disadvantage of this technique is its poor psychological influence
on some students. If the students or players are to help in the
ratings or are to be made acquainted with the tool employed, it may
tend to have a discouraging effect on the lower group members who
are used as standards. Also, such rating devices tend to take the
attention off the standards of achievement desired and place it on
the individual students who are used as models.

Comparison Scales. Another variation of the category-rating
technique is the use of photographs, drawings, or diagrams, to depict
more vividly the varying standards or levels of achievement in the
items being evaluated. This is very similar to the student-to-
student rating in design and implementation. The students in the
group are compared with standards in the form of photos, models,
or stick figures, instead of living models. The number of standards

is usually four or five. There are several posture standards of this type. One of the most well known is shown in Figure 8–9, p. 232.

Graphic Scales. The graphic scale is a category rating in diagram form. This tool generally takes the form of a linear scale which is usually placed immediately below or above a definition or description of the item being measured. In this case, a line is drawn underneath or over the defined item and divided into segments from left to right. These are suggestive of categories as they range from poorest to best. The rater places a check mark at the place on the scale that represents the student's ability or the amount of the quality possessed. Some scales are constructed so that the dividing lines between two categories may be checked, if the rater is undecided about the category in which the student belongs. In a sense, this adds four categories to an already five-category scale and thus provides for a nine-category scale. Sometimes the categories are described by words such as "Good," "Average," or "Poor," or sometimes by concise descriptive phrases. In some cases the numerical or alphabetical scale is used. It is also possible to combine this type scale with the curve of normal probability. These devices in general enable the rater to visualize more easily the range of the scale and they also provide a much better picture for anyone making use of the ratings. A linear scale is shown below.

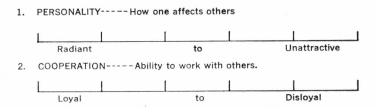

1.   PERSONALITY-----How one affects others

      Radiant   to   Unattractive

2.   COOPERATION-----Ability to work with others.

      Loyal   to   Disloyal

Percentage Scales. The percentage scale is another elaboration of the category technique. This is a scale where one item is rated in terms of percentages from 1 to 100. Since many teachers, parents, and students are familiar with percentiles in mental tests, this technique would have the advantage of being easily understood. However, raters must use 50 as the typically average and rate as many students below the median as above it if they are to be accurate in the use of this device. A variation would be to place students at the bottom, top, 50th, 25th, and 75th percentiles only, or to place them in the various deciles, thus employing a ten category scale. This type of scale is shown below. This scale can be used in profile form by placing all the items to be observed on the scale and after ratings are made by checking the percentiles, the points can be connected by an unbroken line. The weakness of this scale is the fact that raters tend not to use categories below the median.

Items	Score	Percentile
1. Leadership (popular, friendly, & independence)		0 10 20 30 40 50 60 70 80 90 99
2. Sociability (tactful, congenial, poised)		0 10 20 30 40 50 60 70 80 90 99

When the group is an unselected one, categories can be made to conform to the curve of normal probability. This is done by indicating the percentage in each category. For instance, excellent, most, or A, would include the upper 7 per cent; good, many, or B, would include the next lower 24 per cent; average, some, or C, would include the middle 38 per cent; inferior, a few, or D, would include the next lower 24 per cent; and failure, none, or F, would include the lower 7 per cent. As pointed out previously, these various levels or standards should be carefully defined in terms of the quality or trait to be measured. Figure 17–2 shows a rating scale which defines the item to be rated (tennis serve) and then defines the various categories. The percentages of students for each category have been added in case the rater wishes to assure himself that all categories will be used.

Descriptive Scale. A descriptive scale is the type which makes use of descriptive adjectives, phrases, or sentences, to describe the various traits of a given quality or activity. The rater checks the appropriate places which best describe the student.

Elements of the Serve: (1) accuracy, (2) sufficient speed to be effective, (3) rhythmic swing, (4) toss and swing coordination, (5) ball tossed to proper height, (6) racket meets ball at proper height and place, (7) proper weight transference, and (8) body rotation and follow-through.

Score Values:

5. Excellent (7%) Serve meets all elements with no apparent errors. Consistent in accuracy and effectiveness.

4. Good (24%)   Serve gives general impression of good form but minor variations exist. Consistent in accuracy and effectiveness.

3. Average (38%) Serve meets elements of good form but lacks smoothness and ease or lacks control in some one or two respects which affects serve as a whole. Accuracy and effectiveness fairly consistent.

2. Fair (24%)   Acceptable but executes serve with many errors which result in inconsistency in accuracy and effectiveness.

1. Poor (7%)   Serve is inadequate.

Fig. 17–2. Rating scale for tennis serve. (Courtesy Georgia Hulac, Woman's College, University of North Carolina, Greensboro, N.C., 1958.)

A. SPORTSMANSHIP

_____Always displays good sportsmanship
_____Most of the time is a good sport
_____Has tendency toward poor sportsmanship
_____Frequently displays poor sportsmanship
_____Usually displays poor sportsmanship

B. ENTHUSIASM AND INTEREST

_____Enters into all activities with enthusiasm and eagerness
_____Had a few lapses in interest and enthusiasm
_____When motivated is enthusiastic
_____Is seldom enthusiastic
_____Is rarely ever an enthusiastic performer

Numerical Scale. This scale assigns score values to the various levels of the scale. The usual range is from 1 to 5, with 5 indicating the greatest. Sometimes 1 to 10 is used when greater discrimination is needed than the usual five. This is an accepted practice in judging gymnastics and diving. Also, the assigning of weights to the different dives and stunts is a common procedure. The scale in Figure 17–1 has been made into a numerical scale and also the Football Playing Ability and Attitude Rating Scale by Meyer which is shown in Chapter 12, page 451.

Combinations of Scales. Frequently it may be desirable to combine two or more types of rating scales. For example, either the graphic or category scale could be combined with the numerical scale when it is necessary to obtain a composite score and at the same time maintain the values of the other types. Also, the descriptive scale may be combined advantageously with the graphic and all category type could be provided with the percentage of students to be assigned in each category. Several examples of these combinations are shown on the previous page. A combination of the linear graphic, descriptive with given percentages is shown first.

7%	24%	38%	24%	7%
Excellent	Good	Average	Inferior	Poor

A combination of the graphic, descriptive and numerical is sometimes used as follows:

1. EFFORT----Has to do with giving one's best.   Degree of Assurance

10	9	8	7	6	5	4	3	2	1	0		
Always puts forth best effort		Usually puts forth best effort		Tries under motivation		Frequently fails to try		Never tries			positive to guess	

2. DEPENDABILITY----Reliable with a keen sense of integrity.

10	9	8	7	6	5	4	3	2	1	0		
Never neglects duties and responsibilities		Only on occasions neglects duties		Must be followed up frequently		Frequently shirks his duties		Is completely undependable			positive to guess	

19

References

1. Barr, A. S., W. H. Burton, and L. J. Brueckner: *Supervision*. New York, Appleton-Century-Crofts, Inc., 1947, pp. 357–373.
2. Bovard, J. F., F. W. Cozens, and E. P. Hagman: *Tests and Measurements in Physical Education*. 3rd Ed., Philadelphia, W. B. Saunders Co., 1949.
3. Good, C. V., A. S. Barr, and D. E. Scates: *The Methodology of Educational Research*. New York, Appleton-Century-Crofts, 1935, pp. 409–439.
4. Lawshe, C. H.: *Principles of Testing*. New York, McGraw-Hill Book Co., Inc., 1948.
5. Lundberg, G. A.: *Social Research*. New York, Longmans, Green, and Co., 1942.
6. McCall, W. A.: *Measurement*, New York, The Macmillan Co., 1939.
7. McCloy, C. H., and Norma D. Young: *Tests and Measurements in Health and Physical Education*. New York, Appleton-Century-Crofts, Inc., 1954, pp. 21–28.
8. Remmers, H. H., and N. L. Gage: *Educational Measurement and Evaluation*. New York, Harper & Brothers, 1943.
9. Scott, M. Gladys, and Esther French: *Measurement and Evaluation in Physical Education*. Dubuque, Wm. C. Brown Co., Publishers, 1958, pp. 400–427.

GLOSSARY

Ability	—The present level of abilities or characteristics which describe the individual or group mentally, physically, socially, or emotionally.
Ability grouping	—Classifying pupils into homogeneous sections with reference to intelligence, mental or physical achievement, or any known or predicted ability.[5]
Ability test	—A test designed to measure the level of present status or present ability to function.[5]
Absolute grading	—The practice of assigning grades based on performance or achievement only. See "relative grading."[5]
Accreditation	—A professional, regional, state, or national recognition of an educational institution or program for meeting certain standards or evaluative criteria.[5]
Accuracy	—The ability of the individual to control voluntary movements toward an object.
Achievement	—The accomplishment of the individual beyond a defined starting point.
	—The change in ability as shown by the difference between two measurements.
Achievement standards	—Specific levels of attainment to be mastered for a particular purpose; specific requirements for marks or defined levels of attainment.[5]
Achievement test	—A test that measures the extent to which a person has acquired certain information or mastered certain skills, usually as a result of specific instruction.[8]
Activity	—Any learning situation involving change or motion; any mental or motor process in which students participate to derive satisfaction or to attain some desirable goal; in physical education, one of the organized games, sports, or elements in which students demonstrate skill and initiative, and which is selected and conducted for specific outcomes.[5]
Adaptability	—Social—the ability of an individual to adjust his actions or mode of behavior to changes in social situations or general environment; muscular—the ability of the neuromuscular system to activate appropriate motor units in adjusting to muscular efforts to the load requirement.[5]
Adjustment	—The process of changing one's activities or environment to satisfy needs; the changes which an individual undergoes in order to fit environmental conditions; social adjustment usually refers to changes in habits or behavior which must be made by individuals with some deviation or conflict in association with others.[5]
Administration	—All of the techniques and procedures utilized in maintaining and operating the total physical education program according to established principles and policies; that phase of the total organization which assumes final responsibility for the government, regulation, coordination, and provisions for all of the functions, organization, management, supervision, and teaching; briefly, the role of administration is to facilitate program functions.[5]

Administrative evaluation —Refers to the entire process of appraising or judging all of the procedures employed to accomplish the objectives of the program; includes the organization, policies, staff personnel, student achievement, methods and techniques, and facilities and their use.[3]

Aerobic —Requiring the presence of oxygen.[5]

Affective —Concerned with sociopsychological feelings and behavior such as attitudes, values, and adjustment.

Age-Height-Weight tables —Tables showing the average height and the average weight of boys or girls of each chronological age.[5]

Age norms —A score or value which represents the average performance for pupils of the given age in the trait or characteristic measured.[5]

Age scale —A scale in which the units of measurement are the differences between successive age equivalents, each difference is considered as though equal to all other.[11]

Agility —The ability of the body or parts of the body to change directions rapidly and accurately.

Aim —An indication of direction or remote goal which is general in nature.

Aim of Physical Education —The optimum development, integration and adjustment, physically, mentally and socially, of the individual through guided instruction and participation in selected total body sports, rhythmic and gymnastic activities conducted according to social and hygienic standards.[1]

Anecdotal record —A written objective record of an incident in the life of a student as observed by a teacher or leader.

Answer sheet —A form used to make replies to written questions.

Anthropometry —The measurement of the human body.

Apparatus —Gymnastic horses, bucks, bars, ropes, booms, and other devices used as objects on which to exercise in a gymnasium; measurement—any instrument, device, or related group of devices, designed or used to help control or measure skills, abilities, or conditions.[5]

Appraisal —The process of determining the status, quality, quantity, or condition of anything; a process, involving measurement and interpretation; used to determine the extent to which objectives are being achieved.[5]

Appreciation —The ability to realize the value or worth of something which probably had as its beginning an attitude.

Aptitude —A combination of abilities and other characteristics, whether native or acquired, known or believed to be indicative of an individual's ability to learn in some particular area.[8]

Aptitude test —A test which measures the likelihood of an individual's succeeding in given subject area or line of work.[5]

Arbitrary reference point —(assumed mean) Any score or value in a distribution, usually near the center in an ordered series, from which deviations are calculated in a short-cut method of computing the mean; the mid-point of the class or step interval that is assumed to contain the mean.[5]

Arithmetic mean —The sum of a set of scores divided by the number of scores, commonly called average.[8]

Associated learning —That which is learned incidentally or by implication or connection.[5]

Athletic ability	—Motor skills and abilities involved in the performance of athletic sports, measured in terms of achievement; present power to perform in athletic events.[5]
Athletic aptitude	—The inherent and acquired characteristics or traits which indicate an individual's ability to acquire proficiency in athletic skills; the ability of the individual to make future athletic achievement.[5]
Athletic index	—A score or value derived from several prognostic measurements relating to ability in sports and games; useful for classification or homogeneous grouping of pupils.[5]
Athletic type	—A type of body build characterized by broad shoulders, a well-developed chest, thick neck, flat abdomen, and large muscles; refers to mesomorphs.[5]
Atomistic concept	—The view held by some people concerning the unity of physical, mental, spiritual, and social aspects of man; the belief that man exists as separate parts joined together but not really functionally related, and that any aspect, physical or mental, can be highly developed without any resulting change in the other aspect.[5]
Attitude	—The beginning of feelings or ways of thinking about something which result in emotionalized tendencies to respond in certain ways.
Attitude scale	—An attitude measuring instrument with experimentally determined and equated units; gives a quantitative evaluation of an attitude.[5]
Attribute	—A characteristic or a quality.
Audiometer	—An instrument for measuring the power of hearing or the audibility or intensity of sounds.[13]
Average	—A general term applied to measures of central tendency. The three most widely used averages are the arithmetic mean, the median, and the mode.[8]
Avoirdupois	—A system of weights based on a pound of 16 ounces.
Balance	—The ability of the individual to maintain his neuromuscular system in a static condition for an efficient response or to control it in a specific efficient posture while it is moving.
Bar graph	—A graphic presentation utilizing bars of various length to symbolize differences in quantity, size, or other measures.[9]
Basic skill	—(fundamental skill) A motor skill that is basic or essential to the mastery of an activity, such as running, jumping, throwing, kicking, striking, etc.; a coordinated combination of basic movements.[5]
Battery	—A group of several tests standardized on the same population so that results on the several tests are comparable. Sometimes loosely applied to any group of tests administered together, even though not standardized on the same subjects.[8]
Biomechanics	—The study of the motion of living organisms.[5]
Biserial correlation	—A technique used when one variable is quantitative and one is dichotomous.
Body build	—See "Somatotypes."
Body-image	—The way the body and its parts are perceived.
Body types	—See "Somatotypes."
Caliper	—An instrument used to measure the thickness or diameter of something.

Capacity	—The ultimate level of development in the ability or characteristic measured.
Cardiovascular	—Pertaining to the heart and circulatory functions.
Cardiovascular test	—A test which measures the response of the heart to regulated amounts of exercise.[5]
Ceiling	—The upper limit of ability measured by a test.[8]
Centile	—Any one of the 100 groups or divisions separated by percentile scores; *i.e.*, the 1st centile includes all scores below the 1st centile point; the 42nd centile includes all scores between the 41st and 42nd percentile points; the 100 centile includes all scores above the 99th percentile point.[5]
Central tendency	—A single score which is used to represent all the scores in a distribution.
Character	—The phase of personality comprising the more structural or enduring traits or characteristics which give continuity to personality over time, and which are of ethical and social significance; personality viewed in relation to some system of morality, and by which individuals may be compared.[5]
Character test	—A test designed to assess such ethical, volitional, or valuational aspects of a personality as honesty, persistence, loyalty, and values and ideals.[5]
Chart	—A sheet giving information in the form of diagrams, tables, and illustrations.
Check list	—A list of things to look for as observations are being made.
Chronological age	—Age in years and months.
Classification	—The placement of individuals into groups for a particular purpose.
Classification test	—Any test used to group students according to abilities, age, weight, or any common factors for the purposes of instruction or competition.[5]
Class interval	—(step interval, class size) The range of scores, or the number of score units, between the upper and lower limits of a section, or interval, of test scores in a frequency distribution.[5]
Coefficient of correlation	—(r) A measure of the degree of relationship, or "going-togetherness," between two sets of measures for the same group of individuals.[8]
Coefficient of equivalence	—The type of reliability coefficient obtained from the administration of parallel or equivalent forms of a test to the same individuals.[5]
Coefficient of internal consistency	—The type of reliability coefficient obtained when using either the split-halves or Kuder-Richardson formulas for computations.[5]
Coefficient of stability	—The type of reliability coefficient obtained by retesting or the administration of the same test twice to the same persons.[5]
Cognitive	—Concerned with intellectual abilities and skills such as knowledges and comprehension.
Comparable scores	—Scores having characteristics in common.
Completion item	—A test question calling for the filling in of a phrase, sentence, etc., from which one or more parts have been omitted.[8]
Concomitant learning	—Learning in a casual manner, without the intent to learn; learning which occurs while the intent or attention is focused on some other problems.[5]

Concurrent validity —Validity based upon correlation with a criterion variable that is measured at about the same time as the test is administered.[5]

Construct validity —That quality of a test having inferred value because of its demonstrated agreement with a theory; that involved whenever a test is to be interpreted as a measure of a quality or attribute that is not defined operationally.[5]

Content validity —Validity of a test which can be demonstrated by a careful examination of the content of test items.[5]

Continuous data —Data with any number of sub-divisions like distance or time.

Continuum —A line along which a trait, or set of scores, is conceived as being continuously distributed; a variable such that, no matter how close together any two values may be, it is always possible to have a third value between them; a continuous variable.[11]

Coordination —The ability of the performer to integrate types of movements into specific patterns.

Correction for guessing —Subtracting a fraction of the number of wrong answers from the number of right answers.

Correlation —The relation of two or more sets of paired data; perfect positive correlation is expressed as 1.00; perfect negative correlation as -1.00; and the absence of correlation as 0.00.[5]

Criterion —A standard by which a test may be judged or evaluated; a set of scores, ratings, etc., that a test is designed to predict or to correlate with.[8]
—A quality used as a basis for judging the value of something.

Cumulative frequency —A column in a frequency distribution table that shows, for any given interval, how many scores in the distribution lie below the upper limit of that interval.[5]

Cumulative percentage —The percentage of cases falling at or below any given point in a frequency distribution; determined by adding all cases below the given point and determining the percentage of the total cases which this sum constitutes.[5] Its curve permits a quick determination of percentile ranks.[5]

Curricular validity —Validity of a test shown by the extent of agreement between the test content and objectives with curricular content and objectives; demonstrated subjectively when test items cover the curricular content and objectives, are carefully constructed according to accepted rules or criteria, and are proportioned in number according to the percent of emphasis placed upon each objective.[5]

Curriculum —A progressive series of courses and/or experiences in a particular educational level or in a specific field of learning for a definite social purpose; the sum or range of experiences, in or outside of school, whether consciously controlled and guided or undirected, that favorably influences the discovery, unfolding, and development of the personality, abilities, and traits of the individual in accordance with accepted educational aims.[5]

Data —Facts or figures from which conclusions can be drawn.

Decathlon —An athletic contest in which each contestant takes part in ten events.

Decile —Any one of the nine percentile points in a distribution that divide the distribution into ten equal parts.[8]

Development —An increase in power to function; qualitative organization of behavior patterns as a result of heredity and activity supported by normal growth; an unfolding of abilities within the limits of inherent capacity.[5]

Deviation —The amount by which a score differs from some reference value, such as the mean, the norm, or the score on some other test.[8]

Diagnosis —The result of a procedure by which the nature of a problem is determined by a study of its history, signs, and symptoms; the conclusions drawn from facts derived from a process of discovering the nature of problems, or the interests, attitudes, motives, and aptitudes of an individual through tests, interviews, case studies, etc.[5]

Diagnostic test —A test used to locate specific areas of weakness or strength, and to determine the nature of weaknesses or deficiencies; it yields measures of the components or subparts of some larger body of information or skill.[8]

Dichotomous data —Data with a two-fold division like pass-or-fail.

Difficulty rating —The proportion of the students who get an item correct. The higher the difficulty rating the easier the item.

Discriminative index —The extent to which the observation or measures obtained from a group differ from one another or scatter about some measure of central tendency.[5]

Dispersion —The range or variability of a distribution.

Distractors —Any of the incorrect choices in a multiple-choice or matching item.[8]

Distribution —(frequency distribution) A tabulation of scores from high to low, or low to high, showing the number of individuals that obtain each score or fall in each score interval.[8]

Dynamometer —An apparatus for measuring power, especially muscular effort of men or animals. It commonly embodies a spring to be compressed or a weight to be sustained by a force applied combined with an index, or automatic recorder, to show the work performed.

Educability —The ease and thoroughness with which one learns new motor skills.

Education —A change, a modification, or an adjustment on the part of an individual as a result of experience.

Empirical —A method that relies on practical experience and observations alone.[13]

Empirical measures—Measures assigned or obtained from observations or derived from tests constructed on the basis of experience rather than on some well defined theory.[5]

Empirical validity —The worth or value of a test for a given purpose which has been proven through experience.[5]

Endurance —The result of a physiological capacity of the individual to sustain movement over a period of time.

Equivalent form —Any one of several forms of a test that is similar in content and item difficulty, and that yields very similar average scores, variability measures, and reliability estimates when administered to the same group.[5]

Ergograph	—An instrument for recording the work done by a muscle or muscle group, used in studying fatigue.
Ergometer	—Instrument used for measuring the amount of energy used or work done.[5]
Essay test	—A form of test in which only the questions are supplied while the respondents compose the answers.
Ethical character	—An individual's personality traits and behavior evaluated in terms of some moral code or set of ethical principles; usually connotes positive factors.[5]
Evaluation	—The art of judgment scientifically applied according to some predetermined standards.
	—A process of education which makes use of measurement techniques which, when applied to either the product or process of education, results in both qualitative and quantitative data expressed in both subjective and objective manner and used for comparisons with preconceived criteria.
Evaluative criteria	—The bases of standards against which the worth or status of something may be checked or compared; factors used by an accrediting agency to determine if a school or department shall be accredited.[5]
Extrapolation	—The process of estimating values of a variable beyond the range of available data.[5]
Eye-hand coordination	—Ability to use the eyes and hands together in such acts as fixating, grasping, and manipulating objects; important in all activities requiring fine accuracy, such as shooting a basektball or hitting a baseball.[5]
Face validity	—Refers to the acceptability of a test and test situation by the tester in terms of apparent use to be made of a test. The test has face validity when it seemingly measures the variable in question.[9]
Factor	—Any trait or variable considered in an investigation; any trait or characteristic, common to one or several variables, which causes or accounts for the correlations among a set of variables.[5]
Fitness	—That state which characterizes the degree to which the person is able to function.
Flanagan method	—A method of determining the index of discrimination of test items.
Flexibility	—The range of movement in a joint.
Foil	—An incorrect answer, a distractor.
Forced-choice item	—Any test item when the examinee is required to select one or more of the given alternatives.[5]
Free response test	—A test on which the items require the subject to respond at his own volition, in his own words, without selecting from provided alternatives.[5]
Frequency	—The number of actual individual occurrences in a specific class.
Frequency distribution	—A tabulation of scores from high to low, or low to high, showing the number of individuals that obtain each score, and if arranged in intervals, the number that fall into each interval.[5]
Frequency polygon	—A graphic representation of a frequency distribution, constructed by plotting each frequency as an ordinate above the midpoint of its class interval and connecting these plotted points by straight lines.[5]

Functioning of responses	—Extent to which various responses are chosen in multiple-choice, multiple-response, and matching items.[9]
General athletic ability	—(GAA) The present ability to perform in a variety of athletic events or sports; determined by a combination of basic elements such as speed, coordination, power, endurance, flexibility, strength, and agility.[5]
General motor ability	—(GMA) Developed capacity; the present ability of an individual to perform in a variety of sports activities; the ability to successfully perform in most big muscular activities requiring neuromuscular coordinations, such as walking, running, jumping, and playing games involving these and other fundamental skills.[5]
General motor capacity	—(GMC) The potentiality of an individual to perform in many motor (neuromuscular, psychomotor) activities involving large ranges of movement.[5]
Goniometer	—An instrument, consisting of a protractor, a stationary arm, and a movable arm, for measuring angles in determining joint flexibility.[5]
Grade	—Symbols used to denote an estimate of student status, progress, and achievement.
Grade-point	—Numerical evaluation of scholastic achievement based upon a formula of equivalents that grants credit varying with the grade attained, as, for example, 4 points for an A, 3 for B, etc., with zero or negative points for failure.[5]
Graph	—A diagram representing the successive changes in the value of a variable quantity.
Graphic rating scale	—A form of recording a rating (subjective estimates), according to the strength of some quality or trait, along with a straight line (continuum), descriptive phrases of the trait being written below the line; the two extremes represent the highest and lowest degrees of the trait.[11]
Group test	—A test that may be administered to a number of individuals at the same time by one examiner.[8]
Grouped data	—The condensation of scores into step intervals which comprise a frequency distribution.
Growth curve	—A graphic representation of the changes that occur in a trait or function as a result of maturation; may apply to either physical or mental growth.[5]
Habit	—A fixed way of behavior which comes from responding to a social situation in the same way many times.
Hand dynamometer	—(manometer) An instrument used to measure strength of handgrip, in which resistance is usually provided by powerful springs which must be compressed, the number of pounds of pressure exerted being registered on a dial.[5]
Handedness test	—A test or group of tests used to determine right or left hand preference; usually involves handwriting, tapping, throwing, gripping, etc.[5]
Height-weight tables	—Tables showing the average weight of boys or girls having a given height.[5]
Heterogeneity	—The nature of groups, the individuals of which are different or unlike; having wide variability; the tendency of a group to show marked dissimilarity.[5]
Histogram	—A vertical bar graph of a frequency distribution.[9]

Holistic concept —(unity) The view held by some physical educators concerning the unity of man; the belief that man is an integrated whole being and that when one part (physical, mental, etc.) is directly affected, other parts, although indirectly and sometimes of a lesser degree, are also affected.[5]

Homogeneity —The nature of groups the individuals of which are similar or alike with regard to some trait or characteristic; the property of having very small and regular variability.[5]

Homogeneous grouping —Classification by similar or identical elements.

Hull scale —A standard scale which has a mean of 50 and 3.5 standard deviations on each side of the mean.

Human movement —The change in position of the individual in time-space resulting from force developed from the individual's expenditure of energy interacting with his environment; may be expressive, communicative, or developmental, or adaptive (coping with environment).[5]

Hypothesis —A guiding idea, temporary explanation, or statement of probability, used to begin and guide an investigation for relevant data and to predict certain results or consequences; a tentative solution set up for testing as to its tenability.[5]

Ideal —An appreciation on the positive side with a standard which is near perfect or in the upper quartile

Ideal-self —A composite of the expectations of society and the aspirations of the self.

Index —The relation or proportion of one amount or dimension to another.

Index of discrimination —The ability of a test item to differentiate between persons possessing much of some trait and those possessing little.[8]

Index of reliability —The square root of the reliability; used in test construction as a statement of the highest coefficient of validity that can possibly be obtained for a test with a given reliability coefficient; the correlation between true and obtained scores on a test, or the probable correlation between one test and the average of an infinitely large number of parallel tests.[5]

Individual test —A test that can be administered to only one person at a time.[8]

Interest —A subjective-objective attitude, concern, or condition involving a precept or an idea in attention and a combination of intellectual and feeling consciousness; may be temporary or permanent; based on native curiosity and conditioned by experience.[5]

Interpretation —An unbiased, detailed description and explanation of the findings of an investigation, including a statement of the observed facts and their meaning as they related to the source or general population.[5]

Interpolation —Any process of estimating intermediate values between two known points.[8]

Interval —A space between two things.
—The extent of difference between two qualities or conditions.

Interview —An oral questionnaire.

Inventory —Usually a list of qualities, traits, or characteristics.

Item —A single question or exercise in a test.[8]

Item analysis —The process of evaluating single test items by any of several methods. It usually involves determining the difficulty value and the discriminating power of the item, and often its correlation with some criterion.[8]

Item validity —Discriminative value of an item; the correlation between an item and some criterion of performance; correlation between an item and the whole test of which it is a part.[5]

Judgment —The ability to evaluate the facts in a problematic situation and/or ability to relate two or more concepts.[1]

Kinesthetic sense —The sense which gives the individual an awareness of position of the body or parts of body as it moves through space.

Knowledge —Awareness or cognizance of information.

Knowledge test —Any test designed to measure what an individual knows about a particular subject; distinguished from aptitude, attitude, and physical performance tests.[5]

Kuder-Richardson formula(s) —Formulas for estimating the reliability of a test from information about the individual items in the test, or from the mean score, standard deviation, and number of items in the test.[8]

Law of averages —The statistical law that the stability of a statistic tends to increase as the number of observations on which it is based is increased.[5]

Leadership —The ability and readiness to inspire and guide others, individuals or groups, toward specific objectives.[5]

Learning curve —A graphic representation of certain aspects of progress in ability during successive periods of practice, in terms of equal time or of equal accomplishment units.[5]

Leptokurtic —Refers to a frequency curve that is more highly peaked than the normal probability curve.[5]

Level of confidence —A statistical term to indicate the degree of confidence that may be placed upon an interval estimate, generally shown by a probability percentage, such as being 95 per cent certain.[9]

Level of significance —A statistical term describing the percentage that defines the likelihood of concluding that a difference between two means, percentages, or other comparable measures exists when in reality it does not; *e.g.*, if the difference in mean scores of boys and girls is reportedly significant at the .01 level, this means that there is only a 1 in 100 chance that a sample difference as large as or larger than the one observed would occur by chance sampling error if there is in reality no difference between the mean of the population of boys and the mean of the population of girls.[9]

Linear relationship —(rectilinear correlation) A relationship between two or more variables that can be represented by a straight line; as one variable increases or decreases, the other moves likewise or inversely.[5]

Line graph —A line on coordinate paper designed to show the rise and fall of a variable over a period of time or when compared with another variable.[5]

Local norms —Norms that have been made by collecting data in a certain school system and using them, instead of national or regional norms, to evaluate student performance.[5]

Manometer —Hand dynamometer.

Mark —Grade

Matching item	—A test item calling for the correct association of each entry in one list with an entry in a second list.[8]
McCall score	—T-score.
Mean	—The point on a distribution of scores usually referred to as the average. It is the point about which the sum of the plus deviations is equal to the sum of the minus deviations.[13]
	—Sum of all measures divided by their number.
Measurement	—A technique of evaluation which makes use of procedures which are generally precise and objective, which will generally result in quantitative data, and which characteristically can express its results in numerical form.
Median	—The middle score in a distribution; the point that divides the group into two equal parts.[8]
	—That point along the score continuum above which and below which half of the cases fall.
Metric	—Used in measurement based on the meter and the gram.
Midpoint	—The point or value midway between the real upper and real lower limits of a class interval.[5]
Mode	—The score or value that occurs most frequently in a distribution.[8]
Morphology	—Science of form and structure.[5]
Motor ability	—The present acquired and innate ability to perform motor skills of a general or fundamental nature, exclusive of highly specialized sports or gymnastic techniques.
Motor ability test	—A test designed to determine, measure, and evaluate physical abilities, useful as a means of placing game contests on a fair competitive basis and for the classification of pupils for instruction in physical education.[5]
Motor capacity	—The innate or inborn ability to learn complex motor coordinations.[5]
Motor educability	—The ease and thoroughness with which one learns new motor skills.
Motor fitness	—A readiness or preparedness for performance with special regard for big muscle activity without undue fatigue.
	—It concerns the capacity to move the body efficiently with force over a reasonable length of time.
Motor learning	—Learning in which the learner achieves new facility in the performance of bodily movements as a result of specific practice; distinguished from improvement of function resulting from maturation.[5]
	—The integration of movement into a pattern for a purpose as a result of training procedures and environmental conditions.[7]
Movement-image	—The way the moving body is perceived.
Multiple-choice item	—A test item in which the examinee's task is to choose the correct or best answer from several given answers, or options.[8]
Multiple correlation	—The correlation between a dependent or criterion variable and the sum of a number of independent variables, which are weighted so as to give a maximum correlation.[9]
Multiple-response item	—A special type of multiple-choice item in which two or more of the given choices may be correct.[8]
N	—The symbol commonly used to represent the number of cases in a distribution.[8]
National norm	—A norm based on adequate nationwide sampling.[5]

Negative —An inverse relationship between paired variables; as one
   relationship   variable increases the other decreases.[5]

Nomograph —(alignment chart) A chart in which three variables are
   plotted on straight lines so that if any two are known, the
   third can be found with the use of a straight edge.[5]

Nonverbal test —A paper-and-pencil test, usually used with children in the
   primary grades, in which the test items are symbols, figures,
   and pictures rather than words; instructions are given orally.[11]

Normal curve —The bell-shaped curve of a theoretical distribution that de-
   picts a massing of scores or data at the center with gradually
   diminishing numbers toward both extremes; the mean,
   median, and mode coincide.[5]

Normal —A frequency distribution in which the scores or values are so
   distribution   distributed that a normal probability curve is the best fitting
   curve.[5]

Norms —Statistics that describe the test performance of specific
   groups, such as pupils of various ages or grades in the standardization group for a test. Norms are often assumed to be
   representative of some larger population.[8]

—An experimentally derived index which enables teachers to
   compare the achievement or status of their students with
   those of a similar group.

Nutrition —The sum of the processes by which the body takes in, assimilates, and utilizes food substances.

Objective —A precise and definite statement of the steps in the process of
   realization of an aim.

Objective test —A test in the scoring of which there is no possibility of difference of opinion among scorers as to whether responses are to
   be scored right or wrong.[8]

Objectivity —The degree of uniformity with which various persons score
   the same tests. This is often expressed by a correlation
   coefficient.[13]

Observation —The act of watching the behavior, actions, or status of
   students for a specific purpose by a trained observer.

Ogive —The graph of a cumulative percentage frequency distribution.

Organic efficiency —A test of functional efficiency of bodily organic systems,
   test   especially circulatory and respiratory; early name for a test
   of response of the heart to exercise.[5]

Organismic unity —The concept that the body acts and reacts as a functional
   unit rather than by separate parts; the view which opposes
   the dichotomous idea of mind and body as separate functional
   parts.[5]

Outcome —A specific quality or characteristic of one who has participated in selected activities under desirable conditions and
   with effective technique.

Parallel tests —Equivalent forms of a test.[5]

Partial correlation —The correlation between two variables with the influence of
   one or more other variables being eliminated.[9]

Pearson product- —The r method of correlation that seeks a straight-line rela-
   moment coeffi-   tionship from the scatter or spread of two or more groups
   cient of correla-   of scores.[13]
   tion

Pentathlon —An athletic contest in which each contestant takes part in
   five events.

Percentile	—(P) A point in a distribution below which falls the per cent of cases indicated by the given percentile. Thus the 15th percentile denotes the score or point below which 15 per cent of the scores fall.[8]
Percentile graph	—Ogive curve.[5]
Percentile rank	—The per cent of scores in a distribution equal to or lower than the score corresponding to the given rank.[8]
Percentile score	—The score representing the percentage of persons who fall below a given raw score.[5]
Perception	—The total pattern arising from many sensations and resulting in a meaning which is more than the sum of its parts.[4]
Perceptual motor skills	—The skills which enable the individual to perceive (seeing, hearing, understanding, sensing, etc.); all of the mental and sensory attributes which contribute to the state of readiness.[5]
Performance test	—A test requiring motor or manual response on the examinee's part.[8]
Personality	—The total psychological and social reactions of an individual; the synthesis of his subjective, emotional, and mental life; his behavior and his reactions to the environment.[5]
Philosophy	—A basic belief, the result of a systematic and disciplined examination of values and underlying assumptions. This basic belief helps to determine purposes, criteria, and standards.
Physical capacity test	—A test of physical fitness and skill, based on a series of sub-tests of strength, agility and physical achievement, for which standards have been established. Results are often expressed in terms of a strength index.[5]
Physical education	—An education by physical means where many of education's objectives are achieved through movement experiences.
Physical fitness	—Work capacity; the total functional capacity to perform some specified task requiring muscular effort, considers the individual involved, task to be performed, quality and intensity of effort; one aspect of total fitness; involves sound organic development, motor skill and the capacity to perform physical work with biological efficiency.[5]
Physical performance tests	—Those objective tests used to measure learnings which include motor ability, motor fitness, sport skill, posture, and nutrition.
Polygon	—Graphic representation of a frequency distribution, a line graph of a particular frequency distribution.
Posture	—The position of the whole body and its segments.
Potential ability	—The capacity to perform by virtue of some yet undeveloped or unrealized physical or mental attribute.
Potential energy	—Work capacity or energy resulting from relative position instead of motion, such as in a raised object or coiled spring.[5]
Power	—Capacity of the individual to bring into play maximum muscle contraction at the fastest rate of speed.
Power tests	—Knowledge tests in which the student has a reasonable opportunity to read all the items and indicate his answers in the time alloted.
	—A test intended to measure level of performance rather than speed of response; hence one in which there is either no time limit or a very generous one.[8]

Predictive index	—An index used to transform the coefficient of correlation (r) to a better than chance figure; $(1-\sqrt{1-r^2})$, expressed as a percent.[13]
Principle	—A guiding rule for action toward a desired goal and based on scientific facts or philosophic judgments.
Process	—The total physical education curriculum including personnel, program, and environment.
Product	—The student.
Product moment coefficient	—See correlation and coefficient of correlation.
Proficiency test	—A test designed to determine the extent to which a performer can execute some skill or skills with ease and precision; usually involves a single skill or skills involved in a particular activity.[5]
Profile	—A graphic representation of the results on several tests, for either an individual or a group, when the results have been expressed in some uniform or comparable terms.[8]
Prognosis (prognostic test)	—A test used to predict future success or failure in a specific subject or field.[8]
Progress chart	—A graphic representation of achievement in schoolwork, consisting of a series of test scores or other marks taken from time to time and plotted in graphic form.[5]
Progress grade	—A grade based solely on the amount of progress made over a period of time, without regard to the final ability as compared with others in the group.[5]
Projective technique	—A method of personality study which avoids as much as possible any structuring of the situation; the subject responds freely to a series of stimuli such as inkblots, pictures, unfinished sentences, etc., and projects into his responses manifestations of personality characteristics.[5]
Psychomotor	—Concerned with movement and closely related factors which influence it.
Qualitative data	—Data according to kind or quality.
Quantitative data	—Data according to amount or number.
Quartile	—One of three points that divide the cases in a distribution into four equal groups. The lower quartile, or 25th percentile, sets off the lowest fourth of the group; the middle quartile is the same as the 50th percentile, or median; and the third quartile, or 75th percentile, marks off the highest fourth.[8]
Quartile deviation (semi-interquartile range) (Q)	—Half of the range between Q_1 and Q_3.
Question	—An item in a written test.
Questionnaire	—A method of obtaining information directly from an individual about his present status and practices.
Quotient	—The number obtained when one quantity is divided by another, a ratio.
Random sample	—A sample so drawn that every member of a population has an equal chance of being included; excludes bias or selection. Inferences or generalizations may be made on the findings from such a representative sample.[5]
Range	—The difference between the highest and lowest scores obtained on a test by some group.[8]

Ranking	—Arranging the constituents of a group in order in terms of some measure. Rank numbers disclose the relative position of the constituents.[9]
Rank order correlation	—(rho) A method of computing a correlation coefficient by assigning ranks to each pair of scores of individuals, and determining the relationship between them; ranks of the magnitudes are used instead of the magnitudes themselves; usually used with a small number of cases.[5]
Rank scores	—All scores are ordered from the highest to the lowest with the highest score, one, and the lowest, N.
Rating scale	—A subjective estimate which brings order to the processes of observation and self-appraisal and which provides for degrees of the quality, trait, or factor being examined.
Raw score	—The first quantitative result obtained in scoring a test.[8]
Recall item	—An item that requires the examinee to supply the correct answer from his own memory or recollection, as contrasted with a recognition item, in which he need only identify the correct answer.[8]
Recognition item	—An item requiring the examinee to recognize or select the correct answer from among two or more given answers.[8]
Regression equation	—A technique used to predict the most likely measurement in one variable from the known measurement in another.
Relative grading	—The practice of assigning grades on a relative or comparative basis, such as in terms of potentiality or according to how the individual compares with his peers (class or group). See "absolute grading."[5]
Reliability	—The extent to which a test is consistent in measuring whatever it does measure.[8]
Reliability coefficient	—The coefficient of correlation obtained between two forms of a test (alternate-form or parallel-form reliability); between scores on repeated administrations of the same test (test-retest reliability); between halves of a test properly corrected (split-half reliability); or by using the Kuder-Richardson formulas.[11]
Representative sample	—A sample that corresponds to or matches the population of which it is a sample with respect to characteristics important for the purposes under investigation.[8]
Research	—Careful, systematic, patient study and investigation in some field of knowledge to establish facts or principles. —To increase knowledge.
Rho	—Rank order correlation.
Sample	—Scores selected at random from a large group of population so that they have the characteristics of the whole population.[13]
Sampling	—The act or process of selecting a limited number of observations, individuals, or cases to represent a particular universe.[5]
Sampling error	—Errors caused by chance factors in random sampling; usually estimated statistically by the standard error.[5]
Scale	—A qualitative or quantitative graduation of scores used to differentiate the individuals from the group.[6]
Scattergram	—Correlation chart. —A two-dimensional chart affording a basis for computing a correlation coefficient for two variables or scores. Pairs of values are tallied on the chart, giving a visual picture of the relationship between the variables.[9]

Score	—A quantitative or qualitative record of the individual in the traits or characteristics concerned.
Screening test	—A test designed to select from a group those individuals in a specified category; most commonly used for identifying those with exceptional or sub-normal mental capacities or physical deviations.[5]
Self-appraisal	—Self-evaluation; the process of defining one's own status or progress toward specific goals; appraisal may involve measurement and opinion, and is based on the individual's interpretation of his performance and ability.[5]
Self-evaluation	—The process of measuring one's own status or progress toward specific goals.[5]
Self-image	—The way the self is perceived.
Sigma	—(σ) A Greek letter used to represent the standard deviation.[13]
Skewness	—The tendency of a distribution to depart from symmetry of balance around the mean.[8]
Skill	—An art, craft, or science involving the use of the hands or body.
Social development	—Refers to one's adjustment to the group and to other individuals in terms of his and their rights, privileges, and duties.[5]
Socialization	—The process by which individual members of society learn the ways of the group, become functioning members, act according to its standards, accept its rules, and in turn become accepted by the group.[5]
Sociogram	—A chart or diagram that graphically illustrates interactions, usually those desired or not desired, among individuals in a defined group; portrays social relationships within groups in terms of responses to stimulus questions on a sociometric test.[5]
Sociometry	—A technique or method of measuring the amount of organization of a social group in order to show the patterns of relationships and interrelationships.
Somatotype	—A classification of an individual according to body structure.[5]
Somatotype rating	—A series of three numbers, between 1 and 7, indicating the amount of ectomorphy, mesomorphy, and endomorphy in an individual's type of body build.[5]
Spearman Rho	—A method of correlation by rank-difference and designed for use with small numbers.
Spearman-Brown Prophecy formula	—A formula giving the relationship between the reliability of a test and its length. The formula permits estimation of the reliability of a test lengthened or shortened by any amount, from the known reliability of a test of specified length.[8]
Speed	—The capacity of the individual to perform successive movements of the same pattern at a fast rate.
Spirometer	—An instrument for measuring the vital capacity of the lungs, or the volume of air which can be expelled from the chest after the deepest possible inspiration.
Split-half coefficient	—A coefficient of reliability obtained by correlating scores on one-half of a test with scores on the other half. Generally, but not necessarily, the two halves consist of the odd-numbered and the even-numbered items.[8]
Sport skills	—Those physical activities constituting each sport which are distinctive to that sport.

Sportsmanship	—Desirable attitude and actions on the part of sports participants and spectators; qualities and behavior befitting a sportsman; includes such qualities as abiding by the standards of fair play, cooperation, respect for the game, and regard for the rights of others.[5]
Stadiometer	—An instrument for measuring height.
Standard	—The degree of attainment in a criterion and expressed as a quality or quantity.
Standard deviation	—(SD) A measure of the variability or dispersion of a set of scores. The more the scores cluster around the mean, the smaller the standard deviation.[8]
	—The square root of the average of the squared deviations from the mean.
Standard score	—A general term referring to any of a variety of "transformed" scores, in terms of which raw scores may be expressed for reasons of convenience, comparability, ease of interpretation, etc.[8]
	—Scores based on the standard deviation.
Standardized test	—A systematic sample of performance obtained under prescribed conditions, scored according to definite rules, and capable of evaluation by reference to normative information. Some writers restrict the term to tests having the above properties, whose items have been experimentally evaluated, and/or for which evidences of validity and reliability are provided.[8]
Stanine	—One of the steps in a nine-point scale of normalized standard scores. The stanine (short for standard-nine) scale has values from 1 to 9, with a mean of 5, and a standard deviation of 2.[8]
Statistical validity	—Test validity expressed numerically, usually as a coefficient of correlation between scores on the test and another set of measures such as scores on another test, teacher's marks, or ratings by experts.[5]
Statistics	—The science which deals with the collection, organization, analysis, and interpretation of masses of numerical facts.
Status	—Present condition, position, level.[5]
Stencil key	—A scoring key which, when positioned over an examinee's responses either in a test booklet, or more commonly, on an answer sheet, permits rapid identification and counting of all right answers.[8]
Strength	—The capacity of the individual to exert muscular force.
Strength test	—A test designed to measure muscular strength; often designates a test composed of a series of test items which when combined would give a measure of general bodily strength rather than the strength of specific muscles.[5]
Strip key	—A scoring key arranged so that the answers for items on any page or in any column of the test appear in a strip or column that may be placed alongside the examinee's responses for easy scoring.[8]
Subjective	—Resulting from the feelings or temperament of the subject, or person thinking, rather than the attributes of the object thought of.
	—Based on judgment and opinion.

Subjective test	—A test scored on the basis of the scorer's personal judgment of the worth of each answer, rather than by reference to a pre-arranged scoring key or answer sheet; *e.g.*, essay test.[5]
Survey	—A systematic collection analysis, interpretation and report of facts concerning an enterprise.
Taxonomy	—A set of classifications.
Technical learning	—The immediate, specific, and obvious results of teaching; for example, technical learnings in football are how to run, throw, kick, block and tackle. See "associated" and "concomitant" learning.[5]
Test	—A set of questions, problems, or exercises for determining a person's knowledge, abilities, aptitude, or qualifications. —An examination. —A specific tool of measurement for the collection of data and implying a response from the person being measured.
Test battery	—A group of several tests intended to be administered in succession to the same subject or subjects; the tests are usually designed to accomplish a closely related set of measurement objectives.[5]
Testing program	—Any organized plan for systematically carrying out evaluative procedures in a school or school system or among school systems; involves the selection, administering, scoring, and interpretation of tests.[5]
Tetrachoric	—A correlation technique used when both variables are dichotomous.
Trial	—An attempt, endeavor, effort.
True-false item	—A test question or exercise in which the examinee's task is to indicate whether a given statement is true or false.[8]
T-Score	—A derived score based upon the equivalence of percentile values of standard scores, thus avoiding the effects of skewed distributions, and usually having a mean equated to 50 and a standard deviation equated to 10.[9]
Understanding	—The ability to grasp the significance of knowledges, to realize more fully their relationships, and to apply discriminatory powers where they are concerned.
Ungrouped data	—Ranked or raw scores.
Utility	—The ability of a test or measure to be employed for several purposes, such as for classification, assaying achievement, and drill.[5]
Validity	—The extent to which a test does the job for which it is used. Validity is always specific to the purposes for which the test is used, and different kinds of evidence are appropriate for appraising the validity of various types of tests.[8]
Variables	—The traits or factors that change from one case or condition to another; the representations of the traits, usually in quantitative form, such as a measurement or an enumeration.[5]
Variability	—The scatter or spread of scores around a measure of central tendency within a distribution of scores.
Variance	—A measure of variability; the square of the standard deviation; arithmetic mean of the squares of the deviations from the mean.[5]
Weighting	—The relative importance of a single item in a battery of related items.

REFERENCES FOR THE GLOSSARY

1. Bookwalter, Karl W.: *Syllabus in Curriculum in Physical Education*, School of Health, Physical Education and Recreation, Indiana University, Bloomington, 1951.
2. ———: The Tyranny of Words, Journal of Health and Physical Education, *18*, 714–715, 754, December, 1947.
3. Cowell, Charles C., and Wellman L. France: *Philosophy and Principles of Physical Education*. Englewood Cliffs, N.J., Prentice-Hall, Inc., 1963.
4. Cratty, B. J.: *Movement Behavior and Motor Learning*. Philadelphia, Lea & Febiger, 1964.
5. Hunter, Milton D.: *A Dictionary for Physical Educators*, P.E.D., Indiana University, Bloomington, Indiana, 1966. One hundred thirty-three definitions used by permission of the author.
6. Larson, Leonard A., and Rachael Dunaven Yocom: *Measurement and Evaluation in Physical, Health, and Recreation Education*. St. Louis, C. V. Mosby Co., 1951.
7. Lawther, John D.: Directing Motor Skill Learning, Quest, VI:68–76. May, 1966.
8. Lennon, Roger T.: *A Glossary of 100 Measurement Terms*, Test Service Notebook No. 13. New York: Harcourt, Brace & World, Inc. Fifty-three definitions used by permission of the publisher. A few of the definitions used here are abridged. TSN No. 13 may be obtained from the publisher without charge.
9. Meyers, Carlton R., and T. Erwin Blesh: *Measurement in Physical Education*. New York, The Ronald Press, 1962. Nine definitions used by permission of the publisher.
10. Phillips, Marjorie, and Karl W. Bookwalter: Three Little Words, The Physical Educator, *5*, 21, March, 1948.
11. Remmers, H. H., N. L. Gage, and J. F. Rummel: *A Practical Introduction to Measurement and Evaluation*, New York, Harper & Brothers, 1960.
12. Smithells, Philip A., and Peter E. Cameron: *Principles of Evaluation in Physical Education*. New York, Harper & Brothers, 1962.
13. Willgoose, Carl E.: *Evaluation in Health Education and Physical Education*. New York, McGraw-Hill Book Co., Inc., 1961. Seven definitions used by permission of the publisher.

INDEX

Page numbers followed by *fig.* indicate reference to illustrations; those followed by *t* indicate reference to tables.